Neurochemistry of Sleep and Wakefulness

Pharmacological approaches to our understanding of sleep have been at the forefront of sleep research for many years. Traditional techniques have included the use of pharmacological agonists and antagonists, as well as transmitter-specific lesions. These have been enhanced by the introduction of molecular genetics and the use of transgenes and targeted gene deletion. *Neurochemistry of Sleep and Wakefulness* is an exceptional, single source of information on the role of the major mammalian neurotransmitter systems involved in the regulation of sleep and waking. With contributions from internationally recognized experts, this book clearly describes how researchers have made use of the myriad techniques in their armamentarium to characterize the role of a given neurotransmitter in the regulation of sleep and waking. Suitable for experimental and clinical pharmacologists, the book will have wider appeal to sleep researchers, psychiatrists and any professional interested in the interdisciplinary areas of neurobiology and pharmacology.

JAIME M. MONTI has won many awards for his research, including the Claude Bernard Award (Clinical Sleep Research) from the Government of France, and the Schering Award for Basic Sleep Research, in Germany. He is a member of the International College of Neuropsychopharmacology, the Sleep Research Society (USA), the European Sleep Research Society, and the Argentinian Society of Sleep Medicine.

S. R. PANDI-PERUMAL is affiliated with the Division of Clinical Pharmacology and Experimental Therapeutics, Department of Medicine, College of Physicians and Surgeons of Columbia University, New York, USA, which is a major provider of medical education, health-care and research in New York. An internationally recognized sleep researcher, his interests focus on sleep and biological rhythms research.

CHRISTOPHER M. SINTON is Associated Professor of Internal Medicine at the University of Texas Southwestern Medical Center at Dallas. A winner of several awards, including the Phillipe Foundation Fellowship for Neuroscience Research, his current research interests focus on the relationship between sleep and energy homeostasis.

Neurochemistry of Sleep and Wakefulness

Edited by

JAIME M. MONTI

School of Medicine, Clinics Hospital,
Montevideo

S. R. PANDI-PERUMAL

Columbia University

CHRISTOPHER M. SINTON

University of Texas Southwestern Medical
Center

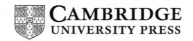

CAMBRIDGE
UNIVERSITY PRESS

CAMBRIDGE UNIVERSITY PRESS
Cambridge, New York, Melbourne, Madrid, Cape Town, Singapore, São Paulo

Cambridge University Press
The Edinburgh Building, Cambridge CB2 8RU, UK

Published in the United States of America by Cambridge University Press, New York

www.cambridge.org
Information on this title: www.cambridge.org/9780521864411

First published 2008

Printed in the United Kingdom at the University Press, Cambridge

A catalogue record for this publication is available from the British Library

ISBN 978-0-521-86441-1 hardback

To our wives, our families, our friends and our teachers,
Who have supported and helped us in all we have accomplished.
And, for one of us, to the memory of
My parents and a summer evening on the Via Appia Antica.

Contents

Color plate section located between pages 368 and 369.

Contributors

Md. Noor Alam
Veterans Administration, Greater Los Angeles Health System and the Department of Psychology, UCLA School of Medicine, Los Angeles, CA 91343, USA

Helen A. Baghdoyan
University of Michigan, Department of Anesthesiology, 7433 Medical Sciences Building I, 1150 West Medical Center Drive, Ann Arbor, MI 48109-0615, USA

Ritchie E. Brown
Laboratory of Neuroscience, Department of Psychiatry, Harvard Medical School, VA Medical Center Brockton, Research 151C, 940, Belmont St., Brockton, MA 02301, USA

Ian G. Campbell
University of California, Davis, UC Davis Sleep Lab, 1712 Picasso Ave, Suite B, Davis, CA 95616, USA

Daniel P. Cardinali
Departamento de Fisiología, Facultad de Medicina, Universidad de Buenos Aires, Paraguay 2155, 1121, Buenos Aires, Argentina

Luis de Lecea
Stanford University, Department of Psychiatry, 701B Welch Road, Palo Alto, CA 94304, USA

Irwin Feinberg
University of California, Davis, UC Davis Sleep Lab, 1712 Picasso Ave, Suite B, Davis, CA 95616, USA

Patrice Fort

UMR5167 CNRS, Institut Fédératif des Neurosciences de Lyon (IFR 19), Université Claude Bernard Lyon I, 7 Rue Guillaume Paradin, 69372 Lyon Cedex 08, France

Amanda A. H. Freeman

Department of Cell Biology, Emory University, 615 Michael Street, Whitehead Building Room # 435, Atlanta, GA 30322, USA

Damien Gervasoni

UMR5167 CNRS, Institut Fédératif des Neurosciences de Lyon (IFR 19), Université Claude Bernard Lyon I, 7 Rue Guillaume Paradin, 69372 Lyon Cedex 08, France

Hui Gong

Veterans Administration, Greater Los Angeles Health System, Sepulveda, 151 A3 Neurophysiology Research, 16111 Plummer Street, North Hills, CA 91343, USA

Romain Goutagny

UMR5167 CNRS, Institut Fédératif des Neurosciences de Lyon (IFR 19), Université Claude Bernard Lyon I, 7 Rue Guillaume Paradin, 69372 Lyon Cedex 08, France

Ruben Guzman-Marin

Veterans Administration, Greater Los Angeles Health System, Sepulveda, 151 A3 Neurophysiology Research, 16111 Plummer Street, North Hills, CA 91343, USA

Osamu Hayaishi

Department of Molecular Behavioral Biology, Osaka Bioscience Institute, 6-2-4 Furuedai, Suita-shi, Osaka 565-0874, Japan

Héctor Jantos

Department of Pharmacology and Therapeutics, Clinics Hospital, Montevideo, Uruguay

Sushil K. Jha

Department of Neuroscience, University of Pennsylvania, Philadelphia, PA 19104, USA

Levente Kapás

Department of Biological Sciences, Fordham University, Bronx, NY 10458, USA

Lucienne Leger
UMR5167 CNRS, Institut Fédératif des Neurosciences de Lyon (IFR 19),
Université Claude Bernard Lyon I, 7 Rue Guillaume Paradin, 69372 Lyon
Cedex 08, France

Pierre-Hervé Luppi
UMR5167 CNRS, Institut Fédératif des Neurosciences de Lyon (IFR 19),
Université Claude Bernard Lyon I, 7 Rue Guillaume Paradin, 69372 Lyon
Cedex 08, France

Ralph Lydic
University of Michigan, Department of Anesthesiology, 7433 Medical
Sciences Building I, 1150 West Medical Center Drive, Ann Arbor, MI
48109–0615, USA

Vibha Madan
School of Life Sciences, Jawaharlal Nehru University, New Delhi 110 067,
India

Birendra N. Mallick
School of Life Sciences, Jawaharlal Nehru University, New Delhi 110 067,
India

Robert W. McCarley
Department of Psychiatry, 116A Harvard Medical School, and VA Medical
Center, 940, Belmont Street, Brockton, MA 02301, USA

Dennis McGinty
Veterans Administration, Greater Los Angeles Health System and
Departments of Psychology, UCLA School of Medicine, Los Angeles, CA
91343, USA

Melvi Methippara
Veterans Administration, Greater Los Angeles Health System and the
Departments of Psychology, UCLA School of Medicine, Los Angeles, CA
91343, USA

Daniel Monti
Mercy Behavioral Health, Pittsburgh, PA 15203, USA

Jaime M. Monti
Department of Pharmacology and Therapeutics, Clinics Hospital,
Montevideo, Uruguay

Lennard P. Niles
McMaster University, Faculty of Health Sciences, Department of Psychiatry
and Behavioural Neurosciences, HSC- 4N77, 1200 Main Street West,
Hamilton, Ontario L8N 3Z5, Canada

S. R. Pandi-Perumal
Division of Clinical Pharmacology and Experimental Therapeutics,
Department of Medicine, College of Physicians and Surgeons of Columbia
University, 630 West 168th Street, New York, NY 10032, USA

Christelle Peyron
UMR5167 CNRS, Institut Fédératif des Neurosciences de Lyon (IFR 19),
Université Claude Bernard Lyon I, 7 Rue Guillaume Paradin, 69372 Lyon
Cedex 08, France

Tarja Porkka-Heiskanen
Institute of Biomedicine/Physiology, Biomedicum, P.O.Box 63, FIN-00014
University of Helsinki, Finland

David B. Rye
Department of Neurology and Program in Sleep, Emory University School
of Medicine, 101 Woodruff Circle, WMRB-Suite 6000, Atlanta, GA 30322,
USA

Rafael J. Salin-Pascual
Departments of Physiology and Psychiatry, School of Medicine, Universidad
Nacional Autónoma de México, Mexico City, P.O.Box 21-238, Mexico City,
Coyoacan 04021, Mexico

Denise Salvert
UMR5167 CNRS, Institut Fédératif des Neurosciences de Lyon (IFR 19),
Université Claude Bernard Lyon I, 7 Rue Guillaume Paradin, 69372 Lyon
Cedex 08, France

Christopher M Sinton
Department of Internal Medicine, University of Texas Southwestern
Medical Center, 5323 Harry Hines Blvd, Dallas, TX 75390-8874, USA

Dag Stenberg
Institute of Biomedicine/Physiology, Biomedicum, P.O.Box 63, FIN-00014
University of Helsinki, Finland

Natalia V. Suntsova
Veterans Administration, Greater Los Angeles Health System, Sepulveda,
151 A3 Neurophysiology Research, 16111 Plummer Street, North Hills, CA
91343, USA

Éva Szentirmai
Department of Physiology, A. Szent-Györgyi Medical and Pharmaceutical Center, University of Szeged, H-6720, Szeged, Domter 10, Hungary, and Department of Veterinary and Comparative Anatomy, Pharmacology and Physiology, Neuroscience Program, Washington State University, Pullman, WA 99164, USA

Ronald Szymusiak
Research Service, Veterans Administration, Greater Los Angeles Health System, 16111 Plummer Street, North Hills, CA 91343, USA

Mahesh Thakkar
Department of Neurology, University of Missouri, Harry S. Truman Memorial Veterans' Hospital, 800 Hospital Drive, Columbia, MO 65201-5297, USA

Yoshihiro Urade
Department of Molecular Behavioral Biology, Osaka Bioscience Institute, 6-2-4 Furuedai, Suita-shi, Osaka 565-0874, Japan

Laure Verret
UMR5167 CNRS, Institut Fédératif des Neurosciences de Lyon (IFR 19), Université Claude Bernard Lyon I, 7 Rue Guillaume Paradin, 69372 Lyon Cedex 08, France

Jon T. Willie
Department of Neurosurgery, Washington University School of Medicine, Campus Box 8057, St. Louis, MO 63110, USA

Preface

Neurochemistry of Sleep and Wakefulness focuses on the actions and inter-actions of neurotransmitters involved in the control and modulation of the behavioral states that we know as waking and sleeping. It presents results and emerging concepts that in recent years have challenged our understanding about the basic brain systems that are involved in sleep and wakefulness. As might be expected, these new findings are also having an effect on the practice of sleep medicine. In fact, once considered a minor sub-specialty, sleep medicine is developing into a significant and growing area of medicine; and much of this growth can be attributed to improved knowledge about brain neurochemistry and the drugs that have been developed as a result.

Thus, inevitably, the relationship between sleep and the chemistry of neuro-transmission has become an area of intense medical, biological, and scientific interest. It seemingly affects all facets of our health and well-being. But this relationship is also complex because it involves fundamental, yet still incompletely understood mechanisms and functions in the brain, most notably the essential difference between sleep and wakefulness. Although this field of research in its current form began with the identification of specific chemical neurotransmitter systems in the brain some forty years ago, we can actually date the beginning of research into sleep neurochemistry to the onset of the twentieth century. At that time sleep factors, or substances in cerebrospinal fluid or blood that build up during wakefulness and dissipate during sleep, were postulated and became the focus of research. Despite some initially promising results that seemed to support the idea, it eventually became evident that this hypothesis was conceptually far more complex than originally conceived. The history of this research is fascinating and is briefly summarized, together with the current consensus, in Chapter 11 of this volume.

Each chapter of *Neurochemistry of Sleep and Wakefulness* has been written by a knowledgeable expert or research team, each of whom is directly involved in the investigations that they describe. This has ensured a text that is readily accessible to both basic and clinical sleep researchers, while covering the breadth of sleep neurochemistry in some detail. This volume thus brings together a collective scholarship in both basic and clinical research with interests that span neuroscience, neurochemistry, neuropharmacology, sleep pharmacology, and biological rhythms.

We have divided the volume into three parts. Part I comprises introductory chapters that summarize the neurochemistry and neurochemical mechanisms of specific states, including a review of the onset of sleep, and of rapid eye movement sleep and wakefulness. Then follows a group of chapters (Part II) that each focus on the relationship between sleep and a specific, well-characterized neurotransmitter system, such as acetylcholine and glutamate. Part III of the volume is devoted to more recent discoveries concerning neurochemical influences on sleep and wakefulness such as melatonin, the prostaglandins, and adenosine. Also in this part are included two chapters on neuropeptides, one of which, Chapter 14, reviews some interesting and potentially critical links between specific neuropeptides and sleep–wakefulness. The uniqueness of the findings described in this chapter is that the neuropeptides involved do not immediately relate to what is currently known about the neuroanatomical circuits of sleep and wakefulness. This suggests future research directions. The close interrelation between sleep and metabolism through hypothalamic neuropeptide circuits that were originally implicated in narcolepsy is underlined in Chapter 15. The volume concludes with a topical review, Chapter 16, which highlights the translation of neurochemical research into therapeutic development.

Neurochemistry of Sleep and Wakefulness is not exhaustive. For example, separate chapters could have been included for G-proteins and signaling cascades, glycine, uridine, lipid signaling, and neuroimaging. Knowledge is evolving rapidly in these areas, but they must await a future edition. However, the volume is current and will therefore be useful to sleep researchers, as well as to neuropharmacologists, neuroanatomists, neurophysiologists, and medical specialists. In addition, this book should prove valuable to medical students and clinicians who require an overall understanding of the field. We trust that the contents and organization of this volume will be both rewarding and interesting for our readers. Our hope is that it will encourage future advances in sleep research and these findings will eventually be themselves summarized in future editions.

As always, we welcome communication from our readers concerning the volume and its organization, and especially concerning any inaccuracies or omissions that remain. We take full responsibility for any such inaccuracies, and we would appreciate having them drawn to our attention.

Acknowledgements

Many individuals played instrumental roles in the conception, development, and completion of *Neurochemistry of Sleep and Wakefulness*. This enterprise was challenging, and the editors received help from many. We are delighted to acknowledge some of them here.

Firstly, we must thank our contributors. Without their involvement and dedication to the research they describe, this volume would not have been possible.

We were very fortunate to experience the warm, professional, and highly enthusiastic support of Martin Griffiths, our Commissioning Editor at Cambridge University Press. His commitment to excellence was a strong guiding force and kept us on track throughout the development of this volume. Indeed, the many talented people at the Press made this project much more enjoyable than it might have been. In particular, we acknowledge the help of Betty Fulford, senior publishing assistant, and Dawn Preston, our production editor.

A particular appreciation is also owed to several anonymous reviewers who made many helpful suggestions. Their perceptive comments and insights were invaluable.

Every effort has been made by the authors, editors, and publishers to contact all the copyright holders to obtain their permission for the reproduction of copyrighted material. Regrettably it remains possible that this process was incomplete. Thus if any copyrights have been overlooked, the publisher will ensure correction at the first opportunity for subsequent reprint of this volume.

Finally, we express our gratitude to our families for their patience and support. Thank you.

Abbreviations

3-MT	3-methoxytryptamine
5-HT	5-hydroxytryptamine (i.e. serotonin)
5-HTP	5-hydroxytryptophan
5-HIAA	5-hydroxyindoleacetic acid
7-NI	7-nitroindazole
8-PST	8-(p-sulfophenyl)-theophylline
ACh	acetylcholine
AChE	acetylcholinesterase
ACSF	artificial cerebrospinal fluid
ADA	adenosine deaminase
AFMK	N-acetyl-N-formyl-5-methoxykynuramine
AH	anterior hypothalamus
AHP	after hyperpolarization
AMP	adenosine monophosphate
AMPA	α-amino-3-hydroxy-5-methyl-4-isoxazole proprionic acid
ARC	arcuate nucleus
ATP	adenosine triphosphate
BF	basal forebrain
BH4	tetrahydrobiopterin
BZD	benzodiazepine
cAMP	cyclic adenosine monophosphate
cDNA	complementary deoxyribonucleic acid
CEA	central nucleus of the amygdala
cGMP	cyclic guanosine monophosphate
CHA	N6-cyclohexyladenosine
ChAT	choline acetyltransferase
ChT	choline transporter

CNS	central nervous system
CNT	concentrating nucleoside transporter
CoA	co-enzyme A
COX	cycloxygenase
CPA	N6-cyclopentyladenosine
CPDX	8-cyclopentyl-1,3-dimethylxanthine
CPT	cyclopentyltheophylline
CRE	cyclic-AMP response element
CREB	cyclic AMP response element binding protein
CRH	corticotrophin-releasing hormone
CSF	cerebrospinal fluid
CSN	cold-sensitive neuron
CST-14	cortistatin-14
CTb	cholera toxin B subunit
CYP	cytochrome P
DAG	diacylglycerol
DARPP	dopamine and cyclic adenoside 3′,5′-monophosphate
DAT	dopamine transporter
DBB	diagonal band of Broca
DL	dorsolateral
DMH	dorsomedial hypothalamic nucleus
DOMA	dihyroxymandelic acid
DOPAC	dihyroxyphenylacetic acid
DPGi	dorsal paragigantocellular reticular nucleus
DPMe	deep mesencephalic reticular nucleus
DR(N)	dorsal raphe (nucleus)
DSIP	delta-sleep-inducing peptide
DSPS	delayed sleep phase syndrome
ECS	electroconvulsive shock
EEG	electroencephalograph
EHNA	erythro-9-(2-hydroxy-3-nonyl)adenine
EMG	electromyogram
eNOS	endothelial nitric oxide synthase
ENT	equilibrative nucleoside transporter
EOG	electrooculogram
EPSP	excitatory postsynaptic potential
FDA	food and drug administration
GABA	γ-aminobutyric acid
GAD	glutamic acid decarboxylase
GHS-R	growth hormone secretagogue receptor

Glu	glutamate
Gly	glycine
GPi	globus pallidus, internal segment
GTP	guanosine triphosphate
HA	histamine
Hcrt	hypocretin
HDC	L-histidine decarboxylase
HIOMT	hydoxyindole *O*-methyltransferase
HLA	human leukocyte antigen
HNMT	histamine *N*-methyltransferase
HPLC	high-performance liquid chromatography
HVA	homovanillic acid
i.p.	intraperitoneal
i.c.v.	intracerebroventricular
IL-1	interleukin-1
IP3	inositol triphosphate
IPSP	inhibitory postsynaptic potential
IR	immunoreactivity
i.v.	intravenous
KO	knockout
L-DOPA	3,4-dihydroxy-L-phenylalanine (i.e. levodopa)
L-NAME	Nω-nitro-L-arginine methyl ester
L-PIA	N6(L-phenylisopropyl)adenosine
L-PGDS	leptomeningeal lipocalin-type prostaglandin D-synthase
LC	locus coeruleus
LD	light/dark
LDT	laterodorsal tegmentum
LH	lateral hypothalamus
LSD	lysergic acid diethylamide
LTS	low-threshold spike
mAChR	muscarnic cholinergic receptor
MAO	monoamine oxidase
MCH	melanin concentrating hormone
MDD	major depressive disorder
MEA	midbrain extrapyramidal area
mGlu(R)	metabotropic glutamate (receptor)
MHC	major histocompatibility complex
MnPN	median preoptic nucleus
mPOA	medial preoptic area
mPRF	medial pontine reticular formation

MPTP	1-methyl-4-phenyl-1,2,3,6-tetrahydropyridine
MRI	magnetic resonance image
MRN	median raphe nucleus
mRNA	messenger ribonucleic acid
MSLT	multiple sleep latency test
MT	melatonin
NA	noradrenaline
NADPH	nicotinamide adenine dinucleotide phosphate, reduced form
NAT	*N*-acetyltransferase
NE	norepinephrine
NECA	5'-*N*-ethylcarboxamide
NERT	norepinephrine reuptake transporter
NMDA	*N*-methyl-*D*-aspartate
NO	nitric oxide
NOS	nitric oxide synthase
NPS	neuropeptide S
NPY	neuropeptide Y
NREM	non-rapid eye movement
NRMc	nucleus reticularis magnocellularis
NRT	nicotine replacement therapy
NTS	nucleus of the solitary tract
OSA	obstructive sleep apnea
OX	orexin
PAG	periaqueductal gray
PCPA	p-chlorophenylalanine
PD	Parkinson's disease
PET	positron emission tomography
PF(L)H	perifornical (lateral) hypothalamus
PG	prostaglandin
PGO	ponto-geniculo-occipital
PH	posterior hypothalamus
PKA	protein kinase A
PKC	protein kinase C
PLC	phospholipase C
PLM	periodic leg movement
PnC	pontis caudalis
PNMT	phenylethanolamine *N*-methyltransferase
PnO	pontis oralis
PnOc	pontis oralis caudal

PnOr	pontis oralis rostral
POA	preoptic area
PP-1	protein phosphatase-1
PPT	pedunculopontine tegmentum
PRN	pontine reticular nucleus
PRO	pontis reticularis oralis
PS	paradoxical sleep
PTK	protein tyrosine kinase
PVN	paraventricular nucleus
PVT	thalamic paraventricular nucleus
RBD	REM sleep behavior disorder
REM	rapid eye movement
RHT	retinohypothalamic tract
RRF	retrorubral field
SCN	suprachiasmatic nucleus
SERT	serotonin reuptake transporter
SHA	S-adenosyl-homocysteine
SHMT	serine hydroxymethytransferase
SIN-1	3-morpholinosydnonimine
SN	substantia nigra
SNAP	S-nitroso-N-acetyl-1,1-penicillamine
SOREM	sleep onset REM
SPS	sleep promoting substance
SSRI	selective serotonin reuptake inhibitor
SWA	slow wave activity
SWS	slow wave sleep
t-MH	tele-methylhistamine
TCA	tricyclic antidepressant
TH	tyrosine hydroxylase
TMN	tuberomammillary nucleus
TNFα	tumor necrosis factor α
TrypH	tryptophan hydroxylase
TSD	total sleep deprivation
TTX	tetrodotoxin
TyH	tyrosine hydroxylase
UII	urotensin II
UV	ultraviolet
VAChaT	vesicular ACh transporter
VLPO	ventrolateral preoptic
VMAT	vesicular monoamine transporter

VTA	ventral tegmental area
WSN	warmth-sensitive neuron
WT	wild-type
α-FMH	α-fluoromethylhistidine
α-MHA	α-methylhistamine

I THE NEUROCHEMISTRY OF THE STATES OF SLEEP AND WAKEFULNESS

1

Neurochemistry of the preoptic hypothalamic hypnogenic mechanism

DENNIS McGINTY, MD. NOOR ALAM, HUI GONG,
MELVI METHIPPARA, NATALIA SUNTSOVA,
RUBEN GUZMAN-MARIN, AND RONALD SZYMUSIAK

The chapter will summarize our current understanding of the neuronal and neurochemical basis of hypnogenesis. The hypothesis of the localization of a hypnogenic mechanism in the mammalian hypothalamic preoptic area (POA) was first proposed by von Economo more than 70 years ago (von Economo, 1930). This hypothesis has been confirmed by findings that experimental POA lesions suppress sleep, and that electrical, chemical, and thermal POA stimulation induce sleep (reviewed by McGinty & Szymusiak, 2001). Unit recording studies have identified POA neurons that exhibit increased activity during NREM sleep, REM sleep, or both. These *sleep-active* neurons are hypothesized to be the substrate of the hypnogenic mechanism. The past decade has seen substantial progress in the further description of this hypnogenic system; we summarize this progress in this chapter.

Localization of sleep-active neurons within the POA

Studies of sleep-active neuronal discharge across the sleep–wake cycle in freely moving animals provide important information about the hypnogenic process (see below) but, because of sampling limitations, are not suitable for systematic mapping of the exact locations of putative hypnogenic neurons. The application of the c-Fos immunoreactivity (IR) method to map sleep-active neurons has stimulated several advances. C-Fos IR is a marker of neuronal activation in most brain sites; immunohistochemically labeled neurons can be mapped systematically. The localization of c-Fos IR following sustained sleep, but not

Neurochemistry of Sleep and Wakefulness, ed. J. M. Monti *et al.* Published by Cambridge University Press.
© Cambridge University Press 2008.

waking at the same circadian time, permits the quantitative mapping of sleep-active neurons.

Initially, it was proposed that sleep-active neurons were concentrated in a small region identified as the ventrolateral POA (VLPO) (Sherin *et al.*, 1996). This finding was based on the fact that, under the conditions of the procedure, few wake-active neurons were present in VLPO. That is, sleep-active neurons were segregated from wake-active neurons, so the presence of c-Fos IR following sleep could be unambiguously attributed to sleep. Subsequently, by using the c-Fos IR method, additional groups of segregated sleep-active neurons were found in the caudal and rostral median preoptic nucleus (MnPN), also a site with little wake-related c-Fos under quiet waking conditions (Gong *et al.*, 2000). The number of cells exhibiting c-Fos IR following sleep was highly correlated with the percentage of sleep during the preceding 2 h. These studies also showed c-Fos IR following sleep throughout dorsal and lateral POA. Sleep-active neurons were also found in these sites with unit recording studies (see below). However, in dorsal and lateral POA, wake-related c-Fos IR was more prominent, so c-Fos IR following sleep might have arisen from some preceding wake-related processes, rather than sleep (but see below).

Phenotype of sleep-active neurons

Most sleep-related c-Fos IR neurons in rostral and caudal MnPN and in VLPO co-localize glutamic acid decarboxylase (GAD), the enzyme marking neurons that synthesize the inhibitory neurotransmitter γ-aminobutyric acid (GABA) (Fig. 1.1). In our initial description, from studies using a polyclonal antibody, 70%–80% of cells expressing c-Fos following high spontaneous sleep co-localized GAD (Gong *et al.*, 2004b). The number of double-labeled cells was highly correlated with percent of sleep in the preceding 2 h in all three sites (Fig. 1.2). In other studies of the MnPN (Modirrousta *et al.*, 2004) and in work from our laboratory using a monoclonal antibody (Gvilia *et al.*, 2006), both the number of c-Fos expressing cells and the percent of c-Fos/GAD double-labeling were somewhat lower, but the co-localization remained significant. Two studies showed that the number of double-labeled cells increased during recovery sleep after sleep deprivation (Gong *et al.*, 2004b; Modirrousta *et al.*, 2004). These studies suggest that additional GABAergic neurons are activated during sleep in association with increased homeostatic drive. This might be one element of a mechanism of sleep homeostasis. Preliminary findings based on retrograde labeling methods showed that many MnPN neurons sending projections to the perifornical lateral hypothalamus (PLH) co-localize GAD (Gong *et al.*, 2004a).

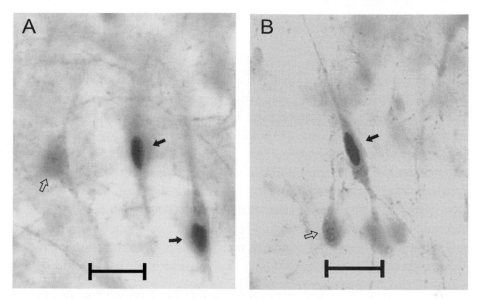

Figure 1.1 Examples of immunostaining for c-Fos IR (dark nuclear staining) and GAD (light cytoplasmic staining) in the MnPN. A higher percentage of GAD-positive cells (arrows) also expressed c-Fos IR (black arrows) following high (A) compared with low spontaneous sleep (B). From Gong *et al.* (2004b). See also Plate 1.

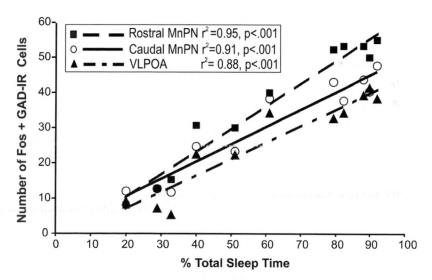

Figure 1.2 Regression analysis between numbers of C-Fos IR + GAD double-labeled neurons and the amount of sleep in the 2 h preceding sacrifice. The numbers of double-labeled cells were highly correlated with the percentage of preceding sleep in VLPO and both rostral and caudal MnPN. From Gong *et al.* (2004b).

Further analysis of the localization of sleep-active neurons within the POA

The numbers of c-Fos/GAD *double-labeled* neurons increased following sleep, compared with waking, in dorsal and lateral POA sites, as well as in MnPN and VLPO (Angara *et al.*, 2004). Sleep-active neurons were also found throughout the lateral POA and in adjacent basal forebrain by using electrophysiological methods (Alam *et al.*, 1995a, 1997; McGinty & Szymusiak, 2001). These findings suggest that the population of sleep-active neurons might be diffusely distributed in the POA, including dorsal and lateral areas, and extend into the basal forebrain. The interpretation is congruent with lesion studies. Some POA lesions that spare the VLPO suppress sleep (Schmidt *et al.*, 2000; John & Kumar, 1998). One study showed a lower correlation between lesion extent and sleep loss after lesions largely sparing VLPO compared with lesions of the VLPO cluster, but this lower correlation seemed to be largely due to cases of *greater* sleep loss than was predicted from lesion extent (see Fig. 1.3 in Lu *et al.*, 2000). Most restricted POA lesions produce partial suppression of sleep. However, very large lesions, encompassing all regions of the POA and adjacent basal forebrain, may produce nearly complete suppression of sleep (McGinty and Sterman, 1968; Sallanon *et al.*, 1989). Thus, most available evidence suggests that sleep-active neurons are distributed in the median, dorsal, lateral, and ventrolateral POA and adjacent basal forebrain.

Details of POA sleep-active neuronal activity

C-Fos IR studies show that increased neuronal activity is correlated with occurrence of sleep, in general. To better evaluate the details of the relationship of neuronal activity and sleep, it is useful to conduct studies of neuronal activity. We have carried out neuronal unit recording studies of VLPO, MnPN, lateral POA, and diagonal band basal forebrain neurons (Suntsova *et al.*, 2002; Szymusiak *et al.*, 1998; Alam *et al.*, 1995a, 1997; Szymusiak & McGinty, 1986). Sleep-active neurons, defined by at least a 20% increase in discharge rate in NREM or REM, constituted 76% of the sample of MnPN neurons and 56% of VLPO neurons, but only about 10% of neurons in lateral POA and DB were sleep-active. These differences are consistent with the differences in the ratios of wake to sleep c-Fos expression in these sites, noted above. Most sleep-active neurons in all sites were slowly discharging during waking, typically doubling discharge rate in NREM sleep (Fig. 1.3). Increases in discharge anticipated EEG synchronization at sleep onset by a few seconds in each site. In MnPN, most sleep active neurons had higher discharge in REM compared with NREM, but in VLPO most neurons had

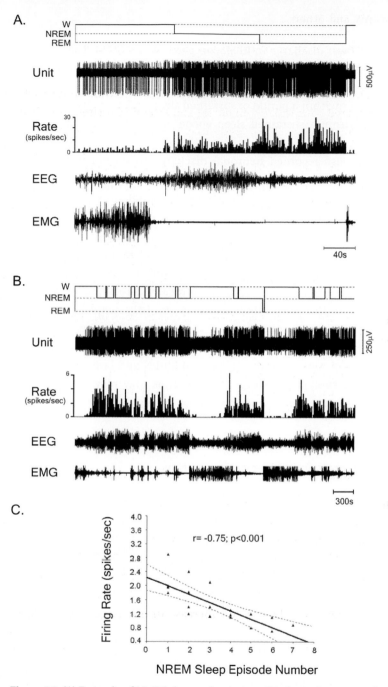

Figure 1.3 (A) Example of MnPN sleep-active neuron. Discharge increases coincident with occurrence of slow wave activity and increases further in REM sleep (right side of sample). (B) Compressed record showing rate histogram across several bouts of NREM sleep. (C) Analysis of a population of such cells showed that MnPN sleep-active neurons exhibited highest discharge during initial NREM episodes and showed progressively declining discharge during subsequent bouts, possibly correlated with sleep drive. From Suntsova *et al.* (2002).

similar or lower discharge in REM, compared with NREM. There were additional differences between the sites. In MnPN, discharge tended to be higher at the beginning of a sustained sleep period, and gradually decline during successive NREM epochs within a period of sustained sleep. In VLPO, discharge progressively increased within a sustained sleep epoch, in association with increasing slow wave activity.

We have also recorded neuronal discharge in several wake-promoting neuronal groups, including the PLH (Alam *et al.*, 2002), histaminergic tuberomammallary nucleus (TMN) of the posterior hypothalamus (PH) (Steininger *et al.*, 1999), dorsal raphe nucleus (Guzman-Marin *et al.*, 2000), and basal forebrain (Szymusiak & McGinty, 1986). The putative histaminergic neurons of the TMN, the putative serotonergic neurons of the dorsal raphe nucleus, and the putative hypocretinergic neurons of the PLH exhibit a wake-active, NREM- *and* REM-off pattern of discharge, changing reciprocally across the W–NREM–REM cycle compared with the typical discharge pattern of the majority of MnPN neurons. Other wake-active neurons in the PH, PLH, and basal forebrain exhibit lower rates in NREM, but higher rates in REM, a discharge pattern that is reciprocal to many VLPO neurons, as well as subsets of MnPN and lateral POA neurons. Thus, the different subtypes of sleep-active neurons may play distinct roles in sleep micro-architecture, and these types may be regionally segregated within the POA.

Efferents from sleep-active neurons

POA neurons are the source of efferents to several established arousal systems. The VLPO is the source of a strong projection to the histaminergic neurons of the ventrolateral posterior hypothalamus (Sherin *et al.*, 1998). The dorsal raphe nucleus receives afferents from the lateral POA and MnPN as well as VLPO (Zardetto-Smith & Johnson, 1885; Peyron *et al.*, 1998; Steininger *et al.*, 2001). The VLPO and dorsolateral POA send projections to the posterior lateral hypothalamus (Steininger *et al.*, 2001; Yoshida *et al.*, 2006; Sakurai *et al.*, 2005). In these semiquantitative analyses, the medial and lateral POA, and MnPN, as well as VLPO, have the highest density of projections to the PLH field. There is evidence that hypocretin/orexin-containing neurons of the PLH receive direct projections from VLPO GABAergic neurons (Sakurai *et al.*, 2005). The locus coeruleus also receives POA projections (Steininger *et al.*, 2001). Thus, it is likely that projections from the POA sleep-active neurons to arousal systems are GABAergic, at least in part. In support of this hypothesis, we have found that stimulation of the MnPN produces short-latency inhibition of PLH neurons (Fig. 1.4). Train stimulation evoked EEG synchronization.

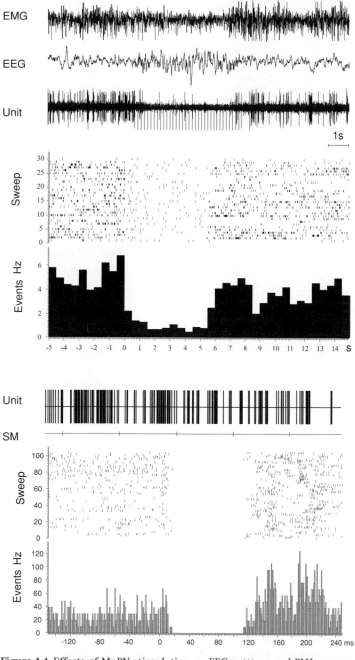

Figure 1.4 Effects of MnPN stimulation on EEG patttern and PLH neuronal activity. Upper: An MnPN 6 s stimulus train suppressed PLH neuronal discharge, evoked EEG synchronization, and reduced EMG activity. The sweep display shows effects of successive stimulus trains. The events display shows averaged PLH neuronal discharge rate in conjunction with train stimulation. Lower: Raster plot showing neuronal discharge during single pulse stimulation. In this example, PLH neuronal activity was inhibited with a latency of about 10 ms; inhibition lasted about 110 ms. Activation of MnPN neurons during NREM sleep would result in suppression of PLH neuronal activity.

GABA release and GABAergic control of arousal systems

Studies using microdialysis showed increased GABA release during sleep, including in REM sleep in the dorsal raphe nucleus (Nitz & Siegel, 1997a) and locus coeruleus (Nitz & Siegel, 1997b), and in NREM sleep in posterior hypothalamus (Nitz & Siegel, 1996). We have studied the role of GABA in control of PLH neurons including hypocretin/orexin-containing neurons in relation to sleep–wake state (Alam *et al.*, 2005). Administration of the GABA antagonist bicuculline (BIC) by microdialysis in PLH suppressed NREM and REM sleep and increased c-Fos IR labeling in hypocretin-positive neurons (Fig. 1.5). These neurons express GABA receptors (Moragues *et al.*, 2003). In the dorsal raphe nucleus, application of the GABA agonist muscimol increased REM sleep, and application of a GABA antagonist, picrotoxin, suppressed REM sleep. These studies suggest that GABA is tonically facilitating both NREM sleep and REM sleep by inhibiting hypocretin neurons, dorsal raphe serotonergic neurons, and other arousal systems. One source of the GABA released during NREM in the PLH as well as the dorsal raphe nucleus and locus coeruleus could be POA and basal forebrain sleep-active GABAergic neurons. In support of this hypothesis are findings that MnPN electrical stimulation inhibits PLH neuronal discharge (Fig. 1.3) and that inactivation of basal forebrain neurons with a GABA agonist, muscimol, increases c-Fos expression in PLH neurons, including orexin-containing neurons (Satoh *et al.*, 2003).

Thermosensitive component of the POA hypnogenic system

Local POA warming by 1–2 °C by means of a water-perfused 'thermode' can trigger NREM sleep onset, increase NREM within sustained sleep, and increase EEG slow wave activity within sustained NREM sleep (reviewed by McGinty & Szymusiak, 2001). Effects of local POA warming are mediated by responses of warmth-sensitive neurons (WSNs) that are identified within the POA. WSNs exhibit brisk increases in discharge in response to small changes in local temperature, more than is expected on the basis of metabolic considerations. WSNs typically constitute 10%–20% of neurons encountered; most POA neurons are unresponsive to small changes in local temperature. We previously showed that a majority of WSNs are sleep-active. Sleep-active WSNs also increase discharge a few seconds before EEG synchronization at sleep onset (Alam *et al.*, 1995a, 1997). Since activation of these neurons by local POA warming is sufficient to initiate and maintain NREM sleep, and these neurons are also activated before and during spontaneous sleep, we can hypothesize that the activation of sleep-active WSNs facilitates spontaneous NREM sleep. The activation of

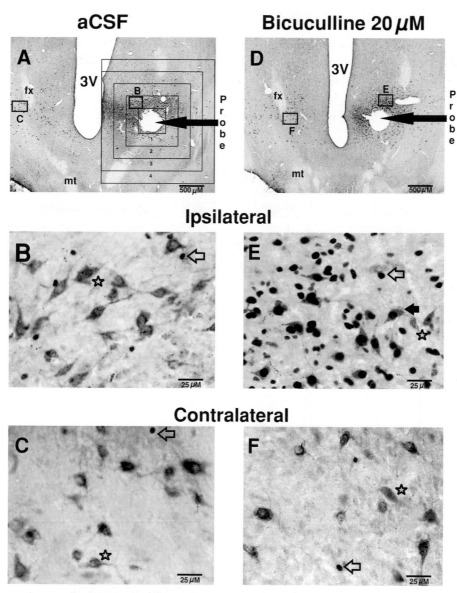

Figure 1.5 Effects of local microdialytic administration of the GABA antagonist bicuculline (BIC) on c-Fos expression in PLH cells. (A, D) Horizontal sections around the hole left by microdialysis membrane. A grid (A) around the probes was used to quantify effects of drug as a function of distance from the membrane. (B, E) Effects of aCSF (B) or BIC (E) on c-Fos IR (small dark spots) and orexin/hypocretin (gray cytoplasmic label) immunostaining. BIC greatly enhanced the numbers of cells exhibiting c-Fos IR. Some orexin/hypocretin-labeled cells were double-labeled. There were no changes contralaterally (C, F), showing that effects were not due to behavioral changes. From Alam *et al.* (2005).

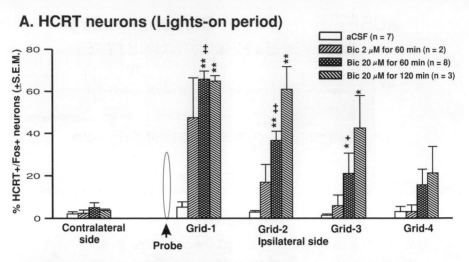

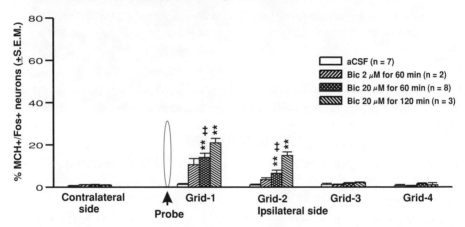

Figure 1.6 (A) Changes in c-Fos IR in hypocretin/orexin(HCRT+)- containing neurons in response to BIC treatment as a function of distance from the microdialysis probe. The percentage of double-labeled cells was greatest closer to the probe (grids 1 and 2, compared with 3 and 4) and was greater with higher concentrations or exposure times. Contralateral cells were not affected. (B) Much lower percentages of melanin-concentrating hormone (MCH+) exhibited c-Fos IR activation in response to BIC. From Alam *et al.* (2005).

POA WSNs also initiates thermolytic autonomic processes with resulting heat loss. It is reasonable to speculate that the activation of these neurons underlies the peripheral vasodilation and evoked lowering of body temperature at sleep onset (reviewed by Heller, 2005) and the association of high sleep propensity with the low-body-temperature phase of the circadian temperature cycle

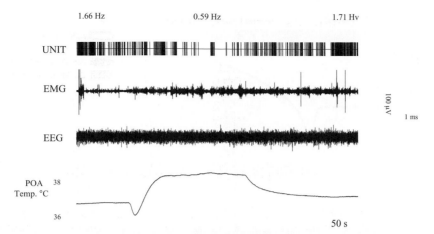

Figure 1.7 Effects of local POA warming on discharges of a DRN, wake-active, REM-off, putative serotonin-containing neuron. POA warming suppressed DRN neuronal discharge, without any change in behavioral state, as shown by EEG spectral analysis. Thus activation of POA WSNs can suppress DRN discharge. The DRN receives direct projections from the POA. From Guzman-Marin *et al.* (2000).

(Dijk & Czeisler, 1995). The association of high sleep propensity with lowering of body temperature could reflect the coincident drive of both processes by the circadian pacemaker. However, we have recently demonstrated close coupling of sleep propensity with falling temperature during ultradian temperature cycles in circadian arrhythmic rats with suprachiasmatic nucleus (SCN) lesions (Baker *et al.*, 2005a). Thus, the association of sleep with falling body temperature likely reflects direct coupling of sleep and thermoregulatory processes rather than circadian control.

Since some sleep-active neurons are WSNs, and sleep-active neurons may distribute inhibitory afferents to arousal-related neurons, we predicted that activation of WSNs by local warming would inhibit arousal systems. We have shown that local POA warming inhibits discharge of putative serotonergic neurons (Guzman-Marin *et al.*, 2000), putative hypocretin-containing neurons in the PLH (Methippara *et al.*, 2003), and other arousal-related PH (Krilowicz *et al.*, 1994) and basal forebrain arousal-related neurons (Alam *et al.*, 1995b) (Figs. 1.7 and 1.8). In these studies, the effects of POA warming were independent of state change as indicated by EEG slowing. Thus, activation of POA WSNs at sleep onset may induce sleep by inhibition of diffuse arousal systems, probably by release of GABA.

The POA also contains cold-sensitive neurons (CSNs), cells activated by local cooling and inhibited by local warming. Most CSNs are wake-active; thus, like arousal-related neurons in PLH, PH, DRN and basal forebrain, they exhibit

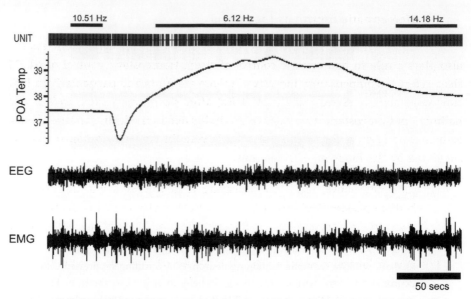

Figure 1.8 Effects of local POA warming on a PLH wake-active, REM-off, putative hypocretin/orexin-containing neuron. POA warming suppressed the waking-related discharge of PLH neurons, in the absence of any state change. The PLH receives strong projections from all subregions of the POA, including GABAergic projections. From Methippara *et al.* (2003).

discharge patterns across the sleep–wake cycle that are reciprocal to sleep-active neurons including WSNs. These neurons are thought to have local connections with WSNs to achieve thermoregulation. These POA wake-active neurons may play a critical role in the response to neurochemical sleep factors to achieve sleep homeostasis.

The sleep–wake switch model

Some arousal-related neurotransmitters, including noradrenaline, serotonin, and acetylcholine, "feed back" to inhibit POA sleep-active neurons. This aspect of the system has been reviewed previously (McGinty & Szymusiak, 2000; Saper *et al.*, 2001). Therefore, once sleep-active neurons are activated, arousal-related neurons are inhibited, and inhibitory control of sleep-active neurons by arousal systems is reduced. In this way, sleep onset is facilitated. That is, the mutually inhibitory systems can switch more quickly from wake to sleep, and back. These mutually inhibitory interactions also promote stability of both waking and sleep.

Homeostatic control by the POA

Some evidence supports a hypothesis that the POA hypnogenic system also plays a role in homeostatic control of sleep. Homeostatic control of NREM sleep refers to compensatory increases in sleep amounts and particularly in EEG slow wave activity (SWA, usually 0.5–4 Hz) after sleep deprivation. SWA is the hallmark of homeostatic control. SWA gradually declines within sustained sleep, as homeostatic drive for sleep is satisfied. A role for the POA in homeostasis is suggested by the following observations.

(1) As noted above, local POA warming increases SWA within sustained NREM episodes (McGinty *et al.*, 1994). SWA is also increased in both rats and humans during sleep following whole body warming (reviewed by Guzman-Marin *et al.*, 2000).

(2) POA lesions suppress the amount of SWA within residual sleep (Lu *et al.*, 2000).

(3) Sleep-related VLPO neurons exhibit increased discharge within NREM during recovery sleep after deprivation, and their discharge rates were correlated with the amount of SWA within sleep episodes (Szymusiak *et al.*, 1998). Thus, VLPO-type sleep-active neurons may directly control the SW content of the NREM EEG, presumably by suppressing arousal systems.

(4) As noted above, MnPN neurons have highest discharge at the beginning of sleep and progressively declining discharge across sustained sleep (Suntsova *et al.*, 2002). This pattern is correlated with homeostatic drive.

(5) Increased numbers of POA GABAergic neurons exhibited c-Fos IR during recovery sleep following deprivation.

These studies are consistent with the concept of POA control of homeostasis, but are not definitive. A definitive study demonstrating the necessity of the POA for homeostatic control of sleep using the lesion method would be difficult to interpret since baseline sleep would be greatly diminished. Instead, recent studies have examined the role of the POA in response to endogenous sleep factors thought to underlie sleep homeostasis.

Hypnogenic sleep factors and the POA

A fundamental question concerns the neurochemical mechanisms that regulate the activity of POA sleep-active neurons. Currently, this problem has been approached through studies of putative "sleep factors", endogenous molecules that could mediate sleep control through (1) accumulation within waking to signal homeostatic drive, and (2) activation of hypnogenic processes. Several such factors have been identified. Here we summarize evidence that these factors may act on the POA.

IL-1β

IL-1β is a well documented sleep factor (reviewed by Obal & Krueger, 2003). Its administration increases sleep, its blockade decreases sleep and sleep rebound, and its transcription increases during waking. IL-1 receptor knock-out mice sleep less. Local application of IL-1β in POA also stimulates NREM sleep. We examined the effects of local administration of IL-1β and an antagonist through microdialytic application adjacent to lateral POA neurons (Alam *et al.*, 2004). Neuronal activity is recorded within 0.5–1.0 mm of a microdialysis membrane in unrestrained rats. IL-1β potently inhibited the activity of 79% of wake-active neurons. The inhibitory response to IL-1β of wake-active neurons could be blocked by pre-treatment with IL-1ra, an IL-1β antagonist. IL-1β application also excited some sleep-active neurons, but this response was inconsistent.

We have also used the c-Fos IR technique to help identify the localization of neurons exhibiting responses to i.c.v. application of IL-1β (Baker *et al.*, 2005b). ICV IL-1β administration induced a delayed increase in NREM sleep, during hours 4 and 5 after administration. However, REM was inhibited during the first 2 hours. These studies showed that IL-1β induced increased c-Fos IR in MnPN, compared with controls, both 2 h and 5 h after administration *in animals allowed to sleep*. These responses were not seen in animals that were not permitted to sleep. Thus, a sleep-permissive process must be in place to reveal the effects of IL-1β in POA. This suggests that IL-1β effects on MnPN are indirect, possibly mediated through actions on wake-active neurons, as suggested by the unit recording study reviewed above.

Adenosine

Adenosine is also a well-documented sleep factor (Porkka-Heiskanen *et al.*, 2002). Systemic or local basal forebrain administration of agonists increases NREM or REM sleep, its blockade decreases sleep, and it accumulates in basal forebrain during sustained waking. The effects of adenosine are mediated by an inhibitory A1 receptor and an excitatory A2a receptor. We have studied the effects of adenosinergic agonists and antagonists in both basal forebrain and POA. Using the microdialysis-unit recording method, we found that adenosine A1 agonists suppressed the activity of arousal-related BF neurons, and A1 antagonists increased their discharge (Alam *et al.*, 1999). Although some individual sleep-related neurons were excited by adenosine, there were no consistent effects on the sample population. We also studied the effects on sleep–wake patterns of more sustained application of A1 and A2a agonists and antagonists by using reverse microdialysis for drug delivery in POA and BF (Methippara *et al.*, 2005). In the POA, in contrast to the BF, delivery of A1 agonists increased waking and A1 antagonists decreased waking. A2a agonists increased sleep and antagonists decreased sleep. We concluded that the effects of adenosinergic agents depend on the predominant cell type in the site of application. In POA, where sleep-active neurons are prominent, the sleep-promoting effects of adenosinergic agonists seem to be mediated by A2a receptors.

Prostaglandin D2 (PGD2)

There is also support for a role of PGD2 in sleep control and homeostasis (Hayaishi, 2002). PGD2 is synthesized in the subarachnoid space ventral to the POA. Administration of PGD2 in the subarachnoid space induces normal sleep, and inhibition of synthesis or receptors suppresses sleep. Sleep rebound after deprivation is reduced in mice in which the synthetic enzyme is knocked out. Administration of PGD2 to the subarachnoid space also induces c-Fos in the VLPO as well as dorsal POA neurons (Scammel *et al.*, 1998). The hypnogenic actions of PGD2 seem to be mediated by an adenosine A2a pathway (Satoh *et al.*, 1966).

The actions of sedative hypnotics

Most hypnotic drugs act on GABA receptors. It is reasonable to hypothesize that hypnotic actions are mediated by the GABA receptors on wake-promoting neurons innervated by POA sleep-active neurons, but there is little study of this problem. However, there is evidence that GABAergic anesthetics induce c-Fos IR in the VLPO and suppress c-Fos IR in histaminergic neurons (Nelson *et al.*, 2002).

Summary

Recent studies have provided detailed information about the properties of the POA hypnogenic system. The POA contains sleep-active neurons, many of which synthesize the inhibitory neurotransmitter GABA. Although there are high densities of these sleep-active neurons in the VLPO and MnPN, some evidence suggests that they are also distributed throughout the POA and extend into the adjacent BF. These POA/BF sleep-active neurons distribute efferents to established arousal-related neurons, including hypocretin/orexin-, histamine-, serotonin-, and noradrenaline-containing neurons in the lateral and posterior hypothalamus, midbrain, and pons. Sleep-active neurons increase discharge prior to EEG slow-wave activity at sleep onset, and maintain elevated discharge throughout NREM and REM sleep, although the patterns of discharge with respect to details of sleep architecture differ among POA sites. On the other hand, arousal-related neurons in lateral and posterior hypothalamus and midbrain exhibit reduced discharge during NREM and, in the subsets of these neurons, reduced discharge during REM sleep, the mirror-image of the activity of sleep-active neurons. In PLH, DRN, and LC, GABA release is increased during NREM or REM sleep. GABA inhibits the activation of PLH arousal-related neurons, including hypocretin/orexin-containing neurons in PLH. Stimulation of the MnPN suppresses the discharge of PLH arousal-related neurons. Some POA sleep-active neurons are locally warmth-sensitive. Local POA warming also suppresses the activity of arousal-related neurons, and facilitates NREM sleep. We summarized the still incomplete evidence that homeostatic mechanisms are also mediated by POA sleep-active neurons. Thermoregulatory processes, as well as some established sleep factors which mediate homeostatic processes, including IL-1, PGD2, and adenosine, act within the POA region and either directly or indirectly excite POA sleep-active neurons. Thus, the current evidence suggests that homeostatic processes facilitate sleep-active neuronal activity. Sleep-active neurons release GABA to inhibit multiple arousal-related neuronal systems which, in turn, control the primary elements of distinguishing NREM sleep and waking, including thalamocortical EEG patterns, muscle tone, and autonomic processes. Systemic drug treatments that affect GABAergic actions often influence all of these functions.

Acknowledgements

Supported by Research Service of the Veterans Administration and PHS grants MH 47480, MH 63323, and HL 60296. The authors thank Feng Xu, Keng-Tee Chew, and Tariq Bashir for support.

References

Alam, Md. N., McGinty, D., & Szymusiak, R. (1995a). Neuronal discharge of preoptic/anterior hypothalamic thermosensitive neurons: relation to NREM sleep. *Am. J. Physiol.* **269**, R1240–9.

Alam, Md. N., Szymusiak, R., & McGinty, D. (1995b). Local preoptic/anterior hypothalamic warming alters spontaneous and evoked neuronal activity in the magno-cellular basal forebrain. *Brain Res.* **696**, 221–30.

Alam, Md. N., McGinty, D., & Szymusiak, R. (1997). Thermosensitive neurons of the diagonal band in rats: relation to wakefulness and non-rapid eye movement sleep. *Brain Res.* **752**, 81–9.

Alam, Md. N., Szymusiak, R., Gong, H., King, J., & McGinty, D. (1999). Adenosinergic modulation of rat basal forebrain neurons during sleep and waking: neuronal recording with microdialysis. *J. Physiol. (Lond.)* **521**(3), 679–90.

Alam, Md. N., Gong, H., Alam, T., Jaganath, R., McGinty, D., & Szymusiak, R. (2002). Sleep-waking discharge patterns of neurons recorded in the rat perifornical lateral hypothalamic area. *J. Physiol.* **538**, 619–31.

Alam, Md. N., McGinty, D., Bashir, T. *et al.* (2004). Interleukin-1β modulates state-dependent discharge of preoptic area and basal forebrain neurons: role in sleep regulation. *Eur. J. Neurosci.* (**in press**).

Alam, Md. N., Kumar, S., Bashir, T. *et al.* (2005). GABA-mediated control of hypocretin- but not melanin-concentrating hormone-immunoreactive neurons during sleep in rats. *J. Physiol.* **563**, 569–82.

Angara, C., Gong, H., Stewart, D. R. *et al.* (2004). Activation of distributed POA GABAergic neurons during recovery sleep. *Soc. Neurosci. Abstr.* **34**, 895.10.

Baker, F. C., Angara, C., Szymusiak, R., & McGinty, D. (2005a). Persistence of sleep-temperature coupling after suprachiasmatic nuclei lesions in rats. *Am. J. Physiol. Regul. Integr. Comp. Physiol.* **289**, R827–38.

Baker, F. C., Shah, S., Stewart, D. *et al.* (2005b). Interleukin 1β enhances non-rapid eye movement sleep and increases c-Fos expression in the median preoptic nucleus of the hypothalamus. *Am. J. Physiol. Regul. Integr. Comp. Physiol.* **288**, R998–1005.

Dijk, D. J. & Czeisler, C. A. (1995). Contribution of the circadian pacemaker and the sleep homeostat to sleep propensity, sleep structure, electroencephalic slow waves, and sleep spindle activity in humans. *J. Neurosci.* **15**, 3526–38.

Gong, H., Szymusiak, R., King, J., Steininger, T., & McGinty, D. (2000). Sleep-related c-Fos expression in the preoptic hypothalamus: effects of ambient warming. *Am. J. Physiol. Regul. Integr. Comp. Physiol.* **279**, R2079–88.

Gong, H., McGinty, D., Angara, C. *et al.* (2004a). Retorgrade labeling in the preoptic area of the hypothalamus following injections of fluor-gold into the perifornical lateral hypothalamus. *Sleep* **27**, A16.

Gong, H., McGinty, D., Guzman-Marin, R. *et al.* (2004b). Activation of GABAergic neurons in the preoptic area during sleep and in response to sleep deprivation. *J. Physiol.* **556**, 935–46.

Guzman-Marin, R., Alam, Md. N., Szymusiak, R. *et al.* (2000). Discharge modulation of rat dorsal raphe neurons during sleep and waking: Effects of preoptic/basal forebrain warming. *Brain Res.* **875**, 23–34.

Gvilia, I., Turner, A., McGinty, D., & Szymusiak, R. (2006). Preoptic area neurons and the homeostatic regulation of rapid eye movement sleep. *J. Neurosci.* **26**, 3037–44.

Hayaishi, O. (2002). Molecular genetic studies on sleep-wake regulation, with special emphasis of the prostaglandin D_2 system. *J. Appl. Physiol.* **92**, 863–8.

Heller, H. C. (2005). Temperature, thermoregulation, and sleep. In *Principles and Practice of Sleep Medicine*, ed. M. H. Kryger, T. Roth, & W. C. Dement, pp. 292–304. Philadelphia, PA: Elsevier Saunders.

John, J. & Kumar, V. (1998). Effect of NMDA lesion of the medial preoptic neurons on sleep and other functions. *Sleep* **21**, 587–98.

Krilowicz, B. L., Szymusiak, R., & McGinty, D. (1994). Regulation of posterior lateral hypothalamic arousal related neuronal discharge by preoptic anterior hypothalamic warming. *Brain Res.* **668**, 30–8.

Lu, J., Greco, M. A., Shiromani, P., & Saper, C. B. (2000). Effect of lesions of the ventrolateral preoptic nucleus on NREM and REM sleep. *J. Neurosci.* **20**, 3830–42.

McGinty, D. and Sterman, M. B. (1968). Sleep suppression after basal forebrain lesions in the cat. *Science* **160**, 1253–5.

McGinty, D. & Szymusiak, R. (2000). The sleep-wake switch: a neuronal alarm clock. *Nature Med.* **6**, 510–11.

McGinty, D. & Szymusiak, R. (2001). Brain structures and mechanisms involved in the generation of NREM sleep: focus on the preoptic hypothalamus. *Sleep Med. Revs* **5**, 323–42.

McGinty, D., Szymusiak, R., & Thomson, D. (1994). Preoptic/anterior hypothalamic warming increases EEG delta frequency activity within non-rapid eye movmement sleep. *Brain Res.* **667**, 273–7.

Methippara, M., Alam, Md. N., Szymusiak, R., & McGinty, D. (2003). Preoptic area warming inhibits wake-active neurons in the perifornical lateral hypothalamus. *Brain Res.* **960**, 165–73.

Methippara, M. M., Kumar, S., Alam, Md. N., Szymusiak, R., & McGinty, D. (2005). Effects on sleep of microdialysis of adenosine A1 and A2A receptor analogs into the lateral preoptic area of rats. *Am. J. Physiol. Regul. Integr. Comp. Physiol.* **289**, 1715–23.

Modirrousta, M., Mainville, L., & Jones, B. E. (2004). GABAergic neurons with α2-adrenergic receptors in basal forebrain and preoptic area express c-Fos during sleep. *Neuroscience* **129**, 803–10.

Moragues, N., Ciofi, P., Lafon, P., Tramu, G., & Garret, M. (2003). GABA$_A$ receptor epsilon subunit expression in identified peptidergic neurons of the rat hypothalamus. *Brain Res.* **967**, 285–9.

Nelson, L. E., Guo, T. Z., Lu, J. *et al.* (2002). The sedative component of anesthesia is mediated by GABA$_A$ receptors in an endogenous sleep pathway. *Nature Med.* **5**, 979–84.

Nitz, D. & Siegel, J. M. (1996). GABA release in posterior hypothalamus across sleep-wake cycle. *Am. J. Physiol.* **271**, R1707–12.

Nitz, D. & Siegel, J. (1997a). GABA release in the dorsal raphe nucleus: role in the control of REM sleep. *Am. J. Physiol.* **273**, R451–5.

Nitz, D. & Siegel, J. M. (1997b). GABA release in the locus coeruleus as a function of sleep/wake state. *Neuroscience* **78**, 795–801.

Obal Jr., F. & Krueger, J. M. (2003). Biochemical regulation of non-rapid-eye-movement sleep. *Frontiers Biosci.* **8**, 520–50.

Peyron, C., Petit, J.-M., Rampon, C., Jouvet, M., & Luppi, P.-H. (1998). Forebrain afferents to the rat dorsal raphe nucleus demonstrated by retrograde and anterograde tracing methods. *Neuroscience* **82**, 443–68.

Porkka-Heiskanen, T., Alanko, L., Kalinchuk, A., & Stenberg, D. (2002). Adenosine and sleep. *Sleep Med. Revis* **6**, 321–32.

Sakurai, T., Nagata, R., Yamanaka, A. *et al.* (2005). Input of orexin/hypocretin neurons revealed by a genetically encoded tracer in mice. *Neuron* **46**, 297–308.

Sallanon, M., Sakai, K., Denoyer, M., Jouvet, M. (1989) Long lasting insomnia induced by preoptic neuron lesions and its transient reversal by muscimol injections into the posterior hypothalamus. *Neuroscience.* **32**, 669–83.

Saper, C. B., Chou, T. C., & Scammel, T. E. (2001). The sleep switch: hypothalamic control of sleep and wakefulness. *Trends Neurosci.* **24**, 726–31.

Satoh, S., Matsumura, H., Suzuki, F., & Hayaishi, O. (1966). Promotion of sleep mediated by the A2a adenosine receptor and possible involvement of this receptor in the sleep induced by prostaglandin D2 in rats. *Proc. Natl. Acad. Sci. USA* **93**, 5980–4.

Satoh, S., Matsumura, H., Nakajima, T. *et al.* (2003). Inhibition of rostral basal forebrain neurons promotes wakefulness and induces FOS in orexin neurons. *Eur. J. Neurosci.* **17**, 1635–45.

Scammel, T., Gerashchenko, D, Urade, Y. *et al.* (1998). Activation of ventrolateral preoptic neurons by the somnogen prostaglandin D2. *Proc. Natl. Acad. Sci. USA* **95**, 7754–9.

Schmidt, M., Valatx, J.-L., Sakai, K., Fort, P., & Jouvet, M. (2000). Role of the lateral preoptic area in sleep-related erectal mechanisms and sleep generation in the rat. *J. Neurosci.* **20**, 6640–7.

Sherin, J. E., Shiromani, P. J., McCarley, R. W., & Saper, C. B. (1996). Activation of ventrolateral preoptic neurons during sleep. *Science* **271**, 216–19.

Sherin, J. E., Elmquist, J. K., Torrealba, F., & Saper, C. B. (1998). Innervation of histaminergic tuberomammillary neurons by GABAergic and galaninergic neurons in the ventrolateral preoptic nucleus of the rat. *J Neurosci.* **18**, 4705–21.

Steininger, T. L., Alam, Md. N., Gong, H., Szymusiak, R., & McGinty, D. (1999). Sleep-waking discharge of neurons in the posterior lateral hypothalamus of the albino rat. *Brain Res.* **840**, 138–47.

Steininger, T. L., Gong, H., McGinty, D., & Szymusiak, R. (2001). Subregional organization of preoptic area/anterior hypothalamic projections to arousal-related monoaminergic cell groups. *J. Comp. Neurol.* **429**, 638–53.

Suntsova, N., Szymusiak, R., Alam, Md. N., Guzman-Marin, R., & McGinty, D. (2002). Sleep-waking discharge patterns of median preoptic nucleus neurons in rats. *J. Physiol.* **543**, 665–77.

Szymusiak, R. & McGinty, D. (1986). Sleep-related neuronal discharge in the basal forebrain of cats. *Brain Res.* **370**, 82–92.

Szymusiak, R., Alam, N., Steininger, T., & McGinty, D. (1998). Sleep-waking discharge patterns of ventrolateral preoptic/anterior hypothalamic neurons in rats. *Brain Res.* **803**, 178–88.

von Economo, C. (1930). Sleep as a problem of localization. *J. Nerv. Ment. Dis.* **71**, 249–59.

Yoshida, K., McCormack, S., Espana, R. A., Crocker, A., & Scammell, T. E. (2006). Afferents to the orexin neurons of the rat brain. *J. Comp. Neurol.* **494**, 845–61.

Zardetto-Smith, A. & Johnson, A. (1885). Chemical topography of efferent projections from the median preoptic nucleus to pontine monoaminergic cell groups in the rat. *Neurosci. Lett.* **199**, 215–19.

2

Neuroanatomical and neurochemical basis of wakefulness and REM sleep systems

RITCHIE E. BROWN AND ROBERT W. McCARLEY

Introduction

The functional states of the central nervous system are determined not only by the inputs received from the external world but also by internally generated electrical and chemical signals. These internally generated signals are responsible for the generation of the states we call sleep and wakefulness and for the transition between states. Neurons generate electrical signals as a result of the uneven distribution of ions across their cell membranes and the passage of ions through pores (ion channels) in these membranes. Neurotransmitters (chemical signaling molecules) are released from the processes of neurons and affect the electrical signaling of target neurons (or muscles) by opening ion channels themselves or by modulating ion channels via second messenger systems. The electrical properties of neurons involved in the control of rapid eye movement (REM) sleep and wakefulness will be described separately. Here we focus on the localization and neurochemistry of neurotransmitters involved in the control of these states.

A variety of different methodologies has been employed to investigate the neurotransmitter systems involved in control of behavioral states. *Biochemical* experiments have elucidated the pathways and enzymes involved in the synthesis, degradation, release and reuptake of different neurotransmitters. *Immunohistochemical* techniques have allowed the visualization of their cellular and subcellular distribution throughout the nervous system as well as the distribution of their receptors and uptake systems. *Chemical sampling* techniques, including

Neurochemistry of Sleep and Wakefulness, ed. J. M. Monti *et al.* Published by Cambridge University Press.
© Cambridge University Press 2008.

microdialysis–electrochemical detection and voltammetry, have allowed the measurement of neurotransmitter concentrations during different behavioral states. *Pharmacological* experiments have investigated the effects of neurotransmitters or compounds affecting their synthesis, release, degradation as well as the effects of specific agonists/antagonists of their receptors. *Electrophysiological* experiments in vivo and in vitro have allowed recording of the discharge of neurons across behavioral state as well as analysis of their intrinsic membrane properties and the ion channels affected by neurotransmitters acting upon them (covered only briefly here). *Electrical or chemical lesion* techniques have allowed the selective destruction of neurotransmitter systems. More recently *genetic engineering/molecular biological* approaches have been used to produce animals lacking particular neurotransmitters or their receptors or to temporarily inactivate them. In humans, *brain imaging* techniques (PET, MRI) are also increasingly being used to monitor brain changes across behavioral states. In combination with many of these other methods *electrographic recording* techniques, i.e. measurement of the electroencephalogram (EEG), electromyogram (EMG) and electrooculogram (EOG), are used to characterize the changes in sleep–wake states that occur.

The majority of our knowledge concerning the neurotransmitters that shape the sleep–wake cycle has been gleaned from experiments in animals, in particular cats, which have large brains and long bouts of wakefulness, slow wave sleep (SWS) and rapid eye movement (REM) sleep and more recently rats and mice which are more amenable to electrophysiological/genetic approaches. Fortunately, the basic neuronal architecture controlling wakefulness and REM sleep appears to be highly conserved throughout evolution so that results in these species can often be applied to humans and other animals. However, interspecies differences are also present, in particular in the amount and timing of sleep episodes.

An excellent description of the discovery of neurotransmitters is provided by Valenstein (2005). Only the essentials of neurotransmitter metabolism are covered here; for more detailed information the reader is directed to textbooks of neurochemistry, e.g. Siegel *et al.* (1994). For a more advanced coverage of the topics discussed here as well as information on the electrical properties of the neurons involved, the interested reader is directed to Steriade & McCarley (2005).

Overview of brain regions controlling wakefulness and REM sleep

A number of clinical and preclinical observations published prior to the era of modern neuroscience gave clues as to the brain areas that are involved in the control of the sleep–wake cycle (Fig. 2.1). The Viennese neurologist Constantin von Economo observed patients suffering from extreme insomnia

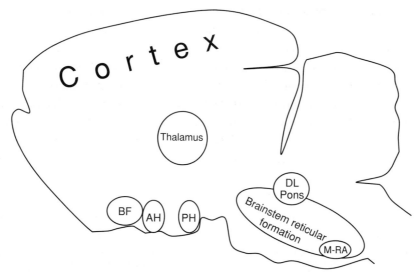

Figure 2.1 Schematic of the rat brain (sagittal section) showing the approximate location of important brain structures controlling wakefulness and REM sleep. Abbreviations: AH, anterior hypothalamus; BF, basal forebrain; DL pons, dorsolateral pons (rapid eye movement sleep control area); M-RA, Magoun/Rhines inhibitory area in the ventral medulla; PH, posterior hypothalamus.

or extreme sleepiness following the worldwide flu pandemic of 1917–20 (von Economo, 1926). Examination of their brains revealed that those patients with insomnia had damage to the anterior part of the hypothalamus, whereas those with excessive sleepiness had damage to the posterior part of the hypothalamus. He concluded that the anterior hypothalamus contains a sleep-inducing center whereas the posterior hypothalamus contains a wake-promoting area. These observations were backed up by lesion experiments in animals by the anatomist Nauta (1946). More recent investigations have revealed that the anterior hypothalamus possesses sleep-active neurons containing the neurotransmitters GABA and galanin whereas the posterior hypothalamus contains the wake-promoting neurotransmitters histamine and the orexins/hypocretins (Saper *et al.*, 2001). Moruzzi and Magoun found that stimulation of the brainstem reticular core led to low-voltage fast EEG activity in the cortex typical of wakefulness (and REM sleep) via activation of non-specific thalamic nuclei projecting to the cortex, leading to the concept of the reticular activating system (Moruzzi & Magoun, 1949). Following the discovery of REM sleep in humans by Kleitman and colleagues (Aserinsky & Kleitman, 1953; Dement & Kleitman, 1957), lesion and transection experiments by Jouvet and colleagues revealed that destruction of a small part of this region, the dorsolateral pons close to the mesopontine junction, was sufficient to abolish this state, which he termed paradoxical sleep (Jouvet, 1962; Mouret *et al.*, 1967b). More recent investigations have revealed that this area contains wake-active noradrenaline and serotonin neurons and wake–REM-active cholinergic and glutamatergic neurons (Jones, 1991a; McCarley, 2004). Both wake-active and REM-active neurons are under the control of GABAergic neurons (Xi *et al.*, 1999; Luppi *et al.*, 2004; Jones, 2004; McCarley, 2004). Magoun and Rhines delineated an inhibitory region in the ventral medulla involved in the inhibition of muscle tone (as occurs during REM sleep) which has since been shown to contain a population of inhibitory neurons releasing the neurotransmitter glycine (Magoun & Rhines, 1946). In the following sections we will examine the function of these and other neurotransmitters in the regulation of wakefulness and REM sleep.

Cholinergic brainstem and basal forebrain neurons

The concept of chemical neurotransmission originated in the 1920s with the classic experiments of Otto Loewi (which were themselves inspired by a dream), who demonstrated that by transferring the ventricular fluid of a stimulated frog heart onto an unstimulated frog heart he could reproduce the effects of a (parasympathetic) nerve stimulus on the unstimulated heart (Loewi & Navratil, 1926). Subsequently, it was found that acetylcholine was the neurotransmitter released from these parasympathetic nerve fibers. As well as playing a critical role in synaptic transmission in the autonomic nervous system and at vertebrate neuromuscular junctions (Dale, 1935), acetylcholine plays a central role in the control of wakefulness and REM sleep. Some have even gone as far as to call acetylcholine "a neurotransmitter correlate of consciousness" (Perry *et al.*, 1999).

Acetylcholine is formed from acetyl CoA (produced as a byproduct of the citric acid and glycolytic pathways) and choline (component of membrane lipids) by the enzyme choline acetyltransferase (ChAT). Following release it is degraded in the extracellular space by the enzyme acetylcholinesterase (AChE) to acetate and choline. The formation of acetylcholine is limited by the intracellular concentration of choline, which is determined by the (re)uptake of choline into the nerve ending (Taylor & Brown, 1994).

The development of antibodies against ChAT allowed the distribution of neurons producing acetylcholine in the nervous system to be revealed (Mesulam *et al.*, 1983; Armstrong *et al.*, 1983; Jones & Beaudet, 1987; Vincent & Reiner, 1987). In the context of control of wakefulness and REM sleep two groups of cholinergic neurons are of primary importance. Neurons located in the basal forebrain and medial septum provide the cholinergic innervation of the cerebral cortex and hippocampus, respectively, whereas neurons located near the junction of midbrain and pons (laterodorsal tegmentum (LDT) and pedunculopontine tegmentum (PPT)) release acetylcholine in the thalamus and brainstem. These LDT/PPT neurons lie within the area shown by lesion and transection experiments to be crucial in the control of REM sleep (Fig. 2.1). Kainate acid lesion of cell bodies in the LDT/PPT region revealed a positive correlation between the extent of cholinergic cell loss and reduction in REM sleep amounts (Webster & Jones, 1988).

Measurements of acetylcholine release across behavioral states in the cerebral cortex and thalamus have shown that acetylcholine concentrations are at their highest during wakefulness and REM sleep, i.e. high acetylcholine levels are correlated with the presence of low-voltage fast activity in the EEG (Jasper & Tessier, 1971; Williams et al., 1994; Leonard & Lydic, 1997). Similarly, recordings of the activity of cholinergic neurons in the basal forebrain and LDT/PPT revealed that they fire at their highest rates during wakefulness or during wakefulness and REM sleep (El Mansari et al., 1989; Steriade et al., 1990a; Manns et al., 2003). Cholinergic neurons can also fire in bursts during these states, which further enhances the release of transmitter in the target regions and may be important in the generation of the synchronized neuronal discharges that occur in the pons, lateral geniculate nucleus of the thalamus and the occipital cortex (PGO waves) during REM sleep (Hu et al., 1988; Steriade et al., 1990b).

The effects of acetylcholine on target organs were divided into nicotinic and muscarinic effects by Henry Dale at the beginning of the twentieth century (Dale, 1914). Subsequently, these same terms were used to describe acetylcholine receptor subtypes. Nicotinic effects were those that could be produced by application of nicotine; nicotinic receptors are ion channels permeable to cations and are responsible for fast synaptic transmission at neuromuscular junctions as well as elsewhere in the nervous system (Changeux et al., 1984). Muscarinic effects were those that could be reproduced by administration of the drug muscarine, which is the principal active component of the poisonous mushroom *Amanita muscaria*. Muscarinic receptors (M_1–M_5) act through GTP-hydrolyzing proteins (G proteins) and second messenger systems to affect ion channels indirectly (Bonner et al., 1987, 1988). M_1-like receptors (M_1, M_3, M_5) are coupled to G_q type G proteins, the activation of which generally leads to excitatory actions on target neurons. M_2-like receptors (M_2, M_4) are coupled to G_i/G_o G proteins. Stimulation of postsynaptic receptors leads to a reduction in the excitability of target neurons, whereas activation of presynaptic receptors leads to inhibition of neurotransmitter release (McCormick, 1992; Roth et al., 1996).

Pharmacological experiments have strongly implicated acetylcholine in the control of REM sleep. In humans, intravenous infusion of the AChE inhibitor physostigmine induced REM sleep when given during slow wave sleep (Sitaram *et al.*, 1976). Injection of the broad-spectrum cholinergic agonist carbachol, selective muscarinic agonists or AChE inhibitors (physostigmine or neostigmine) into the brainstem reticular formation of the cat rapidly induces a long-lasting REM-like state, characterized by low-voltage fast activity in the cortex, muscle atonia, rapid eye movements and PGO waves (Mitler & Dement, 1974; Sitaram *et al.*, 1976; Hobson *et al.*, 1983; Baghdoyan *et al.*, 1984a, b; Vanni-Mercier *et al.*, 1989; Velazquez-Moctezuma *et al.*, 1989; Yamamoto *et al.*, 1990). The most effective region corresponded with the dorsolateral region of the pontine reticular formation shown by Jouvet and colleagues to be critical for REM sleep. In contrast, depletion of acetylcholine by administration of the choline uptake blocker hemicholinium-3 decreases waking and abolishes REM sleep (Hazra, 1970). Furthermore, acetylcholine has prominent effects on the majority of pontine reticular formation neurons, which are thought to be effector neurons for different aspects of the REM state (Greene *et al.*, 1989). The M_2 and M_3 subtypes of muscarinic receptors appear to be the most prominent ones in the brainstem reticular formation (Buckley *et al.*, 1988; Baghdoyan, 1997). Pharmacological and genetic experiments indicate that these are the main subtypes responsible for controlling REM sleep (Datta *et al.*, 1993; Sakai & Onoe, 1997; Baghdoyan & Lydic, 1999; Marks & Birabil, 2001; Goutagny *et al.*, 2005).

Cholinergic LDT/PPT neurons project to the thalamus, causing depolarization of relay and non-specific cortically projecting neurons via M_1-type receptors but hyperpolarization of GABAergic thalamic reticular neurons via M_2-type receptors (McCormick, 1993; Steriade *et al.*, 1993). Both of these actions lead to the abolition of spindles and other EEG phenomena characteristic of deep slow wave sleep. Application of nicotinic antagonists abolishes the thalamic component of PGO waves, indicating that the cholinergic input to the thalamus is required for the generation of these events, which precede and accompany REM sleep (Hu *et al.*, 1988).

Cholinergic neurons in the LDT and PPT produce neuronal nitric oxide synthase (nNOS), the synthesizing enzyme for the gaseous signaling molecule nitric oxide (NO). NO is produced from arginine with nicotinamide adenine dinucleotide phosphate (NADPH) an important cofactor (electron donor) in this reaction (Bredt & Snyder, 1992). Staining for nNOS or NADPH diaphorase (which co-localizes with NOS) selectively labels cholinergic neurons in this area of the brain (Vincent *et al.*, 1983). Recent evidence suggests that NO released from cholinergic brainstem neurons may play a role in the regulation of behavioral state (Leonard *et al.*, 2001; Cespuglio *et al.*, 2004).

Cholinergic neurons in the basal forebrain and medial septum selectively express the low affinity (p75) receptor for nerve growth factor which allows them to be targeted and destroyed by using an antibody against this receptor coupled to the ribosomal toxin saporin. Selective chemical lesions of the basal forebrain cholinergic neurons generally produce relatively minor changes in the distribution of sleep–wake states but consistently reduce faster EEG rhythms, which are thought to be associated with attentional processes and higher levels of consciousness (Kapas et al., 1996; Wenk, 1997; Berntson et al., 2002). Projections of the cholinergic basal forebrain to the rostral pole of the thalamic reticular nucleus and to the cerebral cortex mediate the promotion of fast EEG rhythms through actions on nicotinic and muscarinic receptors (Buzsaki et al., 1988; Parent et al., 1988; McCormick, 1992; Manns et al., 2000). Similarly, selective lesion of the medial septal cholinergic neurons strongly reduces the hippocampal theta rhythm (Lee et al., 1994; Gerashchenko et al., 2001). Both nicotinic and muscarinic receptors play a role in the control of thalamocortical rhythms and EEG low-voltage fast activity through the modulation of glutamatergic projection neurons and GABAergic reticular neurons (Steriade, 2004). Interestingly, drugs that antagonize muscarinic receptors often cause hallucinations and a reduction in the level of consciousness (Perry et al., 1999). Inhibition of cholinergic basal forebrain neurons by adenosine and possibly also serotonin is thought to contribute to the sleepiness produced by prolonged wakefulness (see below).

Serotonin (5-hydroxytryptamine) brainstem raphe neurons

Serotonin was first discovered in the 1930s by Erspamer and colleagues as a factor released from enterochromaffin cells in the gut which caused constriction of smooth muscle (at that time it was called enteramine) (Whitaker-Azmitia, 1999). The name serotonin (1948 on) derives from work on hypertension: thus serotonin is a serum (platelet) derived factor that increases the tone of blood vessels via its action on smooth muscle. Its structure was determined to be a tryptamine molecule with a hydroxyl group at the 5-position (5-hydroxytryptamine (5-HT)) (Rapport et al., 1948). Serotonin was first shown to be a neurotransmitter in the early 1950s, initially in invertebrates and then subsequently also in the mammalian brain (Twarog, 1954; Amin et al., 1954; Twarog & Page, 2005). Shortly after, serotonin was linked to mental illness owing to its similarity in structure to the hallucinogen LSD (Woolley & Shaw, 1954) and also to sleep by the findings that depletion of cerebral serotonin leads to a long-lasting insomnia (Jouvet, 1969). In contrast to these early findings, serotonin is now thought to promote wakefulness and oppose the generation of REM sleep.

The precursor for the synthesis of 5-HT is the amino acid L-tryptophan, which is obtained from dietary protein (Fig. 2.2A). L-tryptophan is converted to 5-hydroxytryptophan (5-HTP) in serotonin neurons by the enzyme tryptophan

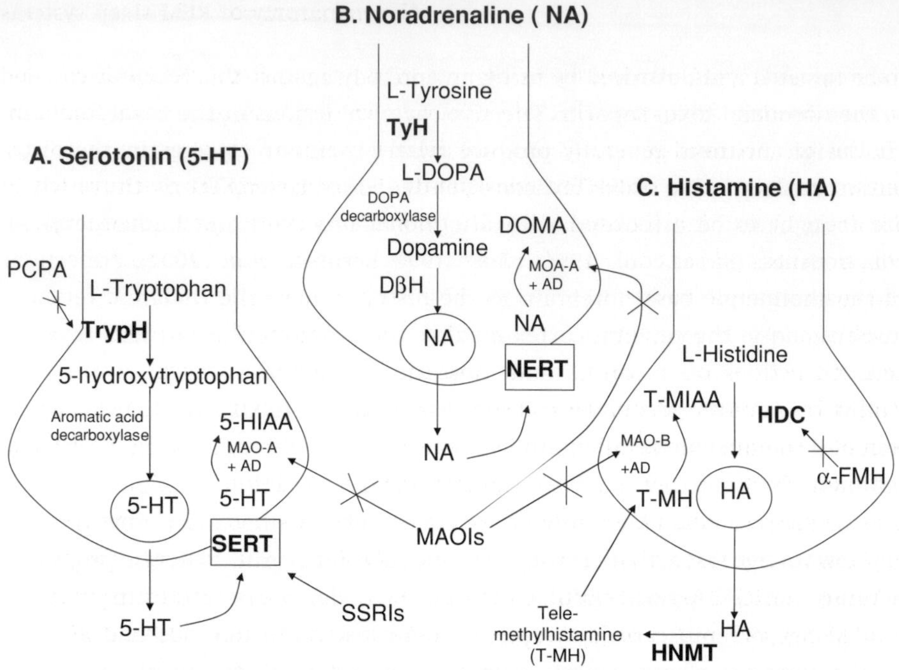

Figure 2.2 Metabolism of the biogenic amines serotonin, noradrenaline, and histamine. Neurons releasing these neurotransmitters show a wake-ON, REM-off firing pattern. (A) The rate-limiting step in the formation of serotonin (5-HT) is the formation of 5-hydroxytryptophan from L-tryptophan by the enzyme tryptophan hydroxylase (TrypH). TrypH can be irreversibly inhibited by p-chlorophenylalanine (PCPA). Subsequently 5-hydroxytryptophan is converted to 5-HT by aromatic acid decarboxylase. The action of serotonin is terminated by reuptake through serotonin reuptake transporters (SERT) on the presynaptic terminal. These transporters can be inhibited by selective serotonin reuptake inhibitors (SSRIs). Intracellularly, serotonin is degraded by the action of monoamine oxidase (MAO, mainly type A) and aldehyde dehydrogenase (AD) to 5-hydroxyindoleacetic acid (5-HIAA). (B) The rate-limiting step in the formation of catecholamines, including noradrenaline (NA) is the formation of L-DOPA from L-tyrosine by the enzyme tyrosine hydroxylase (TyH). Dopamine is formed from L-DOPA by the enzyme DOPA decarboxylase. In noradrenaline neurons dopamine is converted into noradrenaline by dopamine β-hydroxylase (DβH). The action of noradrenaline (norepinephrine, NE) is terminated by selective reuptake transporters (NERT) on the presynaptic terminal. Intracellularly, noradrenaline is degraded by the action of monoamine oxidase (MAO, mainly type A) and aldehyde dehydrogenase (AD) to dihydroxymandelic acid (DOMA). A number of other catabolic pathways are also active (not shown). (C) Histamine (HA) is formed from L-histidine by the enzyme histidine decarboxylase (HDC). HDC can be irreversibly inhibited by α-fluoromethylhistidine (α-FMH). Unlike the other biogenic amines, the action of serotonin is terminated by inactivation by the enzyme histamine-N-methyltransferase (HNMT) to tele-methylhistamine (t-MH). t-MH is in turn degraded by the action of monoamine oxidase (MAO, mainly type B) and aldehyde dehydrogenase (AD) to tele-methylimidazoleacetic acid (5-MIAA). Monoamine oxidase inhibitors (MAOIs) can increase the extracellular concentration of these and other amines (e.g. dopamine) by inhibiting their breakdown.

hydroxylase (TrypH, also known as L-tryptophan-5-monooxygenase). This enzyme is not normally saturated with the substrate (tryptophan) so brain levels of 5-HT can be enhanced by increasing the dietary intake of tryptophan or by systemic administration of 5-HTP. Subsequently 5-hydroxytrophan is converted to 5-hydroxytryptamine (serotonin) by the enzyme aromatic acid decarboxylase, which is also present in catecholamine neurons. Serotonin is catabolized by the enzymes monoamine oxidase (also present in other aminergic neurons) and aldehyde dehydrogenase to form the primary metabolite 5-hydroxyindoleacetic acid (5-HIAA). Once released from neurons, the action of serotonin is controlled by serotonin reuptake transporters (SERT). The extracellular concentration of serotonin can be enhanced by application of selective serotonin reuptake inhibitors (SSRIs, e.g. Prozac^{TM}) or monoamine oxidase inhibitors (MAOIs, which also increase catecholamine levels) which are both used for the treatment of depression and various sleep disorders (Nishino & Mignot, 1997; Argyropoulos & Wilson, 2005). Application of MAOIs or SSRIs causes a profound suppression of REM sleep (Jouvet et al., 1965; Jouvet, 1969; Wilson & Argyropoulos, 2005). A similar effect can be elicited by intravenous or intraperitoneal injection of 5-HTP (Jouvet, 1969).

Histochemical staining techniques were first used to map the distribution of serotonin-producing neurons in the CNS (Dahlstrom & Fuxe, 1964). Major groupings (B1–B9) of serotonin neurons are located along the midline of the mesencephalon and brainstem in the so-called raphe (lit. seam) nuclei (Jacobs & Azmitia, 1992). The largest groupings of serotonin neurons and those which have been most intensively investigated in the context of the sleep–wake cycle are the dorsal and median raphe, which provide the serotonergic innervation of the midbrain and forebrain. Serotonin neurons in the raphe magnus, raphe pallidus, and raphe obscurus provide the majority of the serotonergic innervation of the lower brainstem and spinal cord. Typical of serotonin neurons and several other neurotransmitter systems involved in the control of wakefulness and REM sleep is that they involve a relatively small number of neurons with widespread projections to large areas of the nervous system. Thus, they are ideally constructed to achieve global changes in brain state.

Chemical depletion of serotonin, irreversible inhibition of TrypH with p-chlorophenylalanine (PCPA), or lesion of the area where serotonin-containing perikarya are located was found to cause a long-lasting insomnia (Mouret et al., 1967a; Jouvet, 1969, 1988). Although PCPA is not completely selective for TrypH and has effects on other neurotransmitter systems, intracerebroventricular or intrahypothalamic injection of the serotonin precursor 5-HTP was able to restore sleep to PCPA-treated animals (Jouvet, 1988). These results led Michel Jouvet, one of the pioneers of sleep research, to propose the monoaminergic theory of sleep and waking: 5-HT promotes sleep whereas catecholamines (see below) promote waking (Jouvet, 1969). However, recordings of serotonin neurons and measurements of serotonin release did not reveal the expected results that serotonin neurons are most active during sleep. Instead it was found that serotonin neurons fire at a slow steady rate during waking, reduce their firing during slow wave sleep, and are virtually silent during REM sleep (McGinty & Harper, 1976; Trulson & Jacobs, 1979). Similarly, serotonin release in many brain regions as measured by voltammetry or microdialysis/electrochemical detection reveals that the highest levels are present during wakefulness and the lowest during REM (Wilkinson et al., 1991; Portas et al., 2000). Subsequent data showed that PCPA (or its metabolites) and 5-HTP both have effects on other enzymes as well as on TrypH, e.g. on tyrosine hydroxylase, the enzyme responsible for synthesis of catecholamines and phenylethanolamine N-methyltransferase, the enzyme responsible for converting noradrenaline to adrenaline (Coen et al., 1983). Furthermore, electrolytic lesions of the raphe area are likely to have damaged other neurotransmitter systems in addition to the serotonin system. Thus, it remains unclear to what extent the insomnia caused by PCPA and raphe lesions is due to effects on the serotonin system.

In addition to causing insomnia, PCPA was found to cause PGO spikes to appear continuously during waking. Precise correlations between the firing of serotonin neurons and the timing of PGO spikes have revealed a tight inverse relationship (Lydic et al., 1987). Thus, serotonin is likely to play an important role in the suppression of PGO spikes during waking and early slow wave sleep.

The activity of serotonin neurons and release of serotonin in target regions is controlled by a large number of auto- and heteroreceptors (Jacobs & Azmitia, 1992; Barnes & Sharp, 1999). Particularly important in this regard are somatodendritic 5-HT$_{1A}$ inhibitory autoreceptors. Administration of the 5-HT$_{1A}$ agonist 8-OH-DPAT into the dorsal raphe region leads to an increase in REM sleep (Monti & Jantos, 1992; Portas et al., 1996; Monti et al., 2000). However, this subtype of serotonin receptors is also present postsynaptically on many neurons, including those involved in regulation of wakefulness and REM sleep (e.g. on cholinergic LDT neurons (Luebke et al., 1992)) and on presynaptic terminals. In contrast to the dorsal raphe, activation of 5-HT$_{1A}$ receptors in the LDT causes an inhibition of REM-active cholinergic neurons and a decrease in REM sleep (Horner et al., 1997; Thakkar et al., 1998).

Noradrenaline (norepinephrine) brainstem locus coeruleus neurons

Adrenaline was the first hormone to be isolated. Noradrenaline was discovered in 1907 to be the precursor of adrenaline but it was not until 1946 that von Euler was able to convincingly prove that it acts as a neurotransmitter released by sympathetic nerves. Cytochemical staining techniques developed by Falck and Hillarp in the 1960s revealed that noradrenaline-synthesizing neurons are present in regions of the brainstem known to be involved in the regulation of REM sleep.

The biosynthetic pathways for catecholamines were elucidated by Julius Axelrod, who shared the Nobel Prize for Medicine or Physiology in 1970 with von Euler (Axelrod, 1971). The rate-limiting enzyme in the synthesis of all the catecholamines (dopamine, noradrenaline, and adrenaline) is tyrosine hydroxylase (TyH), which converts L-tyrosine to L-DOPA (Fig. 2.2B). The carboxyl group is removed from L-DOPA by the enzyme DOPA decarboxylase to form dopamine. Noradrenaline is formed from dopamine by the action of dopamine-β-hydroxylase. Noradrenaline is catabolized to adrenaline by phenylethanolamine N-methyltransferase (PNMT). Degradation of catecholamines is achieved by the enzymes monoamine oxidase and catechol-O-methyltransferase. As for serotonin, the action of noradrenaline is controlled by noradrenaline reuptake transporters (NERT). The extracellular concentration of noradrenaline can be enhanced by application of selective inhibitors of noradrenaline transporters or monoamine oxidase inhibitors. These drugs are the primary ones used for the treatment of cataplexy (loss of muscle tone triggered by emotional arousal) in the sleep disorder narcolepsy (Nishino & Mignot, 1997). Depletion of catecholamines and serotonin can be achieved by application of the alkaloid reserpine (produced by the plant *Rauwolfia vomitoria*), which binds to presynaptic vesicles containing these neurotransmitters and prevents their refilling. Reserpine application causes sedation.

Noradrenaline-containing neurons are scattered throughout the brainstem. The largest group of noradrenaline neurons and the one most intensively investigated with respect to the sleep–wake cycle is the locus coeruleus (lit. blue place). These neurons provide the main innervation of the forebrain and midbrain, and even project to the spinal cord. They are located in the dorsolateral pons, in the area that Jouvet and others found to be crucially involved in the control of REM sleep (Jones, 1991b). As with several other cell groups involved in the control of the wakefulness and REM sleep, selective destruction of LC neurons or depletion of noradrenaline produces relatively minor changes in behavioural state (Jones, 1991b). This is likely due to the inherent redundancy of the system: multiple neurotransmitters converge on the same effector systems, for example thalamocortical neurons (McCormick, 1992). Depletion of noradrenaline does, however, prevent the activation of plasticity-related genes in the cerebral cortex during waking (Cirelli *et al.*, 1996; Cirelli & Tononi, 2004).

Depletion of catecholamines by inhibition of their synthesis with α-methylparatyrosine produces an increase in sleep, whereas drugs that enhance the extracellular concentration of catecholamines by enhancing release or blocking reuptake increase wakefulness. Thus, it could be suggested that catecholamine neurons, including noradrenaline neurons, are wake-promoting neurons. Recordings of the activity of locus coeruleus neurons confirmed this suggestion, revealing that locus coeruleus neurons have a pattern of discharge similar to that of serotonin neurons (Hobson *et al.*, 1975; Rasmussen *et al.*, 1986). They fire at a low rate in a pacemaker-like fashion during wakefulness, reduce their firing during slow wave sleep, and cease firing during REM, i.e. they are wake-ON, REM-off neurons. Recordings from LC neurons in genetically narcoleptic dogs revealed that cataplexy is associated with cessation of firing as seen during REM sleep (Wu *et al.*, 1999) whereas other aminergic neurons (serotonergic or histaminergic) do not reduce their firing to the levels seen in REM sleep (John *et al.*, 2004). Thus, noradrenergic LC neurons may be particularly important for the maintenance of muscle tone during waking.

Noradrenaline acts on three types of receptor. The α_1 receptors mediate the main excitatory effects of noradrenaline upon wake-active neurons in the dorsal raphe, basal forebrain, and elsewhere (Vandermaelen & Aghajanian, 1983; Nicoll, 1988; Fort *et al.*, 1995; Brown *et al.*, 2002). The α_2 receptors mediate inhibitory effects of noradrenaline, e.g. on noradrenaline neurons themselves and on cholinergic brainstem neurons (Williams *et al.*, 1985; Williams & Reiner, 1993). The β-receptors modulate neurons in a more subtle fashion, increasing excitability via blockade of afterhyperpolarizations in hippocampal and cortical neurons (Haas & Konnerth, 1983). Activation of β-receptors also promotes synaptic plasticity via activation of the cyclic-AMP-dependent kinase (PKA) and cyclic AMP response element binding protein (CREB) signal transduction pathway (Stanton & Sarvey, 1987; Cirelli *et al.*, 1996).

The reciprocal interaction model of REM sleep

Early pharmacological experiments suggested that acetylcholine and the monoamines interact in the control of REM sleep generation (Karczmar *et al.*, 1970). Thus, potentiation of the action of acetylcholine by systemic application of the AChE inhibitor eserine enhanced waking when applied alone, whereas it produced REM sleep when monoamines had been previously depleted with reserpine. The transection studies carried out by Jouvet (1962) established that the brainstem is sufficient for the generation of cycles of slow wave and rapid eye movement sleep (although their timing and duration is modulated by higher brain structures). More precise lesion studies established that a region of the brainstem surrounding the locus coeruleus was the crucial site for the generation of REM sleep. Recordings of the electrical activity of neurons in this area by

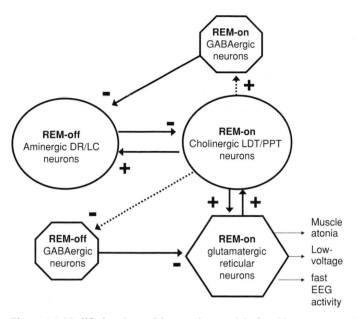

Figure 2.3 Modified reciprocal interaction model of rapid eye movement (REM) sleep control (McCarley/Hobson). The essence of this model is represented in the center of this figure. Cholinergic REM-on neurons in the laterodorsal (LDT) and pedunculopontine (PPT) nuclei of the brainstem are inhibited by REM-off aminergic (serotonergic and noradrenaline) neurons in the dorsal raphe (DR) and locus coeruleus (LC) during other behavioral states. The REM-state is stabilized by mutually excitatory interactions between cholinergic neurons and glutamatergic effector neurons in the reticular formation which are responsible for the different features of REM sleep such as muscle atonia. The REM-state is terminated by renewed activity in aminergic neurons, produced by excitation from the cholinergic neurons. GABAergic neurons control both the aminergic REM-off neurons and the glutamatergic REM-on neurons, and these neurons may in turn be under the control of cholinergic neurons (dotted arrows).

McCarley and Hobson revealed two populations of neurons (Hobson *et al.*, 1975). REM-on neurons increased their firing just prior to and during REM, whereas REM-off neurons showed the reverse pattern. REM-off neurons were proposed to be noradrenaline neurons (serotonin neurons show a similar pattern of firing) whereas REM-on neurons were proposed to be reticular neurons. Subsequently, the REM-on control neurons were proposed to be cholinergic and to direct the firing of glutamatergic effector neurons in the reticular formation responsible for the different aspects of REM sleep (e.g. muscle atonia). McCarley and Hobson proposed an elegant mathematical model, based upon the reciprocal interaction of these two groups of cells, which was able to capture the basic structure of the oscillation between SWS and REM sleep (McCarley & Hobson, 1975) (Fig. 2.3).

The essence of this model is that REM-off neurons (noradrenaline and serotonin neurons) inhibit REM-on neurons (cholinergic neurons) during waking and slow wave sleep but as these neurons reduce their firing (originally thought to be due to activation of inhibitory autoreceptors) during SWS, REM-on neurons are disinhibited and REM sleep is generated. Positive feedback between REM-on neurons (cholinergic and glutamatergic reticular neurons) stabilizes the REM state (Greene *et al.*, 1989; Stevens *et al.*, 1992; Imon *et al.*, 1996). REM-on neurons are also proposed to be excitatory to REM-off neurons so that, as the REM state continues, REM-off neurons gradually become more active, terminating the REM bout. A more sophisticated version of this model has been produced by McCarley and Massaquoi (the limit cycle model) which incorporates circadian influences on the REM oscillator (these may be mediated by the orexins/hypocretins; see below) as well as local GABAergic neurons, which are likely to be important in shutting off REM-off neurons as well as in controlling the activity of REM-on neurons (McCarley & Massaquoi, 1986; McCarley, 2004). Several aspects of the model have been confirmed, including the inhibition of cholinergic neurons by serotonin and noradrenaline (Luebke *et al.*, 1992; Williams & Reiner, 1993; Koyama & Kayama, 1993; Portas *et al.*, 1996; Horner *et al.*, 1997; Thakkar *et al.*, 1998) and the excitation of noradrenaline neurons by acetylcholine (Shen & North, 1992; Koyama & Kayama, 1993; Li *et al.*, 1998).

Histamine neurons in the hypothalamic tuberomammillary nucleus

Histamine was first identified as a biologically active molecule by Henry Dale at the beginning of the twentieth century by examination of the plant fungus ergot (Dale, 1950). In 1927, Dale and colleagues went on to isolate histamine from several different types of animal tissue (histamine is derived from the Greek word *histos*, meaning tissue). The presence of histamine in the brain was demonstrated as early as 1943 by Kwiatowski. Synthesis of histamine in the brain and electrophysiological effects of histamine on neurons were shown in the 1970s (Taylor & Snyder, 1971; Hosli & Haas, 1971; Schwartz *et al.*, 1972; Haas, 1974) but it was not until the 1980s, when histaminergic perikarya could be visualized (Watanabe *et al.*, 1984; Panula *et al.*, 1984), that histamine was accepted as a neurotransmitter. The sedative effects of antihistamines, which cross the blood–brain barrier, originally suggested that histamine is a neurotransmitter promoting wakefulness; more recent experiments support this proposal (Lin, 2000; Brown *et al.*, 2001b).

Histamine is synthesized in the brain from L-histidine by the enzyme histidine decarboxylase (HDC) (Fig. 2.2C). HDC can be inhibited by application of α-fluoromethylhistidine (α-FMH). Unlike serotonin and the catecholamines, no high-affinity uptake system has been discovered and it appears that the action of histamine is terminated through its catabolism to telemethylhistamine by the enzyme histamine N-methyltransferase (HNMT). Telemethylhistamine is further degraded to telemethylimidazoleacetic acid by the combined action of monoamine oxidase B and an aldehyde dehydrogenase. As well as being present in neurons, histamine is also present in some parts of the brain in mast cells (Schwartz et al., 1991).

With the development of antibodies against histamine and histidine decarboxylase in 1984 the localization of histaminergic neurons was revealed (Watanabe et al., 1984; Panula et al., 1984). Histamine neurons are located exclusively in the ventral part of the posterior hypothalamus in the tuberomammillary nucleus (TMN). Histamine neurons send projections from the TMN to essentially the whole brain, including other areas involved in sleep and wakefulness. Histamine is rarely released at synaptic connections between neurons but instead is released from axonal varicosities. Histamine acts upon four subtypes of receptor, three of which are prominently expressed in the brain (Brown et al., 2001b). H_1 and H_2 receptors are expressed postsynaptically whereas H_3 receptors are autoreceptors regulating firing of neurons in the TMN and histamine release in target areas. H_3 receptors also regulate the release of other neurotransmitters. Several subtypes of H_3 receptor have been identified and recent evidence suggests that they can exhibit constitutive activity, i.e. they are active in the absence of agonist (Morisset et al., 2000).

The role of histamine in the sleep–wake cycle has been investigated most closely by Lin, Jouvet and colleagues (Lin, 2000) and by Monti and co-workers (Monti, 1993). Single-unit recordings from histamine neurons in vivo have shown that their pattern of firing across the sleep–wake cycle is similar to that of noradrenaline and serotonin neurons, i.e. they fire in a pacemaker-like fashion at low frequencies during waking, decrease their firing during slow wave sleep, and are silent during REM sleep (Vanni-Mercier et al., 1984; John et al., 2004). Accordingly, a circadian rhythm of histamine release has been demonstrated (Mochizuki et al., 1992). Upregulation of histamine tone by application of histamine itself, H_1 agonists or H_3 antagonists enhances wakefulness and low-voltage fast activity in the cortex. Pharmacological inhibition of HDC, blockade of histamine H_1 receptors (e.g. by the use of antihistamines used in the treatment of allergies) or depression of histamine release with the H_3 autoreceptor agonist R-α-methylhistamine all lead to a reduction in waking and/or fast EEG rhythms and an increase in deep slow wave sleep (Lin et al., 1988, 1990; Monti, 1993). Genetic downregulation of the histamine system in HDC knockout mice does not cause significant changes in the amounts of wakefulness, SWS, and REM, but the ability of these mice to maintain wakefulness in a novel environment is compromised (Parmentier et al.,

2002). Whereas the firing of noradrenaline LC neurons is abolished and that of serotonin neurons is substantially reduced during cataplexy (loss of muscle tone without loss of consciousness), the firing rate of histamine neurons remains high, suggesting that they are important for preserving conscious awareness during this state (John *et al.*, 2004).

Orexin/hypocretin neurons in the perifornical hypothalamus

Orexins/hypocretins were only discovered at the end of the twentieth century but already a large amount is known about their role in control of the sleep–wake cycle and their role in the sleep disorder narcolepsy (Taheri *et al.*, 2002; Brown, 2003). Two groups discovered these peptide neurotransmitters independently (hence the two names). The group of Sakurai and colleagues named these peptides orexins owing to their location in the lateral hypothalamic feeding area (from the Greek *orexis*, appetite) and the finding that intracerebroventricular application of orexin A could stimulate feeding (Sakurai *et al.*, 1998), whereas the group of de Lecea and Sutcliffe named them hypocretins owing to their location in the *hypo*thalamus and their similarity to the hormone se*cretin* (de Lecea *et al.*, 1998).

Orexin A and Orexin B are proteolytically cleaved from a larger precursor protein, preproorexin (131 amino acids in humans), which is encoded by a single gene consisting of two exons. Orexin A is a 33 amino acid peptide consisting of 2 α-helices held together by two disulfide bonds, whereas orexin B consists of 28 amino acids and lacks disulfide linkages (Sakurai *et al.*, 1998). Thirteen of the 28 amino acids are homologous with orexin A. Immunohistochemistry against the orexins revealed that the cell bodies producing these peptides are located exclusively in the posterior lateral hypothalamus around the fornix. Like other systems involved in control of the sleep–wake cycle these neurons send axonal projections to practically the entire CNS, with particularly dense innervation of regions containing aminergic cell groups (Peyron *et al.*, 1998; de Lecea *et al.*, 1998; Sakurai *et al.*, 1998). Orexins activate two types of receptor (OX_1R and OX_2R or HcrtR1 and HcrtR2), the activation of which leads to predominantly excitatory effects on target neurons (van den Pol *et al.*, 1998; Brown, 2003). The type II receptor (which is mutated in narcoleptic canines) is activated by both peptides with similar efficacy whereas the type I receptor is activated at 10–100-fold lower concentrations by orexin A when compared with orexin B (Sakurai *et al.*, 1998).

The sleep disorder narcolepsy, which affects around 1 in every 2000 people, is characterized by a tetrad of symptoms: excessive daytime sleepiness, cataplexy (loss of muscle tone triggered by emotional arousal), hypnagogic hallucinations, and sleep paralysis. Sleep onset REM periods and fragmented night-time sleep are also a characteristic of this disorder (normally the first REM bout of the night occurs following a long period of slow wave sleep). A variety of sophisticated techniques have shown that orexin neurons are involved in narcolepsy (Taheri et al., 2002). The initial impetus for this suggestion was provided by two papers in 1999. One of these papers showed that the genetic defect responsible for narcolepsy in a strain of dogs involved a defect in the orexin type II receptor (Lin et al., 1999). The other paper described mice lacking orexins: orexin knockout mice (Chemelli et al., 1999). These mice had reduced wakefulness and episodes of "behavioral arrest", which typically correlated with direct transitions from wakefulness to REM sleep on the EEG/EMG, and resembled the cataplectic attacks seen in other narcoleptic animals. Subsequently it was shown that mice lacking both orexin receptors or with a lesion of orexin neurons also exhibited the narcoleptic phenotype. Mice lacking OX_2R receptors exhibited a milder narcoleptic phenotype (cf. Chapter 15, this volume). Analysis of orexin neurons in postmortem human narcoleptic brains or measurement of orexin levels in narcoleptic patients has revealed that most human cases of narcolepsy are caused by a loss of orexin neurons (Peyron et al., 2000; Thannickal et al., 2000).

Measurement of orexin levels across behavioral states showed that orexin levels are highest during waking, especially waking associated with movement, and are reduced during sleep (Kiyashchenko et al., 2002). These findings were corroborated by studies using activity of the immediate early gene *fos* as a measure of neuronal activity (Estabrooke et al., 2001). Very recently, single-unit recordings have been made from identified orexin neurons in the perifornical area of the hypothalamus (Mileykovskiy et al., 2005; Lee et al., 2005). These recordings revealed that orexin neurons fire at their highest rate during waking with movement, followed by quiet waking, and decrease their firing during SWS and REM sleep. However, they do exhibit increased firing during phasic periods of REM sleep involving movement (muscle twitches).

Orexins promote wakefulness and oppose REM sleep by acting on and exciting other wake-promoting neurons (Fig. 2.4) such as basal forebrain and brainstem cholinergic neurons, intralaminar thalamic neurons, histaminergic TMN neurons, serotonergic dorsal raphe neurons, and noradrenergic locus coeruleus neurons (Eriksson et al., 2001; Eggermann et al., 2001; Brown et al., 2001a; Burlet et al., 2002; Bayer et al., 2002; Brown, 2003). How orexins control muscle tone and prevent cataplexy and sleep paralysis is incompletely understood but likely involves orexin modulation of neurons within the brainstem, which control the complete loss of muscle tone that occurs during REM sleep (REM muscle atonia).

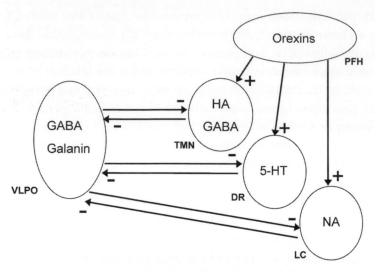

Figure 2.4 Flip–flop switch model of wake and slow wave sleep active systems. Mutually inhibitory connections exist between GABAergic/Galaninergic slow wave sleep active neurons in the ventrolateral preoptic area (VLPO) of the anterior hypothalamus and aminergic neurons in the hypothalamus (histamine (HA) neurons in the tuberomammillary nucleus (TMN)) and brainstem (serotonin (5-HT) neurons in the dorsal raphe (DR) and noradrenaline (NA) neurons in the locus coeruleus (LC)). Orexinergic neurons in the perifornical hypothalamus (PFH) stabilize the waking state via excitation of the waking side of the flip–flop switch (aminergic neurons).

GABAergic neurons in the preoptic area of the hypothalamus and basal forebrain

The major inhibitory neurotransmitter in the brain, γ-aminobutyric acid (GABA) was discovered in 1950 by Roberts and Awapara (Awapara *et al.*, 1950). Experiments in the following decades convincingly showed that it is a neuro-transmitter (Harris-Warrick, 2005). The sedative effects of drugs acting on GABA$_A$ receptors suggested a role for GABA in opposing wakefulness and promoting sleep but the widespread distribution of GABAergic neurons throughout the brain made the identification of those GABAergic neurons involved in control of the sleep–wake cycle problematic. A high concentration of GABAergic neurons was found within the preoptic area of the anterior hypothalamus, the area that von Economo had suggested was a sleep-promoting area. Single-unit recordings in this area revealed a subpopulation of neurons whose firing was enhanced just prior to and during slow wave sleep (Szymusiak & McGinty, 1986). The pre-cise localization of GABAergic neurons promoting sleep was resolved in 1996 through the use of the marker of neuronal activation c-*fos* (an immediate early gene). This technique identified a correlation between neuronal activity (as measured by c-*fos*) and the amount of slow wave sleep in the core region of the ventro-lateral preoptic region (VLPO) and a correlation between c-*fos* and the amount of REM sleep in the area surrounding the VLPO: the extended VLPO (eVLPO) (Sherin *et al.*, 1996; Lu *et al.*, 2002). GABAergic neurons in the core of the VLPO were also found to contain the peptide neurotransmitter galanin (Sherin *et al.*, 1998).

GABA is formed by the so-called GABA shunt. The first step in the GABA shunt is the formation of glutamic acid from α-ketoglutarate (formed from glucose metabolism in the Krebs cycle) by the enzyme GABA α-oxoglutarate transaminase (GABA-T). GABA is formed from glutamic acid by the enzyme glutamic acid decarboxylase (GAD), which has two isoforms, GAD_{67} and GAD_{65}, and is exclusively expressed in neurons utilizing GABA as neurotransmitter. GABA is metabolized to succinic semialdehyde by GABA-T. Succinic semialdehyde is converted to succinic acid, which can re-enter the Krebs cycle, completing the loop. Once released GABA is taken up by a high-affinity plasma membrane transporter.

GABA activates two main types of receptor in the CNS (a third type is located mainly in the retina): $GABA_A$ receptors are ion channels permeable to chloride ions and are made up of a large number of alternative subunits, whereas $GABA_B$ receptors are coupled to potassium channels and calcium channels via the action of G-proteins. The most commonly used sedative drugs (benzodiazepines and barbiturates) act upon the $GABA_A$ receptor and prolong the decay time of currents through the $GABA_A$ receptor. Different subunit combinations of the $GABA_A$ receptor confer sensitivity or resistance to these drugs in different neuronal types (McKernan *et al.*, 2000).

The flip–flop switch controlling wake–sleep transitions

Von Economo originally proposed the existence of an anterior hypothalamic sleep-promoting area and a posterior hypothalamic waking centre. More recent anatomical tracing experiments revealed that neurons in the core of the VLPO project heavily to wake-promoting histamine neurons in the tuberomammillary nucleus (TMN) of the posterior hypothalamus and also to wake-promoting serotonin neurons in the dorsal raphe (DR) and noradrenaline neurons in the locus coeruleus (LC) of the brainstem (Sherin *et al.*, 1998). Electrophysiological experiments showed that GABA and galanin inhibit TMN, DR and LC neurons (Lin *et al.*, 1989; Schönrock *et al.*, 1991; Pieribone *et al.*, 1995; Gervasoni *et al.*, 1998, 2000) whereas serotonin and noradrenaline inhibit VLPO neurons (serotonin also excites a proportion of VLPO neurons) (Gallopin *et al.*, 2000). Histamine does not directly inhibit VLPO neurons but histamine neurons also contain GABA (Kukko-Lukjanov & Panula, 2003), thus TMN neurons can potentially also inhibit VLPO neurons. These mutually inhibitory interactions between VLPO neurons and TMN/DR/LC neurons were conceptualized in the form of a flip–flop switch by Saper and colleagues (2001) such that activation of VLPO leads to inactivity of TMN/DR/LC neurons and sleep whereas activation of TMN/DR/LC leads to inactivity of VLPO neurons and wakefulness (Fig. 2.4). A crucial aspect of this model is that the two halves of the switch, by strongly inhibiting each other, create a feedback loop that is stable in only two states such that intermediate states of sleep and wakefulness are very brief. A further component to the model was the proposal that orexins stabilize behavioral state via their strong excitatory actions on wake-promoting neurons. Analysis of orexin knockout mice revealed that they have many more transitions between wake, SWS, and REM states than do wild-type mice, supporting this model (Mochizuki *et al.*, 2004).

GABAergic brainstem neurons

GABA not only plays an important (inhibitory) role in the control of wakefulness but also gates REM sleep via two distinct actions (Figure 2.3). Application of $GABA_A$ receptor antagonists into the brainstem sites shown to be involved in the generation of REM sleep leads to enhanced amounts of REM sleep (Xi *et al.*, 1999; Boissard *et al.*, 2002; Sanford *et al.*, 2003). Furthermore, GABA levels in these same regions decrease during REM with respect to wakefulness and SWS. Thus, GABAergic neurons (probably located within the brainstem) suppress the firing of REM-on neurons during other states. In contrast, GABA levels in the dorsal raphe and locus coeruleus increase during REM (Nitz & Siegel, 1997a, b) and contribute to the silencing of serotonin and noradrenaline neurons that occurs during this state (Gervasoni *et al.*, 1998, 2000). Thus, other GABAergic neurons (located within the brainstem and in the extended VLPO) help turn off REM-off neurons.

Other GABAergic neurons

GABA is the most important inhibitory neurotransmitter in the brain so it is perhaps not surprising that it plays myriad roles in the control of wakefulness and REM sleep. The thalamic reticular nucleus consists exclusively of GABAergic neurons and plays a critical role in the generation of the different thalamocortical rhythms observed in the electroencephalogram during the sleep–wake cycle through modulation of thalamocortical neurons (Steriade & McCarley, 2005). Interneurons within the cortex and hippocampus are also crucial for shaping the firing of principal neurons and especially for the generation of fast EEG rhythms (Freund & Buzsaki, 1996). GABAergic neurons located in the basal forebrain, hypothalamus, and midbrain project to the cortex (Manns et al., 2000; Lee et al., 2001). Their role in the control of wakefulness and fast EEG rhythms is a topic that requires much further investigation.

Glycine

The amino acid glycine was proposed to be a neurotransmitter in the mammalian spinal cord in 1965 (Aprison & Werman, 1965). Glycine is involved primarily in one aspect of the sleep–wake cycle, namely regulation of muscle tone and in particular the muscle atonia that occurs during REM sleep (Werman et al., 1967; Chase & Morales, 1990). Glycine is formed from serine by the enzyme serine hydroxymethyltransferase (SHMT) (Daly & Aprison, 1974). The action of glycine is terminated by a high-affinity transporter system (Zeilhofer et al., 2005). Glycine activates a chloride-permeable ion channel, similar in structure to the GABA$_A$ receptor, which can be blocked by strychnine (Davidoff et al., 1969; Young & Snyder, 1973; Betz et al., 1999). Recordings from spinal motor neurons revealed that they receive a barrage of inhibitory synaptic potentials, which silence them during REM sleep, and that these inhibitory potentials can be blocked by application of strychnine (Morales & Chase, 1978). Glycine-containing neurons are located throughout the spinal cord and medulla (Davidoff et al., 1967; Zeilhofer et al., 2005). A population of large glycinergic neurons in the Magoun and Rhines area of the ventromedial medulla, which receive glutamatergic inputs from REM muscle atonia-ON neurons in the dorsolateral (subcoerulean) pontine reticular formation, has been most closely linked to REM muscle atonia (Magoun & Rhines, 1946; Lai & Siegel, 1988; Boissard et al., 2002). However, spinal glycinergic neurons may also be contacted by the same glutamatergic REM muscle atonia-ON neurons.

Glutamate

The amino acid glutamate is the most widely used excitatory neurotransmitter in the central nervous system of mammals. Glutamate is the primary neurotransmitter used by the vast majority of reticular formation, thalamic and cortical neurons, which play a crucial role in the generation of the characteristic electrical activity as recorded in the electroencephalogram (for details see Steriade & McCarley (2005)). The activity of these neurons is tightly regulated by the other neurotransmitters described in this chapter.

The metabolism of glutamate is regulated by an interaction between neurons and glial cells and is closely linked to changes in brain energy utilization. Changes in brain oxygen use, blood flow, and glucose utilization observed in human brain imaging studies (PET, MRI) are closely related to activity at gluta-matergic synapses (Magistretti & Pellerin, 1999).

Glutamate activates three classes of receptor: AMPA/kainate, NMDA, and metabotropic glutamate receptors (mGluRs). AMPA/kainate receptors mediate synaptic transmission at glutamatergic synapses stimulated at low frequencies, whereas NMDA and mGluRs are responsible for changes in the strength of these synapses (synaptic plasticity). Pharmacological agents that potentiate ion flow through AMPA/kainate receptors (AMPAkines) are under investigation as possible cognitive enhancers. Several anesthetic agents and drugs of abuse (PCP, ketamine) act on NMDA receptors.

Dopamine

The role of dopamine in the control of wakefulness is intriguing and at the same time confusing. The most potent wake-promoting substances known (amphetamines, modafinil) have a common site of action in inhibiting the dopamine reuptake transporter (DAT), thus increasing extracellular levels of dopamine (Wisor *et al.*, 2001). However, single-unit recordings from dopamine neurons in the two largest dopaminergic cell groups projecting to the forebrain, the substantia nigra (SN) and ventral tegmental area (VTA), revealed that their average firing rate did not change across the sleep–wake cycle (Miller *et al.*, 1983). Thus, although pharmacological enhancement of dopaminergic neurotransmission can enhance waking it is unclear whether dopamine systems in the SN/VTA are actually involved in causing changes in behavioral state. Neurons in the VTA increase their firing rate and fire in bursts in response to environmental cues signaling the availability of primary rewards (Schultz, 1998); thus, they may be important in increasing arousal transiently in association with these biologically important signals rather than playing a role in the sleep–wake cycle as such.

Adenosine

The purines adenosine triphosphate (ATP) and adenosine are involved in energy metabolism in all tissues of the body. The effects of adenyl purines on cardiac function were first described in 1929 (Drury & Szent-Gyorgyi, 1929). In 1970, it was reported that adenosine stimulates cyclic AMP formation in the brain and subsequently Burnstock proposed that purines can act as neurotransmitters. Prominent electrophysiological effects of adenosine on neurons were shown in the 1980s (Phillis & Wu, 1981; Haas & Greene, 1984; Dunwiddie, 1985; Greene & Haas, 1991). A role for adenosine in the homeostatic regulation of wakefulness was proposed by Benington & Heller in 1995 (Benington & Heller,

1995). Subsequent work by our laboratory and others has shown that adenosine accumulation in the basal forebrain is particularly important in this homeostatic regulation (Strecker *et al.*, 2000; Basheer *et al.*, 2004).

Extracellular adenosine concentrations are intimately connected with intracellular concentrations of ATP, the universal energy currency of the cell, such that low ATP concentrations (low ATP/AMP ratio) result in increased transport of adenosine out of the cell (Dunwiddie & Masino, 2001). Neuronal metabolism in most parts of the brain is higher during waking than during sleep so it is not surprising that extracellular adenosine levels are higher during waking than during sleep (Porkka-Heiskanen *et al.*, 1997). Interestingly, with prolonged wakefulness (sleep deprivation), adenosine levels do not continue to rise in all brain areas but instead a rise in adenosine appears relatively selectively in the wake-promoting basal forebrain area (and to a lesser extent in the cortex) (Porkka-Heiskanen *et al.*, 2000). Adenosine inhibits cholinergic neurons and likely also other wake-promoting neurons in this area (Thakkar *et al.*, 2003a). Thus, adenosine may enhance sleepiness by inhibiting these wake-active basal forebrain neurons.

The most widely used stimulants in the world are the methylxanthines caffeine and theophylline, which are widely consumed in coffee, tea, and other drinks (Fredholm *et al.*, 1999). It has long been known that the primary pharmacological target of methylxanthines is adenosine receptors (Snyder *et al.*, 1981). Four adenosine receptors have been characterized: A_1, A_{2a}, A_{2b}, and A_3. Of these, the most important in the brain and for the action of methylxanthines are A_1 and A_{2a} receptors (Fredholm *et al.*, 1999). A_1 receptor activation leads to inhibition of neurons and blockade of synaptic transmission whereas A_{2a} receptors are generally excitatory at the single-cell level (Greene & Haas, 1991). The relative contribution of A_1 versus A_{2a} receptors in the somnogenic actions of adenosine is controversial. Adenosine inhibits wake-promoting cholinergic basal forebrain (and brainstem) neurons via A_1 receptors and infusion of antisense oligonucleotides into this region blocks the rebound in sleep occurring following sleep deprivation (Thakkar *et al.*, 2003a, b). On the other hand, mice lacking adenosine A_1 receptors still show a sleep rebound following sleep deprivation, indicating that this response can be elicited through other mechanisms (Stenberg *et al.*, 2003). Mice lacking A_{2a} receptors lack the increase in arousal produced by caffeine in wild-type and A_1 knockout animals but this action of caffeine may be confounded by the strong locomotor activation produced by stimulation of striatal A_{2a} receptors (Fredholm *et al.*, 1999; Huang *et al.*, 2005). It has also been reported that activation of A_{2a} receptors located in the subarachnoid space underlying the basal forebrain/preoptic area has a sleep-promoting effect, although the mechanisms involved are at present unclear (Scammell *et al.*, 2001).

Conclusions

Wakefulness is produced by the concerted action of diffuse activating systems in the basal forebrain (acetylcholine), hypothalamus (histamine and orexins), and brainstem (acetylcholine, noradrenaline, serotonin, glutamate) which together promote low-voltage fast activity in the cortex, depolarization of thalamocortical neurons, and excitation of motor neurons, leading to enhanced muscle tone. Most of these systems have mutually excitatory connections with each other and converge upon common effector mechanisms in target neurons (McCormick, 1992; Brown *et al.*, 2002) so that the loss of one of them produces only minor changes in sleep and waking. The major exception to this is the orexin/hypocretin system, whose dysfunction leads to the sleep disorder narcolepsy. Shut-off of wake-active neurons and induction of slow wave sleep is achieved by increased activity in preoptic-area GABAergic neurons.

REM sleep is produced by activation of cholinergic and glutamatergic brainstem neurons together with inactivation of aminergic neurons (serotonin, noradrenaline, and histamine). Different subpopulations of GABAergic brainstem neurons play a role in controlling the activity of both REM-on and REM-off neurons. Stabilization of wakefulness and suppression of REM sleep is produced by the activity of the orexin/hypocretin system, which may also be important for consolidating wakefulness in the active period of the day. Suppression of wakefulness after prolonged periods without sleep is mediated to a large extent by adenosine accumulation in the basal forebrain and preoptic area.

Acknowledgements

Supported by Veterans Affairs Medical Research Service (Middleton Award, RWM), and NIMH awards R01 MH62522 and R37 MH39683 (RWM)

References

Amin, A. H., Crawford, B. B. & Gaddum, J. H. (1954). Distribution of 5-hydroxytryptamine and substance P in central nervous system. *J Physiol. Lond.* **126**, 596–618.

Aprison, M. H. & Werman, R. (1965). The distribution of glycine in cat spinal cord and roots. *Life Sci.* **4**, 2075–83.

Argyropoulos, S. V. & Wilson, SJ. (2005). Sleep disturbances in depression and the effects of antidepressants. *Int. Rev. Psychiatr.* **17**, 237–5.

Armstrong, D. M., Saper, C. B., Levey, A. I., Wainer, B. H. & Terry R. D. (1983). Distribution of cholinergic neurons in rat brain: demonstrated by the immunocytochemical localization of choline acetyltransferase. *J. Comp. Neurol.* **216**, 53–68.

Aserinsky, E. & Kleitman, N. (1953). Regularly occurring periods of eye motility, and concomitant phenomena, during sleep. *Science* **118**, 273–4.

Awapara, J., Landau, A. J., Fuerst, R. & Seale, B. (1950). Free gamma-aminobutyric acid in brain. *J. Biol. Chem.* **187**, 35–9.

Axelrod, J. (1971). Noradrenaline: fate and control of its biosynthesis. *Science* **173**, 598–606.

Baghdoyan, H. A. (1997). Location and quantification of muscarinic receptor subtypes in rat pons: implications for REM sleep generation. *Am. J. Physiol.* **273**, R896–R904.

Baghdoyan, H. A. & Lydic, R. (1999). M2 muscarinic receptor subtype in the feline medial pontine reticular formation modulates the amount of rapid eye movement sleep. *Sleep* **22**, 835–47.

Baghdoyan H. A., Monaco, A. P., Rodrigo-Angulo, M. L. *et al.* (1984a). Microinjection of neostigmine into the pontine reticular formation of cats enhances desynchronized sleep signs. *J. Pharmacol. Exp. Ther.* **231**, 173–80.

Baghdoyan, H. A., Rodrigo-Angulo, M. L., McCarley, R. W. & Hobson J. A. (1984b). Site-specific enhancement and suppression of desynchronized sleep signs following cholinergic stimulation of three brainstem regions. *Brain Res.* **306**, 39–52.

Barnes, N. M. & Sharp, T. (1999). A review of central 5-HT receptors and their function. *Neuropharmacology* **38**, 1083–52.

Basheer, R., Strecker, R. E., Thakkar, M. M. & McCarley, R. W. (2004). Adenosine and sleep-wake regulation. *Prog. Neurobiol.* **73**, 379–6.

Bayer, L., Eggermann, E., Saint-Mleux, B. *et al.* (2002). Selective action of orexin (hypocretin) on nonspecific thalamocortical projection neurons. *J. Neurosci.* **22**, 7835–9.

Benington J. H. & Heller, H. C. (1995). Restoration of brain energy metabolism as the function of sleep. *Prog. Neurobiol.* **45**, 347–60.

Berntson, G. G., Shafi, R. & Sarter, M. (2002). Specific contributions of the basal forebrain corticopetal cholinergic system to electroencephalographic activity and sleep/waking behaviour. *Eur. J. Neurosci.* **16**, 2453–61.

Betz, H., Kuhse, J., Schmieden, V. *et al.* (1999). Structure and functions of inhibitory and excitatory glycine receptors. *Ann. N. Y. Acad. Sci.* **868**, 667–76.

Boissard, R., Gervasoni, D., Schmidt, M. H. *et al.* (2002). The rat ponto-medullary network responsible for paradoxical sleep onset and maintenance: a combined microinjection and functional neuroanatomical study. *Eur. J. Neurosci.* **16**, 1959–73.

Bonner, T. I., Buckley, N. J., Young, A. C. & Brann, M. R. (1987). Identification of a family of muscarinic acetylcholine receptor genes. *Science* **237**, 527–32.

Bonner, T. I., Young, A. C., Brann, M. R. & Buckley N. J. (1988). Cloning and expression of the human and rat m5 muscarinic acetylcholine receptor genes. *Neuron* **1**, 403–10.

Bredt, D. S. & Snyder, S. H. (1992). Nitric oxide, a novel neuronal messenger. *Neuron* **8**, 3–11.

Brown, R. E. (2003). Involvement of hypocretins/orexins in sleep disorders and narcolepsy. *Drug News Perspect.* **16**, 75–9.

Brown, RE., Sergeeva, O., Eriksson, K. S. & Haas, H. L. (2001a). Orexin A excites serotonergic neurons in the dorsal raphe nucleus of the rat. *Neuropharmacology* **40**, 457–9.

Brown, R. E., Stevens, D. R. & Haas, H. L. (2001b). The physiology of brain histamine. *Prog. Neurobiol.* **63**, 637–72.

Brown, R. E., Sergeeva, O. A., Eriksson, K. S. & Haas, H. L. (2002). Convergent excitation of dorsal raphe serotonin neurons by multiple arousal systems (orexin/hypocretin, histamine and noradrenaline). *J. Neurosci.* **22**, 8850–9.

Buckley, N. J., Bonner, T. I. & Brann, M. R. (1988). Localization of a family of muscarinic receptor mRNAs in rat brain. *J. Neurosci.* **8**, 4646–52.

Burlet, S., Tyler, C. J. & Leonard, C. S. (2002). Direct and indirect excitation of laterodorsal tegmental neurons by Hypocretin/Orexin peptides: implications for wakefulness and narcolepsy. *J. Neurosci.* **22**, 2862–72.

Buzsaki, G., Bickford, R. G., Ponomareff, G. *et al.* (1988). Nucleus basalis and thalamic control of neocortical activity in the freely moving rat. *J. Neurosci.* **8**, 4007–26.

Cespuglio, R., Debilly, G. & Burlet, S. (2004). Cortical and pontine variations occurring in the voltammetric no signal throughout the sleep-wake cycle in the rat. *Arch. Ital. Biol.* **142**, 551–6.

Changeux, J. P., Devillers-Thiery, A & Chemouilli, P. (1984). Acetylcholine receptor: an allosteric protein. *Science* **225**, 1335–45.

Chase, M. H. & Morales, F. R. (1990). The atonia and myoclonia of active (REM) sleep. *A. Rev. Psychol.* **41**, 557–84.

Chemelli, R. M., Willie, J. T., Sinton, C. M. *et al.* (1999). Narcolepsy in orexin knockout mice: molecular genetics of sleep regulation. *Cell* **98**, 437–51.

Cirelli, C. & Tononi, G. (2004). Locus ceruleus control of state-dependent gene expression. *J. Neurosci.* **24**, 5410–19.

Cirelli, C., Pompeiano, M. & Tononi, G. (1996). Neuronal gene expression in the waking state: a role for the locus coeruleus. *Science* **274**, 1211–15.

Coen, C. W., Coombs, M. C., Wilson, P. M. & Clement, E. M. & MacKinnon, P. C. (1983). Possible resolution of a paradox concerning the use of p-chlorophenylalanine and 5-hydroxytryptophan: evidence for a mode of action involving adrenaline in manipulating the surge of luteinizing hormone in rats. *Neuroscience* **8**, 583–91.

Dahlstrom, A.. and Fuxe, K. (1964). Evidence for the existence of monoamine containing neurons in the central nervous system. I. Demonstration of monoamines in the cell bodies of brainstem neurons. *Acta. Physiol. Scand.* **62** (suppl. 232), 1–55.

Dale, H. (1935). Pharmacology and nerve endings. *Proc. R. Soc. Med.* **28**, 319–32.

Dale, H. (1950). The pharmacology of histamine: with a brief survey of evidence for its occurrence, liberation, and participation in natural reactions. *Ann. N. Y. Acad. Sci.* **50**, 1017–28.

Dale, H. H. (1914). The action of certain esters and ethers of choline and their relation to muscarine. *J Pharmacol* **6**, 147–90.

Daly, E. C. & Aprison, M. H. (1974). Distribution of serine hydroxymethyltransferase and glycine transaminase in several areas of the central nervous system of the rat. *J. Neurochem.* **22**, 877–85.

Datta, S., Quattrochi, J. J. & Hobson, J. A. (1993). Effect of specific muscarinic M2 receptor antagonist on carbachol induced long-term REM sleep. *Sleep* **16**, 8–14.

Davidoff, R. A., Shank, R. P., Graham, L. T. Jr., Aprison, M. H. & Werman, R. (1967). Association of glycine with spinal interneurones. *Nature* **214**, 680–1.

Davidoff, R. A., Aprison, M. H. & Werman, R. (1969). The effects of strychnine on the inhibition of interneurons by glycine and gamma-aminobutyric acid. *Int. J. Neuropharmacol.* **8**, 191–4.

de Lecea, L., Kilduff, T. S., Peyron, C. *et al.* (1998). The hypocretins: hypothalamus-specific peptides with neuroexcitatory activity. *Proc. Natl. Acad. Sci. USA* **95**, 322–7.

Dement, W. & Kleitman, N. (1957). Cyclic variations in EEG during sleep and their relation to eye movements, body motility, and dreaming. *Electroencephalogr. Clin. Neurophysiol. Suppl.* **9**, 673–90.

Drury, A. N. & Szent-Gyorgyi, A. (1929). The physiological activity of adenine compounds with special reference to their action upon mammalian heart. *J. Physiol. Lond.* **68**, 213–7.

Dunwiddie, T. V. (1985). The physiological role of adenosine in the central nervous system. *Int. Rev. Neurobiol.* **27**, 63–139.

Dunwiddie, T. V. & Masino, S. A. (2001). The role and regulation of adenosine in the central nervous system. *An. Rev. Neurosci.* **24**, 31–55.

Eggermann, E., Serafin, M., Bayer, L. *et al.* (2001). Orexins/hypocretins excite basal forebrain cholinergic neurones. *Neuroscience* **108**, 177–81.

El Mansari, M., Sakai, K. & Jouvet, M. (1989). Unitary characteristics of presumptive cholinergic tegmental neurons during the sleep-waking cycle in freely moving cats. *Exp. Brain. Res.* **76**, 519–29.

Eriksson, K. S., Sergeeva, O., Brown, R. E. & Haas, H. L. (2001). Orexin/Hypocretin excites the histaminergic neurons of the tuberomammillary nucleus. *J. Neurosci.* **21**, 9273–9.

Estabrooke, I. V., McCarthy, M. T., Ko, E. *et al.* (2001). Fos expression in orexin neurons varies with behavioral state. *J. Neurosci.* **21**, 1656–62.

Fort, P., Khateb, A., Pegna, A., Muhlethaler, M. & Jones, B. E. (1995). Noradrenergic modulation of cholinergic nucleus basalis neurons demonstrated by in vitro pharmacological and immunohistochemical evidence in the guinea-pig brain. *Eur. J. Neurosci.* **7**, 1502–11.

Fredholm, B. B., Battig, K., Holmen, J., Nehlig, A. & Zvartau, E. E. (1999). Actions of caffeine in the brain with special reference to factors that contribute to its widespread use. *Pharmacol. Rev.* **51**, 83–133.

Freund, T. F. & Buzsaki, G. (1996). Interneurons of the hippocampus. *Hippocampus* **6**, 347–470.

Gallopin, T., Fort, P., Eggermann, E. *et al.* (2000). Identification of sleep-promoting neurons in vitro. *Nature* **404**, 992–5.

Gerashchenko, D., Salin-Pascual, R. & Shiromani, P. J. (2001). Effects of hypocretin-saporin injections into the medial septum on sleep and hippocampal theta. *Brain Res.* **913**, 106–15.

Gervasoni, D., Darracq, L., Fort, P. *et al.* (1998). Electrophysiological evidence that noradrenergic neurons of the rat locus coeruleus are tonically inhibited by GABA during sleep. *Eur. J. Neurosci.* **10**, 964–70.

Gervasoni, D., Peyron, C., Rampon, C., *et al.* (2000). Role and origin of the GABAergic innervation of dorsal raphe serotonergic neurons. *J. Neurosci.* **20**, 4217–25.

Goutagny, R., Comte, J. C., Salvert, D. *et al.* (2005). Paradoxical sleep in mice lacking M3 and M2/M4 muscarinic receptors. *Neuropsychobiology* **52**, 140–6.

Greene, R. W. & Haas, H. L. (1991). The electrophysiology of adenosine in the mammalian central nervous system. *Prog. Neurobiol.* **36**, 329–41.

Greene, R. W., Gerber, U. & McCarley, R. W. (1989). Cholinergic activation of medial pontine reticular formation neurons in vitro. *Brain Res.* **476**, 154–9.

Haas, H. L. (1974). Histamine: action on single hypothalamic neurones. *Brain Res.* **76**, 363–6.

Haas, H. L. & Greene, R. W. (1984). Adenosine enhances afterhyperpolarization and accommodation in hippocampal pyramidal cells. *Pflugers Arch.* **402**, 244–7.

Haas, H. L. & Konnerth, A. (1983). Histamine and noradrenaline decrease calcium-activated potassium conductance in hippocampal pyramidal cells. *Nature* **302**, 432–4.

Harris-Warrick R. (2005). Synaptic chemistry in single neurons: GABA is identified as an inhibitory neurotransmitter. *J. Neurophysiol.* **93**, 3029–31.

Hazra, J. (1970). Effect of hemicholinium-3 on slow wave and paradoxical sleep of cat. *Eur. J. Pharmacol.* **11**, 395–7.

Hobson, J. A., McCarley, R. W. & Wyzinski, P. W. (1975). Sleep cycle oscillation: reciprocal discharge by two brainstem neuronal groups. *Science* **189**, 55–8.

Hobson, J. A., Goldberg, M., Vivaldi, E. & Riew, D. (1983). Enhancement of desynchronized sleep signs after pontine microinjection of the muscarinic agonist bethanechol. *Brain Res.* **275**, 127–36.

Horner, R. L., Sanford, L. D., Annis, D., Pack, A. I. & Morrison, A. R. (1997). Serotonin at the laterodorsal tegmental nucleus suppresses rapid-eye-movement sleep in freely behaving rats. *J. Neurosci.* **17**, 7541–52.

Hosli, L. & Haas, H. L. (1971). Effects of histamine, histidine and imidazole acetic acid on neurones of the medulla oblongata of the cat. *Experientia* **27**, 1311–12.

Hu, B., Bouhassira, D., Steriade, M. & Deschenes, M. (1988). The blockage of ponto-geniculo-occipital waves in the cat lateral geniculate nucleus by nicotinic antagonists. *Brain Res.* **473**, 394–7.

Huang, Z. L., Qu, W.M., Eguchi, N. *et al.* (2005). Adenosine A2A, but not A1, receptors mediate the arousal effect of caffeine. *Nat. Neurosci.* **8**, 858–9.

Imon, H., Ito, K., Dauphin, L. & McCarley, R. W. (1996). Electrical stimulation of the cholinergic laterodorsal tegmental nucleus elicits scopolamine-sensitive excitatory postsynaptic potentials in medial pontine reticular formation neurons. *Neuroscience* **74**, 393–401.

Jacobs, B. L. & Azmitia, E. C. (1992). Structure and function of the brain serotonin system. *Physiol. Rev.* **72**, 165–229.

Jasper, H. H. & Tessier, J. (1971). Acetylcholine liberation from cerebral cortex during paradoxical (REM) sleep. *Science* **172**, 601–2.

John, J., Wu, M. F., Boehmer, L. N. & Siegel, J. M. (2004). Cataplexy-active neurons in the hypothalamus; implications for the role of histamine in sleep and waking behavior. *Neuron* **42**, 619–4.

Jones, B. E. (1991a). Paradoxical sleep and its chemical/structural substrates in the brain. *Neuroscience* **40**, 637–56.

Jones, B. E. (1991b). The role of noradrenergic locus coeruleus neurons and neighboring cholinergic neurons of the pontomesencephalic tegmentum in sleep-wake states. *Prog. Brain. Res.* **88**, 533–43.

Jones, B. E. (2004). Paradoxical REM sleep promoting and permitting neuronal networks. *Arch. Ital. Biol.* **142** 379–96.

Jones, B. E. & Beaudet, A. (1987). Distribution of acetylcholine and catecholamine neurons in the cat brainstem: a choline acetyltransferase and tyrosine hydroxylase immunohistochemical study. *J. Comp. Neurol.* **261**, 15–32.

Jouvet, M. (1962). [Research on the neural structures and responsible mechanisms in different phases of physiological sleep.] *Arch. Ital. Biol.* **100**, 125–206.

Jouvet, M. (1969). Biogenic amines and the states of sleep. *Science* **163**, 32–41.

Jouvet, M. (1988). The regulation of paradoxical sleep by the hypothalamo-hypophysis. *Arch. Ital. Biol.* **126**, 259–74.

Jouvet, M., Vimont, P. & Delorme, F. (1965). [Elective suppression of paradoxical sleep in the cat by monoamine oxidase inhibitors.]. *C. R. Seances. Soc. Biol. Fil.* **159**, 1595–9.

Kapas, L., Obal, F. Jr., Book, A. A. *et al.* (1996). The effects of immunolesions of nerve growth factor-receptive neurons by 192 IgG-saporin on sleep. *Brain Res.* **712**, 53–9.

Karczmar, A. G., Longo, V. G. & De Carolis, A. S. (1970). A pharmacological model of paradoxical sleep: the role of cholinergic and monoamine systems. *Physiol. Behav.* **5**, 175–82.

Kiyashchenko, L. I., Mileykovskiy, B. Y., Maidment, N. *et al.* (2002). Release of hypocretin (orexin) during waking and sleep states. *J. Neurosci.* **22**, 5282–6.

Koyama, Y. & Kayama, Y. (1993). Mutual interactions among cholinergic, noradrenergic and serotonergic neurons studied by ionophoresis of these transmitters in rat brainstem nuclei. *Neuroscience* **55**, 1117–26.

Kukko-Lukjanov, T. K. & Panula, P. (2003). Subcellular distribution of histamine, GABA and galanin in tuberomamillary neurons in vitro. *J. Chem. Neuroanat.* **25**, 279–92.

Lai, Y. Y. & Siegel, J. M. (1988). Medullary regions mediating atonia. *J. Neurosci.* **8**, 4790–6.

Lee, M. G., Chrobak, J. J., Sik, A., Wiley, R. G. & Buzsaki, G. (1994). Hippocampal theta activity following selective lesion of the septal cholinergic system. *Neuroscience* **62**, 1033–47.

Lee, M. G., Hassani, O. K. & Jones, B. E. (2005). Discharge of identified orexin/hypocretin neurons across the sleep-waking cycle. *J. Neurosci.* **25**, 6716–20.

Lee, R. S., Steffensen, S. C. & Henriksen, S. J. (2001). Discharge profiles of ventral tegmental area GABA neurons during movement, anesthesia, and the sleep-wake cycle. *J. Neurosci.* **21**, 1757–66.

Leonard, C. S., Michaelis, E. K. & Mitchell, K. M. (2001). Activity-dependent nitric oxide concentration dynamics in the laterodorsal tegmental nucleus in vitro. *J. Neurophysiol.* **86**, 2159–72.

Leonard, T. O. & Lydic, R. (1997). Pontine nitric oxide modulates acetylcholine release, rapid eye movement sleep generation, and respiratory rate. *J. Neurosci.* **17**, 774–85.

Li, X., Rainnie, D. G., McCarley, R. W. & Greene, R. W. (1998). Presynaptic nicotinic receptors facilitate monoaminergic transmission. *J. Neurosci.* **18**, 1904–12.

Lin, J. S. (2000). Brain structures and mechanisms involved in the control of cortical activation and wakefulness, with emphasis on the posterior hypothalamus and histaminergic neurons. *Sleep Med. Revi.* **4**, 471–503.

Lin, J. S., Sakai, K. & Jouvet, M. (1988). Evidence for histaminergic arousal mechanisms in the hypothalamus of cat. *Neuropharmacology* **27**, 111–22.

Lin, J. S., Sakai, K., Vanni, M. G. & Jouvet, M. (1989). A critical role of the posterior hypothalamus in the mechanisms of wakefulness determined by microinjection of muscimol in freely moving cats. *Brain Res.* **479**, 225–40.

Lin, J. S., Sakai, K., Vanni-Mercier, G. *et al.* (1990). Involvement of histaminergic neurons in arousal mechanisms demonstrated with H3-receptor ligands in the cat. *Brain Res.* **523**, 325–30.

Lin, L., Faraco, J., Li, R. *et al.* (1999). The sleep disorder canine narcolepsy is caused by a mutation in the hypocretin (orexin) receptor 2 gene. *Cell* **98**, 365–76.

Loewi, O. & Navratil, E. (1926). Ueber humorale Uebertragbarkeit der Herznervenwirkung. X. Ueber das Schicksal des Vagusstoffs. *Pflugers Arch.* **214**, 678–88.

Lu, J., Bjorkum, A. A., Xu, M. *et al.* (2002). Selective activation of the extended ventrolateral preoptic nucleus during rapid eye movement sleep. *J. Neurosci.* **22**, 4568–76.

Luebke, J. I., Greene, R. W., Semba, K. *et al.* (1992). Serotonin hyperpolarizes cholinergic low-threshold burst neurons in the rat laterodorsal tegmental nucleus in vitro. *Proc. Natl. Acad. Sci. USA* **89**, 743–7.

Luppi, P. H., Gervasoni, D., Boissard, R. *et al.* (2004). Brainstem structures responsible for paradoxical sleep onset and maintenance. *Arch. Ital. Biol.* **142**, 397–411.

Lydic, R., McCarley, R. W. & Hobson, J. A. (1987). Serotonin neurons and sleep. II. Time course of dorsal raphe discharge, PGO waves, and behavioral states. *Arch. Ital. Biol.* **126**, 1–28.

Magistretti, P. J. & Pellerin, L. (1999). Cellular mechanisms of brain energy metabolism and their relevance to functional brain imaging. *Phil. Trans. R. Soc. Lond. B* **354**, 1155–63.

Magoun, H. W. & Rhines, R. (1946). An inhibitory mechanism in the bulbar reticular formation. *J. Neurophysiol.* **9**, 165–71.

Manns, I. D., Alonso, A. & Jones, B. E. (2000). Discharge profiles of juxtacellularly labeled and immunohistochemically identified GABAergic basal forebrain neurons recorded in association with the electroencephalogram in anesthetized rats. *J. Neurosci.* **20**, 9252–63.

Manns, I. D., Alonso, A. & Jones, B. E. (2003). Rhythmically discharging basal forebrain units comprise cholinergic, GABAergic, and putative glutamatergic cells. *J. Neurophysiol.* **89**, 1057–66.

Marks, G. A. & Birabil, C. G. (2001). Comparison of three muscarinic agonists injected into the medial pontine reticular formation of rats to enhance REM sleep. *Sleep. Res. Online* **4**, 17–24.

McCarley, R. W. (2004). Mechanisms and models of REM sleep control. *Arch. Ital. Biol.* **142**, 429–67.

McCarley, R. W. & Hobson, J. A. (1975). Neuronal excitability modulation over the sleep cycle: a structural and mathematical model. *Science* **189**, 58–60.

McCarley, R. W. & Massaquoi, S. G. (1986). A limit cycle mathematical model of the REM sleep oscillator system. *Am. J. Physiol.* **251**, R1011–R29.

McCormick, D. A. (1992). Neurotransmitter actions in the thalamus and cerebral cortex and their role in neuromodulation of thalamocortical activity. *Prog. Neurobiol.* **39**, 337–88.

McCormick, D. A. (1993). Actions of acetylcholine in the cerebral cortex and thalamus and implications for function. *Prog. Brain. Res.* **98**, 303–8.

McGinty, D. J. & Harper, R. M. (1976). Dorsal raphe neurons: depression of firing during sleep in cats. *Brain Res.* **101**, 569–75.

McKernan, R. M., Rosahl, T. W., Reynolds, D. S. *et al.* (2000). Sedative but not anxiolytic properties of benzodiazepines are mediated by the GABA(A) receptor alpha1 subtype. *Nat. Neurosci.* **3**, 587–92.

Mesulam, M. M., Mufson, E. J., Wainer, B. H. & Levey, A. I. (1983). Central cholinergic pathways in the rat: an overview based on an alternative nomenclature (Ch1-Ch6). *Neuroscience* **10**, 1185–201.

Mileykovskiy, B. Y., Kiyashchenko, L. I. & Siegel, J. M. (2005). Behavioral correlates of activity in identified hypocretin/orexin neurons. *Neuron* **46**, 787–98.

Miller, J. D., Farber, J., Gatz, P., Roffwarg, H. & German, D. C. (1983). Activity of mesencephalic dopamine and non-dopamine neurons across stages of sleep and waking in the rat. *Brain Res.* **273**, 133–41.

Mitler, M. M. & Dement, W. C. (1974). Cataplectic-like behavior in cats after micro-injections of carbachol in pontine reticular formation. *Brain Res.* **68**, 335–43.

Mochizuki, T., Yamatodani, A., Okakura, K. *et al.* (1992). Circadian rhythm of histamine release from the hypothalamus of freely moving rats. *Physiol. Behav.* **51**, 391–4.

Mochizuki, T., Crocker, A., McCormack, S. *et al.* (2004). Behavioral state instability in orexin knock-out mice. *J. Neurosci.* **24**, 6291–300.

Monti, J. M. (1993). Involvement of histamine in the control of the waking state. *Life Sci.* **53**, 1331–8.

Monti, J. M. & Jantos, H. (1992). Dose-dependent effects of the 5-HT1A receptor agonist 8-OH-DPAT on sleep and wakefulness in the rat. *J. Sleep Res.* **1**, 169–75.

Monti, J. M., Jantos, H., Monti, D. & Alvarino, F. (2000). Dorsal raphe nucleus administration of 5-HT1A receptor agonist and antagonists: effect on rapid eye movement sleep in the rat. *Sleep Res. Online* **3**, 29–34.

Morales, F. R. & Chase, M. H. (1978). Intracellular recording of lumbar motoneuron membrane potential during sleep and wakefulness. *Exp. Neurol.* **62**, 821–7.

Morisset, S., Rouleau, A., Ligneau, X. *et al.* (2000). High constitutive activity of native H3 receptors regulates histamine neurons in brain. *Nature* **408**, 860–4.

Moruzzi, G. & Magoun, H. W. (1949). Brainstem reticular formation and activation of the EEG. *Electroencephalogr. Clin. Neurophysiol.* **1**, 455–73.

Mouret, J., Bobillier, P. & Jouvet, M. (1967a). [Effect of parachlorophenylalanine on sleep in rats.] *C. R. Seances Soc. Biol. Fil.* **161**, 1600–3.

Mouret, J., Delorme, F. & Jouvet, M. (1967b). [Lesions of the pontine tegmentum and sleep in rats.] *C. R. Seances Soc. Biol. Fil.* **161**, 1603–6.

Nauta, W. J. H.. (1946). Hypothalamic regulation of sleep in rats. An experimental study. *J. Neurophysiol.* **9**, 285–361.

Nicoll, R. A. (1988). The coupling of neurotransmitter receptors to ion channels in the brain. *Science* **241**, 545–51.

Nishino, S. & Mignot, E. (1997). Pharmacological aspects of human and canine narcolepsy. *Prog. Neurobiol.* **52**, 27–78.

Nitz, D. & Siegel, J. (1997a). GABA release in the dorsal raphe nucleus: role in the control of REM sleep. *Am. J. Physiol.* **273**, R451–5.

Nitz, D. & Siegel, J. M. (1997b). GABA release in the locus coeruleus as a function of sleep/wake state. *Neuroscience* **78**, 795–801.

Panula, P., Yang, H. Y. & Costa, E. (1984). Histamine-containing neurons in the rat hypothalamus. *Proc. Natl. Acad. Sci. USA* **81**, 2572–6.

Parent, A., Pare, D., Smith, Y. & Steriade, M. (1988). Basal forebrain cholinergic and noncholinergic projections to the thalamus and brainstem in cats and monkeys. *J. Comp. Neurol.* **277**, 281–301.

Parmentier, R., Ohtsu, H., Djebbara-Hannas, Z. *et al.* (2002). Anatomical, physiological, and pharmacological characteristics of histidine decarboxylase knock-out mice: evidence for the role of brain histamine in behavioral and sleep-wake control. *J. Neurosci.* **22**, 7695–711.

Perry, E., Walker, M., Grace, J. & Perry, R. (1999). Acetylcholine in mind: a neurotransmitter correlate of consciousness? *Trends Neurosci.* **22**, 273–80.

Peyron, C., Tighe, D. K., van-den Pol, A. N. *et al.* (1998). Neurons containing hypocretin (orexin) project to multiple neuronal systems. *J. Neurosci.* **18**, 9 996–10 015.

Peyron, C., Faraco, J., Rogers, W. *et al.* (2000). A mutation in a case of early onset narcolepsy and a generalized absence of hypocretin peptides in human narcoleptic brains. *Nat. Med.* **6**, 991–7.

Phillis, J. W. & Wu, P. H. (1981). The role of adenosine and its nucleotides in central synaptic transmission. *Prog. Neurobiol.* **16**, 187–239.

Pieribone, V. A., Xu, Z. Q., Zhang, X. *et al.* (1995). Galanin induces a hyperpolarization of norepinephrine-containing locus coeruleus neurons in the brainstem slice. *Neuroscience* **64**, 861–74.

Porkka-Heiskanen, T., Strecker, R. E., Thakkar, M. *et al.* (1997). Adenosine: a mediator of the sleep-inducing effects of prolonged wakefulness. *Science* **276**, 1265–8.

Porkka-Heiskanen, T., Strecker, R. E. & McCarley, R. W. (2000). Brain site-specificity of extracellular adenosine concentration changes during sleep deprivation and spontaneous sleep: an in vivo microdialysis study. *Neuroscience* **99**, 507–17.

Portas, C. M., Thakkar, M., Rainnie, D. & McCarley, R. W. (1996). Microdialysis perfusion of 8-hydroxy-2-(di-n-propylamino)tetralin (8-OH-DPAT) in the dorsal raphe nucleus decreases serotonin release and increases rapid eye movement sleep in the freely moving cat. *J. Neurosci.* **16**, 2820–8.

Portas, C. M., Bjorvatn, B. & Ursin, R. (2000). Serotonin and the sleep/wake cycle: special emphasis on microdialysis studies. *Prog. Neurobiol.* **60**, 13–35.

Rapport, M. M., Green, A. A. & Page, I. H. (1948). Serum vasoconstrictor (serotonin). IV. Isolation and characterization. *J. Biol. Chem.* **176**, 1243–51.

Rasmussen, K., Morilak, D. A. & Jacobs, B. L. (1986). Single unit activity of locus coeruleus neurons in the freely moving cat. I. During naturalistic behaviors and in response to simple and complex stimuli. *Brain Res.* **371**, 324–34.

Roth, M. T., Fleegal, M. A., Lydic, R. & Baghdoyan, H. A. (1996). Pontine acetylcholine release is regulated by muscarinic autoreceptors. *Neuroreport* **7**, 3069–72.

Sakai, K. & Onoe, H. (1997). Critical role for M3 muscarinic receptors in paradoxical sleep generation in the cat. *Eur. J. Neurosci.* **9**, 415–23.

Sakurai, T., Amemiya, A., Ishii, M. *et al.* (1998). Orexins and orexin receptors: a family of hypothalamic neuropeptides and G protein-coupled receptors that regulate feeding behavior. *Cell* **92**, 573–85.

Sanford, L. D., Tang, X., Xiao, J., Ross, R. J. & Morrison, A. R. (2003). GABAergic regulation of REM sleep in reticularis pontis oralis and caudalis in rats. *J. Neurophysiol.* **90**, 938–45.

Saper, C. B., Chou, T. C. & Scammell, T. E. (2001). The sleep switch: hypothalamic control of sleep and wakefulness. *Trends Neurosci.* **24**, 726–31.

Scammell, T. E., Gerashchenko, D. Y., Mochizuki, T. *et al.* (2001). An adenosine A2a agonist increases sleep and induces Fos in ventrolateral preoptic neurons. *Neuroscience* **107**, 653–63.

Schönrock, B., Busselberg, D. & Haas, H. L. (1991). Properties of tuberomammillary histamine neurones and their response to galanin. *Agents Actions* **33**, 135–7.

Schultz, W. (1998). Predictive reward signal of dopamine neurons. *J. Neurophysiol.* **80**, 1–27.

Schwartz, J.-C., Lampart, C. & Rose, C. (1972). Histamine formation in rat brain in vivo: effects of histidine loads. *J. Neurochem.* **19**, 801–10.

Schwartz, J. C., Arrang, J. M., Garbarg, M., Pollard, H. & Ruat, M. (1991). Histaminergic transmission in the mammalian brain. *Physiol. Rev.* **71**, 1–51.

Shen, K. Z. & North, R. A. (1992). Muscarine increases cation conductance and decreases potassium conductance in rat locus coeruleus neurones. *J. Physiol.* **455**, 471–85.

Sherin, J. E., Shiromani, P. J., McCarley, R. W. & Saper, C. B. (1996). Activation of ventrolateral preoptic neurons during sleep. *Science* **271**, 216–19.

Sherin, J. E., Elmquist, J. K., Torrealba, F. & Saper, C. B. (1998). Innervation of histaminergic tuberomammillary neurons by GABAergic and galaninergic neurons in the ventrolateral preoptic nucleus of the rat. *J. Neurosci.* **18**, 4705–21.

Siegel, G. J., Agranoff, B. W., Albers, R. W. & Molinoff, P. B. (1994). *Basic Neurochemistry*. New York, NY: Raven Press.

Sitaram, N., Wyatt, R. J., Dawson, S. & Gillin, J. C. (1976). REM sleep induction by physostigmine infusion during sleep. *Science* **191**, 1281–3.

Snyder, S. H., Katims, J. J., Annau, Z., Bruns, R. F. & Daly, J. W. (1981). Adenosine receptors and behavioral actions of methylxanthines. *Proc. Natl. Acad. Sci. USA* **78**, 3260–4.

Stanton, P. K. & Sarvey, J. M. (1987). Norepinephrine regulates long-term potentiation of both the population spike and dendritic EPSP in hippocampal dentate gyrus. *Brain Res. Bull.* **18**, 115–19.

Stenberg, D., Litonius, E., Halldner, L. *et al.* (2003). Sleep and its homeostatic regulation in mice lacking the adenosine A1 receptor. *J. Sleep Res.* **12**, 283–90.

Steriade, M. (2004). Acetylcholine systems and rhythmic activities during the waking – sleep cycle. *Prog. Brain Res.* **145**, 179–6.

Steriade, M. & McCarley, R. W. (2005). *Brain Control of Wakefulness and Sleep*. New York; NY: Plenum Publishers.

Steriade, M., Datta, S., Pare, D., Oakson, G. & Curro Dossi, R. C. (1990a). Neuronal activities in brain-stem cholinergic nuclei related to tonic activation processes in thalamocortical systems. *J. Neurosci.* **10**, 2541–59.

Steriade, M., Pare, D., Datta, S., Oakson, G. & Curro, D. R. (1990b). Different cellular types in mesopontine cholinergic nuclei related to ponto-geniculo-occipital waves. *J. Neurosci.* **10**, 2560–79.

Steriade, M., McCormick, D. A. & Sejnowski, T. J. (1993). Thalamocortical oscillations in the sleeping and aroused brain. *Science* **262**, 679–85.

Stevens, D. R., McCarley, R. W. & Greene, R. W. (1992). Excitatory amino acid-mediated responses and synaptic potentials in medial pontine reticular formation neurons of the rat in vitro. *J. Neurosci.* **12**, 4188–94.

Strecker, R. E., Moriarty, S., Thakkar, M. M. *et al.* (2000). Adenosinergic modulation of basal forebrain and preoptic/anterior hypothalamic neuronal activity in the control of behavioral state. *Behav. Brain Res.* **115**, 183–204.

Szymusiak, R. & McGinty, D. (1986). Sleep-related neuronal discharge in the basal forebrain of cats. *Brain Res.* **370**, 82–92.

Taheri, S., Zeitzer, J. M. & Mignot, E. (2002). The role of hypocretins (orexins) in sleep regulation and narcolepsy. *A. Rev. Neurosci.* **25**, 283–313.

Taylor, K. M. & Snyder, S. H. (1971). Brain histamine: rapid apparent turnover altered by restraint and cold stress. *Science* **172**, 1037–9.

Taylor, P. & Brown, J. H. (1994). Acetylcholine. In *Basic Neurochemistry*, ed. G. J. Siegel, B. W. Agranoff, R. W. Albers & P. B. Molinoff, pp. 231–60. New York, NY: Raven Press.

Thakkar, M. M., Strecker, R. E. & McCarley, R. W. (1998). Behavioral state control through differential serotonergic inhibition in the mesopontine cholinergic nuclei: a simultaneous unit recording and microdialysis study. *J. Neurosci.* **18**, 5490–7.

Thakkar, M. M., Delgiacco, R. A., Strecker, R. E. & McCarley, R. W. (2003a). Adenosinergic inhibition of basal forebrain wakefulness-active neurons: a simultaneous unit recording and microdialysis study in freely behaving cats. *Neuroscience* **122**, 1107–13.

Thakkar, M. M., Winston, S. & McCarley, R. W. (2003b). A1 receptor and adenosinergic homeostatic regulation of sleep-wakefulness: effects of antisense to the A1 receptor in the cholinergic basal forebrain. *J. Neurosci.* **23**, 4278–87.

Thannickal, T. C., Moore, R. Y., Nienhuis, R. *et al.* (2000). Reduced number of hypocretin neurons in human narcolepsy. *Neuron* **27**, 469–74.

Trulson, M. E. & Jacobs, B. L. (1979). Raphe unit activity in freely moving cats: correlation with level of behavioral arousal. *Brain Res.* **163**, 135–50.

Twarog, B. M. (1954). Responses of a molluscan smooth muscle to acetylcholine and 5-hydroxytryptamine. *J. Cell. Comp. Physiol.* **44**, 141–63.

Twarog, B. M. & Page, I. H. (2005). Serotonin content of some mammalian tissues and urine and a method for its determination. *Am. J. Physiol.* **175**, 157–61.

Valenstein, E. S. (2005). *The War of the Soups and the Sparks*. New York, NY: Columbia University Press.

van den Pol, A. N., Gao, X. B., Obrietan, K., Kilduff, T. S. & Belousov, A. B. (1998). Presynaptic and postsynaptic actions and modulation of neuroendocrine neurons by a new hypothalamic peptide, hypocretin/orexin. *J. Neurosci.* **18**, 7962–71.

Vandermaelen, C. P. & Aghajanian, G. K. (1983). Electrophysiological and pharmacological characterization of serotonergic dorsal raphe neurons recorded extracellularly and intracellularly in rat brain slices. *Brain Res.* **289**, 109–19.

Vanni-Mercier, G., Sakai, K. & Jouvet, M. (1984). [Specific neurons for wakefulness in the posterior hypothalamus in the cat.] *C. R. Acad. Sci. III* **298**, 195–200.

Vanni-Mercier, G., Sakai, K., Lin, J. S. & Jouvet, M. (1989). Mapping of cholinoceptive brainstem structures responsible for the generation of paradoxical sleep in the cat. *Arch. Ital. Biol.* **127**, 133–64.

Velazquez-Moctezuma, J., Gillin, J. C. & Shiromani, P. J. (1989). Effect of specific M1, M2 muscarinic receptor agonists on REM sleep generation. *Brain Res.* **503**, 128–31.

Vincent, S. R. & Reiner, P. B. (1987). The immunohistochemical localization of choline acetyltransferase in the cat brain. *Brain Res. Bull.* **18**, 371–415.

Vincent, S. R., Satoh, K., Armstrong, D. M. & Fibiger, H. C. (1983). NADPH-diaphorase: a selective histochemical marker for the cholinergic neurons of the pontine reticular formation. *Neurosci. Lett.* **43**, 31–6.

Von Economo, C. (1926). Die Pathologie des Schlafes. In *Handbuch des Normalen und Pathologischen Physiologie*, ed. A. Von Bethe, G. Von Bergmann, G. Embden, & A. Ellinger, pp. 591–610. Berlin: Springer.

Watanabe, T., Taguchi, Y., Shiosaka, S. *et al.* (1984). Distribution of the histaminergic neuron system in the central nervous system of rats: a fluorescent immunohistochemical analysis with histidine decarboxylase as a marker. *Brain Res.* **295**, 13–25.

Webster, H. H. & Jones, B. E. (1988). Neurotoxic lesions of the dorsolateral pontomesencephalic tegmentum-cholinergic cell area in the cat. II. Effects upon sleep-waking states. *Brain Res.* **458**, 285–302.

Wenk, G. L. (1997). The nucleus basalis magnocellularis cholinergic system: one hundred years of progress. *Neurobiol. Learn. Mem.* **67**, 85–95.

Werman, R., Davidoff, R. A. & Aprison, M. H. (1967). Inhibition of motoneurones by iontophoresis of glycine. *Nature* **214**, 681–3.

Whitaker-Azmitia, P. M. (1999). The discovery of serotonin and its role in neuroscience. *Neuropsychopharmacology*, **21**, 2S–8S.

Wilkinson, L. O., Auerbach, S. B. & Jacobs, B. L. (1991). Extracellular serotonin levels change with behavioral state but not with pyrogen-induced hyperthermia. *J. Neurosci.* **11**, 2732–41.

Williams, J. A. & Reiner, P. B. (1993). Noradrenaline hyperpolarizes identified rat mesopontine cholinergic neurons in vitro. *J. Neurosci.* **13**, 3878–83.

Williams, J. A., Comisarow, J., Day, J., Fibiger, H. C. & Reiner, P. B. (1994). State-dependent release of acetylcholine in rat thalamus measured by in vivo microdialysis. *J. Neurosci.* **14**, 5236–42.

Williams, J. T., Henderson, G. & North, R. A. (1985). Characterization of alpha 2-adrenoceptors which increase potassium conductance in rat locus coeruleus neurones. *Neuroscience* **14**, 95–101.

Wilson, S. & Argyropoulos, S. (2005). Antidepressants and sleep: a qualitative review of the literature. *Drugs* **65**, 927–7.

Wisor, J. P., Nishino, S., Sora, I. *et al.* (2001). Dopaminergic role in stimulant-induced wakefulness. *J. Neurosci.* **21**, 1787–94.

Woolley, D. W. & Shaw, E. (1954). A biochemical and pharmacological suggestion about certain mental disorders. *Proc. Natl. Acad. Sci. USA* **40**, 228–31.

Wu, M. F., Gulyani, S. A., Yau, E. *et al.* (1999). Locus coeruleus neurons: cessation of activity during cataplexy. *Neuroscience* **91**, 1389–99.

Xi, M. C., Morales, F. R. & Chase, M. H. (1999). Evidence that wakefulness and REM sleep are controlled by a GABAergic pontine mechanism. *J. Neurophysiol.* **82**, 2015–19.

Yamamoto, K., Mamelak, A. N., Quattrochi, J. J. & Hobson, J. A. (1990). A cholinoceptive desynchronized sleep induction zone in the anterodorsal pontine tegmentum: locus of the sensitive region. *Neuroscience* **39**, 279–93.

Young, A. B. & Snyder, S. H. (1973). Strychnine binding associated with glycine receptors of the central nervous system. *Proc. Natl. Acad. Sci. USA* **70**, 2832–6.

Zeilhofer, H. U., Studler, B., Arabadzisz, D. *et al.* (2005). Glycinergic neurons expressing enhanced green fluorescent protein in bacterial artificial chromosome transgenic mice. *J. Comp. Neurol.* **482**, 123–41.

3

Rapid eye movement sleep regulation by modulation of the noradrenergic system

BIRENDRA N. MALLICK, VIBHA MADAN AND SUSHIL K. JHA

Abstract

Aserinsky & Kleitman (1953) identified within sleep a physiological state that expresses several signs apparently similar to those that occur during wakefulness. This state was termed rapid eye movement (REM) sleep. REM sleep may play a significant role in maintaining normal physiological functions, as its loss has serious detrimental psychopathological effects. The mechanism of REM sleep regulation is still unknown. The pontine cholinergic and noradrenergic transmissions in the brain undergo reciprocal variations in activity associated with the transformation from non-REM sleep to a REM sleep state and vice versa. The cessation of noradrenergic neuronal firing in the locus coeruleus (LC) plays a crucial role in the regulation of REM sleep. Disinhibition of the LC neurons may result in increased levels of noradrenaline (NA) in the brain, and this increased brain NA is likely to be responsible for the pathophysiological effects associated with REM sleep deprivation. Based on recent findings, we discuss the modulation as well as the role of LC neurons and NA in the modulation of REM sleep and the pathophysiological conditions associated with its deprivation. We propose that LC NA neurons are negative executive neurons for the regulation of REM sleep.

Introduction

One of the important characteristics of living beings is to alternate between active and rest phases, but the underlying mechanism/s and functions

Neurochemistry of Sleep and Wakefulness, ed. J. M. Monti *et al*. Published by Cambridge University Press.
© Cambridge University Press 2008.

are not yet known. An active phenomenon may induce, actively or passively, a state of rest from that of activity, owing to withdrawal of alertness. However, it is still a paradox whether the rest or inactive state is an absolute quiescent state and, if so, could it revert to an active state by itself? One of the possibilities could be that the brain areas regulating active state may induce a state of rest, which is terminated or reversed to its previous state by an external command; the other possibility, however, could be its intrinsic regulation. An active state may be preset temporally to an internal timer/clock or a phenomenon that may be analogous to charging and discharging a capacitor, with variable time constants to terminate the rest period after a certain interval. During the rest period some part/s within the living organism remain/s active and these could terminate the state of rest or inactivity. There are still some unanswered questions as to why living beings shift from one state to another even without an external influence, how the switching is regulated, and whether there is a specific biochemical machinery working hand in hand with the switch center/s for such regulation. Although much progress has been made during the past half century, the reality is that we are yet to understand completely these biological phenomena, including those relating to sleep and wakefulness.

Animals spend their lives in two distinct vigilant states: sleep or rest phase and wakefulness or alert phase. These states are apparently subjective behaviors, but their electrophysiological correlates, for example electroencephalogram (EEG), electro-occulogram (EOG) and electromyogram (EMG) during different vigilant states, are similar among all mammalian species (Tobler, 1995; Zepelin, 2000). Wakefulness and sleep are associated with variations in the state of consciousness and may be divided into qualitatively different states, e.g. high and low alertness, more attentive, less attentive, inattentive and so on. These classifications may still hold for different purposes, but the electrophysiological signals from the brain, the neck, and the eye muscles have helped classify sleep–wakefulness behaviors objectively into different stages. While studying sleep, Aserinsky and Kleitman (1953) found that, unlike the classical belief at that time, sleep was not a homogenous state. They identified a state within the sleep period when the brain electrical activity, the EEG, was similar to that of wakefulness, together with bursts of rapid eye movements, but unlike wakefulness, there was also postural muscle atonia. Based on the eye movements bursts, they named this state *rapid eye movement* (REM) sleep. Since that time, researchers have studied the phenomenon of sleep under REM sleep and non-REM sleep states. Non-REM sleep is also called slow wave sleep as it is associated with an increase in brain slow wave activity accompanied with spindling in most mammalian species (Tobler, 1995; Borbely & Achermann, 2000). REM sleep, also termed paradoxical sleep or active sleep, is distinguished by desynchronized, low-amplitude activity recorded from the brain, accompanied by hippocampal theta waves in association with eye movements, muscle twitching, and postural muscle atonia. The rest state of various non-mammalian species is thought to be analogous to mammalian non-REM sleep. For example, the rest state in amphibians and reptiles is usually associated with spikes or sharp waves recorded from the brain (Hobson *et al.*, 1968; Flanigan, 1973). However, REM sleep, as defined electrophysiologically, appears to be present only in birds and mammals (Amlaner, 1994; Siegel, 1995; Zepelin, 2000).

REM sleep appears to serve imperative functions, although some may still be unknown, and the detailed mechanism/s of its generation and action are also unknown. It is maximum in babies and decreases with ageing; prey spend proportionately less time in REM sleep when compared with predators, and altricial species have more REM sleep than precocial species (Zepelin, 2000). REM sleep is severely affected by certain diseases such as Alzheimer's, narcolepsy, and psychiatric disorders (Petit *et al.*, 2004; Siegel, 2004; Pawlyk *et al.*, 2005). It is still not known why there is so much variation in REM sleep in various species under different conditions. REM sleep loss by selective deprivation methods induces various pathophysiological behaviors. For example, selective REM sleep deprivation for short periods induces aggressiveness, hypersexuality, an increase in neuronal excitability, and impairment of memory processing and memory consolidation (Vogel, 1975; Gulyani *et al.*, 2000; Stickgold, 2005). Prolonged REM sleep deprivation leads to loss of body heat and body mass, despite an increase in energy expenditure, and then even to death under extreme situations (Rechtschaffen *et al.*, 1989). Although not understood in detail, REM sleep seemingly plays a vital role in the maintenance of normal physiological processes. Hence, it is very important to understand its mechanism of regulation.

REM sleep generating areas

It has been known since the work of the English physiologist Charles Sherrington that animals can survive removal of the entire forebrain. Using similar forebrain transection techniques, Jouvet analyzed the sleep and waking states in decerebrate cats. He found that these decerebrate preparations had periods of muscle tone suppression with rapid eye movements resembling those seen during REM sleep (Jouvet, 1965, 1999). In addition, a REM-sleep-like state recurred periodically and had a duration somewhat similar to that in intact animals. In related studies, brain transections between the pons and the midbrain resulted in the appearance of REM sleep signs only caudal to the cut (Villablanca, 1965, 1966). This demonstrated that the forebrain and midbrain might not be essential for the appearance of REM sleep. Several other studies showed that damage to the pons altered REM sleep. It was found that lesion to the pontis reticularis oralis permanently eliminated all the signs of REM sleep (Carli & Zanchetti, 1965). There were some reports that the medial pontine reticular formation (within 2 mm of the midline) was critical for REM sleep (Jones, 1979); other studies (Sastre *et al.*, 1981; Drucker-Colin & Pedraza, 1983; Friedman & Jones, 1984) led to conclusions that the lateral areas of pontine structures, rather than the medial, were critical. Several other studies showed that damage to the pons altered REM sleep and the key region essential for REM sleep generation was in the lateral part of the reticular formation, in the nucleus 'pontis reticularis oralis' (PRO) and locus coeruleus (LC).

In an attempt to further define the brainstem region responsible for REM sleep regulation, transections were made along various planes in the brain stem. REM-sleep-associated signs could be observed only in the brain region that remained connected to the pons and it was concluded that the pontine region in the brainstem was both necessary and sufficient to generate the basic phenomenon of REM sleep (Siegel *et al.*, 1986). Lesions of the LC significantly induced REM sleep (Caballero & De Andres, 1986) and destruction of neurons around the LC led to an irreversible disappearance of atonia during REM sleep (Jouvet & Delorme, 1965; Henley and Morrison, 1974; Sakai, 1980; Braun & Pivik, 1981). However, the results of some other studies did not completely agree with those findings. Lesions restricted to the LC-principal did not have lasting effects (i.e. more than 48 h) on slow wave sleep or REM sleep (Jones *et al.*, 1977) and it was suggested that the gigantocellular tegmental neurons rather than the NA-containing LC neurons were responsible for the REM sleep (Jones, 1979). Depletion of NA from the NA-containing neurons of the LC by local injection of 6-hydroxydopamine did not prevent REM sleep (Laguzzi *et al.*, 1979). Nevertheless, local cooling of the LC-principal increased sleep as well as REM sleep and local cooling of the LC and peri-LC induced wakefulness, thus supporting the role of the LC in REM sleep (Cespuglio *et al.*, 1982). These findings suggested that the LC and PRO play an important role in REM sleep regulation.

The pontine region possesses anatomically distinct nuclear groups: noradrenoline-(NA-ergic) neurons in the LC, acetylcholine-(ACh-ergic) neurons in the laterodorsal tegmentum (LDT) and pedunculopontine tegmentum (PPT), serotonin-(5-HT-ergic) neurons in the dorsal raphe nucleus (DRN), and GABA-ergic, glutamatergic, and various peptidergic neurons distributed throughout the region (Jones, 1991; Semba, 1993; Honda & Semba, 1995; Rye, 1997; Jones, 2004; Verret *et al.*, 2005). These heterogenous populations of neurons in the pons project onto each other and also receive projections from other brain areas containing dopaminergic and orexinergic neurotransmitters (Winsky-Sommerer *et al.*, 2003). As mentioned above, since REM sleep is affected by lesions within the pontine area, it is likely that among these heterogenous pontine nuclei some are REM-sleep-specific.

REM-ON and REM-OFF neurons

Single unit recording studies identified two distinct populations of REM-sleep-specific neurons in the pontine region. One, which is continuously active in waking, slows during non-REM sleep, and is virtually silent during REM sleep, is the "*REM-OFF*" group of neurons (Chu & Bloom, 1973; Aston-Jones & Bloom, 1981; Heym *et al.*, 1982; Jacobs, 1986). Another group of neurons, which is almost inactive during waking and non-REM sleep and is active almost exclusively during REM sleep, is the "*REM-ON*" group of neurons (Hobson *et al.*, 1975). The REM-OFF neurons are aminergic: NA-ergic (Aston-Jones & Bloom, 1981), likely to be involved in muscle atonia, 5-HT-ergic, likely to be involved in the generation of the PGO waves (McGinty & Harper, 1976; Heym *et al.*, 1982; Fornal *et al.*, 1985), and histaminergic (Jones, 2005; Saper *et al.*, 2005). The REM-ON cells are presumably cholinergic (Sakai, 1980; el Mansari *et al.*, 1989; Baghdoyan & Lydic, 2002) and are likely to be involved in EEG desynchronization. However, the presence of some non-cholinergic REM-ON neurons has also been proposed (Sakai, 1980; el Mansari *et al.*, 1989; Baghdoyan & Lydic, 2002). These cells are mainly located in the paragigantocellular reticular formation and the LDT/PPT. The interactions between neurotransmitters play a significant role in modulating the neuronal behavior that results in transition from one state to another, namely from wakefulness to non-REM sleep to REM sleep.

Neurotransmitters and REM sleep regulation

Several neurotransmitters and neuropeptides influence sleep–wakefulness, including REM sleep. Although NA-ergic and ACh-ergic influences have been studied more extensively, other neurotransmitters also play an important role in the modulation of REM sleep (Sakai, 1986; Mallick *et al.*, 1999; Jones, 2005).

Noradrenaline and REM sleep regulation

The brain receives substantial NA-ergic innervation from the diffused ascending and descending projections of the LC, located just posterior to the periaqueductal gray in the dorsorostral pons (Moore & Bloom, 1979). Several reports showed that systemic and local microinjection of NA agonists and antagonists altered the expression of REM sleep, suggesting an important role of NA in the generation and maintenance of REM sleep. The β-2-adrenoceptor-stimulating drug salbutamol decreased REM sleep (Hilakivi, 1983). Stimulation of α-1 adrenoceptors by methoxamine decreased, but moderate inhibition by prazosin facilitated, REM sleep (Hilakivi & Leppavuori, 1984; Pellejero et al., 1984). Local injection of clonidine, an α-2 adrenoceptor agonist, into the LC reduced REM sleep (Tononi et al., 1991). In another study, NA was shown to cause a dose-dependent inhibition of REM sleep when applied unilaterally to the caudal peri-LCα, which contains mainly non-cholinergic and non-noradrenergic neurons. This effect was also mimicked by clonidine and antagonized by the selective α-2 adrenoceptor antagonists rauwolscine and RX 821002 (Crochet & Sakai, 1999). At the cellular level, NA has been found to hyperpolarize mesopontine cholinergic neurons (Williams & Reiner, 1993), which are of the REM-ON type, a possible mechanism by which NA could prevent the appearance of REM sleep.

The NA-ergic REM-OFF neurons in the LC cease firing during REM sleep and fire continuously during REM sleep deprivation (Mallick et al., 1990). Increased activity of the LC NA-ergic neurons has been reported by immunohistochemical detection of c-Fos after spontaneous, and a short enforced period of, sleep deprivation (Tononi et al., 1994). To confirm whether the cessation of the NA-ergic REM-OFF neurons in the LC is a prerequisite for the generation of REM sleep, the cells were continuously kept active by mild, low-frequency electrical stimulation (at 2 Hz, a condition simulating their spontaneous firing rate). This manipulation significantly reduced REM sleep, primarily by reducing the frequency of REM sleep bouts (Singh & Mallick, 1996); however, this response was abolished by blocking β-adrenoceptors with systemic propranolol (Mallick et al., 2005). Hence, it is reasonable to postulate that disinhibition of the LC NA-ergic neurons during REM sleep deprivation would increase the concentration of brain NA. Consistent with this hypothesis, an increased turnover of brain NA was observed after REM sleep deprivation (Pujol et al., 1968; Stern et al., 1971; Porkka-Heiskanen et al., 1995). Furthermore, there was an increase in the activity (Sinha et al., 1973) as well as in the mRNA (Basheer et al., 1998) of the NA-synthesizing enzyme tyrosine hydroxylase (TH) in brain. The levels of TH in NA-ergic specific neurons were also found to be increased after REM sleep deprivation (Majumdar & Mallick, 2003). In contrast, the activity of the NA-degrading enzyme monoamine oxidase-A decreased (Thakkar & Mallick, 1993; Perez & Benedito, 1997) after REM sleep deprivation. Finally, the concentration of NA in different brain areas has been shown to change across the sleep–waking cycle. The level is highest during waking and lowest during REM sleep (Shouse et al., 2000). Taken together, these findings show that brain NA levels decrease during REM sleep, but increase after REM sleep deprivation, suggesting that REM sleep plays a significant role in maintaining the level of brain NA.

Serotonin and REM sleep regulation

In the mammalian brain, the majority of 5-HT-ergic neurons are found within the DRN (Dahlstrom & Fuxe, 1964). By means of widespread projections throughout the neuraxis, these neurons are thought to play a crucial role in sleep regulation (Jouvet, 1972; Jacobs et al., 1990a,b; Jacobs & Azmitia, 1992). DRN 5-HT-ergic neurons fire tonically during wakefulness, decrease their activity during non-REM sleep, and are nearly quiescent during REM sleep; they thus behave similarly to NA-ergic REM-OFF neurons. High-frequency (20 Hz) electrical stimulation of the DRN in the rat induces wakefulness, with a significant REM sleep rebound three hours after stimulation (Houdouin et al., 1991). Recent microdialysis experiments provide evidence of a significant selective increase in the level of 5-HT during wakefulness and a decrease during non-REM and REM sleep in the pontine tegmentum and in cortical and subcortical areas receiving 5-HT-ergic projections, such as the amygdala, hippocampus, prefrontal and frontal cortices, and hypothalamus (Portas et al., 2000). The role of 5-HT in REM sleep regulation is supported by the recent finding that stimulation of 5-HT-ergic neurons in the DRN inhibits neurons in the central nucleus of the amygdala, an area that shows increased neuronal activity during REM sleep (Jha et al., 2005).

Dopamine and REM sleep regulation

In general, among the monoaminergic neurons, dopaminergic neurons do not exhibit any correlation between firing pattern and sleep–wakefulness states (Miller et al., 1983; Trulson & Preussler, 1984). Some indirect evidence, however, suggests state-related changes in the dopaminergic systems originating from the substantia nigra and the ventral tegmental area (VTA). REM sleep is a state of increased activity of the cholinergic system and ACh excites the VTA dopaminergic neurons (Gronier & Rasmussen, 1998; Forster & Blaha, 2000). Dopamine release in certain brain areas is higher during REM sleep and waking when compared with non-REM sleep (Lena et al., 2005). Administration of L-dopa, which increases central dopamine levels, significantly increased the frequency and intensity of dreaming without affecting the frequency of REM sleep. This effect was prevented by antipsychotics that are known to block the transmission of dopamine (Solms, 2000). Hence, it is possible that dopamine could be involved in dreaming during REM sleep.

Histamine and REM sleep regulation

Histamine-containing neurons, located in the tuberomammillary nuclei (TMN) of the posterior hypothalamus, stimulate cortical activation through diffuse projections. Like NA-ergic and 5-HT-ergic neurons, histaminergic neurons also discharge at higher rate during wakefulness, decrease firing during non-REM sleep, and cease firing during REM sleep (Jones, 2005). Facilitation of TMN histaminergic neurons, presumably through the withdrawal of a GABA-ergic influence from the mPOAH, induces wakefulness, whereas disfacilitation, through the activation of mPOAH GABA-ergic transmission, induces non-REM and REM sleep (Saper et al., 2005).

Acetylcholine and REM sleep regulation

Administration of ACh-ergic receptor agonists and antagonists in cats, rats, and mice alters REM sleep (for review, see Hobson et al., 1993). In humans, intramuscular administration of the ACh antagonist scopolamine significantly delays REM sleep onset (Sagales et al., 1969), whereas intraventricular administration of ACh agonists or acetylcholinesterase inhibitors, which increase ACh levels, increases REM sleep by shortening the onset latency and increasing the duration of REM sleep episodes (Sitaram et al., 1976, 1978). In the cat, rat, and mouse, microinjection of a cholinergic agonist in the pontine reticular formation (PRF) caused a REM-sleep-like state that was blocked by the cholinergic antagonist atropine (for review, see Baghdoyan & Lydic, 2002). Microdialysates collected from the same region showed significant increases in the level of ACh during REM sleep and the release was modulated by manipulating GABA-A receptors (Vazquez & Baghdoyan, 2004). ACh in the PRF comes from the cholinergic neurons located in the LDT/PPT (Lydic & Baghdoyan, 1993). The REM sleep-dependent increase in ACh release was consistent with the findings that a subpopulation of LDT/PPT neurons, the REM-ON neurons, show high discharge rates during REM sleep (el Mansari et al., 1989). Injections of cholinergic agonists and antagonists into the PRO, mimicking or blocking the actions of ACh, trigger or prevent REM sleep, respectively (Baghdoyan et al., 1989; Velazquez-Moctezuma et al., 1991; Yamuy et al., 1993; Garzon et al., 1998). These findings suggest that increased ACh in the pontine region, possibly due to increased activity of the cholinergic REM-ON neurons, increases REM sleep (for review, see Rye, 1997). REM-ON neuronal activity has been found to increase in cats with REM sleep deprivation (Mallick et al., 1990) suggesting a compensatory activity, whereas electrical stimulation in the LDT increases REM sleep (Thakkar et al., 1996). Additionally, acetylcholinesterase activity increases in rat brain after REM sleep deprivation, an effect that would reduce the effect of ACh, possibly as a compensatory mechanism (Mallick & Thakkar, 1991, 1992; Thakkar & Mallick, 1991).

GABA and REM sleep regulation

The inhibition and disinhibition of the REM sleep-related REM-OFF and REM-ON neurons possibly hold the key to the regulation of REM sleep. Since

GABA is a major inhibitory neurotransmitter and GABA-ergic neurons are located throughout the brain, the role of GABA in REM sleep regulation has been extensively studied in recent years. Several independent studies suggest that the pontine and basal forebrain GABA-ergic neurons are actively involved in the modulation of REM sleep. GABA-ergic neurons and terminals are present in the brain stem, where REM-ON and REM-OFF neurons are also found. Such GABA-ergic projections originate from anatomically distant regions as well as from local interneurons (for review, see Mallick *et al.*, 1999; Jones, 2005). Iontophoretic application of GABA strongly inhibits DRN 5-HT-ergic neurons, and co-iontophoresis of the GABA-A antagonist bicuculline or picrotoxin antagonizes this effect (Gallager, 1978). During REM sleep, GABA levels increase in the DRN (Nitz & Siegel, 1997b) and it has been reported that the decrease in activity of DRN neurons during REM sleep could be caused by a tonic inhibition from the GABA-ergic neurons (Gervasoni *et al.*, 2000). Microinjection of a GABA-A antagonist and agonist in the LC increase and decrease REM sleep, respectively (Kaur *et al.*, 1997; Mallick *et al.*, 2001), and GABA levels increase in the LC during REM sleep (Nitz & Siegel, 1997a). Pontine microinjection of GABA or a GABA agonist induces prolonged periods of wakefulness, and REM sleep is also affected (Lin *et al.*, 1989; Xi *et al.*, 1999). Conversely, pontine application of bicuculline, a GABA-A antagonist, results in the occurrence of episodes of REM sleep of long duration (Xi *et al.*, 1999). On the other hand, localized microinjection of picrotoxin into the PPT significantly reduces REM sleep (Pal & Mallick, 2004).

Microinjections of the GABA-A agonist muscimol within the histaminergic group of neurons in the posterior hypothalamus result in a complete loss of REM sleep (Lin *et al.*, 1989), whereas microinjection of the GABA-A antagonist picrotoxin into the medial preoptico-anterior hypothalamic area modulates REM sleep and body temperature (Ali *et al.*, 1999; Jha *et al.*, 2001). GABA-A receptors have been shown to affect ACh release in the brainstem, which in turn might regulate REM sleep (Vazquez & Baghdoyan, 2004). However, there are some contradictory results in the literature. For example, systemic administration of the GABA-A agonist gabaxodol (THIP) induces non-REM sleep but not REM sleep (Lancel, 1999), whereas the GABA-B antagonist CGP 35348 increases the amount of REM sleep (Gauthier *et al.*, 1997). A role for GABA in REM sleep regulation may also be supported by the fact that the level of glutamic acid decarboxylase (GAD), the enzyme responsible for the synthesis of GABA, increases significantly in GABA neurons after REM sleep deprivation (Majumdar & Mallick, 2003). This result suggests increased synthesis of GABA after REM sleep deprivation, although this might be a compensatory phenomenon, or the increased GABA levels could be functionally related to REM sleep deprivation. Thus, from these results, although it is evident that GABA modulates REM sleep, the mechanism of action is not clear, but a reasonable hypothesis is that the interaction of an inhibitory neurotransmitter, GABA, with other neurotransmitters is likely to play a significant role in REM sleep regulation. It has been suggested that the GABA-ergic inputs to the REM-ON and REM-OFF neurons could play a permissive role in the regulation of REM sleep (Mallick *et al.*, 1999) and this is discussed in detail below, although involvement of other peptides cannot be ruled out at this stage.

Hypocretins/orexin and REM sleep regulation

The recently identified hypothalamic neuropeptide system, containing hypocretin (Hcrt)/orexin, has been implicated in the sleep disorder narcolepsy (Lin *et al.*, 1999). These neurons directly and strongly innervate, and potently excite, NA-ergic, dopaminergic, 5-HT-ergic, and histaminergic neurons and suppress REM sleep (Winsky-Sommerer *et al.*, 2003). Stimulation of the brainstem wakefulness-inducing area excites REM-OFF neurons and inhibits REM-ON neurons (Thankachan *et al.*, 2001); some of these actions may be mediated by Hcrt/orexin. It has been proposed that a major role of Hcrt/orexin could be facilitatory to motor activity in association with motivated behaviors (Kiyashchenko *et al.*, 2001). An additional role for Hcrt/orexin in REM sleep is supported by the fact that degeneration of Hcrt/orexin neurons or receptors is associated with human and animal narcolepsy, a disorder characterized by an impaired ability to maintain alertness for long periods and by sudden loss of muscle tone (i.e. cataplexy) (Siegel, 2004).

Interaction between neurotransmitters for REM sleep regulation

The findings presented above suggest that several neuronal circuits and several neurotransmitters interact for the coordinated expression of REM sleep and its components. The NA-ergic REM-OFF neurons are continuously active except during REM sleep, whereas the ACh-ergic REM-ON neurons behave in a reciprocal manner, and the levels of the respective neurotransmitters decrease and increase during REM sleep (Shouse *et al.*, 2000; Vazquez & Baghdoyan, 2004). Hence, as a first step, attention was drawn towards an understanding of the coordination and interaction between these two neurotransmitters for REM sleep regulation.

The existence of such an interaction was first proposed by Hobson *et al.* (1975) in the form of their *Reciprocal Interaction Model*. According to these authors, the REM-OFF neurons in the LC are inhibitory to the REM-ON neuronal population, whereas the REM-ON neurons exert an excitatory effect on the LC REM-OFF neurons. Cessation of neuronal activity of the LC neurons during REM sleep thus results in the withdrawal of the tonic inhibition from the REM-ON neurons, whereas activation of REM-ON neurons exerts an excitatory effect on the LC neurons, resulting in inhibition of REM-ON neurons and termination of the REM sleep episode (Hobson et al., 1975). This model, however, failed to explain the mechanism of activation of the REM-ON neurons.

A relatively modified view was subsequently proposed by Sakai in the form of a *Mutual Inhibitory Model*. In this model, the REM-ON and the REM-OFF neurons inhibit each other. During REM sleep there is a progressive decrease in firing rate of the LC NA-ergic neurons and a consequent withdrawal of inhibition from the REM-ON neurons. Accordingly, the state of REM sleep can occur either by direct excitation of REM-ON neurons or by disinhibition of REM-OFF neurons (Sakai, 1988). These views were based on isolated single unit recording studies: REM-OFF and REM-ON neurons were simultaneously recorded in freely moving cats, and the temporal relation of their firing patterns during REM sleep supported this hypothesis (Mallick et al., 1998).

The above mentioned models were a reasonable explanation of the neuro-physiological mechanisms regulating REM sleep, but they did not consider the neurochemical involvement in such regulation. ACh release increases around the LC during REM sleep; microinjection of an ACh agonist or antagonist in and around the LC increases or decreases REM sleep, respectively (for review, see Baghdoyan & Lydic, 2002). The validity of the model/s would depend on the fact that NA and ACh should inhibit the REM-ON and the REM-OFF neurons. But the fact that iontophoretic application of ACh excited NA-ergic LC neurons, the site of REM-OFF neurons (Egan & North, 1986), did not support the proposed models. Hence, it was necessary to review the model/s for the neural mechanism of REM sleep regulation.

GABA-ergic inhibition-based model

It was noted above that the NA-ergic neurons in the LC are REM-executive. They have to be "shut off" for REM sleep facilitation, but cholinergic stimulation of the dorsolateral pontine area, including the LC, by a cholinergic agonist increases REM sleep. These findings suggest that this cholinergic stimulation must somehow, directly or indirectly, inhibit LC neurons for the initiation of REM sleep. Hence, we hypothesized that inhibitory interneuron/s, such as those containing GABA, could convert the cholinergic excitatory influence from the REM-ON neurons, into an inhibition of the LC REM-OFF neurons for the regulation of REM sleep. This view was supported by the fact that the concentration of GABA increases in the LC during REM sleep, the LC receives GABA-ergic inputs from local interneurons as well as from projection neurons, LC neurons possess GABA-ergic receptors, and ACh and GABA agonists and antagonists administered in the LC modulate REM sleep (for review, see Mallick et al., 2002b). In order to confirm our hypothesis, we performed a series of studies in behaving rats in which combinations of the various agonists and antagonists were microinjected into the LC (Mallick *et al.*, 2001), or electrical stimulation of one area (prepositus hypoglossus in this case) was paired with simultaneous microinjection of the GABA antagonist picrotoxin into the LC (Kaur *et al.*, 2001). The studies were completed with postexperimental histological confirmation. The combined results of these experiments led us to propose *GABA-ergic inhibitory* neural connections for inhibition of the REM-OFF neurons for REM sleep regulation (Mallick *et al.*, 2001, 2002b). The working hypothesis of this model is that an increase in the activity of the cholinergic REM-ON neurons would activate the GABA-ergic interneurons in and around the LC and in the prepositus hypoglossus, which in turn would inhibit the NA-ergic REM-OFF neurons. Also, even in the presence of cholinergic inputs which directly innervate the REM-OFF neurons and excite them, the increased collateral release of NA would hyperpolarize the REM-OFF neurons and thus inhibit them. This cessation of LC REM-OFF neuronal activity would in turn withdraw the collateral inhibitory influence, but the neurons would remain inhibited owing to the continued presence of GABA. Hence, this inhibition of the REM-OFF neurons would withdraw the inhibition from the REM-ON neurons, resulting in continuation of the REM sleep episode, the duration of which would then be determined by the period for which sufficient GABA would be available around the LC (Mallick *et al.*, 2001).

However, the question remained as to how the respective states of the REM-OFF and REM-ON neurons during non-REM sleep would initiate the switch between states. Our recent findings throw some light on this issue in that the wakefulness-promoting area in the brainstem maintains the REM-OFF neurons active but inhibits the REM-ON neurons (Thankachan *et al.*, 2001), and the sleep-inducing area in the brainstem excites the REM-ON neurons (Mallick *et al.*, 2004a). Based on these findings it has been proposed that during wakefulness the REM-OFF neurons remain active, which maintains the inhibitory drive on the REM-ON neurons. After a certain duration of non-REM sleep, when some yet unknown conditions are fulfilled, the sleep-active neurons in the brainstem actively excite the REM-ON neurons, resulting in initiation of REM sleep (Fig. 3.1). Finally, it is evident that the NA-ergic REM-OFF neurons must cease firing, as a result of GABA release, for the initiation and maintenance of REM sleep. If the NA-ergic neurons do not cease firing, the increased NA in the brain causes REM sleep deprivation-associated effects and pathologies. As a corollary, continuous activity of the REM-OFF neurons would lead to REM sleep deprivation, and conversely, during REM sleep deprivation these neurons would be continuously active. As noted above, both of these results have been reported in independent studies.

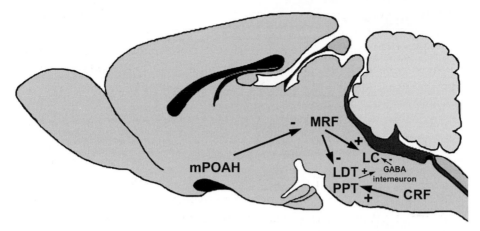

Figure 3.1   Schematic representation of communication between pontine cholinergic REM-ON, NA-ergic REM-OFF and GABA-ergic neurons in the brainstem and influence of brainstem wake- and sleep-inducing areas on REM-ON and REM-OFF neurons for the regulation of REM sleep. Refer to the text for details. The abbreviations are same as in the text; (+) indicates excitation and (−) indicates inhibition.

Physiological validation

REM sleep is a state in which the electrophysiological characteristics of the brain resemble the state of wakefulness while behaviorally the subject is asleep. Several physiological processes also remain activated during REM sleep, suggesting its function in the reactivation of systems from the quiescence of non-REM sleep. The cessation of firing of LC REM-OFF neurons, possibly through the influence of GABA, is a necessity for REM sleep to appear. Conversely, continuous firing of these neurons would inhibit REM sleep and increase central NA levels. The functional importance of REM sleep could be determined by studying the effects of its loss on behavioral and physiological processes (Vogel, 1975; Gulyani et al., 2000; Stickgold, 2005), and we hypothesize that the increased NA level in the brain is one of the major factors responsible for inducing the adverse effects associated with REM sleep deprivation (Fig. 3.2).

Pharmacological blockade of NA-ergic receptors inhibits the appearance of several physiological and behavioral signs associated with REM sleep deprivation. For example, REM sleep deprivation increased Na/K ATPase (Gulyani & Mallick, 1993), a key enzyme responsible for maintaining neuronal excitability, and the effect was prevented by an α-1 adrenoceptor blocker (Gulyani & Mallick, 1995). Increased Na/K ATPase activity was also observed during a pharmacologically induced REM sleep deprivation-like state following continuous infusion of picrotoxin into the LC, which is assumed to prevent the cessation of firing of REM-OFF

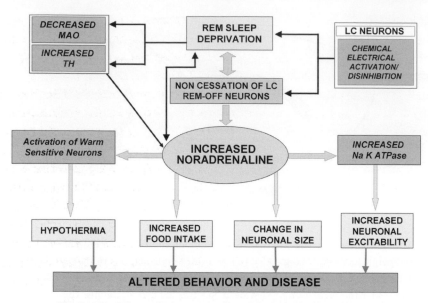

Figure 3.2   Schematic representation of the mechanism of increasing noradrenaline levels in the brain associated with REM sleep loss, and the putative role and mechanism of action of these increased levels in the induction of altered pathophysiological states.

neurons (Kaur *et al.*, 2004). REM sleep deprivation also altered the morphometry of neurons in several brain areas; the change was prevented by the adrenoceptor antagonist prazosin (Majumdar & Mallick, 2005). Furthermore, during REM sleep deprivation, despite a progressive increase in heat production and food intake, brain and body temperatures and body mass show a progressive decline (Rechtschaffen *et al.*, 1989), a sign of an unbalanced metabolic state. Although the detailed mechanism of action for such changes is not known, these changes could be attributed to the increased level of NA in the brain. The main thermoregulatory centre in the brain is the medial preoptic area (McGinty & Szymusiak, 1990), which also receives NA-ergic inputs from the brainstem (Tanaka *et al.*, 1992) and the LC is the primary nucleus for NA-ergic projections throughout the brain (Moore & Bloom, 1979). It is proposed that, since LC REM-OFF neurons do not cease firing during REM sleep deprivation, NA levels increase in the brain, including in the medial preoptic area, and this acts on the thermosensitive neurons and causes hypothermia. We have shown that, in the preoptic area, the thermosensitive neurons possess α-1 adrenoceptors (Mallick *et al.*, 2002a), and NA acts at α-1 adrenoceptors to induce hypothermia (Mallick & Alam, 1992). Also, since adrenoceptor number is altered in relation to changes in NA concentration (Dausse *et al.*, 1982), it is also possible that the altered NA levels may modulate thermosensitivity by altering the number of adrenoceptors on the medial preoptic area thermosensitive neurons. This could be the mechanism for induction of heat dissipation during REM sleep deprivation. Additionally, the increased concentration of NA in the hypothalamus is likely to be the cause of the response to glucose utilization and energy production induced by REM sleep deprivation. Circulating glucose and glucose-mobilizing hormones are increased in response to microinjection of NA into the medial hypothalamus (Chafetz et al., 1986; Steffens et al., 1988). Also, injection of a NA receptor agonist into the ventromedial nucleus of the hypothalamus stimulated food intake (Grandison & Guidotti, 1977; Kelly et al., 1979). Hence, as previously hypothesized (Mallick et al., 2004b), the increased concentration of NA is a possible cause of both the increased food intake and hypothermia during REM sleep deprivation. The mechanism by which NA mediates the changes in pathophysiological regulation induced by REM sleep deprivation has been summarized schematically in Fig. 3.2.

Conclusions

REM sleep is a unique behavioral state present in homoeothermic vertebrates. Neurons in the brainstem pontine area are implicated in its regulation. The LC NA-ergic neurons are continuously active during waking, decrease activity gradually during non-REM sleep, and cease firing during REM sleep, an effect that is possibly mediated by GABA. In contrast, NA-ergic neurons fire continuously during REM sleep deprivation. If the activity of these neurons is maintained by electrical stimulation or by local application of the GABA antagonist picrotoxin, REM sleep is significantly reduced. Continuous activation of these neurons would increase NA levels in the brain, which in turn induce physiological effects similar to those observed after REM sleep deprivation. These findings thus suggest that the LC NA-ergic REM-OFF neurons are negative REM-sleep-executive neurons and that the cessation of their discharge, mediated by GABA, is a prerequisite for the appearance of REM sleep. However, these neurons do not cease firing during REM sleep deprivation, resulting in increased NA in the brain. Increased NA is the principal cause of the pathophysiological conditions associated with REM sleep deprivation.

Acknowledgements

Funding from CSIR, DBT, DST, ICMR, and UGC, India, to BNM is acknowledged.

References

Ali, M., Jha, S. K., Kaur, S. & Mallick, B. N. (1999). Role of GABA-A receptor in the preoptic area in the regulation of sleep-wakefulness and rapid eye movement sleep. *Neurosci. Res.* **33**, 245–50.

Amlaner, C. J. J. (1994). Avian sleep. In *Principles and Practice of Sleep Medicine*, ed. M. H. Kryger, T. Roth, & W. C. Dement, pp. 81–94. Philadelphia, PA: W. B. Saunders Company.

Aserinsky, E. & Kleitman, N. (1953) Regularly occurring periods of eye motility, and concomitant phenomena, during sleep. *Science* **118**, 273–4.

Aston-Jones, G. & Bloom, F. E. (1981). Activity of norepinephrine-containing locus coeruleus neurons in behaving rats anticipates fluctuations in the sleep-waking cycle. *J. Neurosci.* **1**, 876–86.

Baghdoyan, H. A. & Lydic, R. (2002). Neurotransmitters and neuromodulators regulating sleep. In *Sleep and Epilepsy: The Clinical Spectrum*, ed. C. W. Bazil, pp. 17–44. New York, NY: Elsevier Science.

Baghdoyan, H. A., Lydic, R., Callaway, C. W. & Hobson, J. A. (1989). The carbachol-induced enhancement of desynchronized sleep signs is dose dependent and antagonized by centrally administered atropine. *Neuropsychopharmacology* **2**, 67–79.

Basheer, R., Magner, M., McCarley, R. W. & Shiromani, P. J. (1998). REM sleep deprivation increases the levels of tyrosine hydroxylase and norepinephrine transporter mRNA in the locus coeruleus. *Brain Res. Mol. Brain Res.* **57**, 235–40.

Borbely, A. A. & Achermann, P. (2000). Sleep homeostasis and model of sleep regulation. In *Principles and Practice of Sleep Medicine*, ed. M. H. Kryger, T. Roth & W. C. Dement, pp. 377–90. Philadelphia, PA: W. B. Saunders Company.

Braun, C. M. & Pivik, R. T. (1981). Effects of locus coeruleus lesions upon sleeping and waking in the rabbit. *Brain Res.* **230**, 133–51.

Caballero, A. & De Andres, I. (1986). Unilateral lesions in locus coeruleus area enhance paradoxical sleep. *Electroencephalogr. Clin. Neurophysiol.* **64**, 339–46.

Carli, G. & Zanchetti, A. (1965). A study of pontine lesions suppressing deep sleep in the cat. *Arch. Ital. Biol.* **103**, 751–88.

Cespuglio, R., Gomez, M. E., Faradji, H. & Jouvet, M. (1982). Alterations in the sleep-waking cycle induced by cooling of the locus coeruleus area. *Electroencephalogr. Clin. Neurophysiol.* **54**, 570–8.

Chafetz, M. D., Parko, K., Diaz, S. & Leibowitz, S. F. (1986). Relationships between medial hypothalamic alpha 2-receptor binding, norepinephrine, and circulating glucose. *Brain Res.* **384**, 404–8.

Chu, N. & Bloom, F. E. (1973). Norepinephrine-containing neurons: changes in spontaneous discharge patterns during sleeping and waking. *Science* **179**, 908–10.

Crochet, S. & Sakai, K. (1999). Alpha-2 adrenoceptor mediated paradoxical (REM) sleep inhibition in the cat. *Neuroreport* **10**, 2199–204.

Dahlstrom, A. & Fuxe, K. (1964). Localization of monoamines in the lower brain stem. *Experientia* **20**, 398–9.

Dausse, J. P., Le Quan-Bui, K. H. & Meyer, P. (1982). Alpha 1- and alpha 2-adrenoceptors in rat cerebral cortex: effects of neonatal treatment with 6-hydroxydopamine. *Eur. J. Pharmacol.* **78**, 15–20.

Drucker-Colin R. & Pedraza JG. (1983). Kainic acid lesions of gigantocellular tegmental field (FTG) neurons does not abolish REM sleep. *Brain Res.* **272**, 387–91.

Egan, T. M. & North, R. A. (1986). Actions of acetylcholine and nicotine on rat locus coeruleus neurons in vitro. *Neuroscience* **19**, 565–71.

el Mansari, M., Sakai, K. & Jouvet, M. (1989). Unitary characteristics of presumptive cholinergic tegmental neurons during the sleep-waking cycle in freely moving cats. *Exp. Brain Res.* **76**, 519–29.

Flanigan, W. F. (1973). Sleep and wakefulness in iguanid lizards, *Ctenosaura pectinata* and *Iguana iguana. Brain Behav. Evol.* **8**, 401–36.

Fornal, C., Auerbach, S. & Jacobs, B. L. (1985). Activity of serotonin-containing neurons in nucleus raphe magnus in freely moving cats. *Exp. Neurol.* **88**, 590–608.

Forster, G. L. & Blaha, C. D. (2000). Laterodorsal tegmental stimulation elicits dopamine efflux in the rat nucleus accumbens by activation of acetylcholine and glutamate receptors in the ventral tegmental area. *Eur. J. Neurosci.* **12**, 3596–604.

Friedman, L. & Jones, B. E. (1984). Computer graphics analysis of sleep-wakefulness state changes after pontine lesions. *Brain Res. Bull.* **13**, 53–68.

Gallager, D. W. (1978). Benzodiazepines: potentiation of a GABA inhibitory response in the dorsal raphe nucleus. *Eur. J. Pharmacol.* **49**, 133–43.

Garzon, M., De Andres, I. & Reinoso-Suarez, F. (1998). Sleep patterns after carbachol delivery in the ventral oral pontine tegmentum of the cat. *Neuroscience* **83**, 1137–44.

Gauthier, P., Arnaud, C., Gandolfo, G. & Gottesmann, C. (1997). Influence of a GABA(B) receptor antagonist on the sleep-waking cycle in the rat. *Brain Res.* **773**, 8–14.

Gervasoni, D., Peyron, C., Rampon, C. *et al.* (2000). Role and origin of the GABAergic innervation of dorsal raphe serotonergic neurons. *J. Neurosci.* **20**, 4217–25.

Grandison, L. & Guidotti, A. (1977). Stimulation of food intake by muscimol and beta endorphin. *Neuropharmacology* **16**, 533–6.

Gronier, B. & Rasmussen, K. (1998). Activation of midbrain presumed dopaminergic neurones by muscarinic cholinergic receptors: an in vivo electrophysiological study in the rat. *Br. J. Pharmacol.* **124**, 455–64.

Gulyani, S. & Mallick, B. N. (1993). Effect of rapid eye movement sleep deprivation on rat brain Na-K ATPase activity. *J. Sleep Res.* **2**, 45–50.

Gulyani, S. & Mallick, B. N. (1995). Possible mechanism of rapid eye movement sleep deprivation induced increase in Na-K ATPase activity. *Neuroscience* **64**, 255–60.

Gulyani, S., Majumdar, S. & Mallick, B. N. (2000). Rapid eye movement sleep and significance of its deprivation studies – a review. *Sleep and Hypnosis* **2**, 49–68.

Henley, K. & Morrison, A. R. (1974). A re-evaluation of the effects of lesions of the pontine tegmentum and locus coeruleus on phenomena of paradoxical sleep in the cat. *Acta Neurobiol. Exp. (Wars).* **34**, 215–32.

Heym, J., Steinfels, G. F. & Jacobs, B. L. (1982). Activity of serotonin-containing neurons in the nucleus raphe pallidus of freely moving cats. *Brain Res.* **251**, 259–76.

Hilakivi, I. (1983). The role of beta- and alpha-adrenoceptors in the regulation of the stages of the sleep-waking cycle in the cat. *Brain Res.* **277**, 109–18.

Hilakivi, I. & Leppavuori, A. (1984). Effects of methoxamine, and alpha-1 adrenoceptor agonist, and prazosin, an alpha-1 antagonist, on the stages of the sleep-waking cycle in the cat. *Acta Physiol. Scand.* **120**, 363–72.

Hobson, J. A., Goin, O. B. & Goin, C. J. (1968). Electrographic correlates of behaviour in tree frogs. *Nature* **220**, 386–7.

Hobson, J. A., McCarley R. W. & Wyzinski, P. W. (1975). Sleep cycle oscillation: reciprocal discharge by two brainstem neuronal groups. *Science* **189**, 55–8.

Hobson, J. A., Datta, S., Calvo, J. M. & Quattrochi, J. (1993). Acetylcholine as a brain state modulator: triggering and long-term regulation of REM sleep. *Prog. Brain Res.* **98**, 389–404.

Honda, T. & Semba, K. (1995). An ultrastructural study of cholinergic and non-cholinergic neurons in the laterodorsal and pedunculopontine tegmental nuclei in the rat. *Neuroscience* **68**, 837–53.

Houdouin, F., Cespuglio, R. & Jouvet, M. (1991). Effects induced by the electrical stimulation of the nucleus raphe dorsalis upon hypothalamic release of 5-hydroxyindole compounds and sleep parameters in the rat. *Brain Res.* **565**, 48–56.

Jacobs, B. L. (1986). Single unit activity of locus coeruleus neurons in behaving animals. *Prog. Neurobiol.* **27**, 183–94.

Jacobs, B. L. & Azmitia, E. C. (1992). Structure and function of the brain serotonin system. *Physiol. Rev.* **72**, 165–229.

Jacobs, B. L., Wilkinson, L. O. & Fornal, C. A. (1990a). The role of brain serotonin. A neurophysiologic perspective. *Neuropsychopharmacology* **3**, 473–9.

Jacobs, B. L., Fornal, C. A. & Wilkinson, L. O. (1990b). Neurophysiological and neurochemical studies of brain serotonergic neurons in behaving animals. *Ann. NY Acad. Sci.* **600**, 260–8; discussion 268–71.

Jha, S. K., Yadav, V. & Mallick, B. N. (2001). GABA-A receptors in mPOAH simultaneously regulate sleep and body temperature in freely moving rats. *Pharmacol. Biochem. Behav.* **70**, 115–21.

Jha, S. K., Ross, R. J. & Morrison, A. R. (2005). Sleep-related neurons in the central nucleus of the amygdala of rats and their modulation by the dorsal raphe nucleus. *Physiol. Behav.* **86**, 415–26.

Jones, B. E. (1979). Elimination of paradoxical sleep by lesions of the pontine gigantocellular tegmental field in the cat. *Neurosci. Lett.* **13**, 285–93.

Jones, B. E. (1991). Paradoxical sleep and its chemical/structural substrates in the brain. *Neuroscience* **40**, 637–56.

Jones, B. E. (2004). Paradoxical REM sleep promoting and permitting neuronal networks. *Arch. Ital. Biol.* **142**, 379–96.

Jones, B. E. (2005). From waking to sleeping: neuronal and chemical substrates. *Trends Pharmacol. Sci.* **26**, 578–86.

Jones, B. E., Harper, S. T. & Halaris, A. E. (1977). Effects of locus coeruleus lesions upon cerebral monoamine content, sleep-wakefulness states and the response to amphetamine in the cat. *Brain Res.* **124**, 473–96.

Jouvet, M. (1965). Paradoxical sleep – a study of its nature and mechanisms. *Prog. Brain Res.* **18**, 20–62.

Jouvet, M. (1972). The role of monoamines and acetylcholine-containing neurons in the regulation of the sleep-waking cycle. *Ergeb. Physiol.* **64**, 166–307.

Jouvet, M. (1999). Around the discovery of REM sleep in cats. In *Rapid Eye Movement Sleep*, ed. B. N. Mallick & S. Inoue, pp. v–ix. New York, NY: Marcel Dekker.

Jouvet, M. & Delorme, F. (1965). Locus coeruleus et sommeil paradoxal. *C. R. Soc. Biol.* **159**, 895–9.

Kaur, S., Saxena, R. N. & Mallick, B. N. (1997). GABA in locus coeruleus regulates spontaneous rapid eye movement sleep by acting on GABAA receptors in freely moving rats. *Neurosci. Lett.* **223**, 105–8.

Kaur, S., Saxena, R. N. & Mallick, B. N. (2001). GABAergic neurons in prepositus hypoglossi regulate REM sleep by its action on locus coeruleus in freely moving rats. *Synapse* **42**, 141–50.

Kaur, S., Panchal, M., Faisal, M. *et al.* (2004). Long term blocking of GABA-A receptor in locus coeruleus by bilateral microinfusion of picrotoxin reduced rapid eye movement sleep and increased brain Na-K ATPase activity in freely moving normally behaving rats. *Behav. Brain Res.* **151**, 185–90.

Kelly, J., Rothstein, J. & Grossman, S. P. (1979). GABA and hypothalamic feeding systems. I. Topographic analysis of the effects of microinjections of muscimol. *Physiol. Behav.* **23**, 1123–34.

Kiyashchenko, L. I., Mileykovskiy, B. Y., Lai, Y. Y. & Siegel, J. M. (2001). Increased and decreased muscle tone with orexin (hypocretin) microinjections in the locus coeruleus and pontine inhibitory area. *J. Neurophysiol.* **85**, 2008–16.

Laguzzi, R. F., Adrien, J., Bourgoin, S. & Hamon, M. (1979). Effects of intraventricular injection of 6-hydroxydopamine in the developing kitten. 1. On the sleepwaking cycles. *Brain Res.* **160**, 445–59.

Lancel, M. (1999). Role of GABAA receptors in the regulation of sleep: initial sleep responses to peripherally administered modulators and agonists. *Sleep* **22**, 33–42.

Lena, I., Parrot, S., Deschaux, O. *et al.* (2005). Variations in extracellular levels of dopamine, noradrenaline, glutamate, and aspartate across the sleep – wake cycle in the medial prefrontal cortex and nucleus accumbens of freely moving rats. *J. Neurosci. Res.* **81**, 891–9.

Lin, J. S., Sakai, K., Vanni-Mercier, G. & Jouvet, M. (1989). A critical role of the posterior hypothalamus in the mechanisms of wakefulness determined by microinjection of muscimol in freely moving cats. *Brain Res.* **479**, 225–40.

Lin, L., Faraco, J., Li, R. *et al.* (1999). The sleep disorder canine narcolepsy is caused by a mutation in the hypocretin (orexin) receptor 2 gene. *Cell* **98**, 365–76.

Lydic, R. & Baghdoyan, H. A. (1993). Pedunculopontine stimulation alters respiration and increases ACh release in the pontine reticular formation. *Am. J. Physiol.* **264**, R544–54.

Majumdar, S. & Mallick, B. N. (2003). Increased levels of tyrosine hydroxylase and glutamic acid decarboxylase in locus coeruleus neurons after rapid eye movement sleep deprivation in rats. *Neurosci. Lett.* **338**, 193–6.

Majumdar, S. & Mallick, B. N. (2005). Cytomorphometric changes in rat brain neurons after rapid eye movement sleep deprivation. *Neuroscience* **135**, 679–90.

Mallick, B. N. & Alam, M. N. (1992). Different types of norepinephrinergic receptors are involved in preoptic area mediated independent modulation of sleep-wakefulness and body temperature. *Brain Res.* **591**, 8–19.

Mallick, B. N. & Thakkar, M. (1991). Short-term REM sleep deprivation increases acetylcholinesterase activity in the medulla of rats. *Neurosci. Lett.* **130**, 221–4.

Mallick, B. N. & Thakkar, M. (1992). Effect of REM sleep deprivation on molecular forms of acetylcholinesterase in rats. *Neuroreport* **3**, 676–8.

Mallick, B. N., Siegel, J. M. & Fahringer, H. (1990). Changes in pontine unit activity with REM sleep deprivation. *Brain Res.* **515**, 94–8.

Mallick, B. N., Thankachan, S. & Islam, F. (1998). Differential responses of brain stem neurons during spontaneous and stimulation-induced desynchronization of the cortical eeg in freely moving cats. *Sleep Res. Online* **1**, 132–46.

Mallick, B. N., Kaur, S., Jha, S. K. & Siegel, J. M. (1999). Possible role of GABA in the regulation of REM sleep with special reference to REM-OFF neurons. In *Rapid Eye Movement Sleep*, ed. B. N. Mallick & S. Inoue, pp. 153–66. New York, NY: Marcel Dekker.

Mallick, B. N., Kaur, S. & Saxena, R. N. (2001). Interactions between cholinergic and GABAergic neurotransmitters in and around the locus coeruleus for the induction and maintenance of rapid eye movement sleep in rats. *Neuroscience* **104**, 467–85.

Mallick, B. N., Jha, S. K. & Islam, F. (2002a). Presence of alpha-1 adrenoreceptors on thermosensitive neurons in the medial preoptico-anterior hypothalamic area in rats. *Neuropharmacology* **42**, 697–705.

Mallick, B. N., Majumdar, S., Faisal, M. *et al.* (2002b). Role of norepinephrine in the regulation of rapid eye movement sleep. *J. Biosci.* **27**, 539–51.

Mallick, B. N., Thankachan, S. & Islam, F. (2004a). Influence of hypnogenic brain areas on wakefulness- and rapid-eye-movement sleep-related neurons in the brainstem of freely moving cats. *J. Neurosci. Res.* **75**, 133–42.

Mallick, B. N., Jha, S. K. & Madan, V. (2004b). Role of norepinephrine in thermoregulation during rapid eye movement sleep and its deprivation. In *Neurobiology in the Post-Genomic Era*, ed. M. K. Thakur. New Delhi: Narosa.

Mallick, B. N., Singh, S. & Pal, D. (2005). Role of alpha and beta adrenoceptors in locus coeruleus stimulation-induced reduction in rapid eye movement sleep in freely moving rats. *Behav. Brain Res.* **158**, 9–21.

McGinty, D. & Szymusiak, R. (1990). Keeping cool: a hypothesis about the mechanisms and functions of slow-wave sleep. *Trends Neurosci.* **13**, 480–7.

McGinty, D. J. & Harper, R. M. (1976). Dorsal raphe neurons: depression of firing during sleep in cats. *Brain Res.* **101**, 569–75.

Miller, J. D., Farber, J., Gatz, P., Roffwarg, H. & German, D. C. (1983). Activity of mesencephalic dopamine and non-dopamine neurons across stages of sleep and waking in the rat. *Brain Res.* **273**, 133–41.

Moore, R. Y. & Bloom, F. E. (1979). Central catecholamine neuron systems: anatomy and physiology of the norepinephrine and epinephrine systems. *A. Rev. Neurosci.* **2**, 113–68.

Nitz, D. & Siegel, J. M. (1997a). GABA release in the locus coeruleus as a function of sleep/wake state. *Neuroscience* **78**, 795–801.

Nitz, D. & Siegel, J. (1997b). GABA release in the dorsal raphe nucleus: role in the control of REM sleep. *Am. J. Physiol.* **273**, R451–5.

Pal, D. & Mallick, B. N. (2004). GABA in pedunculopontine tegmentum regulates spontaneous rapid eye movement sleep by acting on GABAA receptors in freely moving rats. *Neurosci. Lett.* **365**, 200–4.

Pawlyk, A. C., Jha, S. K., Brennan, F. X., Morrison, A. R. & Ross, R. J. (2005). A rodent model of sleep disturbances in posttraumatic stress disorder: the role of context after fear conditioning. *Biol. Psychiatry* **57**, 268–77.

Pellejero, T., Monti, J. M., Baglietto, J. *et al.* (1984). Effects of methoxamine and alpha-adrenoceptor antagonists, prazosin and yohimbine, on the sleep-wake cycle of the rat. *Sleep* **7**, 365–72.

Perez, N. M. & Benedito, M. A. (1997). Activities of monoamine oxidase (MAO) A and B in discrete regions of rat brain after rapid eye movement (REM) sleep deprivation. *Pharmacol. Biochem. Behav.* **58**, 605–8.

Petit, D., Gagnon, J. F., Fantini, M. L., Ferini-Strambi, L. & Montplaisir, J. (2004). Sleep and quantitative EEG in neurodegenerative disorders. *J. Psychosom. Res.* **56**, 487–96.

Porkka-Heiskanen, T., Smith, S. E., Taira, T. *et al.* (1995). Noradrenergic activity in rat brain during rapid eye movement sleep deprivation and rebound sleep. *Am. J. Physiol.* **268**, R1456–63.

Portas, C. M., Bjorvatn, B. & Ursin, R. (2000). Serotonin and the sleep/wake cycle: special emphasis on microdialysis studies. *Prog. Neurobiol.* **60**, 13–35.

Pujol, J. F., Mouret, J., Jouvet, M. & Glowinski, J. (1968). Increased turnover of cerebral norepinephrine during rebound of paradoxical sleep in the rat. *Science* **159**, 112–14.

Rechtschaffen, A., Bergmann, B. M., Everson, C. A., Kushida, C. A. & Gilliland, M. A. (1989). Sleep deprivation in the rat: X. Integration and discussion of the findings. *Sleep* **12**, 68–87.

Rye, D. B. (1997). Contributions of the pedunculopontine region to normal and altered REM sleep. *Sleep* **20**, 757–88.

Sagales, T., Erill, S. & Domino, E. F. (1969). Differential effects of scopolamine and chlorpromazine on REM and NREM sleep in normal male subjects. *Clin. Pharmacol. Ther.* **10**, 522–9.

Sakai, K. (1980). Some anatomical and physiological properties of ponto-mesencephalic tegmental neurons with special reference to the PGO waves and postural atonia during paradoxical sleep in cat. In *The Reticular*

Formation Revisited, ed. J. A. Hobson & M. A. B. Brazier, pp. 427–47. New York, NY: Raven Press.

Sakai, K. (1986). Central mechanisms of paradoxical sleep. *Brain Dev.* **8**, 402–7.

Sakai, K. (1988). Executive mechanisms of paradoxical sleep. *Arch. Ital. Biol.* **126**, 239–57.

Saper, C. B., Scammell, T. E. & Lu, J. (2005). Hypothalamic regulation of sleep and circadian rhythms. *Nature* **437**, 1257–63.

Sastre, J. P., Sakai, K. & Jouvet, M. (1981). Are the gigantocellular tegmental field neurons responsible for paradoxical sleep? *Brain Res.* **229**, 147–61.

Semba, K. (1993). Aminergic and cholinergic afferents to REM sleep induction regions of the pontine reticular formation in the rat. *J. Comp. Neurol.* **330**, 543–56.

Shouse, M. N., Staba, R. J., Saquib, S. F. & Farber, P. R. (2000). Monoamines and sleep: microdialysis findings in pons and amygdala. *Brain Res.* **860**, 181–9.

Siegel, J. M. (1995). Phylogeny and the function of REM sleep. *Behav. Brain. Res.* **69**, 29–34.

Siegel, J. M. (2004). Hypocretin (orexin): role in normal behavior and neuropathology. *A. Rev. Psychol.* **55**, 125–48.

Siegel, J. M., Tomaszewski, K. S. & Nienhuis, R. (1986). Behavioral states in the chronic medullary and midpontine cat. *Electroencephalogr. Clin. Neurophysiol.* **63**, 274–88.

Singh, S. & Mallick, B. N. (1996). Mild electrical stimulation of pontine tegmentum around locus coeruleus reduces rapid eye movement sleep in rats. *Neurosci. Res.* **24**, 227–35.

Sinha, A. K., Ciaranello, R. D., Dement, W. C. & Barchas, J. D. (1973). Tyrosine hydroxylase activity in rat brain following "REM" sleep deprivation. *J. Neurochem.* **20**, 1289–90.

Sitaram, N., Wyatt, R. J., Dawson, S. & Gillin, J. C. (1976). REM sleep induction by physostigmine infusion during sleep. *Science* **191**, 1281–3.

Sitaram, N., Moore, A. M. & Gillin, J. C. (1978). Induction and resetting of REM sleep rhythm in normal man by arecholine: blockade by scopolamine. *Sleep* **1**, 83–90.

Solms, M. (2000). Dreaming and REM sleep are controlled by different brain mechanisms. *Behav. Brain Sci.* **23**, 843–50; discussion 904–1121.

Steffens, A. B., Scheurink, A. J., Luiten, P. G. & Bohus, B. (1988). Hypothalamic food intake regulating areas are involved in the homeostasis of blood glucose and plasma FFA levels. *Physiol. Behav.* **44**, 581–9.

Stern, W. C., Miller, F. P., Cox, R. H. & Maickel, R. P. (1971). Brain norepinephrine and serotonin levels following REM sleep deprivation in the rat. *Psychopharmacologia* **22**, 50–5.

Stickgold, R. (2005). Sleep-dependent memory consolidation. *Nature* **437**, 1272–8.

Tanaka, J., Nishimura, J., Kimura, F. & Nomura, M. (1992). Noradrenergic excitatory inputs to median preoptic neurons in rats. *Neuroreport* **3**, 95–106.

Thakkar, M. & Mallick, B. N. (1991). Effect of REM sleep deprivation on rat brain acetylcholinesterase. *Pharmacol. Biochem. Behav.* **39**, 211–14.

Thakkar, M. & Mallick, B. N. (1993). Effect of rapid eye movement sleep deprivation on rat brain monoamine oxidases. *Neuroscience* **55**, 677–83.

Thakkar, M., Portas, C. & McCarley, R. W. (1996). Chronic low-amplitude electrical stimulation of the laterodorsal tegmental nucleus of freely moving cats increases REM sleep. *Brain Res.* **723**, 223–7.

Thankachan, S., Islam, F. & Mallick, B. N. (2001). Role of wake inducing brain stem area on rapid eye movement sleep regulation in freely moving cats. *Brain Res. Bull.* **55**, 43–9.

Tobler, I. (1995). Is sleep fundamentally different between mammalian species? *Behav. Brain Res.* **69**, 35–41.

Tononi, G., Pompeiano, M. & Cirelli, C. (1991). Effects of local pontine injection of noradrenergic agents on desynchronized sleep of the cat. *Prog. Brain Res.* **88**, 545–53.

Tononi, G., Pompeiano, M. & Cirelli, C. (1994). The locus coeruleus and immediate-early genes in spontaneous and forced wakefulness. *Brain Res. Bull.* **35**, 589–96.

Trulson, M. E. & Preussler, D. W. (1984). Dopamine-containing ventral tegmental area neurons in freely moving cats: activity during the sleep-waking cycle and effects of stress. *Exp. Neurol.* **83**, 367–77.

Vazquez, J. & Baghdoyan, H. A. (2004). GABAA receptors inhibit acetylcholine release in cat pontine reticular formation: implications for REM sleep regulation. *J. Neurophysiol.* **92**, 2198–206.

Velazquez-Moctezuma, J., Shalauta, M., Gillin, J. C. & Shiromani, P. J. (1991). Cholinergic antagonists and REM sleep generation. *Brain Res.* **543**, 175–9.

Verret, L., Leger, L., Fort, P. & Luppi, P. H. (2005). Cholinergic and noncholinergic brainstem neurons expressing Fos after paradoxical (REM) sleep deprivation and recovery. *Eur. J. Neurosci.* **21**, 2488–504.

Villablanca, J. (1965). The electrocorticogram in the chronic cerveau isole cat. *Electroencephalogr. Clin. Neurophysiol.* **19**, 576–86.

Villablanca, J. (1966). Behavioral and polygraphic study of "sleep" and "wakefulness" in chronic decerebrate cats. *Electroencephalogr. Clin. Neurophysiol.* **21**, 562–77.

Vogel, G. W. (1975). A review of REM sleep deprivation. *Arch. Gen. Psychiatry* **32**, 749–61.

Williams, J. A. & Reiner, P. B. (1993). Noradrenaline hyperpolarizes identified rat mesopontine cholinergic neurons in vitro. *J. Neurosci.* **13**, 3878–83.

Winsky-Sommerer, R., Boutrel, B. & De, Lecea L. (2003). The role of the hypocretinergic system in the integration of networks that dictate the states of arousal. *Drug News Perspect.* **16**, 504–12.

Xi, M. C., Morales, F. R. & Chase, M. H. (1999). Evidence that wakefulness and REM sleep are controlled by a GABAergic pontine mechanism. *J. Neurophysiol.* **82**, 2015–19.

Yamuy, J., Mancillas, J. R., Morales, F. R. & Chase, M. H. (1993). C-fos expression in the pons and medulla of the cat during carbachol-induced active sleep. *J. Neurosci.* **13**, 2703–18.

Zepelin, H. (2000). Mammalian sleep. In *Principles and Practice of Sleep Medicine*, ed. M. H. Kryger, T. Roth & W. C. Dement, pp. 82–92. Philadelphia, PA: W. B. Saunders Company.

II THE INFLUENCE OF NEUROTRANSMITTERS ON SLEEP AND WAKEFULNESS

4

Gamma-aminobutyric acid and the regulation of paradoxical, or rapid eye movement, sleep

PIERRE-HERVÉ LUPPI, DAMIEN GERVASONI, LAURE
VERRET, ROMAIN GOUTAGNY, CHRISTELLE PEYRON,
DENISE SALVERT, LUCIENNE LEGER, AND PATRICE FORT

Paradoxical sleep: the early years

In 1959, Michel Jouvet and François Michel discovered in cats a phase of sleep characterized by a complete disappearance of the muscle tone, and paradoxically associated with a cortical activation and rapid eye movements (REM) (Jouvet & Michel, 1959). In view of its singularity, they proposed to call this state paradoxical sleep (PS). It corresponded to REM sleep, the state described in 1953 by Aserinsky and Kleitman and that correlates with dream activity in humans (Aserinsky & Kleitman, 1953; Dement & Kleitman, 1957). In view of the occurrence of muscle atonia, Jouvet proposed that PS was a distinct sleep state and a true vigilance state independent of slow wave sleep (SWS) and waking (W). Over the 40 years following its discovery, Jouvet and co-workers pursued the study of PS. Supporting the theory of the duality of sleep, they showed that PS, in contrast to SWS, was present in mammals and birds but absent from amphibians and reptiles. Jouvet also demonstrated that PS onset and maintenance depended upon structures different from those regulating SWS and W. He first showed that PS persists after decortication, after cerebellar ablation or transections of the brainstem rostral to the pons. In contrast, transections at the posterior limit of the pons suppressed PS (Jouvet, 1962a). He also demonstrated that a state resembling PS is still visible in the "pontine cat", a preparation in which all the structures rostral to the pons are removed (Jouvet, 1962a). These results indicated

Neurochemistry of Sleep and Wakefulness, ed. J. M. Monti *et al.* Published by Cambridge University Press.
© Cambridge University Press 2008.

that brainstem structures were necessary and sufficient to cause and maintain the state of PS, a concept that is still valid today. Subsequently, Jouvet and others showed that electrolytic and chemical lesions of the dorsal part of the pontis oralis (PnO) and caudalis (PnC) nuclei specifically suppress PS (Carli & Zanchetti, 1965; Jouvet & Delorme, 1965; Webster & Jones, 1988; Sastre *et al.*, 1981; Jouvet, 1962b) indicating that these nuclei contain the neurons responsible for PS onset and maintenance.

The reciprocal interaction model

The 1960s and 1970s were a period marked by the introduction of histochemical methods to identify cholinergic and monoaminergic neurons, of drugs specifically increasing or decreasing the action of their neurotransmitters, and by the development of electrophysiological methods allowing the recordings of single neuron activity. During this time, Jouvet and his colleagues, in parallel with several teams in the world, soon reached the conclusion that reciprocal interactions between cholinergic and monoaminergic neurons underlie the onset of PS (Jouvet, 1969, 1975).

On the one hand, Jouvet (1962b) was the first to demonstrate that cholinergic mechanisms play a major role in PS generation since peripheral atropine administration suppressed PS, whereas anticholinesterase compounds increased PS. Then, George *et al.* (1964) discovered that bilateral injections of carbachol, a cholinergic agonist, into the PnO and PnC promote PS. It was later shown that PS is induced with the shortest latency when carbachol is injected in a small area of the dorsal PnO and PnC (Baghdoyan, 1997; Vanni-Mercier *et al.*, 1989; Lai & Siegel, 1990; Yamamoto *et al.*, 1990; Garzon *et al.*, 1998), named peri-locus coeruleus α (peri-LCα) by Sakai *et al.* (1979b, 1981). Sakai and co-workers from Jouvet's laboratory (Sakai, 1985; Sakai *et al.*, 1981, 2001; Sakai & Koyama, 1996) found that the great majority of the pontine neurons with a tonic activity specific during PS (PS-on neurons) were located in the peri-LCα. They divided these neurons into two populations (Sakai & Koyama, 1996). A first population consisted of neurons (i) located in the dorsal and rostral peri-LCα, (ii) inhibited by carbachol, a cholinergic agonist, and (iii) projecting rostrally to the intralaminar thalamic nuclei of the thalamus, the posterior hypothalamus, and the basal forebrain. A second population was formed of PS-on neurons (i) excited by carbachol, (ii) distributed in all parts of the peri-LCα, and (iii) projecting caudally to the nucleus reticularis magnocellularis (Mc) localized in the ventromedial bulbar reticular formation (Sakai *et al.*, 1979b, 1981). Based on these and other results, it was proposed that neurons of the first type were cholinergic and responsible for the cortical activation during PS, whereas neurons of the second type were glutamatergic and induced muscle atonia via descending excitatory projections to glycinergic pre-motoneurons within the Mc (Sakai & Koyama, 1996; Sakai et al., 2001; Chase et al., 1989; Luppi et al., 1988; Fort et al., 1990, 1993; Jones, 1991b). Supporting this hypothesis, the great majority of neurons in the peri-LCα projecting to the Mc are not cholinergic (Luppi et al., 1988), glutamate release in the Mc increases specifically during PS (Kodama et al., 1998), and injection of non-NMDA glutamate agonists in the Mc suppresses muscle tone (Lai & Siegel, 1991). In addition, the Mc contains spinal-projecting PS-on neurons (Siegel et al., 1979; Sakai et al., 1979a) and its cytotoxic lesion induces a decrease in PS amounts and an increase in muscle tone during PS (Holmes & Jones, 1994). Further, intracellular recordings of motoneurons during strychnine application demonstrated that glycine is responsible for the tonic hyperpolarization of the spinal, hypoglossal, and trigeminal motoneurons (Chase et al., 1989; Soja et al., 1991; Kohlmeier et al., 1996; Yamuy et al., 1999), and we have shown that the Mc contains a large number of glycinergic neurons (Fort et al., 1990, 1993; Rampon et al., 1996a). These glycinergic neurons project directly to spinal motoneurons (Holstege & Bongers, 1991) whereas those of the parvocellular and parvocellular alpha nuclei project directly to the trigeminal motor nucleus (Li et al., 1996; Rampon et al., 1996b). The release of both glycine and GABA increases in the spinal cord and the hypoglossal motor nucleus during the atonia produced by a cholinergic stimulation of the peri-LCα (Kodama et al., 2003). In addition, we recently showed that glycinergic neurons from these nuclei express Fos after a pharmacological induction of PS (Boissard et al., 2002). Moreover, following the induction of PS by carbachol injections in the peri-LCα, Fos-labeled cells were found in the Mc, and were shown to project to the trigeminal motor nucleus (Morales et al., 1999).

On the other hand, a number of results indicated that the onset of PS was due to a reciprocal inhibitory interaction between the PS-on neurons and monoaminergic PS-off neurons. McCarley & Hobson (1975) were the first to detail this hypothesis in the mid 1970s. They were soon followed by Sakai, who proposed a slightly revised model (Sakai et al., 1981). This well-accepted hypothesis was formulated following the findings that serotonergic neurons from the raphe nuclei and noradrenergic neurons from the locus coeruleus cease firing specifically during PS, i.e. have a mirror activity to PS-on neurons (Hobson et al., 1975; Aston-Jones & Bloom, 1981; McGinty & Harper, 1976; Aghajanian & Vandermaelen, 1982). Supporting this theory, drugs enhancing serotonin and noradrenergic transmission, in particular monoamine oxidase inhibitors and serotonin/norepinephrine reuptake blockers, specifically suppress PS (Jones, 1991b; Jouvet, 1969; Gervasoni et al., 2002). However, the sites where the monoamines and particularly serotonin exert their PS-suppressant effect remain unclear.

Indeed, injections of norepinephrine, epinephrine, or benoxathian (an α2 ago-nist) into the peri-LCα inhibit PS, but injections of serotonin have no effect (Tononi et al., 1991; Crochet & Sakai, 1999a,b). Besides, norepinephrine inhibits the non-cholinergic PS-on neurons via α2-adrenoceptors, and has no effect on the cholinergic PS-on neurons from the peri-LCα, whereas serotonin has no effect on either type of neuron (Sakai & Koyama, 1996). Monoamines could also act on PS-on neurons localized in structures other than the peri-LCα, such as the Mc (Luppi et al., 1988) or the pedunculopontine tegmental (PPT) and laterodorsal tegmental cholinergic nuclei (LDT) (Horner & Kubin, 1999). The PPT and LDT con-tain PS-on neurons although the great majority of the neurons in these nuclei are tonically active during both waking and PS (Kayama et al., 1992; Datta et al., 2001; Datta & Siwek, 2002; Datta & Hobson, 1994).

In conclusion, a considerable amount of data supports the hypothesis that the onset and maintenance of PS is due to reciprocal inhibitory interactions between PS-on neurons and PS-off monoaminergic neurons. However, we recently obtained results in rats indicating that GABAergic and glutamatergic neurons might be more important players than cholinergic and monoaminergic neurons. These results were obtained by combining single unit recordings, local adminis-tration of pharmacological agents by micro-iontophoresis in the unanesthetized, head-restrained rat, and anterograde and retrograde tracing combined with Fos and neurochemical identification of labeled cells (Darracq et al., 1996; Gervasoni et al., 1998, 2000; Boissard et al., 2002, 2003; Verret et al., 2005, 2006). In the next sections, we present these results and propose a new theory on the neuronal network responsible for PS.

The GABAergic neurons gating the onset of PS

We recently reported that a long-lasting PS-like hypersomnia can be induced with a short latency in the head-restrained rat by a microiontophoretic application of bicuculline or gabazine, both GABA$_A$ antagonists, within a small area of the dorsolateral pontine tegmentum (Boissard et al., 2002). We also recorded in the same area neurons that are specifically active during PS and excited by bicuculline or gabazine iontophoresis (Boissard et al., 2000). This region matches exactly the sublaterodorsal nucleus (SLD) defined by Swanson (1998). It corresponds approximately to the dorsal subcoeruleus nucleus of Paxinos & Watson (1997) and to the peri-LCα in the cat. Studies in freely moving rats have confirmed our results (Pollock & Mistlberger, 2003; Sanford et al., 2003). In cats, the pressure injection of bicuculline – and to a lesser extent of phaclofen (a GABA$_B$ antagonist) – in the dorsal portion of the PnO (which roughly corre-sponds to the peri-LCα) induces a marked increase in PS with a short latency. In contrast, the application of muscimol (a GABA$_A$ agonist) or baclofen (a GABA$_B$ agonist) induced W (Xi *et al.*, 1999, 2001). Furthermore, the microinjection of scopolamine (a muscarinic receptor antagonist) does not block the induction of PS by bicuculline (Xi *et al.*, 2004), indicating that acetylcholine is not involved in the effect of bicuculline. Together, these data indicate that the removal of a tonic GABAergic input present on SLD PS-on neurons during both W and SWS is the key event for the onset of PS. By combining retrograde tracing with cholera toxin B subunit (CTb) and glutamic acid dehydrogenase (GAD) immunostaining, we recently showed that the GABAergic innervation of SLD neurons arises from both interneurons and distant neurons located in the pontine and deep mesencephalic reticular nuclei and to a minor extent from hypothalamic and medullary structures (Boissard *et al.*, 2003). Furthermore, Xi *et al.* (1999) found in cats that administration of antisense oligonucleotides against GAD mRNA in the nucleus pontis oralis (NPO), a region corresponding to the peri-LCα, produced a significant decrease in W and an increase in PS. However, Maloney *et al.* (2000) found in rats that the number of Fos expressing GABAergic neurons in the rostral pontine reticular nucleus decreased following PS rebound, suggesting that GABAergic neurons from this structure are active during W and SWS and inactive during PS. Finally, it has been shown in cats (Sastre *et al.*, 1996, 2000) and rats (Boissard *et al.*, 2000) that muscimol injections in the most ventrolateral part of the periaqueductal gray, and in the region of the deep mesencephalic reticular nucleus just ventral to it, induce a marked increase in PS. More recently, Sakai *et al.* (2001) reported that muscimol applications limited to the region of the deep mesencephalic reticular nucleus just ventral to the periaqueductal gray induced an increase in PS, whereas those in the ventrolateral periaqueductal gray had no effect. In our study, we reported a notable non-GABAergic projection to the SLD from the ventrolateral periaqueductal gray and a mixed GABAergic and non-GABAergic projection from the region of the deep mesencephalic reticular nucleus just ventral to the periaqueductal gray (Boissard *et al.*, 2003). From these results, we propose that GABAergic neurons located in the dorsal part of the deep mesencephalic reticular nucleus, the pontine reticular nucleus, and/or in the SLD itself, project to and directly inhibit the PS-on neurons from the SLD specifically during W and SWS.

The role of glutamate

We recently showed that the iontophoretic injection of kainic acid (a glutamate agonist) in the SLD excites the PS-on neurons and induces a PS-like state (Boissard *et al.*, 2002). Furthermore, the PS-like state induced by bicuculline iontophoresis in the SLD is reversed by the application of kynurenate, a wide-spectrum antagonist of excitatory amino acids (Boissard et al., 2002). In agreement with these results, the microdialysis application of kainic acid in the cat peri-LCα induces a PS-like state (Onoe & Sakai, 1995). Together, these results suggest that PS-on neurons in the SLD receive a tonic glutamatergic input during all sleep–waking states. They further suggest that, following the removal of the tonic GABAergic input at the onset of PS, an unmasked glutamatergic input is responsible for the tonic activity of the SLD PS-on neurons throughout PS. The glutamatergic neurons providing this constant excitatory input to SLD PS-on neurons are likely located in the brainstem, although forebrain glutamatergic neurons could also participate. Indeed, as shown by the persistence of a PS-non PS cycle in the "pontine cat", the structures responsible for the genesis of PS are restricted to the brainstem (Jouvet, 1962a). Accordingly, such glutamatergic inputs can arise from the numerous non-GABAergic neurons projecting to the SLD and localized in the ventrolateral periaqueductal gray and the mesencephalic, pontine, and parvocellular reticular nuclei. Inputs to the SLD originating in the primary motor area of the frontal cortex, the bed nucleus of the stria terminalis, and the central nucleus of the amygdala might also participate in the activation of the SLD PS-on neurons. Indeed, corticofugal pyramidal cells are glutamatergic. Using fMRI, Maquet et al. (1996) found that the regional blood flow in the amygdaloid complex is positively correlated with PS. Furthermore, the electrical stimulation of the central nucleus of the amygdala increases the frequency of pontine waves recorded in or just above the SLD during PS (Deboer et al., 1998). From these results, we hypothesized that the frontal cortex and the central nucleus of the amygdala and functionally related bed nucleus of the stria terminalis provide excitatory glutamatergic projections to PS-on neurons from the SLD. Additional studies are needed to verify this hypothesis.

Role of acetylcholine

Carbachol iontophoresis into the rat SLD induces a W state with increased muscle activity and no effect on SLD PS-on neurons (Boissard et al., 2002). These results indicate significant differences between rats and cats in the pharmacological sensitivity of the pontine PS-on neurons. In agreement with our results, carbachol injections into the rat pontine reticular formation only slightly enhance PS (Gnadt & Pegram, 1986; Shiromani & Fishbein, 1986; Velazquez-Moctezuma et al., 1989; Bourgin et al., 1995) or have no reliable effect (Deurveilher et al., 1997). In cats, however, PS occurs almost immediately after a carbachol injection and the episodes last longer than in control PS. The carbachol-effective sites in rats are widely distributed in the pontine reticular formation. In contrast, the most effective site in cats is the peri-LCα that corresponds to the rat SLD (Vanni-Mercier *et al.*, 1989). The absence of effect of carbachol injections in the SLD does not rule out a role of acetylcholine in the onset and maintenance of PS in the rat. Indeed, it is possible that PS-on neurons in the SLD have muscarinic and/or nicotinic receptors, but that carbachol is unable to modify their activity because of the strong GABAergic tonic inhibition revealed in our studies. Supporting this hypothesis, carbachol injections in the region of the SLD can induce, with a short latency, a long period of atonia in anesthetized or decerebrate rat models in which the GABAergic inhibitory tone on SLD neurons is decreased or even absent (Taguchi *et al.*, 1992; Fenik *et al.*, 1999). Another possibility is that the cholinergic system plays an important role in PS in rats via an action on populations of neurons controlling PS localized in pontine regions other than the SLD. Supporting this idea, pressure injections of carbachol in the most ventral part of the oral pontine reticular formation markedly enhance PS time in cats (De Andres *et al.*, 1985; Garzon *et al.*, 1998). An increase in the number of PPT and LDT cholinergic neurons containing Fos has been observed in PS recovery following PS deprivation (Maloney *et al.*, 1999), although in our recent study reproducing these experiments, only a few cholinergic neurons containing Fos were observed in these nuclei (Verret *et al.*, 2005). In addition, M2 and M4 muscarinic receptors KO mice displayed no change in PS, whereas M3 KO mice showed only a small decrease in PS (Goutagny *et al.*, 2005a).

GABAergic neurons responsible for the inactivation of monoaminergic neurons during PS

According to the classical "reciprocal interaction" model (McCarley & Hobson, 1975; Sakai *et al.*, 1981), the cessation of firing of the noradrenergic and serotonergic neurons at the onset of PS is the result of active PS-specific inhibitory processes originating from PS-on cells. These neurons were first hypothesized to be cholinergic and localized in the peri-LCα, LDT, and PPT. However, acetylcholine excites LC noradrenergic neurons and is only weakly inhibitory on serotonergic DRN neurons (Guyenet & Aghajanian, 1979; Koyama & Kayama, 1993). It was therefore suggested that they might use GABA or glycine instead as an inhibitory neurotransmitter (Luppi *et al.*, 1991; Jones, 1991a). To test this hypothesis, we investigated the effect of bicuculline or gabazine and strychnine (a glycine antagonist) on the activity of LC noradrenergic and DRN serotonergic cells. The antagonists were applied by micro-iontophoresis during W, SWS, and PS on monoaminergic neurons recorded in the head-restrained unanesthetized rat (Darracq *et al.*, 1996; Gervasoni *et al.*, 1998, 2000).

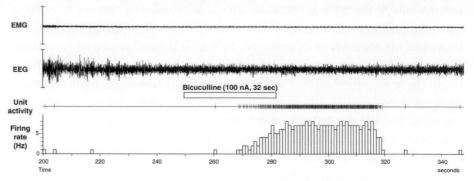

Figure 4.1 Effect of an iontophoretic injection of bicuculline, a GABA$_A$ antagonist, on a locus coeruleus noradrenergic neuron. With reduced activity during slow wave sleep, this neuron then becomes silent during paradoxical sleep (PS). The application of bicuculline reversibly restores tonic discharge, indicating the role of GABA in the cessation of activity of this neuron during PS.

Iontophoretic applications of bicuculline, gabazine, or strychnine during SWS or PS restored a tonic firing in LC noradrenergic (Fig. 4.1) and DRN serotonergic neurons (Darracq *et al.*, 1996; Gervasoni *et al.*, 1998, 2000). Application of these antagonists during W induced a sustained increase in discharge rate. These experiments revealed the existence of tonic GABA and glycinergic inputs to the LC and DRN that are effective during all vigilance states. Importantly, we found that when the effect of strychnine occurred during transitions between PS and W, the discharge rate of the LC or DRN neurons further increased at the onset of W. In contrast, during bicuculline administration, the discharge rate of a LC or DRN neuron did not change at the transition between PS and W. These results strongly suggested that the release of GABA but not that of glycine is responsible for the inactivation of LC noradrenergic neurons and DRN serotonergic during PS. At variance with our results, Levine & Jacobs (1992) have found in cats that the iontophoretic application of bicuculline reversed the typical suppression of neuronal activity of DRN serotonergic neurons during SWS but not during PS. In addition, Sakai & Crochet (2000) found that the microdialysis infusion of bicuculline in cats had no effect on DRN serotonergic neurons during PS and suspected a non-specific excitatory effect of bicuculline in our experiments. This latter proposal appeared unlikely since we reproduced the effect of bicuculline with gabazine, another specific GABA$_A$ antagonist (unpublished results). Our results are further supported by the microdialysis studies of Nitz & Siegel (1997a,b), showing in cats a significant increase in GABA release in the DRN and LC during PS compared with W and SWS and, in contrast, no detectable changes in glycine concentrations. Based on these and our results, we suggest that, during W, the LC and DRN cells are under a tonic GABAergic inhibition that increases during SWS and even further during PS, and that such increase in GABAergic inhibition is responsible for the inactivation of these neurons during the sleep states. In contrast, the glycinergic tonic inhibition would be constant across the sleep–waking cycle and thus control the general excitability of LC and DRN neurons.

Double-staining experiments combining GAD and CTb immunostaining also showed that the LC and DRN receive GABAergic inputs from neurons located in a large number of distant regions, from the forebrain to the medulla (Luppi et al., 1999; Gervasoni et al., 2000). Indeed, we observed a substantial number of GAD-immunoreactive neurons in the preoptic area, the lateral hypothalamic area, the mesencephalic and pontine periaqueductal gray, and the dorsal paragigantocellular reticular nucleus that project to the LC and DRN (Luppi et al., 1999; Gervasoni et al., 2000). Based on physiological and electrophysiological data (see above), we expect that one or several of these GABAergic afferents are "switched on" specifically at the onset of and during PS episodes and are responsible for the inhibition of brainstem monoaminergic neurons during PS. It was recently proposed that GABAergic neurons located in the extended ventrolateral preoptic nucleus might be responsible (Lu et al., 2002). However, PS-like episodes continue to occur in pontine or decerebrate cats (Jouvet, 1972). Moreover, PS episodes induced by carbachol injections in the pons of decerebrate animals are still associated with a cessation of activity of serotonergic neurons of the raphe obscurus and pallidus nuclei (Woch et al., 1996). Therefore, it is likely that the ventrolateral periaqueductal gray and/or the dorsal paragigantocellular nucleus contain the GABAergic neurons responsible for the inhibition of monoaminergic neurons during PS (Luppi et al., 1999; Gervasoni et al., 2000). Supporting this hypothesis, local applications of bicuculline block the dorsal paragigantocellular-evoked inhibition of LC neurons (Ennis & Aston-Jones, 1989) and focal iontophoretic applications of NMDA in the ventral periaqueductal gray induce bicuculline-sensitive IPSPs in DRN serotonergic neurons (Liu et al., 2000). Further, Yamuy et al. (1995) showed that, after a long period of PS induced by a pontine injection of carbachol, a large number of Fos-positive cells are visible in the DRN and a region lateral to it. Moreover, Maloney et al. (1999) observed in the periaqueductal gray an increase in Fos-positive GAD immunoreactive neurons after a PS rebound induced by deprivation. To directly determine the GABAergic afferents to the LC that are active during PS, we recently combined iontophoretic application of CTb in the LC with Fos staining in rats deprived of PS, rats with enhanced recovery PS after selective deprivation, and control rats. Using this method, we observed a large number of CTb and Fos double-immunostained neurons in the dorsal paragigantocellular reticular nucleus and a substantial number in the ventrolateral periaqueductal gray and the lateral paragigantocellular reticular nucleus specifically after PS rebound (Verret *et al.*, 2003). From these results, we propose that the GABAergic neurons responsible for the inhibition of the LC noradrenergic neurons during PS are mainly, but not exclusively, located in the dorsal paragigantocellular reticular nucleus. In order to further test this hypothesis, we recorded the spontaneous activity of neurons from the dorsal paragigantocellular reticular nucleus across the sleep–waking cycle in head-restrained rats. Neurons with an activity specific to PS (PS-on neurons) were found within this nucleus (Goutagny *et al.*, 2005b), supporting the idea that it contains the GABAergic neurons responsible for the cessation of activity of the noradrenergic neurons of the LC during PS. This hypothesis is also supported by a recent study showing that electrical stimulation of the area of the dorsal paragigantocellular reticular nucleus induces an increase in PS quantities (Kaur *et al.*, 2001). It is, however, likely that the GABAergic neurons inhibiting the serotonergic neurons of the DRN are localized in the ventrolateral periaqueductal gray rather than the dorsal paragigantocellular reticular nucleus since the latter structure provides only a weak GABAergic projection to the DRN (Gervasoni *et al.*, 2000).

The role of additional structures and neurotransmitters

To localize the structures involved in the onset and maintenance of PS, we recently compared the distribution of Fos-labelled neurons in the brainstem of control rats, of rats selectively deprived of PS for approximately 72 h, and of rats allowed to recover from such deprivation (Verret *et al.*, 2003, 2005, 2006). A large number of Fos-labeled cells, positively correlated with the percentage of time spent in PS, was observed in the structures containing neurons involved in PS such as the LDT sublaterodorsal, alpha and ventral gigantocellular reticular nuclei. In addition, a large number of Fos-labeled cells was seen after PS rebound in the extended VLPO, posterior hypothalamus, lateral, ventrolateral, and dorsal periaqueductal gray, dorsal and lateral paragigantocellular reticular nuclei, and nucleus raphe obscurus. Interestingly, half of the cells in the latter nucleus were immunoreactive to choline acetyltransferase (Verret *et al.*, 2005). These findings demonstrate that many brainstem structures not previously identified contain neurons active during PS and might therefore play a key role during this state. Among them, the posterior hypothalamus particularly retained our attention since a number of studies indicate that it plays an important role in sleep–wake control.

The posterior hypothalamus

A considerable amount of data indicates that the posterior hypothalamus (PH) plays a crucial role in vigilance states regulation. First, von Economo reported that posterior hypothalamic and midbrain junction lesions resulted in sleepiness based on observations of patients from the encephalitis lethargica epidemic during World War 1 (Von Economo, 1926). In subsequent years, insomnia was reported in monkeys (Ranson, 1939), rats (Nauta, 1946), and cats (Swett & Hobson, 1968) following electrolytic lesions of the PH. Transient hyperinsomnia was also observed after lesions with ibotenic acid (Sallanon et al., 1988; Swett & Hobson, 1968) or inactivation by local application of muscimol, a GABAa agonist (Lin et al., 1989; Sallanon et al., 1989). Furthermore, it was shown that the waking effect of modafinil and amphetamine is suppressed by the injection of muscimol in the cat posterior hypothalamus (Lin et al., 1992, 1996). Vanni-Mercier et al. (1984) also found neurons active only or mainly during waking in the PH of the cat during extracellular recordings.

After a careful review of the literature, we found evidence that the PH also plays a role in PS regulation. First, despite the fact that a PS-like state still occurred in "pontine cats", showing that the brainstem was sufficient to produce PS, PS recovery following PS deprivation was abolished in these animals (Jouvet, 1988). These results suggest that the brainstem contains the structures responsible for PS but not those responsible for its homeostatic regulation. In support of these observations, several studies reported that a small proportion of the neurons recorded in the PH are specifically active during PS (Alam et al., 2002; Koyama et al., 2003; Steininger et al., 1999). Recent data summarized below confirm that the PH contains populations of neurons involved in PS control.

The hypocretin (orexin) neuronal population

Narcolepsy, a sleep disorder characterized by excessive daytime sleepiness and cataplexy, may be caused by the lack of hypocretin mRNA and peptides in humans (Peyron et al., 2000) or a disruption of the hypocretin receptor 2 or its ligand in dogs and mice (Lin et al., 1999; Chemelli et al., 1999). Hypocretin-containing neurons are located exclusively in the dorsomedial, lateral, and perifornical hypothalamic areas (Peyron et al., 1998). Two hypocretin sequences, Hcrt-1 (orexin-A) and Hcrt-2 (orexin-B), are generated from a single preprohypocretin (De Lecea et al., 1998; Peyron et al., 1998; Sakurai et al., 1998). Axons from these neurons are found in the hypothalamus, locus coeruleus (LC), raphe nuclei, tuberomamillary nucleus, midline thalamus, all levels of spinal cord, sympathetic and parasympathetic centers, and many other brain regions (van den Pol, 1999; Peyron *et al.*, 1998). The two G-protein-coupled hypocretin receptors (HcrtR-1 and HcrtR-2) (Sakurai *et al.*, 1998) also show a widespread and heterogenous pattern of expression throughout the CNS (Hervieu *et al.*, 2001; Marcus *et al.*, 2001; Trivedi *et al.*, 1998). Interestingly, HcrtR-1 and HcrtR-2 are densely packed in monoaminergic and cholinergic nuclei involved in the regulation of sleep and wakefulness (Jones, 1993). Thus, hypocretins may control vigilance by modulating the activity of monoaminergic and cholinergic neurons. Pharmacological studies indicate potent wake-promoting and PS-reducing effects following ICV administration and local injections in the LC of Hcrt (Hagan *et al.*, 1999; Bourgin *et al.*, 2000). Furthermore, the waking effect of Hcrt-1 when injected in the lateral ventricle can be blocked by systemic injections of antagonist of the H1 histaminergic receptors (Yamanaka *et al.*, 2002), not present in H1 knockout mice (Huang *et al.*, 2001). In vitro, Hcrt applications strongly increase the firing rate of LC noradrenergic neurons (Horvath *et al.*, 1999; Hagan *et al.*, 1999), of dopaminergic VTA neurons (Nakamura *et al.*, 2000), of serotonergic dorsal raphe neurons (Liu *et al.*, 2002; Brown *et al.*, 2001), and of histaminergic neurons of the tuberomammillary nucleus (Bayer *et al.*, 2001; Eriksson *et al.*, 2001). These data are therefore consistent with a global stimulatory effect of Hcrt on monoaminergic tone in the maintenance of wakefulness.

In addition, Hcrt cells are c-Fos-positive after a period of natural or pharmacologically induced waking, such as treatments with stimulants like amphetamine or modafinil. On the contrary, they are not c-Fos positive after PS rebound, indicating that Hcrt neurons are inactive during PS (Torterolo *et al.*, 2003; Verret *et al.*, 2003). Consistent with these observations, it has been shown by continuous microdialysis or 24 h CSF sampling that the level of Hcrt released *in situ* or in the CSF is higher during the active period than the quiet period in the rat (Yoshida *et al.*, 2001) and monkey (Zeitzer *et al.*, 2003). Hcrt cells are silent during SWS and tonic periods of PS, with occasional burst discharges during phasic PS. They discharge during active waking, they have moderate and approximately equal levels of activity during grooming and eating, and they show maximal activity during exploratory behavior (Mileykovskiy *et al.*, 2005; Lee *et al.*, 2005). With regard to monoaminergic neurons (see above), the cessation of activity of Hcrt cells during sleep is likely caused by a tonic GABAergic inhibition. Indeed, local application of bicuculline in the perifornical region induces waking and c-Fos labeling of the hypocretin but not of the intermingled MCH neurons (Goutagny *et al.*, 2005c; Alam *et al.*, 2005).

The MCH peptidergic neuronal population

We recently demonstrated that the PH contains a very large number of Fos-labeled neurons in rats perfused after a 3 h PS rebound compared with those perfused at the end of the deprivation (Verret *et al.*, 2003). We further demonstrated that the majority of these neurons were immunoreactive to MCH. These results suggest that MCH neurons are specifically and strongly active during PS. They are in agreement with electrophysiological studies showing the presence of neurons strongly active during PS in the PH (Alam *et al.*, 2002; Koyama *et al.*, 2003; Steininger *et al.*, 1999).

To determine whether MCH plays a role in PS regulation, we performed i.c.v. administrations of MCH. Injections of 0.2, 1 and 5 µg induced a dose-dependent increase in PS compared with saline, due to an increase in the number of PS bouts but not of their duration. To a minor extent, an increase in the amount of SWS was also observed after MCH administration. Since MCH neurons are active during PS and MCH is primarily an inhibitory peptide (Gao & van den Pol, 2001), MCH neurons likely promote PS indirectly by inhibiting neurons, themselves inhibiting the PS executive neurons during W and SWS. The monoaminergic neurons in the brainstem, the histaminergic neurons in the caudal hypothalamus, and the hypocretin neurons all belong to this category. They are active during W, decrease or nearly cease their activity during SWS, and are silent during PS (Gervasoni *et al.*, 1998, 2000; Steininger *et al.*, 1999; Mileykovskiy *et al.*, 2005; Lee *et al.*, 2005). Further, based on electron and light microscopic observations, it has been shown that MCH and hypocretin neurons are interconnected (Bayer *et al.*, 2002; Guan *et al.*, 2002). We therefore propose that MCH neurons primarily modulate SWS and PS via an inhibitory action on the intermingled hypocretin neurons. They could also increase PS via a direct inhibitory projection on the mesencephalic and pontine GABAergic neurons that tonically inhibit the pontine PS executive neurons located in the sublaterodorsal nucleus (see above)(Boissard *et al.*, 2002, 2003). In contrast, hypocretin neurons would provide excitatory projections to these GABAergic neurons and hence inhibit PS.

Conclusion: a new network model for the onset and maintenance of PS

Based on our results, we propose the following model (Fig. 4.2). The activation of PS-on glutamatergic neurons from the SLD underlies the onset and maintenance of PS. During W and SWS, these neurons are inhibited by a tonic GABAergic input arising from GABAergic PS-off neurons localized in the SLD and in the deep mesencephalic and pontine reticular nuclei. Noradrenergic and serotonergic PS-off neurons, although not essential, also participate in the inactivation of SLD neurons, particularly during W. At the onset of, and throughout, PS the monoaminergic neurons cease firing because of an active GABAergic inhibition from PS-on neurons located in the dorsal

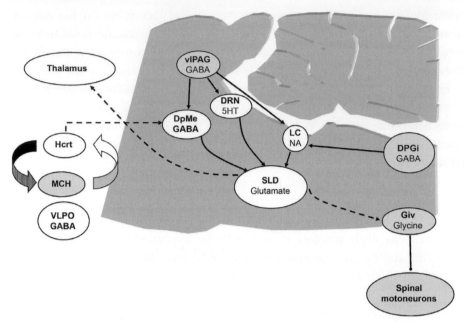

Figure 4.2 Model of the network responsible for paradoxical sleep onset and maintenance Abbreviations: DRN, dorsal raphe nucleus; 5-HT, serotonin; LC, locus coeruleus; NA, noradrenaline; LDT, laterodorsal tegmental nucleus; Ach, acetylcholine; Mc, magnocellular reticular nucleus; Gly; glycine; DPMe, deep mesencephalic reticular nucleus; PAG, periaqueductal gray; DPGi, dorsal paragigantocellular reticular nucleus; PPT, pedunculopontine nucleus; PRN, pontine reticular nucleus; SLD, sublaterodorsal nucleus; Glu, glutamate; Pef/HLA periformical/lateral hypothalamic area; Hcrt, hypocretin (i.e. orexin).

paragigantocellular reticular nucleus and the periaqueductal gray. Although the exact mechanism of the cessation of activity of the GABAergic PS-off neurons remains unknown, we propose that the GABAergic PS-on neurons inhibiting the monoaminergic neurons could, at the same time, inhibit the GABAergic PS-off neurons.

The activation of the SLD PS-on neurons at the onset of PS would be due to the masked glutamatergic excitatory input present during all vigilance states, but blocked during W and SWS by the inhibitory inputs from the GABAergic and monoaminergic PS-off neurons. It would arise from one or several non-GABAergic brainstem afferents to the SLD (e.g. the periaqueductal gray, the deep mesencephalic and pontine reticular nuclei, and the parvocellular reticular nucleus).

Ascending SLD PS-on glutamatergic neurons would induce cortical activation via their projections to intralaminar thalamic relay neurons in conjunction with W/PS-on cholinergic and glutamatergic neurons from the LDT and PPT, mesencephalic and pontine reticular nuclei, and the basal forebrain. Descending PS-on glutamatergic SLD neurons would induce muscle atonia via their excitatory projections to glycinergic premotoneurons localized in the magnocellular and parvocellular reticular nuclei.

Forebrain neurons would not be necessary for PS onset and maintenance. However, hypocretin and MCH hypothalamic neurons would participate in the homeostasis of PS through reciprocal connections and their respective excitatory and inhibitory projections on the brainstem monoaminergic and GABAergic PS-off neurons.

Acknowledgements

This work was supported by CNRS (UMR 5167 and FRE 2469) and Université Claude Bernard Lyon 1.

References

Aghajanian, G. K. & Vandermaelen, C. P. (1982). Intracellular identification of central noradrenergic and serotonergic neurons by a new double labeling procedure. *J. Neurosci.* **2**, 1786–92.

Alam, M. N., Gong, H., Alam, T. *et al.* (2002). Sleep-waking discharge patterns of neurons recorded in the rat perifornical lateral hypothalamic area. *J. Physiol.* **538**, 619–31.

Alam, M. N., Kumar, S., Bashir, T. *et al.* (2005). GABA-mediated control of hypocretin- but not melanin-concentrating hormone-immunoreactive neurones during sleep in rats. *J. Physiol.* **563**, 569–82.

Aserinsky, E. & Kleitman, N. (1953). Regularly occurring periods of eye motility and concomitant phenomena during sleep. *Science* **118**, 273–4.

Aston-Jones, G. & Bloom, F. E. (1981). Activity of norepinephrine-containing locus coeruleus neurons in behaving rats anticipates fluctuations in the sleep-waking cycle. *J. Neurosci.* **1**, 876–86.

Baghdoyan, H. A. (1997). Cholinergic mechanisms regulating REM sleep. In *Sleep Science: Integrating Basic Research and Clinical Practice*, ed. W. J. Schwartz. Basle: S. Karger Publishing.

Bayer, L., Eggermann, E., Serafin, M. *et al.* (2001). Orexins (hypocretins) directly excite tuberomammillary neurons. *Eur. J. Neurosci.* **14**, 1571–5.

Bayer, L., Mairet-Coello, G., Risold, P. Y. & Griffond, B. (2002). Orexin/hypocretin neurons: chemical phenotype and possible interactions with melanin-concentrating hormone neurons. *Regul. Pept.* **104**, 33–9.

Boissard, R., Gervasoni, D., Fort, P. *et al.* (2000). Neuronal networks responsible for paradoxical sleep onset and maintenance in rats: a new hypothesis. *Sleep* **23** (suppl.), 107.

Boissard, R., Gervasoni, D., Schmidt, M. H. *et al.* (2002). The rat ponto-medullary network responsible for paradoxical sleep onset and maintenance: a combined microinjection and functional neuroanatomical study. *Eur. J. Neurosci.* **16**, 1959–73.

Boissard, R., Fort, P., Gervasoni, D., Barbagli, B. & Luppi, P. H. (2003). Localization of the GABAergic and non-GABAergic neurons projecting to the sublaterodorsal nucleus and potentially gating paradoxical sleep onset. *Eur. J. Neurosci.* **18**, 1627–39.

Bourgin, P., Escourrou, P., Gaultier, C. & Adrien, J. (1995). Induction of rapid eye movement sleep by carbachol infusion into the pontine reticular formation in the rat. *Neuroreport* **6**, 532–6.

Bourgin, P., Huitron-Resendiz, S., Spier, A. D. *et al.* (2000). Hypocretin-1 modulates rapid eye movement sleep through activation of locus coeruleus neurons. *J. Neurosci.* **20**, 7760–5.

Brown, R. E., Sergeeva, O., Eriksson, K. S. & Haas, H. L. (2001). Orexin A excites serotonergic neurons in the dorsal raphe nucleus of the rat. *Neuropharmacology* **40**, 457–9.

Carli, G. & Zanchetti, A. (1965). A study of pontine lesions suppressing deep sleep in the cat. *Arch. Ital. Biol.* **103**, 751–88.

Chase, M. H., Soja, P. J. & Morales, F. R. (1989). Evidence that glycine mediates the postsynaptic potentials that inhibit lumbar motoneurons during the atonia of active sleep. *J. Neurosci.* **9**, 743–51.

Chemelli, R. M., Willie, J. T., Sinton, C. M. *et al.* (1999). Narcolepsy in orexin knockout mice: molecular genetics of sleep regulation. *Cell* **98**, 437–51.

Crochet, S. & Sakai, K. (1999a). Alpha-2 adrenoceptor mediated paradoxical (REM) sleep inhibition in the cat. *Neuroreport* **10**, 2199–204.

Crochet, S. & Sakai, K. (1999b). Effects of microdialysis application of monoamines on the EEG and behavioural states in the cat mesopontine tegmentum. *Eur. J. Neurosci.* **11**, 3738–52.

Darracq, L., Gervasoni, D., Souliere, F. *et al.* (1996). Effect of strychnine on rat locus coeruleus neurones during sleep and wakefulness. *Neuroreport* **8**, 351–5.

Datta, S. & Hobson, J. A. (1994). Neuronal activity in the caudo-lateral peribrachial pons: Relationship to PGO waves and rapid eye movement. *J. Neurophysiol.* **71**, 95–109.

Datta, S. & Siwek, D. F. (2002). Single cell activity patterns of pedunculopontine tegmentum neurons across the sleep-wake cycle in the freely moving rats. *J. Neurosci. Res.* **70**, 611–21.

Datta, S., Spoley, E. E. & Patterson, E. H. (2001). Microinjection of glutamate into the pedunculopontine tegmentum induces REM sleep and wakefulness in the rat. *Am. J. Physiol. Regul. Integr. Comp. Physiol.* **280**, 752–9.

De Andres, I., Gomez-Montoya, J., Gutierrez-Rivas, E. & Reinoso-Suarez, F. (1985). Differential action upon sleep states of ventrolateral and central areas of pontine tegmental field. *Arch. Ital. Biol.* **123**, 1–11.

De Lecea, L., Kilduff, T. S., Peyron, C. *et al.* (1998). The hypocretins: hypothalamus-specific peptides with neuroexcitatory activity. *Proc. Natl. Acad. Sci. USA* **95**, 322–7.

Deboer, T., Sanford, L. D., Ross, R. J. & Morrison, A. R. (1998). Effects of electrical stimulation in the amygdala on ponto-geniculo-occipital waves in rats. *Brain Res.* **793**, 305–10.

Dement, W. & Kleitman, N. (1957). The relation of eye movements during sleep to dream activity: an objective method for the study of dreaming. *J. Exp. Psychol. Learn. Mem. Cogn.* **53**, 339–46.

Deurveilher, S., Hars, B. & Hennevin, E. (1997). Pontine microinjection of carbachol does not reliably enhance paradoxical sleep in rats. *Sleep* **20**, 593–607.

Ennis, M. & Aston-Jones, G. (1989). GABA-mediated inhibition of locus coeruleus from the dorsomedial rostral medulla. *J. Neurosci.* **9**, 2973–81.

Eriksson, K. S., Sergeeva, O., Brown, R. E. & Haas, H. L. (2001). Orexin/hypocretin excites the histaminergic neurons of the tuberomammillary nucleus. *J. Neurosci.* **21**, 9273–9.

Fenik, V., Ogawa, H., Davies, R. O. & Kubin, L. (1999). Pontine carbachol produces a spectrum of REM sleep-like and arousal-like electrocortical responses in urethane-anesthetized rats. *Sleep Res. Online* **2** (suppl.), 30.

Fort, P., Luppi, P. H., Wenthold, R. & Jouvet, M. (1990). [Glycine immunoreactive neurons in the medulla oblongata in cats.] *C. R. Acad. Sci. III*, **311**, 205–12.

Fort, P., Luppi, P. H. & Jouvet, M. (1993). Glycine-immunoreactive neurones in the cat brain stem reticular formation. *Neuroreport* **4**, 1123–6.

Gao, X. B. & van den Pol, A. N. (2001). Melanin concentrating hormone depresses synaptic activity of glutamate and GABA neurons from rat lateral hypothalamus. *J. Physiol.* **533**, 237–52.

Garzon, M., De Andres, I. & Reinoso-Suarez, F. (1998). Sleep patterns after carbachol delivery in the ventral oral pontine tegmentum of the cat. *Neuroscience* **83**, 1137–44.

George, R., Haslett, W. L. & Jenden, D. J. (1964). A cholinergic mechanism in the brainstem reticular formation: induction of paradoxixal sleep. *Int. J. Neuropharmacol.* **3**, 541–52.

Gervasoni, D., Darracq, L., Fort, P. *et al.* (1998). Electrophysiological evidence that noradrenergic neurons of the rat locus coeruleus are tonically inhibited by GABA during sleep. *Eur. J. Neurosci.* **10**, 964–70.

Gervasoni, D., Peyron, C., Rampon, C. *et al.* (2000). Role and origin of the GABAergic innervation of dorsal raphe serotonergic neurons. *J. Neurosci.* **20**, 4217–25.

Gervasoni, D., Panconi, E., Henninot, V. *et al.* (2002). Effect of chronic treatment with milnacipran on sleep architecture in rats compared with paroxetine and imipramine. *Pharmacol. Biochem. Behav.* **73**, 557–63.

Gnadt, J. W. & Pegram, G. V. (1986). Cholinergic brainstem mechanisms of REM sleep in the rat. *Brain Res.* **384**, 29–41.

Goutagny, R., Comte, J. C., Salvert, D. *et al.* (2005a). Paradoxical sleep in mice lacking M(3) and M(2)/M(4) muscarinic receptors. *Neuropsychobiology* **52**, 140–6.

Goutagny, R., Fort, P., Lapray, D. & Luppi, P. H. (2005b). Role of dorsal paragigantocellular nucleus in paradoxical sleep regulation: a study combining electrophysiology and pharmacology across vigilance states in the rat. *Soc. Neurosci. Abstr.* **00**, 000–000.

Goutagny, R., Luppi, P. H., Salvert, D., Gervasoni, D. & Fort, P. (2005c). GABAergic control of hypothalamic melanin-concentrating hormone-containing neurons across the sleep-waking cycle. *Neuroreport* **16**, 1069–73.

Guan, J. L., Uehara, K., Lu, S. *et al.* (2002). Reciprocal synaptic relationships between orexin- and melanin-concentrating hormone-containing neurons in the rat lateral hypothalamus: a novel circuit implicated in feeding regulation. *Int. J. Obes. Relat. Metab. Disord.* **26**, 1523–32.

Guyenet, P. G. & Aghajanian, G. K. (1979). ACh, substance P and met-enkephalin in the locus coeruleus: pharmacological evidence for independent sites of action. *Eur. J. Pharmacol.* **53**, 319–28.

Hagan, J. J., Leslie, R. A., Patel, S. *et al.* (1999). Orexin A activates locus coeruleus cell firing and increases arousal in the rat. *Proc. Natl. Acad. Sci. USA* **96**, 10911–16.

Hervieu, G. J., Cluderay, J. E., Harrison, D. C., Roberts, J. C. & Leslie, R. A. (2001). Gene expression and protein distribution of the orexin-1 receptor in the rat brain and spinal cord. *Neuroscience* **103**, 777–97.

Hobson, J. A., Mccarley, R. W. & Wyzinski, P. W. (1975). Sleep cycle oscillation: reciprocal discharge by two brainstem neuronal groups. *Science* **189**, 55–8.

Holmes, C. J. & Jones, B. E. (1994). Importance of cholinergic, GABAergic, serotonergic and other neurons in the medial medullary reticular formation for sleep-wake states studied by cytotoxic lesions in the cat. *Neuroscience* **62**, 1179–200.

Holstege, J. C. & Bongers, C. M. (1991). A glycinergic projection from the ventromedial lower brainstem to spinal motoneurons. An ultrastructural double labeling study in rat. *Brain Res.* **566**, 308–15.

Horner, R. L. & Kubin, L. (1999). Pontine carbachol elicits multiple rapid eye movement sleep-like neural events in urethane-anaesthetized rats. *Neuroscience* **93**, 215–26.

Horvath, T. L., Peyron, C., Diano, S. *et al.* (1999). Hypocretin (orexin) activation and synaptic innervation of the locus coeruleus noradrenergic system. *J. Comp. Neurol.* **415**, 145–59.

Huang, Z. L., Qu, W. M., Li, W. D. *et al.* (2001). Arousal effect of orexin A depends on activation of the histaminergic system. *Proc. Natl. Acad. Sci. USA* **98**, 9965–70.

Jones, B. (1993). The organization of central cholinergic systems and their functional importance in sleep-waking states. In *Cholinergic Function and Dysfunction. Progress in Brain Research*, ed. A. Cuello. Amsterdam: Elsevier.

Jones, B. E. (1991a). Noradrenergic locus coeruleus neurons: their distant connections and their relationship to neighboring (including cholinergic and GABAergic) neurons of the central gray and reticular formation. *Prog. Brain Res.* **88**, 15–30.

Jones, B. E. (1991b). Paradoxical sleep and its chemical/structural substrates in the brain. *Neuroscience* **40**, 637–56.

Jouvet, M. (1962a). Recherches sur les structures nerveuses et les mécanismes responsables des différentes phases du sommeil physiologique. *Arch. Ital. Biol.* **100**, 125–206.

Jouvet, M. (1962b). Sur l'existence d'un systeme hypnique ponto-limbique. Ses rapports avec l'activité onirique. In *Symposium sur la Physiologie de l'Hippocampe*, ed. P. Passouant, pp. 00–00. Paris: CNRS.

Jouvet, M. (1969). Biogenic amines and the states of sleep. *Science* **163**, 32–41.

Jouvet, M. (1972). The role of monoamines and acetylcholine-containing neurons in the regulation of the sleep-waking cycle. *Ergeb. Physiol.* **64**, 166–307.

Jouvet, M. (1975). Cholinergic mechanisms and sleep. In *Cholinergic Mechanisms*, ed. P. G. Waser. New York, NY: Raven Press.

Jouvet, M. (1988). The regulation of paradoxical sleep by the hypothalamo-hypophysis. *Arch. Ital. Biol.* **126**, 259–74.

Jouvet, M. & Delorme, F. (1965). Locus coeruleus et sommeil paradoxal. *C. R. Seanc. Soc. Biol.* **159**, 895–9.

Jouvet, M. & Michel, F. (1959). Corrélations électromyographiques du sommeil chez le chat décortiqué et mésencéphalique chronique. *C. R. Soc. Biol.* **153**, 422–5.

Kaur, S., Saxena, R. N. & Mallick, B. N. (2001). GABAergic neurons in prepositus hypoglossi regulate REM sleep by its action on locus coeruleus in freely moving rats. *Synapse* **42**, 141–50.

Kayama, Y., Ohta, M. & Jodo, E. (1992). Firing of 'possibly' cholinergic neurons in the rat laterodorsal tegmental nucleus during sleep and wakefulness. *Brain Res.* **569**, 210–20.

Kodama, T., Lai, Y. Y. & Siegel, J. M. (1998). Enhanced glutamate release during REM sleep in the rostromedial medulla as measured by in vivo microdialysis. *Brain Res.* **780**, 178–81.

Kodama, T., Lai, Y. Y. & Siegel, J. M. (2003). Changes in inhibitory amino acid release linked to pontine-induced atonia: an in vivo microdialysis study. *J. Neurosci.* **23**, 1548–54.

Kohlmeier, K. A., Lopez-Rodriguez, F., Liu, R. H., Morales, F. R. & Chase, M. H. (1996). State-dependent phenomena in cat masseter motoneurons. *Brain Res.* **722**, 30–8.

Koyama, Y. & Kayama, Y. (1993). Mutual interactions among cholinergic, noradrenergic and serotonergic neurons studied by ionophoresis of these transmitters in rat brainstem nuclei. *Neuroscience* **55**, 1117–26.

Koyama, Y., Takahashi, K., Kodama, T. & Kayama, Y. (2003). State-dependent activity of neurons in the perifornical hypothalamic area during sleep and waking. *Neuroscience* **119**, 1209–19.

Lai, Y. Y. & Siegel, J. M. (1990). Cardiovascular and muscle tone changes produced by microinjection of cholinergic and glutamatergic agonists in dorsolateral pons and medial medulla. *Brain Res.* **514**, 27–36.

Lai, Y. Y. & Siegel, J. M. (1991). Pontomedullary glutamate receptors mediating locomotion and muscle tone suppression. *J. Neurosci.* **11**, 2931–7.

Lee, M. G., Hassani, O. K. & Jones, B. E. (2005). Discharge of identified orexin/hypocretin neurons across the sleep-waking cycle. *J. Neurosci.* **25**, 6716–20.

Levine, E. S. & Jacobs, B. L. (1992). Neurochemical afferents controlling the activity of serotonergic neurons in the dorsal raphe nucleus: microiontophoretic studies in the awake cat. *J. Neurosci.* **12**, 4037–44.

Li, Y. Q., Takada, M., Kaneko, T. & Mizuno, N. (1996). GABAergic and glycinergic neurons projecting to the trigeminal motor nucleus: a double labeling study in the rat. *J. Comp. Neurol.* **373**, 498–510.

Lin, J. S., Sakai, K., Vanni-Mercier, G. & Jouvet, M. (1989). A critical role of the posterior hypothalamus in the mechanisms of wakefulness determined by microinjection of muscimol in freely moving cats. *Brain Res.* **479**, 225–40.

Lin, J. S., Roussel, B., Akaoka, H. *et al.* (1992). Role of catecholamines in the modafinil and amphetamine induced wakefulness, a comparative pharmacological study in the cat. *Brain Res.* **591**, 319–26.

Lin, J. S., Hou, Y., Sakai, K. & Jouvet, M. (1996). Histaminergic descending inputs to the mesopontine tegmentum and their role in the control of cortical activation and wakefulness in the cat. *J. Neurosci.* **16**, 1523–37.

Lin, L., Faraco, J., Li, R. *et al.* (1999). The sleep disorder canine narcolepsy is caused by a mutation in the hypocretin (orexin) receptor 2 gene. *Cell* **98**, 365–76.

Liu, R., Jolas, T. & Aghajanian, G. (2000). Serotonin 5-HT(2) receptors activate local GABA inhibitory inputs to serotonergic neurons of the dorsal raphe nucleus. *Brain Res.* **873**, 34–45.

Liu, R. J., Van Den Pol, A. N. & Aghajanian, G. K. (2002). Hypocretins (orexins) regulate serotonin neurons in the dorsal raphe nucleus by excitatory direct and inhibitory indirect actions. *J. Neurosci.* **22**, 9453–64.

Lu, J., Bjorkum, A. A., Xu, M. *et al.* (2002). Selective activation of the extended ventrolateral preoptic nucleus during rapid eye movement sleep. *J. Neurosci.* **22**, 4568–76.

Luppi, P. H., Sakai, K., Fort, P., Salvert, D. & Jouvet, M. (1988). The nuclei of origin of monoaminergic, peptidergic, and cholinergic afferents to the cat nucleus reticularis magnocellularis: a double-labeling study with cholera toxin as a retrograde tracer. *J. Comp. Neurol.* **277**, 1–20.

Luppi, P. H., Charlety, P. J., Fort, P. *et al.* (1991). Anatomical and electrophysiological evidence for a glycinergic inhibitory innervation of the rat locus coeruleus. *Neurosci. Lett.* **128**, 33–6.

Luppi, P. H., Gervasoni, D., Peyron, C. *et al.* (1999). Norepinephrine and REM Sleep. In *Rapid Eye Movement Sleep*, ed. B. N. Mallick & S. Inoue. New Delhi: Norosa Publishing House.

Maloney, K. J., Mainville, L. & Jones, B. E. (1999). Differential c-Fos expression in cholinergic, monoaminergic, and GABAergic cell groups of the pontomesencephalic tegmentum after paradoxical sleep deprivation and recovery. *J. Neurosci.* **19**, 3057–72.

Maloney, K. J., Mainville, L. & Jones, B. E. (2000). c-Fos expression in GABAergic, serotonergic, and other neurons of the pontomedullary reticular formation and raphe after paradoxical sleep deprivation and recovery. *J. Neurosci.* **20**, 4669–79.

Maquet, P., Peters, J., Aerts, J. *et al.* (1996). Functional neuroanatomy of human rapid-eye-movement sleep and dreaming. *Nature* **383**, 163–6.

Marcus, J. N., Aschkenasi, C. J., Lee, C. E. *et al.* (2001). Differential expression of orexin receptors 1 and 2 in the rat brain. *J. Comp. Neurol.* **435**, 6–25.

McCarley, R. W. & Hobson, J. A. (1975). Neuronal excitability modulation over the sleep cycle: a structural and mathematical model. *Science* **189**, 58–60.

McGinty, D. J. & Harper, R. M. (1976). Dorsal raphe neurons: depression of firing during sleep in cats. *Brain Res.* **101**, 569–75.

Mileykovskiy, B. Y., Kiyashchenko, L. I. & Siegel, J. M. (2005). Behavioral correlates of activity in identified hypocretin/orexin neurons. *Neuron* **46**, 787–98.

Morales, F. R., Sampogna, S., Yamuy, J. & Chase, M. H. (1999). c-fos expression in brainstem premotor interneurons during cholinergically induced active sleep in the cat. *J. Neurosci.* **19**, 9508–18.

Nakamura, T., Uramura, K., Nambu, T. *et al.* (2000). Orexin-induced hyperlocomotion and stereotypy are mediated by the dopaminergic system. *Brain Res.* **873**, 181–7.

Nauta, W. J. (1946). Hypothalamic regulation of sleep in rats. Experimental Study. *J. Neurophysiol.* **9**, 285–316.

Nitz, D. & Siegel, J. (1997a). GABA release in the dorsal raphe nucleus: role in the control of REM sleep. *Am. J. Physiol.* **273**, R451–5.

Nitz, D. & Siegel, J. M. (1997b). GABA release in the locus coeruleus as a function of sleep/wake state. *Neuroscience* **78**, 795–801.

Onoe, H. & Sakai, K. (1995). Kainate receptors: a novel mechanism in paradoxical (REM) sleep generation. *Neuroreport* **6**, 353–6.

Paxinos, G. & Watson, C. (1997). *The Rat Brain in Stereotaxic Coordinates*. Orlando, FL: Academic Press.

Peyron, C., Tighe, D. K., Van Den Pol, A. N. *et al.* (1998). Neurons containing hypocretin (orexin) project to multiple neuronal systems. *J. Neurosci.* **18**, 9996–10 015.

Peyron, C., Faraco, J., Rogers, W. *et al.* (2000). A mutation in a case of early onset narcolepsy and a generalized absence of hypocretin peptides in human narcoleptic brains. *Nat. Med.* **6**, 991–7.

Pollock, M. S. & Mistlberger, R. E. (2003). Rapid eye movement sleep induction by microinjection of the GABA-A antagonist bicuculline into the dorsal subcoeruleus area of the rat. *Brain Res.* **962**, 68–77.

Rampon, C., Luppi, P. H., Fort, P., Peyron, C. & Jouvet, M. (1996a). Distribution of glycine-immunoreactive cell bodies and fibers in the rat brain. *Neuroscience* **75**, 737–55.

Rampon, C., Peyron, C., Petit, J. M. *et al.* (1996b). Origin of the glycinergic innervation of the rat trigeminal motor nucleus. *Neuroreport* **7**, 3081–5.

Ranson, S. W. (1939). Somnolence caused by hypothalamic lesions in the monkey. *Arch. Neurol. Psychiatr.* **41**, 1–23.

Sakai, K. (1985). Neurons responsible for paradoxical sleep. In *Sleep: Neurotransmitters and Neuromodulators*, ed. A. Wauquier and Janssen Research Foundation. New York: Raven Press.

Sakai, K. & Crochet, S. (2000). Serotonergic dorsal raphe neurons cease firing by disfacilitation during paradoxical sleep. *Neuroreport* **11**, 3237–41.

Sakai, K. & Koyama, Y. (1996). Are there cholinergic and non-cholinergic paradoxical sleep-on neurones in the pons? *Neuroreport* **7**, 2449–53.

Sakai, K., Kanamori, N. & Jouvet, M. (1979a). [Neuronal activity specific to paradoxical sleep in the bulbar reticular formation in the unrestrained cat.] *C. R. Seanc. Acad. Sci.* D **289**, 557–61.

Sakai, K., Sastre, J. P., Salvert, D. *et al.* (1979b). Tegmentoreticular projections with special reference to the muscular atonia during paradoxical sleep in the cat: an HRP study. *Brain Res.* **176**, 233–54.

Sakai, K., Sastre, J. P., Kanamori, N. & Jouvet, M. (1981). State-specific neurones in the ponto-medullary reticular formation with special reference to the postural atonia during paradoxical sleep in the cat. In *Brain Mechanisms of Perceptual Awareness and Purposeful Behavior*, ed. O. Pompeiano & C. Aimone Marsan. New York, NY: Raven Press.

Sakai, K., Crochet, S. & Onoe, H. (2001). Pontine structures and mechanisms involved in the generation of paradoxical (REM) sleep. *Arch. Ital. Biol.* **139**, 93–107.

Sakurai, T., Amemiya, A., Ishii, M. *et al.* (1998). Orexins and orexin receptors: a family of hypothalamic neuropeptides and G protein-coupled receptors that regulate feeding behavior. *Cell* **92**, 573–85.

Sallanon, M., Sakai, K., Buda, C., Puymartin, M. & Jouvet, M. (1988). Increase of paradoxical sleep induced by microinjections of ibotenic acid into the ventrolateral part of the posterior hypothalamus in the cat. *Arch. Ital. Biol.* **126**, 87–97.

Sallanon, M., Denoyer, M., Kitahama, K. *et al.* (1989). Long-lasting insomnia induced by preoptic neuron lesions and its transient reversal by muscimol injection into the posterior hypothalamus in the cat. *Neuroscience* **32**, 669–83.

Sanford, L. D., Tang, X., Xiao, J., Ross, R. J. & Morrison, A. R. (2003). GABAergic regulation of REM sleep in reticularis pontis oralis and caudalis in rats. *J. Neurophysiol.* **90**, 938–45.

Sastre, J. P., Sakai, K. & Jouvet, M. (1981). Are the gigantocellular tegmental field neurons responsible for paradoxical sleep? *Brain Res.* **229**, 147–61.

Sastre, J. P., Buda, C., Kitahama, K. & Jouvet, M. (1996). Importance of the ventrolateral region of the periaqueductal gray and adjacent tegmentum in the control of paradoxical sleep as studied by muscimol microinjections in the cat. *Neuroscience* **74**, 415–26.

Sastre, J. P., Buda, C., Lin, J. S. & Jouvet, M. (2000). Differential c-fos expression in the rhinencephalon and striatum after enhanced sleep-wake states in the cat. *Eur. J. Neurosci.* **12**, 1397–410.

Shiromani, P. J. & Fishbein, W. (1986). Continuous pontine cholinergic microinfusion via mini-pump induces sustained alterations in rapid eye movement (REM) sleep. *Pharmacol. Biochem. Behav.* **25**, 1253–61.

Siegel, J. M., Wheeler, R. L. & McGinty, D. J. (1979). Activity of medullary reticular formation neurons in the unrestrained cat during waking and sleep. *Brain Res.* **179**, 49–60.

Soja, P. J., Lopez-Rodriguez, F., Morales, F. R. & Chase, M. H. (1991). The postsynaptic inhibitory control of lumbar motoneurons during the atonia of active sleep: effect of strychnine on motoneuron properties. *J. Neurosci.* **11**, 2804–11.

Steininger, T. L., Alam, M. N., Gong, H., Szymusiak, R. & McGinty, D. (1999). Sleep-waking discharge of neurons in the posterior lateral hypothalamus of the albino rat. *Brain Res.* **840**, 138–47.

Swanson, L. W. (1998). *Brain Maps: Structure of the Rat Brain: a Laboratory Guide with Printed and Electronic Templates for Data, Models, and Schematics*. New York, NY: Elsevier.

Swett, C. P. & Hobson, J. A. (1968). The effects of posterior hypothalamic lesions on behavioral and electrographic manifestations of sleep and waking in cats. *Arch. Ital. Biol.* **106**, 283–93.

Taguchi, O., Kubin, L. & Pack, A. I. (1992). Evocation of postural atonia and respiratory depression by pontine carbachol in the decerebrate rat. *Brain Res.* **595**, 107–15.

Tononi, G., Pompeiano, M. & Cirelli, C. (1991). Suppression of desynchronized sleep through microinjection of the alpha 2-adrenergic agonist clonidine in the dorsal pontine tegmentum of the cat. *Pflugers Arch.* **418**, 512–18.

Torterolo, P., Yamuy, J., Sampogna, S., Morales, F. R. & Chase, M. H. (2003). Hypocretinergic neurons are primarily involved in activation of the somatomotor system. *Sleep* **26**, 25–8.

Trivedi, P., Yu, H., Macneil, D. J., Van Der Ploeg, L. H. & Guan, X. M. (1998). Distribution of orexin receptor mRNA in the rat brain. *FEBS Lett.* **438**, 71–5.

van den Pol, A. N. (1999). Hypothalamic hypocretin (orexin): robust innervation of the spinal cord. *J. Neurosci.* **19**, 3171–82.

Vanni-Mercier, G., Sakai, K. & Jouvet, M. (1984). [Specific neurons for wakefulness in the posterior hypothalamus in the cat.] *C. R. Acad. Sci. III*, **298**, 195–200.

Vanni-Mercier, G., Sakai, K., Lin, J. S. & Jouvet, M. (1989). Mapping of cholinoceptive brainstem structures responsible for the generation of paradoxical sleep in the cat. *Arch. Ital. Biol.* **127**, 133–64.

Velazquez-Moctezuma, J., Gillin, J. C. & Shiromani, P. J. (1989). Effect of specific M1, M2 muscarinic receptor agonists on REM sleep generation. *Brain Res.* **503**, 128–31.

Verret, L., Goutagny, R., Fort, P. *et al.* (2003). A role of melanin-concentrating hormone producing neurons in the central regulation of paradoxical sleep. *BMC Neurosci.* **4**, 19.

Verret, L., Leger, L., Fort, P. & Luppi, P. H. (2005). Cholinergic and noncholinergic brainstem neurons expressing Fos after paradoxical (REM) sleep deprivation and recovery. *Eur. J. Neurosci.* **21**, 2488–504.

Verret, L., Fort, P., Gervasoni, D., Leger, L. & Luppi, P. H. (2006). Localization of the neurons active during paradoxical (REM) sleep and projecting to the locus coeruleus noradrenergic neurons in the rat. *J. Comp. Neurol.* **495**, 573–86.

Von Economo, C. (1926). *Die Pathologie des Schlafes. Handbuch des Normalen und Pathologischen Physiologie*. Berlin: A. Von Bethe, G. V. Bergman, G. Embden, U. A. Ellinger (Eds).

Webster, H. H. & Jones, B. E. (1988). Neurotoxic lesions of the dorsolateral pontomesencephalic tegmentum-cholinergic cell area in the cat. II. Effects upon sleep-waking states. *Brain Res.* **458**, 285–302.

Woch, G., Davies, R. O., Pack, A. I. & Kubin, L. (1996). Behaviour of raphe cells projecting to the dorsomedial medulla during carbachol-induced atonia in the cat. *J. Physiol.* **490**(3), 745–58.

Xi, M. C., Morales, F. R. & Chase, M. H. (1999). Evidence that wakefulness and REM sleep are controlled by a GABAergic pontine mechanism. *J. Neurophysiol.* **82**, 2015–19.

Xi, M. C., Morales, F. R. & Chase, M. H. (2001). The motor inhibitory system operating during active sleep is tonically suppressed by GABAergic mechanisms during other states. *J. Neurophysiol.* **86**, 1908–15.

Xi, M. C., Morales, F. R. & Chase, M. H. (2004). Interactions between GABAergic and cholinergic processes in the nucleus pontis oralis: neuronal mechanisms controlling active (rapid eye movement) sleep and wakefulness. *J. Neurosci.* **24**, 10670–8.

Yamamoto, K., Mamelak, A. N., Quattrochi, J. J. & Hobson, J. A. (1990). A cholinoceptive desynchronized sleep induction zone in the anterodorsal pontine tegmentum: locus of the sensitive region. *Neuroscience* **39**, 279–93.

Yamanaka, A., Tsujino, N., Funahashi, H. *et al.* (2002). Orexins activate histaminergic neurons via the orexin 2 receptor. *Biochem. Biophys. Res. Commun.* **290**, 1237–45.

Yamuy, J., Sampogna, S., Lopez-Rodriguez, F. *et al.* (1995). Fos and serotonin immunoreactivity in the raphe nuclei of the cat during carbachol-induced active sleep: a double-labeling study. *Neuroscience* **67**, 211–23.

Yamuy, J., Fung, S. J., Xi, M., Morales, F. R. & Chase, M. H. (1999). Hypoglossal motoneurons are postsynaptically inhibited during carbachol-induced rapid eye movement sleep. *Neuroscience* **94**, 11–15.

Yoshida, Y., Fujiki, N., Nakajima, T. *et al.* (2001). Fluctuation of extracellular hypocretin-1 (orexin A) levels in the rat in relation to the light-dark cycle and sleep-wake activities. *Eur. J. Neurosci.* **14**, 1075–81.

Zeitzer, J. M., Buckmaster, C. L., Parker, K. J. *et al.* (2003). Circadian and homeostatic regulation of hypocretin in a primate model: implications for the consolidation of wakefulness. *J. Neurosci.* **23**, 3555–60.

5

Acetylcholine modulates sleep and wakefulness: a synaptic perspective

RALPH LYDIC AND HELEN A. BAGHDOYAN

Seventy years ago Otto Loewi and Henry Dale shared the 1936 Nobel Prize for the discovery that acetylcholine (ACh) is a neurotransmitter. Loewi's Nobel Lecture provided the following historical context for their discovery (Loewi, 1936): "Up until the year 1921 it was not known how the stimulation of a nerve influenced the effector organ's function, in other words, in what way the stimulation was transmitted to the effector organ from the nerve-ending." The significance of Loewi's and Dale's discovery is emphasized by the profound relevance of ACh for sensorimotor, autonomic, and arousal state control. At all neuromuscular junctions ACh is the transmitter. For the autonomic nervous system, all preganglionic sympathetic and parasympathetic nerves use ACh, as do postganglionic fibers of the parasympathetic nervous system. In the context of the present volume, the effector organ of sleep is the brain. Therefore, this chapter focuses on the role of cholinergic "nerve endings" through which "the effector organ" generates states of sleep and wakefulness. This chapter uses Loewi's synaptic perspective to review data from many laboratories demonstrating that cholinergic synaptic mechanisms (Fig. 5.1) regulate levels of arousal.

Blocking degradation of ACh activates the EEG and enhances REM sleep

The discovery of rapid eye movement (REM) sleep (Aserinsky & Kleitman, 1953) as a state of enhanced electroencephalographic (EEG) activity implied

Neurochemistry of Sleep and Wakefulness, ed. J. M. Monti *et al.* Published by Cambridge University Press. © Cambridge University Press 2008.

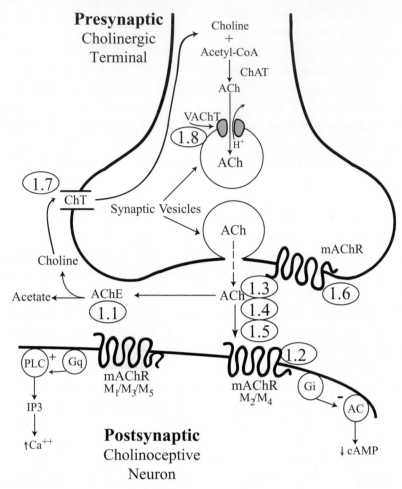

Figure 5.1 Schematic model of a cholinergic synapse in the brain. The presynaptic terminal is drawn at the top. Cholinergic neurons are phenotypically defined by the ACh-synthetic enzyme choline acetyltransferase (ChAT) and by the presynaptic vesicular ACh transporter (VAChT) where ACh is packaged into synaptic vesicles. These cholinergic vesicles fuse with the presynaptic membrane and release ACh into the synaptic cleft. In some brain regions, there is evidence that cholinergic presynaptic terminals contain muscarinic cholinergic receptors (mAChR) that function as autoreceptors to modulate the release of ACh. Within the synaptic cleft the enzyme acetylcholinesterase (AChE) rapidly degrades ACh to choline and acetate. The presynaptic terminal can also contain a choline transporter (ChT) that is involved in the reuptake of choline. The bottom half of the drawing illustrates the membrane of a postsynaptic neuron containing postsynaptic muscarinic receptors (mAChR), which exist as five subtypes (M_1–M_5). Numbers 1.1–1.8 are amplified in the text to show that manipulating VAChT, ChT, ACh, presynaptic muscarinic receptors, postsynaptic muscarinic receptors, and AChE significantly alters REM sleep.

the existence of endogenous neurochemical mechanisms underlying rhythmic oscillations in brain excitability. This newly documented sleep state was shown to have broad biological significance by the discovery that cats also exhibited REM sleep characterized by an activated EEG (Dement, 1958). Only a year earlier, Italian investigators had reported that electrical excitability of rabbit brain was significantly increased by the acetylcholinesterase inhibitor eserine (physostigmine) (Longo & Silvestrini, 1957). This finding hinted that ACh might be one of the endogenous brain molecules contributing to REM sleep generation. During the early 1960s preclinical studies from multiple laboratories provided direct support for the view that ACh contributes to REM sleep generation (Jouvet, 1962; Cordeau et al., 1963; Hernández-Peón et al., 1963; George et al., 1964; Baxter, 1969). Support for the role of ACh as an endogenous molecule involved in REM sleep generation was strong enough by the 1970s to prompt the development of formal hypotheses (Karczmar et al., 1970; Jouvet, 1972) involving synaptic and mathematical models of sleep cycle control (Hobson et al., 1975; McCarley & Hobson, 1975).

The now accepted view that brain ACh plays a major role in regulating states of sleep and wakefulness was particularly promoted by the excellent agreement between human and non-human data. These studies hypothesized that if ACh contributes to the generation of REM sleep, then administering drugs known to block the breakdown of ACh should trigger or increase REM sleep. An anticipated effect of blocking the enzymatic degradation of ACh (1.1 on Fig. 5.1) is to increase the synaptic concentration of endogenous ACh. Intravenous administration of the acetylcholinesterase inhibitor physostigmine increased REM sleep in cat (Domino et al., 1968). In humans, intravenous injection of cholinergic agonists or acetylcholine esterase inhibitors shortened latency to onset and increased duration of REM sleep (Sitaram et al., 1976, 1978). Therefore, the finding that REM sleep in human and cat is significantly increased by systemic administration of the acetylcholine esterase inhibitor physostigmine provides compelling support for the view that endogenously released ACh contributes to REM sleep generation. In light of the fact that brain function is localized to specific brain regions (Haymaker, 1953), the finding that REM sleep is increased by systemic physostigmine raised a key question: in which brain regions is ACh critically important for causing REM sleep? Emphasis on the pontine brain stem as a major substrate for REM sleep generation came from experiments showing the loss of normal REM sleep signs following surgical transections that separated the pons from more rostral brain regions (Jouvet, 1962, 1972).

Pontine cholinergic agonists and acetylcholine esterase inhibitors enhance REM sleep

If ACh contributes to REM sleep generation via brain regions known to be essential for normal generation of REM sleep, then administering cholinomimetics into these same brain regions should increase REM sleep (Fig. 5.2). Many laboratories have shown that administering cholinergic agonists (such as carbachol or bethanechol) or ACh-esterase inhibitors (such as neostigmine) into the pontine reticular formation of cat and rat causes a REM sleep-like state (Mitler & Dement, 1974; Baghdoyan et al., 1984a,b 1987, 1989; Gnadt & Pegram, 1986; Shiromani & Fishbein, 1986; Vanni-Mercier et al., 1989; Hobson et al., 1993; Imeri et al., 1994; Bourgin et al., 1995; Datta, 1995; Lee et al., 1995; Tononi & Pompeiano, 1996; Garzon et al., 1997; Marks & Birabil, 1998; Baghdoyan & Lydic, 1999; Capece et al., 1999; Kubin, 2001; Kumar & Raju, 2001; Reinoso-Suárez et al., 2001; Mavanji & Datta, 2003; Wetzel et al., 2003). Figure 5.2 illustrates the finding that microinjecting the acetylcholine esterase inhibitor neostigmine into the medial pontine reticular formation of intact, unanesthetized cat causes a state that behaviorally and electrographically mimics REM sleep.

In cat and rat, the cholinergically evoked REM sleep-like state was shown to be anatomically site-dependent (Baghdoyan et al., 1984b, 1987; Gnadt & Pegram, 1986; Vanni-Mercier et al., 1989; Yamamoto et al., 1990; Bourgin et al., 1995; Reinoso-Suárez et al., 2001). Studies of cat have localized the most effective sites to rostral portions of the medial pontine reticular formation. In rat, the cholinergically evoked REM sleep-like state is most effectively produced by microinjecting carbachol into the caudal region of the oral pontine reticular nucleus (Bourgin et al., 1995). Microinjections of carbachol into the rostral region of the oral pontine reticular nucleus or into the caudal pontine reticular nucleus were ineffective for evoking the REM sleep-like state (Bourgin et al., 1995). Some investigators have taken issue with the finding that although pontine carbachol in rat causes a statistically significant increase in REM sleep of about 50%, this increase is much less than the 300% increase in REM sleep caused by pontine administration of carbachol in cat (Baghdoyan & Lydic, 1999; Reinoso-Suárez et al., 2001). The mechanisms underlying these species-specific differences remain unclear. It is known, however, that the neural networks generating physiological traits characteristic of REM sleep can be cholinergically activated even in anesthetized rat (Horner & Kubin, 1999) and cat (Xi et al., 1997).

The most recent species to be studied with respect to cholinergic REM sleep enhancement is mouse (Lydic et al., 2002). Microinjection of neostigmine into the pontine reticular formation of C57BL/6J (B6) mouse has now been shown to cause a REM sleep-like state (Fig. 5.3). REM sleep also can be enhanced in B6.v-lep[ob]

A.

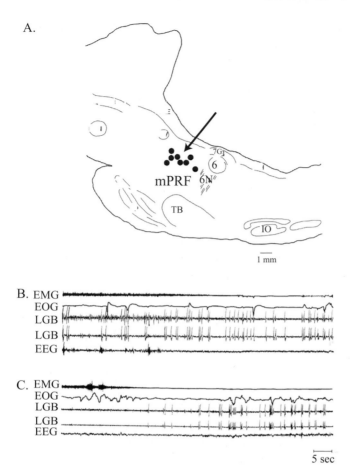

B. EMG
   EOG
   LGB
   LGB
   EEG

C. EMG
   EOG
   LGB
   LGB
   EEG

5 sec

Figure 5.2 REM sleep is enhanced by preventing the degradation of ACh in a restricted region of the medial pontine reticular formation (mPRF). Sagittal view of the cat brain stem (A) with rostral to the left. The black circles (arrow) show locations where microinjecting the acetylcholinesterase inhibitor neostigmine caused a behavioral state and electrographic events (C) that mimic the electrographic characteristics of spontaneous REM sleep (B). Note that microinjecting neostigmine into the mPRF of awake cat caused the onset of skeletal muscle atonia recorded from the neck electromyogram (EMG), rapid eye movements in the electro-oculogram (EOG), large amplitude field potentials called ponto-geniculo-occipital waves recorded bilaterally from the lateral geniculate bodies (LGB), and activation of the cortical electroencephalogram (EEG). (A) from Baghdoyan *et al.* (1984a): (B, C) from Baghdoyan *et al.*, 1987.

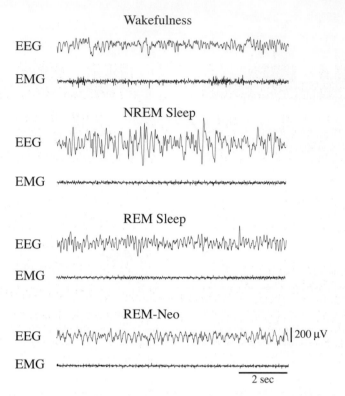

Figure 5.3 Ten-second electroencephalogram (EEG) and neck muscle electromyogram (EMG) recordings from one C57BL/6J mouse show cortical electrographic features during states of wakefulness, NREM sleep, REM sleep, and the neostigmine-induced REM-sleep-like state (REM-Neo). The bottom row of EEG and EMG recordings were obtained during REM-Neo caused by delivering neostigmine (133 ng/50 nl) into the pontine reticular formation. Microinjection of neostigmine caused mice to display the electrographic traits of EEG activation and EMG hypotonia. From Douglas *et al.* (2005).

(ob/ob) mouse by pontine reticular formation microinjection of neostigmine (Fig. 5.4) (Douglas *et al.*, 2005). Systematic mapping studies of the most effective sites for cholinergic REM sleep enhancement in mouse have not yet been published. REM sleep enhancement caused by microinjecting neostigmine into the mouse pontine reticular formation (Lydic *et al.*, 2002; Coleman *et al.*, 2004; Douglas *et al.*, 2005), however, is consistent with data from human, cat, and rat. The finding that microinjection of neostigmine into mouse pontine reticular formation enhances REM sleep is supported by data showing that systemic exposure to sublethal levels of organophosphates, such as the irreversible acetylcholinesterase inhibitor soman, increases REM sleep in mice (Crouzier

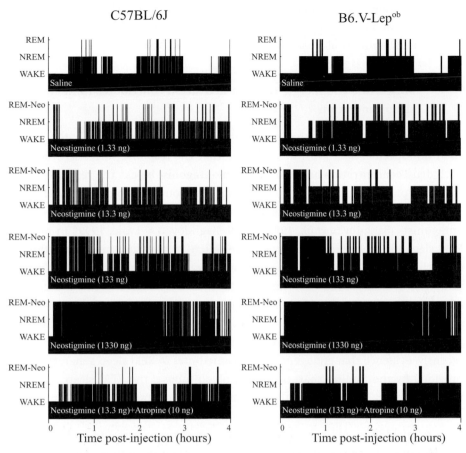

Figure 5.4 Representative time course of sleep and wakefulness recorded from a C57BL/6J mouse (left column) and an obese mouse (B6.V-Lep^ob, right column) for four hours following microinjection of neostigmine into the pontine reticular formation. These figures demonstrate the REM sleep enhancement caused by microinjecting increasing concentrations of neostigmine. The bottom two plots further illustrate that the neostigmine-induced REM-sleep-like state (REM-Neo) was blocked by co-administration of the muscarinic receptor antagonist atropine. Note the similarity in the distribution of sleep and wakefulness following microinjection of atropine (bottom two plots) and microinjection of saline (top two plots). From Douglas *et al.* (2005).

et al., 2004). Thus cholinergic enhancement of REM sleep in mouse (Lydic *et al.*, 2002; Coleman *et al.*, 2004; Douglas *et al.*, 2005) faithfully models spontaneous REM sleep (Crouzier *et al.*, 2004). It should also be clear that the enhancement of REM sleep in mouse caused by central (Lydic *et al.*, 2002; Coleman *et al.*, 2004; Douglas *et al.*, 2005) and systemic (Crouzier *et al.*, 2004) administration of acetylcholinesterase inhibitors directly parallels the REM sleep enhancement in cat and human caused by systemic administration of acetylcholinesterase inhibitors (Domino et al., 1968; Sitaram et al., 1976, 1978).

Muscarinic cholinergic receptor activation contributes to REM sleep generation

In order to assert that any drug response is receptor-mediated rather than non-specific, data must demonstrate that the response varies significantly with drug concentration and show that an antagonist blocks the response. Data from cat provided the first demonstration that pontine cholinergic REM sleep enhancement is concentration-dependent and blocked by muscarinic receptor antagonists (Baghdoyan et al., 1984a, 1989; Baghdoyan & Lydic, 1999). In rat, the REM sleep-like state produced by pontine reticular formation microinjection of carbachol (Gnadt & Pegram, 1986) is concentration-dependent and blocked by atropine, demonstrating that the state is caused by activation of muscarinic receptors (Bourgin et al., 1995). These findings are consistent with studies in rat showing that natural REM sleep is mediated by muscarinic receptors in the oral pontine reticular nucleus (Shiromani & Fishbein, 1986; Imeri et al., 1994). Most recently, evidence that endogenous ACh contributes to REM sleep generation was provided by the finding that, in B6 and ob/ob mouse, the REM sleep enhancement caused by pontine reticular formation administration of neostigmine is concentration-dependent and blocked by atropine (Fig. 5.4).

Agreement that muscarinic cholinergic receptors contribute to REM sleep generation encouraged studies aiming to clarify the role of muscarinic receptor subtypes. Molecular cloning studies have identified five subtypes of muscarinic receptors (Buckley, 1990; Jones et al., 1992). Muscarinic receptor subtypes also can be distinguished pharmacologically on the basis of differential antagonist binding affinities (Hulme et al., 1990; Caulfield, 1993). As emphasized previously (Baghdoyan & Lydic, 1999) there are no truly subtype-selective muscarinic receptor antagonists, because no single antagonist shows both high affinity for one cloned subtype and low affinity for the other four molecularly identified subtypes. In vivo studies aiming to define the role of muscarinic receptor subtypes must also contend with a lack of subtype-selective muscarinic receptor agonists (Caulfield & Birdsall, 1998). Despite this limitation, use of competition binding assays has made it possible to obtain in vitro autoradiographic data (Fig. 5.5) showing that the M2 muscarinic receptor is the predominant subtype in the medial pontine reticular formation of cat (Baghdoyan et al., 1994) and the homologous oral pontine reticular nucleus of rat (Baghdoyan, 1997). These findings are consistent with in vivo microinjection data in cat (Velazquez-Moctezuma et al., 1990b; Baghdoyan & Lydic, 1999) and rat (Imeri et al., 1994) showing that the

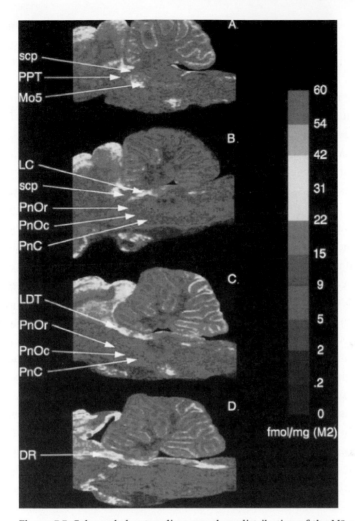

Figure 5.5 Color-coded autoradiograms show distribution of the M2 muscarinic receptor subtype in sagittal views of rat brain stem. M2 binding was quantified as fmol/mg tissue equivalent. Color bar at right indicates higher (red) to lower (purple) M2 binding. Images labeled (A)–(D) show a section every 0.5 mm and progress from lateral (A, approximately 1.9 mm from the midline) to medial (D, approximately 0.4 mm from the midline), according to a rat brain atlas (Paxinos & Watson, 1998). Abbreviations: PPT, pedunculopontine tegmental nucleus; Mo5, motor trigeminal nucleus; scp, superior cerebellar peduncle; LC, locus coeruleus; PnOr, rostral portion of the oral pontine reticular nucleus (PnO); PnOc, caudal portion of the PnO; PnC, caudal pontine reticular nucleus; LDT, laterodorsal tegmental nucleus; DR, dorsal raphe nucleus. From Baghdoyan (1997). (See also Plate 3.)

M2 subtype modulates the amount of REM sleep. If postsynaptic muscarinic receptors of the M2 subtype contribute to REM sleep generation, then pharmacological manipulation of M2-activated signal transduction cascades would be anticipated to alter REM sleep (1.2 on Fig. 5.1).

Muscarinic receptors are coupled to guanine nucleotide binding (G) proteins. M2 and M4 muscarinic receptor subtypes are linked to inhibitory G proteins (Gi), which decrease adenylate cyclase, leading to a decrease in cAMP. Pertussis toxin catalyzes the ADP-ribosylation of the α-subunit of Gi proteins (Carty, 1994), and thereby inhibits intracellular signaling mechanisms normally caused by activating Gi proteins. Pertussis toxin prevents coupling between M2/M4 receptors and Gi proteins. Injecting pertussis toxin directly into medial regions of the pontine reticular formation blocks cholinergic REM sleep enhancement in cat (Shuman et al., 1995) and B6 mouse (Coleman et al., 2004a). These data support the interpretation that agonist activation of M2 and/or M4 muscarinic receptors increases REM sleep, increases inhibition of adenylate cyclase by Gi, and decreases cAMP (1.2 on Fig. 5.1). Injecting molecules that stimulate adenylate cyclase, cAMP, or protein kinase-A into the pontine reticular formation of cat significantly decreases cholinergic enhancement of REM sleep (Capece & Lydic, 1997). Consistent results were obtained from experiments in which REM sleep was increased by administering inhibitors of adenylate cyclase to homologous regions of rat pontine reticular formation (Marks & Birabil, 2000). As reviewed below, ACh in medial regions of the pontine reticular formation originates from cholinergic neurons in the laterodorsal and pedunculopontine tegmental nuclei. In freely moving rat, pedunculopontine tegmental neurons discharge during the brain-activated states of wakefulness and REM sleep (Datta & Siwek, 2002). Administering an inhibitor of adenylate cyclase into the pedunculopontine tegmental nuclei of rat decreased REM sleep (Datta & Prutzman, 2005).

M1, M3, and M5 muscarinic receptors likely also contribute to the neurochemical modulation of sleep, and the foregoing results do not imply sleep regulation by only M2 and/or M4 subtypes. REM sleep is disrupted by pharmacological blockade of M3 muscarinic receptors in the perilocus coeruleus region of cat pons, suggesting a role for the M3 subtype in REM sleep regulation (Sakai & Onoe, 1997). Activation of M1, M3, or M5 receptors stimulates phospholipase C (PLC) via Gq protein(s). PLC cleaves phosphatidylinositol-4,5-bisphosphate (PIP2) into membrane-bound diacylglycerol (DAG) and inositol triphosphate (IP3), which leads to release of intracellular Ca^{2+} stores and activation of protein kinase C (PKC). Both the cAMP and PKC signal transduction pathways alter protein phosphorylation and neuronal responses. Thus, all muscarinic receptor subtypes are coupled to signal transduction cascades that enable cholinergic neurotransmission to alter cell excitability and, ultimately, states of sleep and wakefulness.

ACh release in the pontine reticular formation is maximal during REM sleep

The finding that cholinergic agonists and acetylcholinesterase inhibitors enhance REM sleep, and that muscarinic cholinergic antagonists inhibit REM sleep, supports the view that endogenous ACh contributes to REM sleep generation. Although logical and remarkably consistent across species, from a neurochemical perspective these findings are indirect. If the endogenous molecule ACh contributes to REM sleep generation, then ACh should increase during REM sleep in brain regions where injecting cholinomimetics enhances REM sleep (1.3 on Fig. 5.1).

ACh content of whole brain was reported as early as 1949 to vary as a function of arousal state (Richter & Crossland, 1949). Increasingly deeper states of general anesthesia were shown in the early 1960s to cause a progressive decrease in ACh levels within the cortex (Mitchell, 1963; Krnjevic, 1967). The introduction to this chapter noted that ACh was the first neurotransmitter identified, and ACh was the first neurotransmitter in the cortex to be shown to vary as a function of sleep and wakefulness (Celesia & Jasper, 1966; Jasper & Tessier, 1971). Cortical ACh was collected during states of wakefulness, NREM sleep, and REM sleep by using a cup technique (Jasper & Tessier, 1971). Levels of cortical ACh during REM sleep were not significantly different from ACh measures during wakefulness, and 45% greater than ACh measures during non-REM sleep (Jasper & Tessier, 1971). These initial findings in cortex were subsequently replicated by using in vivo microdialysis (Marrosu et al., 1995).

ACh measured from cortex, and the fact that cortical activation arises from the reticular formation (Moruzzi & Magoun, 1949), encouraged measurement of ACh in the pontine reticular formation. The results of these studies demonstrated that in the dorsal tegmental field of cat ACh release was significantly increased during REM sleep (Kodama et al., 1990). If the REM-sleep-like state caused by pontine injection of cholinomimetics is similar to spontaneous REM sleep, then ACh release in the medial regions of the pontine reticular formation during the cholinergically evoked state should show a similar REM-state-dependent increase (1.4 on Fig. 5.1). This hypothesis was tested by using intact, unanesthetized cats in which it was possible to record states of sleep and wakefulness while measuring ACh on one side of the medial pontine reticular formation before and after the cholinergic agonist carbachol was microinjected into the contralateral medial pontine reticular formation (Lydic et al., 1991). The results (Fig. 5.6), comparing ACh measures during wakefulness with ACh measures during the cholinergically induced REM-sleep-like state, showed that microinjection of carbachol into the medial pontine reticular formation caused a 75% increase in ACh release (Lydic et al., 1991). Thus, during both spontaneous

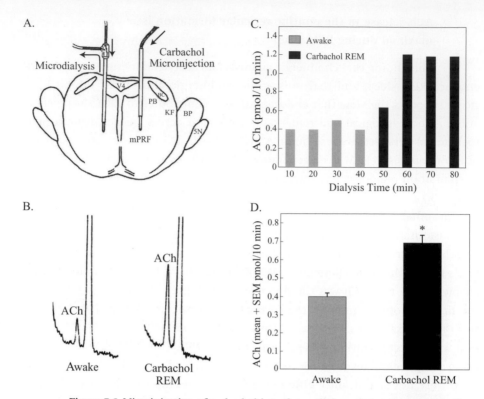

Figure 5.6 Microinjection of carbachol into the medial pontine reticular formation (mPRF) causes a significant increase in ACh release in the contralateral medial pontine reticular formation. (A) A microdialysis probe (left mPRF) and a microinjector (right mPRF) are illustrated at stereotaxic coordinates of posterior (P) = 3.0, lateral (L) = 1.5, and horizontal (H) = −5.0 according to an atlas of the cat brain stem (Berman, 1968). Abbreviations: V4, fourth ventricle; BC, brachium conjunctivum; PB, parabrachial nucleus; KF, Kolliker–Füse nucleus; BP, brachium pontis; 5N, trigeminal nerve. (B) Representative chromatograms used to quantify ACh release as pmol/10 min of dialysis during wakefulness and during the REM-sleep-like state caused by medial pontine reticular formation microinjection of carbachol. (C) The time course of a typical experiment in which ACh level is plotted as a function of arousal state. Each histogram represents the amount of ACh in a 10 min dialysis sample. The carbachol-induced REM-sleep-like state lasted for 40 min. (D) ACh release measured in four cats during 440 min of wakefulness and 440 min of the REM sleep-like state caused by medial pontine reticular formation microinjection of carbachol. Modified from Lydic et al. (1991).

REM sleep (Kodama *et al.*, 1990; Leonard & Lydic, 1995, 1997) and cholinergic REM sleep enhancement (Lydic *et al.*, 1991), ACh release is significantly increased in the same regions of the pontine reticular formation where microinjection of cholinomimetics enhances REM sleep (1.3 and 1.4 on Fig. 5.1). These results support the conclusion that at the level of ACh release, the cholinergic enhancement of REM sleep is a faithful model of spontaneous REM sleep.

Pontine cholinergic neurons are located in the laterodorsal and pedunculopontine tegmental (LDT/PPT) nuclei (Jones & Beaudet, 1987). The presynaptic element schematized by Fig. 5.1 can be visualized as an axon terminal within the medial pontine reticular formation arising from a cholinergic neuron within the LDT/PPT. Figure 5.7 shows LDT/PPT neurons that project to medial regions of the cat pontine reticular formation (Mitani *et al.*, 1988; Shiromani *et al.*, 1988). Applying progressively increasing levels of electrical stimulation to LDT/PPT neurons causes a monotonic increase in ACh release from presynaptic cholinergic terminals (1.5 on Fig. 5.1), demonstrating that LDT/PPT neurons regulate ACh release within the medial pontine reticular formation (Lydic & Baghdoyan, 1993). Subsequent studies emphasize the functional significance of this ACh release by the finding that electrical stimulation of the LDT/PPT causes a significant increase in REM sleep (Thakkar *et al.*, 1996). The findings that LDT/PPT stimulation increases ACh release in the medial pontine reticular formation and increases REM sleep are in good agreement with neuropharmacological data (Fig. 5.2) and with electrophysiological data showing that LDT/PPT neurons begin to discharge just before REM sleep onset and fire maximally throughout REM sleep (El Mansari *et al.*, 1989; Kayama *et al.*, 1992). ACh release in the pontine reticular formation is critical for REM sleep generation, as is clear from the finding that experimental lesions of cholinergic LDT/PPT neurons significantly disrupt REM sleep (Webster & Jones, 1988).

Autoreceptor modulation of ACh release, REM sleep, and EEG excitability

ACh regulates the cortical arousal characteristic of both REM sleep and wakefulness (Semba, 1991, 2000; Sarter & Bruno, 1997, 2000). Medial regions of the pontine reticular formation (Figs. 5.2 and 5.7) contribute to regulating both the state of REM sleep and the trait of EEG activation. Within the medial pontine reticular formation, presynaptic cholinergic terminals (Fig. 5.1) that release ACh also are endowed with muscarinic cholinergic receptors (Roth *et al.*, 1996). Autoreceptors are defined as presynaptic receptors that bind the neurotransmitter that is released from the presynaptic terminal (Kalsner, 1990). Autoreceptors provide feedback modulation of transmitter release. Autoreceptor activation

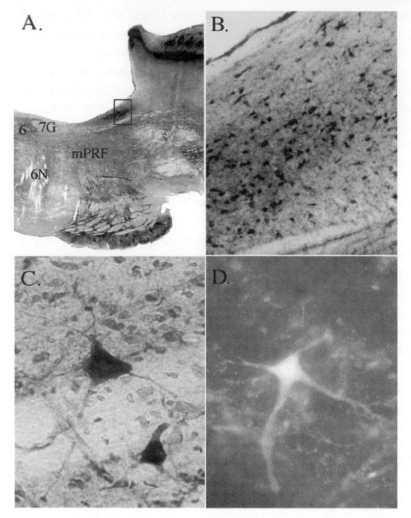

Figure 5.7 Cholinergic and cholinoceptive regions of the pons that contribute to the regulation of sleep and wakefulness. (A) A sagittal view of cat pons with caudal to the left. Abbreviations: 6, abducens nucleus; 7G, the genu of the facial nerve; 6N, the sixth cranial nerve; mPRF, medial pontine reticular formation. The boxed area in (A) includes laterodorsal and pedunculopontine tegmental (LDT/PPT) neurons that synthesize acetylcholine (Jones & Beaudet, 1987). The region of the black box is enlarged in (B) to show cells stained positively for NADPH-diaphorase (black dots). In the LDT/PPT, 100% of the cholinergic neurons stain positively for NADPH-diaphorase (Vincent et al., 1983; Steriade and McCarley, 2005). These LDT/PPT cells project to cholinoceptive cells in the medial pontine reticular formation that contain muscarinic cholinergic receptors. Muscarinic receptors are present in medial regions of the pontine reticular formation of cat (Baghdoyan et al., 1994), rat (Baghdoyan, 1997; Capece et al., 1998), and C57BL/6J mouse (DeMarco et al., 2003). (C) and (D) highlight a cholinergic LDT/PPT neuron (C) that was identified via retrograde fluorescent tracer (D) as projecting to the medial pontine reticular formation. (Modified from Lydic & Baghdoyan, 2005). (See also Plate 4.)

decreases transmitter release and autoreceptor blockade increases transmitter release. Previous sections of this chapter have presented evidence demonstrating cholinergic modulation of REM sleep and EEG excitability. If muscarinic cholinergic autoreceptors in the medial pontine reticular formation (1.6 on Fig. 5.1) are functionally important for cholinergic neurotransmission, then autoreceptor blockade within the medial pontine reticular formation should cause enhanced release of ACh in the medial pontine reticular formation.

Scopolamine is a muscarinic antagonist with equal and high affinity for all five muscarinic cholinergic receptor subtypes. Microdialysis delivery of scopolamine to the cat medial pontine reticular formation causes a concentration-dependent increase in ACh release, demonstrating that ACh release is modulated by muscarinic cholinergic autoreceptors (Roth et al., 1996). The finding that microdialysis delivery of scopolamine to the medial pontine reticular formation significantly increases local ACh release (Fig. 5.8A) encouraged efforts to specify the muscarinic cholinergic receptor subtype functioning as an autoreceptor. Additional dialysis experiments compared the relative potency of different muscarinic receptor antagonists for increasing ACh release in cat pontine reticular formation (Baghdoyan et al., 1998). The antagonists tested, AF-DX 116 and pirenzepine, have different affinity profiles for the different muscarinic receptor subtypes. AF-DX 116 has greater affinity for the M2 and M4 subtypes than for the M1, M3, and M5 subtypes, whereas pirenzepine has equal and high affinity for the M1 and M4 subtypes, and lower affinity for the M2, M3, and M5 subtypes. The demonstration that AF-DX 116 was more potent than pirenzepine for increasing ACh release supported the conclusion that in cat pontine reticular formation, the M2 subtype functions as an autoreceptor to modulate ACh release from LDT/PPT terminals (1.6 on Fig. 5.1).

The functional significance of autoreceptor modulation of ACh release in the medial pontine reticular formation is illustrated by the discovery that muscarinic autoreceptor blockade causes cortical EEG activation (Fig. 5.8B). The brainstem reticular formation has been known for many years to regulate cortical excitability (Moruzzi & Magoun, 1949). Cortical excitation causes the high-frequency, low-amplitude EEG activation characteristic of wakefulness and REM sleep. In contrast, cortical inhibition is characterized by high-amplitude, low-frequency (8–14 Hz) spindles. The EEG spindles of NREM sleep are similar to the inactivated EEG observed during general anesthesia caused by halothane (Keifer et al., 1994). The discovery (Fig. 5.8B) that dialysis delivery of scopolamine to the medial pontine reticular formation of anesthetized cat causes a concentration-dependent activation of the cortical EEG indicates that muscarinic autoreceptors in the medial pontine reticular formation form one synaptic mechanism contributing to arousal. As illustrated in Fig. 5.1, because ACh release in the medial

A.

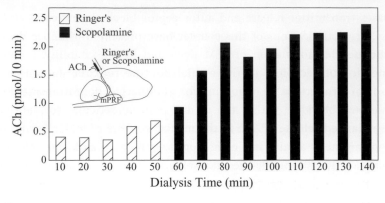

B.

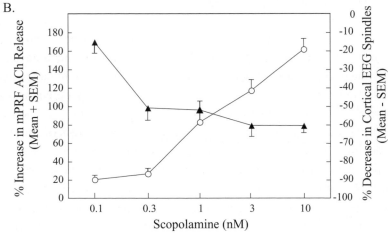

Figure 5.8 Muscarinic cholinergic autoreceptors in the medial pontine reticular formation modulate ACh release in the medial pontine reticular formation and cortical electroencephalographic (EEG) activity. (A) Time course of ACh release in the medial pontine reticular formation before (hatched bars) and during (solid bars) dialysis delivery of the muscarinic receptor antagonist scopolamine. Each histogram represents the amount of ACh in one 10 min dialysis sample. The first five histograms show ACh release in the medial pontine reticular formation during 50 min of dialysis with Ringer's (control). Solid histograms indicate medial pontine reticular formation ACh release during dialysis with Ringer's containing scopolamine. The scopolamine-induced increase indicates that ACh release is mediated by muscarinic autoreceptors. Similar experiments using dialysis delivery of muscarinic antagonists with differential affinity and relative selectivity for the five muscarinic cholinergic receptor subtypes support the conclusion that the autoreceptor mediating ACh release in cat medial pontine reticular formation is the M2 subtype. Modified from Baghdoyan *et al.* (1998). (B) Dialysis delivery to the medial pontine reticular formation of increasing concentrations of scopolamine (abscissa) caused a significant increase in ACh release (left ordinate) while decreasing the number of cortical EEG spindles per min (right ordinate). Regression analyses indicated that 97% of the variance in ACh release and EEG spindle frequency was accounted for by the concentration of scopolamine. Modified from Roth *et al.* (1996).

pontine reticular formation arises from presynaptic terminals of LDT/PPT neurons, the Fig. 5.8 data suggest that muscarinic autoreceptors reside on these LDT/PPT terminals (1.6 on Fig. 5.1).

The finding that blocking presynaptic muscarinic autoreceptors causes cortical EEG activation (Fig. 5.8) is not limited to the medial pontine reticular formation or to halothane-anesthetized cat. Muscarinic autoreceptors also modulate ACh release in prefrontal cortex of C57BL/6J (B6) mouse (Douglas *et al.*, 2001). Microdialysis was used to deliver the muscarinic receptor antagonist AF-DX 116 to one prefrontal cortex while measuring EEG in the contralateral prefrontal cortex (Douglas *et al.*, 2002b). AF-DX 116 has a greater affinity for the M2 and M4 subtypes than for the M1, M3, and M5 subtypes. The results (Fig. 5.9) demonstrated that cortical delivery of AF-DX 116 significantly increased ACh release and decreased the number of EEG spindles (Fig. 5.9B). Fourier analysis of the digitized EEG showed that dialysis delivery of AF-DX 116 to the prefrontal cortex caused a significant decrease in the EEG power of slow wave (delta) activity (Douglas *et al.*, 2002b). The data summarized by Fig. 5.9 are consistent with the interpretation that, in prefrontal cortex of B6 mouse, EEG activation can be elicited by antagonizing muscarinic autoreceptors of the M2 and/or M4 subtype (Douglas *et al.*, 2002b). The sleep-related relevance of the Fig. 5.9 data relates to the finding that during NREM sleep the generation of slow wave EEG activity requires decreased cholinergic input (Steriade, 1999). In addition, the prefrontal cortex has particular significance for regulation of arousal (Muzur *et al.*, 2002). Deactivation of the prefrontal cortex is a defining characteristic of sleep (reviewed in Stickgold *et al.*, 2001). Brain energy metabolism in regions of human prefrontal cortex is deactivated in NREM sleep (Braun *et al.*, 1997; Andersson *et al.*, 1998). The prefrontal cortex is particularly vulnerable to the effects of both sleep deprivation (Horne, 1993; Harrison & Horne, 1997) and anesthesia (Andrade, 1996; Casele-Rondi, 1996). The prefrontal cortex contributes to cardiopulmonary control (Groenewegen & Uylings, 2000) and states of sleep and anesthesia are characterized by autonomic dysregulation.

By what synaptic mechanisms might dialysis delivery of AF-DX 116 increase ACh release in the prefrontal cortex (Fig. 5.9) while activating the EEG in the contralateral prefrontal cortex? Cortical neurons are excited by ACh (Krnjevic, 1967) but an explanation for the Fig. 5.9 data requires information concerning the postsynaptic receptors in the cortex from which the activated EEG was recorded. Figure 5.10 summarizes evidence that ACh alters prefrontal cortical EEG activity via an interaction between presynaptic muscarinic autoreceptors of the M2 subtype and postsynaptic muscarinic receptors of the M1 subtype (Douglas *et al.*, 2002a). Microdialysis delivery of AF-DX 116, a muscarinic antagonist with highest affinity for the M2 and M4 subtypes, increased prefrontal cortical ACh release,

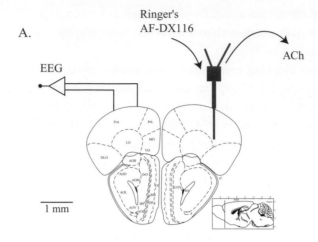

A.

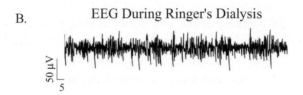

B.   EEG During Ringer's Dialysis

C.   EEG During Dialysis Delivery of AF-DX116

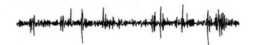

Figure 5.9 Microdialysis drug delivery to one side of prefrontal cortex alters the electroencephalographic (EEG) activity in the contralateral prefrontal cortex of C57BL/6J mouse. (A) Schematic coronal section from a mouse brain atlas (Paxinos & Franklin, 2001) showing the technique for simultaneous measures of EEG from the left prefrontal cortex and ACh release from the right prefrontal cortex. Insert at lower right gives a mid-sagittal perspective, with a vertical line showing the level of the coronal schematic drawing along the rostral (left) to caudal (right) axis. (B) EEG spindles during dialysis with Ringer's (control); (C) a representative EEG recording showing that dialysis delivery of AF-DX116 caused a decrease in the number of EEG spindles. From Douglas *et al.* (2002b).

and activated the EEG in the contralateral prefrontal cortex. EEG activation was characterized by a significant decrease in number of EEG spindles and EEG slow wave power (Vrms). Microdialysis delivery of AF-DX 116 plus pirenzepine, a relatively selective M1 and M4 muscarinic antagonist, also significantly increased ACh release but did not decrease the number of EEG spindles and did not change

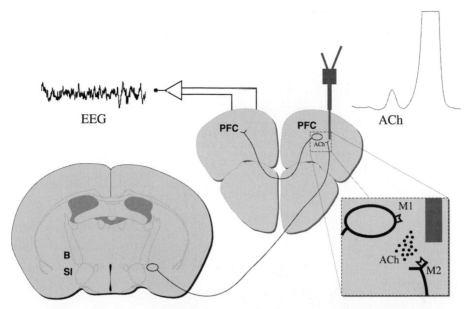

Figure 5.10 Presynaptic muscarinic autoreceptors in one prefrontal cortex alter EEG via postsynaptic muscarinic receptors in the contralateral cortex. Muscarinic cholinergic autoreceptors in prefrontal cortex modulating ACh release are likely to include the M2 subtype (Douglas *et al.*, 2001, 2002b; Zhang *et al.*, 2002). The primary source of ACh in mouse cortex is from cortically projecting cholinergic neurons in the substantia innominata and basal nucleus of Meynert (Kitt *et al.*, 1994). The inset illustrates that dialysis delivery of M2/M4 versus M1/M4 muscarinic antagonists dissociated enhanced ACh release in one cortex from EEG activation in the contralateral cortex. This finding supports the interpretation that postsynaptic muscarinic receptors of the M1 subtype are a primary site by which ACh activates the EEG. From Douglas *et al.* (2002a).

EEG slow waves. The differential EEG and ACh responses to dialysis delivery of AF-DX 116 (M2/M4) versus pirenzepine (M1/M4) supports the conclusion that, in B6 mouse, postsynaptic muscarinic receptors of the M1 subtype form one receptor mechanism by which ACh activates the EEG (Douglas *et al.*, 2002a). The data summarized in Fig. 5.11 provide direct measures of G protein activation in basal forebrain and prefrontal cortex by muscarinic cholinergic receptors (DeMarco *et al.*, 2004). The in vitro data of Fig. 5.11A indicate the presence of functional muscarinic receptors in regions of B6 mouse prefrontal cortex where in vivo microdialysis studies (Douglas *et al.*, 2002a, b) revealed modulation of ACh release and EEG by pre- and postsynaptic muscarinic receptors (Figs. 5.9 and 5.10).

Evidence that cortical ACh regulates EEG of prefrontal cortex (Figs. 5.9 and 5.10) implies that manipulating pontine cholinergic neurotransmission alters

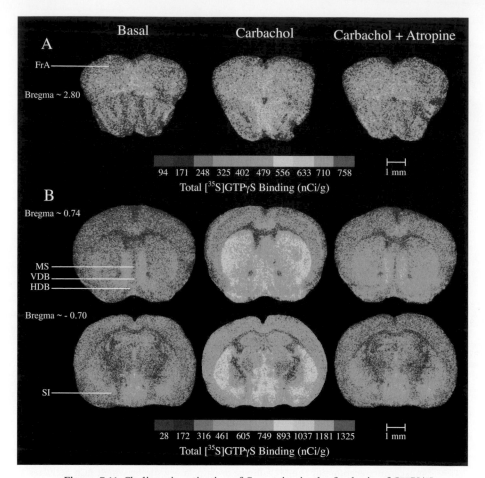

Figure 5.11 Cholinergic activation of G proteins in the forebrain of C57BL/6J mouse. Color-coded G protein activation is shown (A) for the frontal association cortex (FrA), which is the mouse homolog of prefrontal cortex, and for (B) basal forebrain. Color-coded autoradiograms of coronal sections show total [^{35}S]GTPγS binding (representing activation of G proteins) for three conditions (columns). Note the difference in the color scale between the FrA (A) and the basal forebrain (B), indicating higher total binding in the basal forebrain. In sections treated with carbachol plus atropine, [^{35}S]GTPγS binding was similar to basal levels. Additional data showed that carbachol caused a concentration-dependent increase in G protein activation. Together, these data demonstrate that G protein activation was mediated by muscarinic receptors. Abbreviations: FrA, frontal association cortex; MS, medial septum; VDB, vertical and HDB, horizontal limbs of the diagonal band of Broca; SI, substantia innominata. From DeMarco *et al.* (2004). (See also Plate 5.)

ACh release in prefrontal cortex. In B6 mouse, dialysis delivery of the cholinergic agonist carbachol to the pontine reticular formation causes a significant decrease in ACh release within the prefrontal cortex (DeMarco *et al.*, 2004). Earlier sections of this chapter reviewed data indicating that cortical ACh increases during REM sleep (Jasper & Tessier, 1971) and that microinjection of carbachol into one side of the medial pontine reticular formation increases ACh release in the contralateral pontine reticular formation (Lydic *et al.*, 1991). How is one to resolve the finding that dialysis delivery of carbachol to the pontine reticular formation causes decreased ACh release in the prefrontal cortex? The answer emphasizes regional specificity of responses to neurotransmitters and the heterogeneity of the cortex. The early studies of sleep-dependent changes in cortical ACh used a technique that made it possible to accumulate exudate from the plial surface of the anterior suprasylvian and postcruciate cortex (Jasper & Tessier, 1971). The microdialysis data showing that pontine administration of carbachol decreased ACh release in prefrontal cortex (DeMarco *et al.*, 2004) are consistent with studies showing that the prefrontal cortex is deactivated during REM sleep (Braun *et al.*, 1997; Maquet *et al.*, 1997; Nofzinger *et al.*, 1997; Muzur *et al.*, 2002). The finding that pontine carbachol decreased ACh release in mouse homolog to prefrontal cortex (DeMarco *et al.*, 2004) suggests that the REM sleep-dependent increase in ACh release within the pontine reticular formation (Kodama *et al.*, 1990; Lydic *et al.*, 1991; Leonard & Lydic, 1995, 1997) may be one mechanism causing deactivation of prefrontal cortex. This idea is supported by ongoing research indicating that ACh release in prefrontal cortex of cat decreases during REM sleep and during the REM-sleep-like state caused by pontine administration of carbachol.

Blocking transporter proteins for choline and ACh disrupts REM sleep

Acetylcholine synthesis and neurotransmission requires normal functioning of two active transport mechanisms. Choline acetyltransferase (ChAT) is the enzyme responsible for ACh synthesis from the precursor molecules acetyl coenzyme A and choline. ChAT is the neurochemical phenotype used to define cholinergic neurons; although ChAT is present in cell bodies, it is concentrated in cholinergic terminals. The ability of ChAT to produce ACh is critically dependent on an adequate level of choline. Cholinergic neurons possess a high-affinity choline uptake mechanism referred to as the choline transporter (ChT in Fig. 5.1). The choline transporter can be blocked by the molecule hemicholinium-3. Blockade of the choline transporter by hemicholinium-3 decreases ACh release, demonstrating that one rate-limiting mechanism in the production of ACh is neuronal uptake of choline (reviewed in Ferguson *et al.*, 2004). If ACh is critically important for generating REM sleep, and if choline is key for ACh synthesis, then hemicholinium-3 blockade of the choline transporter would be anticipated to decrease REM sleep (1.7 in Fig 5.1). Around the same time that ACh levels were found to be maximal in anterior suprasylvian and postcruciate cortex during REM sleep (Jasper & Tessier, 1971), Domino and colleagues reported that blocking the choline transporter with hemicholinium-3 decreases brain ACh, deactivates the EEG, and inhibits REM sleep (Dren & Domino, 1968; Domino & Stawiski, 1971). The fundamental role of choline and the ChT for production of ACh is now clear from the finding in knockout mice that disrupting the gene coding for hemicholinium-3-sensitive Ch is a lethal deletion (Ferguson *et al.*, 2004).

ACh is packaged for release from presynaptic terminals by an active transport process involving the vesicular ACh transporter (VAChT) (Prior *et al.*, 1992; Parsons *et al.*, 1993a,b). The membrane of cholinergic synaptic vesicles contains a vesicular ACh transporter that pumps ACh into the vesicle in exchange for hydrogen ions that are provided to the vesicle by an ATP-driven proton pump. The synaptic vesicle membrane possesses a cytoplasmically oriented protein that provides a binding site for vesamicol (2-(4-phenylpipendinyl) cyclohexanol), an exogenous molecule that blocks presynaptic packaging of ACh. If endogenous ACh plays a causal role in the regulation of REM sleep, then blocking vesicular packaging with vesamicol should decrease ACh release and, ultimately, decrease REM sleep (1.8 in Fig. 5.1). In rat, intracerebroventricular injections of vesamicol cause a dose-dependent decrease in REM sleep (Salin-Pascual & Jimenez-Anguiano, 1995). Blocking the vesamicol receptor also decreases REM sleep enhancement (Fig. 5.12) caused by microinjecting neostigmine into medial regions of cat pontine reticular formation (Capece *et al.*, 1997). The studies in cat demonstrated that disrupting the vesicular packaging of ACh decreased the duration of individual REM sleep epochs. Vesamicol receptor blockade caused a significant decrease in REM sleep duration but not in the number of REM sleep epochs. These results can be contrasted with data showing that the number of cholinergically induced REM sleep epochs is modulated by muscarinic cholinergic signal transduction pathways (Shuman *et al.*, 1995; Capece & Lydic, 1997) presumed to be localized to postsynaptic neurons in the medial pontine reticular formation (Fig. 5.1). Considered together, these data demonstrate that altering specific components of pre- and postsynaptic cholinergic neurotransmission in the medial pontine reticular formation has specific effects on the temporal organization of REM sleep (Capece *et al.*, 1999).

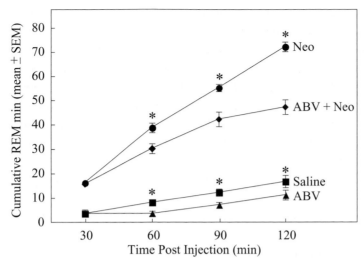

Figure 5.12 REM sleep is decreased by blocking the vesamicol receptor. The time course of REM sleep is shown during two hours of polygraphic recordings that followed microinjection into cat medial pontine reticular formation of the acetylcholine esterase inhibitor neostigmine (Neo), the vesamicol receptor blocker ($\pm$)-4-aminobenzovesamicol (ABV, a derivative of vesamicol), or saline (vehicle control). The top function shows the enhancement of REM sleep caused by neostigmine. ABV injection into the medial pontine reticular formation 15 min before neostigmine (ABV+Neo) caused a significant decrease in REM sleep. The lower two functions compare the time course of spontaneous REM sleep following saline microinjection with the time course of REM sleep after microinjecting ABV into the medial pontine reticular formation. Note that during the first 90 min of these 2 h recordings the vesamicol receptor blocker ABV decreased natural REM sleep. These data, therefore, illustrate a similarity between spontaneous REM sleep and the REM sleep-like state caused by neostigmine. From Capece *et al.* (1997).

Limitations, future directions, and conclusions

This review is limited to a primary focus on ACh in relation to muscarinic cholinergic receptors. Nicotinic cholinergic receptors also contribute to arousal state control. The nicotinic receptor is a ligand-gated channel consisting of five primary subunits. When activated by ACh or nicotine, the pore of the nicotinic cholinergic receptor opens, allowing influx of Na^+ and Ca^{2+} and efflux of K^+. These subunits have multiple combinatorial configurations around the ion channel. The ligand-gated ion-channel database lists 16 nicotinic cholinergic receptor subtypes that have been identified in human (Le Novère & Changeux, 2001).

The role of nicotinic cholinergic receptors in sleep cycle control has been examined in animals and humans. Domino and colleagues were the first to report that administration of nicotine to cat causes EEG activation (Domino & Yamamoto, 1965). Many studies have shown that cigarette smoking disrupts sleep (Soldatos *et al.*, 1980; Htoo *et al.*, 2004) and that nicotine enhances arousal (Lawrence *et al.*, 2002). Cigarette smoke is a complex admixture containing more than 4,000 different molecules, of which at least 50 are known carcinogens. More pharmacologically specific studies have shown that transdermal administration of nicotine to non-smoking humans also decreases REM sleep (Gillin *et al.*, 1994).

An important research direction concerns efforts to specify the synaptic mechanisms and brain regions through which nicotinic cholinergic transmission modulates sleep. As reviewed elsewhere (Jones *et al.*, 1999), nicotinic cholinergic receptors are typically localized to presynaptic nerve terminals in brain regions known to mediate the behavioral effects of nicotine and ACh. This generalization appears directly relevant to sleep-promoting neurons in the ventrolateral preoptic (VLPO) area. ACh inhibits putative sleep-promoting VLPO neurons via a nicotinic, presynaptic action that enhances noradrenaline release (Saint-Mleux *et al.*, 2004). Another opportunity for future research includes specifying the nicotinic cholinergic receptor subtypes and the brain regions through which nicotine acts to modulate levels of arousal. Progress in this area is illustrated by the finding that mice in which the gene coding for the β2 subunit of the nicotinic cholinergic receptor has been deleted show sleep patterns consistent with the interpretation that the β2 component of the nicotinic cholinergic receptor contributes to organization of the sleep–wakefulness cycle (Léna *et al.*, 2004).

These data naturally lead to the question of whether nicotinic cholinergic receptors in the pons influence the traits that define REM sleep. For studies using cat, there is a lack of agreement between reports that microinjection of nicotine into the pontine reticular formation fails to cause (George *et al.*, 1964) versus causes (Velazquez-Moctezuma *et al.*, 1990a) REM sleep. On the one hand, there is evidence from one in vitro electrophysiological study for the existence of nicotinic receptors that depolarize a subpopulation of neurons in the pontine reticular formation (Stevens *et al.*, 1993). On the other hand, nicotine delivered systemically to cat via transdermal patch enhances wakefulness and decreases REM sleep (Vazquez *et al.*, 1996). Studies in rat concur that acute administration of nicotine causes a dose-dependent decrease in REM sleep (Salin-Pascual *et al.*, 1999). Nicotine increases the discharge of neurons in the wakefulness-promoting dorsal raphe nucleus (Guzman-Marin *et al.*, 2001) and decreases discharge in LDT/PPT regions known to provide ACh to the pontine reticular formation (Mihailescu *et al.*, 2001).

The conclusion that ACh contributes to EEG activation and REM sleep generation is supported by more than 50 years of research. Figure 5.1 illustrates the remarkable agreement between eight lines of evidence at the synaptic level, all showing that ACh and muscarinic cholinergic receptors generate REM sleep and modulate EEG excitability. Many molecules in addition to ACh contribute to arousal state control, and the *textus receptus* on the neurochemistry of sleep and anesthesia remains incomplete. Synaptic models of the cholinergic regulation of sleep must be expanded to incorporate multiple brain regions (Saper *et al.*, 2001; Steriade & McCarley, 2005) and neurotransmitter systems (Lydic & Baghdoyan, 2005; Verret *et al.*, 2005). For example, the arousal-promoting peptides hypocretin-1 and hypocretin-2 (orexin A and orexin B) increase ACh release in rat pontine reticular formation (Bernard *et al.*, 2003, 2006). Nitric oxide alters sleep; there is evidence that nitric oxide modulates ACh release in pontine reticular formation of cat (Leonard & Lydic, 1995, 1997) and mouse (Lydic *et al.*, 2006). In mouse, dialysis delivery of an adenosine A_{2A} receptor agonist to the pontine reticular formation increases sleep and increases ACh release (Coleman *et al.*, 2006). Microinjection of adenosine receptor agonists into rat pontine reticular formation also has been shown to enhance REM sleep (Marks *et al.*, 2003).

There are many questions that remain unanswered concerning ACh and arousal state control. The functional roles of the five subtypes of muscarinic receptor remain poorly understood. The potential interaction between nicotinic and muscarinic cholinergic receptors in the context of sleep is not clear. Almost no data exist specifying the functional role in sleep cycle control for the multiple presynaptic proteins known to reside in cholinergic terminals. The broad physiological relevance of ACh noted at the beginning of this chapter implies a potential clinical significance of ACh for disorders directly and indirectly related to sleep. The clinical relevance of ACh insures an active future for research on cholinergic pharmacology. Pain is a particularly compelling clinical concern that demands rapid clinical intervention. Pain disrupts sleep and pain is now viewed as a vital sign to be evaluated in every patient. Opioids provide good pain relief but have the unwanted side effects of depressing ACh release in the pontine reticular formation (Lydic *et al.*, 1993; Mortazavi *et al.*, 1999) and prefrontal cortex (Osman *et al.*, 2005), decreasing REM sleep (Keifer *et al.*, 1992; Kshatri *et al.*, 1998; Lydic, 2001; Baghdoyan, 2006) and disrupting the temporal organization of sleep (Walder *et al.*, 2001; Reymond Shaw *et al.*, 2005; Roehrs & Roth, 2005; Shaw *et al.*, 2005). Drugs used to generate states of sedation or general anesthesia also disrupt cholinergic neurotransmission (Meuret *et al.*, 2000; Backman *et al.*, 2004). The unwanted side effects of opioids, sedative, and anesthetic molecules are more severe in older patients. The Centers for Disease Control and Prevention web site (www.cdc.gov/aging) refers to the aging of the U.S. population as "one of the major public health challenges of the 21st century." Many of the dementias of aging involve disruption of cholinergic neurotransmission (Whitehouse, 2004) and disordered sleep (Foley *et al.*, 1995; Ancoli-Israel & Alessi, 2005). Pressing clinical concerns will promote research on ACh for many years to come.

Acknowledgements

Supported by National Institutes of Health Grants HL40881, MH45361, HL57120, HL65272, and the Department of Anesthesiology. We thank M.A. Norat and N. Goldberg for editorial assistance.

References

Ancoli-Israel, S. & Alessi, C. (2005). Sleep and aging. *Am. J. Geriatr. Psychiatry* **13**, 341–3.

Andersson, J. L., Onoe, H., Hetta, J. *et al.* (1998). Brain networks affected by synchronized sleep visualized by positron emission tomography. *J. Cereb. Blood Flow Metab.* **18**, 701–15.

Andrade, J. (1996). Investigations of hypesthesia: using anesthetics to explore relationships between consciousness, learning, and memory. *Conscious Cogn.* **5**, 562–80.

Aserinsky, E. & Kleitman, N. (1953). Regularly occurring periods of eye motility, and concomitant phenomena, during sleep. *Science* **118**, 273–4.

Backman, S. B., Fiset, P. & Plourde, G. (2004). Cholinergic mechanisms mediating anesthetic induced altered states of consciousness. *Prog. Brain Res.* **145**, 197–206.

Baghdoyan, H. A. (1997). Location and quantification of muscarinic receptor subtypes in rat pons: implications for REM sleep generation. *Am. J. Physiol.* **273**, R896–R904.

Baghdoyan, H. A. (2006). Hyperalgesia induced by REM sleep loss: a phenomenon in search of a mechanism. *Sleep* **29**, 137–9.

Baghdoyan, H. A. & Lydic, R. (1999). M2 muscarinic receptor subtype in the feline medial pontine reticular formation modulates the amount of rapid eye movement sleep. *Sleep* **22**, 835–47.

Baghdoyan, H. A., Monaco, A. P., Rodrigo-Angulo, M. L. *et al.* (1984a). Microinjection of neostigmine into the pontine reticular formation of cats enhances desynchronized sleep signs. *J. Pharmacol. Exp. Ther.* **231**, 173–80.

Baghdoyan, H. A., Rodrigo-Angulo, M. L., McCarley, R. W. & Hobson, J. A. (1984b). Site-specific enhancement and suppression of desynchronized sleep signs following cholinergic stimulation of three brain stem regions. *Brain Res.* **306**, 39–52.

Baghdoyan, H. A., Rodrigo-Angulo, M. L., McCarley, R. W. & Hobson, J. A. (1987). A neuroanatomical gradient in the pontine tegmentum for the cholinoceptive induction of desynchronized sleep signs. *Brain Res.* **414**, 245–61.

Baghdoyan, H. A., Lydic, R., Callaway, C. W. & Hobson, J. A. (1989). The carbachol-induced enhancement of desynchronized sleep signs is dose dependent and antagonized by centrally administered atropine. *Neuropsychopharmacology* **2**, 67–79.

Baghdoyan, H. A., Mallios, V. J., Duckrow, R. B. & Mash, D. C. (1994). Localization of muscarinic receptor subtypes in brain stem areas regulating sleep. *Neuroreport* **5**, 1631–4.

Baghdoyan, H. A., Lydic, R. & Fleegal, M. A. (1998). M2 muscarinic autoreceptors modulate acetylcholine release in the medial pontine reticular formation. *J. Pharmacol. Exp. Ther.* **286**, 1446–52.

Baxter, B. L. (1969). Induction of both emotional behavior and a novel form of REM sleep by chemical stimulation applied to cat mesencephalon. *Exp. Neurol.* **23**, 220–9.

Berman, A. L. (1968). *The Brain Stem of the Cat.* Madison, WI: University of Wisconsin Press.

Bernard, R., Lydic, R. & Baghdoyan, H. A. (2003). Hypocretin-1 causes G protein activation and increases ACh release in rat pons. *Eur. J. Neurosci.* **18**, 1775–85.

Bernard, R., Lydic, R. & Baghdoyan, H. A. (2006). Hypocretin (orexin) receptor subtypes differentially enhance acetylcholine release and activate G protein subtypes in rat pontine reticular formation. *J. Pharmacol. Exp. Ther.* **317**, 163–71.

Bourgin, P., Escourrou, P., Gaultier, C. & Adrien, J. (1995). Induction of rapid eye movement sleep by carbachol infusion into the pontine reticular formation in the rat. *Neuroreport* **6**, 532–6.

Braun, A. R., Balkin, T. J., Wesensten, N. J. *et al.* (1997). Regional cerebral blood flow throughout the sleep-wake cycle: an H2 15O PET study. *Brain* **120**, 1173–97.

Buckley, N. J. (1990). Molecular pharmacology of cloned muscarinic receptors. In *Transmembrane Signalling, Intracellular Messengers and Implications for Drug Development*, ed. S. R. Nahorski, pp. 11–30. Chichester: John Wiley & Sons.

Capece, M. L. & Lydic, R. (1997). Cyclic AMP and protein kinase A modulate cholinergic rapid eye movement sleep generation. *Am. J. Physiol.* **273**, R1430–40.

Capece, M. L., Efange, S. M. & Lydic, R. (1997). Vesicular acetylcholine transport inhibitor suppresses REM sleep. *Neuroreport* **8**, 481–4.

Capece, M. L., Baghdoyan, H. A. & Lydic, R. (1998). Carbachol stimulates [^{35}S]guanylyl 5'-(γ-thio)triphosphate binding in rapid eye movement sleep-related brain stem nuclei of rat. *J. Neurosci.* **18**, 3779–85.

Capece, M. L., Baghdoyan, H. A. & Lydic, R. (1999). New directions for the study of cholinergic REM sleep generation: Specifying presynaptic and postsynaptic mechanisms. In *REM Sleep*, ed. B. N. Mallick & S. Inoué, pp. 123–41. London: Narosa Press.

Carty, D. J. (1994). Pertussis toxin-catalyzed ADP-ribosylation of G proteins. *Meth. Enzymol.* **237**, 63–70.

Casele-Rondi, G. (1996). Perceptual processing during general anaesthesia reconsidered within a neuro-psychological framework. In *Memory and Awareness in Anesthesia*, vol. 3, ed. B. Bonke, J. Bovill & N. Moerman, pp 102–7, Assen: Van Gorcum.

Caulfield, M. P. (1993). Muscarinic receptors – characterization, coupling and function. *Pharmacol. Ther.* **58**, 319–79.

Caulfield, M. P. & Birdsall, N. J. (1998). International union of pharmacology. XVIII. Classification of muscarinic acetylcholine receptors. *Pharmacol. Rev.* **50**, 279–90.

Celesia, G. G. & Jasper, H. H. (1966). Acetylcholine released from cerebral cortex in relation to state of activation. *Neurology* **16**, 1053–64.

Coleman, C. G., Lydic, R. & Baghdoyan, H. A. (2004). M2 muscarinic receptors in pontine reticular formation of C57BL/6J mouse contribute to rapid eye movement sleep generation. *Neuroscience* **126**, 821–30.

Coleman, C. G., Baghdoyan, H. A. & Lydic, R. (2006). Dialysis delivery of an adenosine A_{2A} agonist into the pontine reticular formation of C57BL/6J mouse increases pontine acetylcholine release and sleep. *J. Neurochem.* **96**, 1750–9.

Cordeau, J., Moreau, A., Beaulnes, A. & Laurin, C. (1963). EEG and behavioral changes following microinjections of acetylcholine and adrenaline in the brain stem of cats. *Arch. Ital. Biol.* **101**, 30–47.

Crouzier, D., Le Crom, V. B., Four, E., Lallement, G. & Testylier, G. (2004). Disruption of mice sleep stages induced by low doses of organophosphorus compound soman. *Toxicology* **199**, 59–71.

Datta, S. (1995). Neuronal activity in the peribrachial area: relationship to behavioral state control. *Neurosci. Biobehav. Rev.* **19**, 67–84.

Datta, S. & Prutzman, S. L. (2005). Novel role of brain stem pedunculopontine tegmental adenylyl cyclase in the regulation of spontaneous REM sleep in the freely moving rat. *J. Neurophysiol.* **94**, 1928–37.

Datta, S. & Siwek, D. F. (2002). Single cell activity patterns of pedunculopontine tegmentum neurons across the sleep-wake cycle in the freely moving rats. *J. Neurosci. Res.* **70**, 611–21.

DeMarco, G. J., Baghdoyan, H. A. & Lydic, R. (2003). Differential cholinergic activation of G proteins in rat and mouse brainstem: relevance for sleep and nociception. *J. Comp. Neurol.* **457**, 175–84.

DeMarco, G. J., Baghdoyan, H. A. & Lydic, R. (2004). Carbachol in the pontine reticular formation of C57BL/6J mouse decreases acetylcholine release in prefrontal cortex. *Neuroscience* **123**, 17–29.

Dement, W. (1958). The occurrence of low voltage, fast, electroencephalogram patterns during behavioral sleep in the cat. *Electroencephalogr. Clin. Neurophysiol.* **10**, 291–6.

Domino, E. F. & Stawiski, M. (1971). Modification of the cat sleep cycle by hemicholinium-3, a cholinergic antisynthesis agent. *Res. Commun. Chem. Pathol. Pharmacol.* **2**, 461–7.

Domino, E. F. & Yamamoto, K. I. (1965). Nicotine: effect on the sleep cycle of the cat. *Science* **150**, 637–8.

Domino, E. F., Yamamoto, K. & Dren, A. T. (1968). Role of cholinergic mechanisms in states of wakefulness and sleep. *Prog. Brain. Res.* **28**, 113–33.

Douglas, C. L., Baghdoyan, H. A. & Lydic, R. (2001). M2 muscarinic autoreceptors modulate acetylcholine release in prefrontal cortex of C57BL/6J mouse. *J. Pharmacol. Exp. Ther.* **299**, 960–6.

Douglas, C. L., Baghdoyan, H. A. & Lydic, R. (2002a). Postsynaptic muscarinic M1 receptors activate prefrontal cortical EEG of C57BL/6J mouse. *J. Neurophysiol.* **88**, 3003–9.

Douglas, C. L., Baghdoyan, H. A. & Lydic, R. (2002b). Prefrontal cortex acetylcholine release, EEG slow waves, and spindles are modulated by M2 autoreceptors in C57BL/6J mouse. *J. Neurophysiol.* **87**, 2817–22.

Douglas, C. L., Bowman, G. N., Baghdoyan, H. A. & Lydic, R. (2005). C57BL/6J and B6.v-lep[ob] mice differ in the cholinergic modulation of sleep and breathing. *J. Appl. Physiol.* **98**, 918–29.

Dren, A. T. & Domino, E. F. (1968). Effects of hemicholinium (HC-3) on EEG activation and brain acetylcholine in the dog. *J. Pharmacol. Exp. Ther.* **161**, 141–54.

El Mansari, M., Sakai, K. & Jouvet, M. (1989). Unitary characteristics of presumptive cholinergic tegmental neurons during the sleep-waking cycle in freely moving cats. *Exp. Brain. Res.* **76**, 519–29.

Ferguson, S. M., Bazalakova, M., Savchenko, V. *et al.* (2004). Lethal impairment of cholinergic neurotransmission in hemicholinium-3-sensitive transporter knockout mice. *Proc. Natl. Acad. Sci. USA* **101**, 8762–7.

Foley, D. J., Monjan, A. A., Brown, S. L. *et al.* (1995). Sleep complaints among elderly persons: an epidemiologic study of three communities. *Sleep* **18**, 425–32.

Garzon, M., de Andres, I. & Reinoso-Suarez, F. (1997). Neocortical and hippocampal electrical activities are similar in spontaneous and cholinergic-induced REM sleep. *Brain Res.* **766**, 266–70.

George, R., Haslett, W. L. & Jenden, D. J. (1964). A cholinergic mechanism in the brainstem reticular formation: induction of paradoxical sleep. *Int. J. Neuropharmacol.* **72**, 541–52.

Gillin, J. C., Lardon, M., Ruiz, C., Golshan, S. & Salin-Pascual, R. (1994). Dose-dependent effects of transdermal nicotine on early morning awakening and rapid eye movement sleep time in nonsmoking normal volunteers. *J. Clin. Psychopharmacol.* **14**, 264–7.

Gnadt, J. W. & Pegram, G. (1986). Cholinergic brainstem mechanisms of REM sleep in the rat. *Brain Res.* **384**, 29–41.

Groenewegen, H. & Uylings, H. (2000). The prefrontal cortex and the integration of sensory, limbic and autonomic information. *Prog. Brain Res.* **126**, 3–28.

Guzman-Marin, R., Alam, M. N., Mihailescu, S. *et al.* (2001). Subcutaneous administration of nicotine changes dorsal raphe serotonergic neurons discharge rate during REM sleep. *Brain Res.* **888**, 321–5.

Harrison, Y. & Horne, J. A. (1997). Sleep deprivation affects speech. *Sleep* **20**, 871–7.

Haymaker, W. (1953). *The Founders of Neurology.* Springfield, IL: Springfield.

Hernández-Peón, R., Chávez-Ibarra, G., Morgane, P. J. & Timo-Iaria, C. (1963). Limbic cholinergic pathways involved in sleep and emotional behavior. *Exp. Neurol.* **8**, 93–111.

Hobson, J. A., McCarley, R. W. & Wyzinski, P. W. (1975). Sleep cycle oscillation: reciprocal discharge by two brainstem neuronal groups. *Science* **189**, 55–8.

Hobson, J. A., Datta, S., Calvo, J. M. & Quattrochi, J. (1993). Acetylcholine as a brain state modulator: triggering and long-term regulation of REM sleep. *Prog. Brain Res.* **98**, 389–404.

Horne, J. A. (1993). Human sleep, sleep loss and behaviour: implications for the prefrontal cortex and psychiatric disorder. *Br. J. Psychiatry* **162**, 413–19.

Horner, R. L. & Kubin, L. (1999). Pontine carbachol elicits multiple rapid eye movement sleep-like neural events in urethane-anaesthetized rats. *Neuroscience* **93**, 215–26.

Htoo, A., Talwar, A., Feinsilver, S. H. & Greenberg, H. (2004). Smoking and sleep disorders. *Med. Clin. N. Am.* **88**, 1575–91.

Hulme, E. C., Birdsall, N. J. M. & Buckley, N. J. (1990). Muscarinic receptor subtypes. *A. Rev. Pharmacol. Toxicol.* **30**, 633–73.

Imeri, L., Bianchi, S., Angeli, P. & Mancia, M. (1994). Selective blockade of different brain stem muscarinic receptor subtypes: effects on the sleep-wake cycle. *Brain Res.* **636**, 68–72.

Jasper, H. H. & Tessier, J. (1971). Acetylcholine liberation from cerebral cortex during paradoxical (REM) sleep. *Science* **172**, 601–2.

Jones, B. E. & Beaudet, A. (1987). Distribution of acetylcholine and catecholamine neurons in the cat brainstem: a choline acetyltransferase and tyrosine hydroxylase immunohistochemical study. *J. Comp. Neurol.* **261**, 15–32.

Jones, S., Sudweeks, S. & Yakel, J. L. (1999). Nicotinic receptors in the brain: correlating physiology with function. *Trends Neurosci.* **22**, 555–61.

Jones, S. V. P., Levey, A. I., Weiner, D. M. *et al.* (1992). Muscarinic acetylcholine receptors. In *Molecular Biology of G-Protein-Coupled Receptors*, ed. M. R. Brann, pp. 170–97, Boston, MA: Birkhäuser.

Jouvet, M. (1962). Recherches sur les structures nerveuses et les mechanismes responsables des differentes phases du sommeil physiologique. *Arch. Ital. Biol.* **100**, 125–206.

Jouvet, M. (1972). The role of monoamines and acetylcholine containing neurons in the regulation of the sleep-waking cycle. *Ergeb. Physiol.* **64**, 166–307.

Kalsner, S. (1990). Heteroreceptors, autoreceptors, and other terminal sites. In *Presynaptic Receptors and the Question of Autoregulation of Neurotransmitter Release*, ed. S. Kalsner & T. C. Westfall, pp. 1–6. New York, NY: New York Academy of Sciences.

Karczmar, A. G., Longo, V. G. & De Carolis, A. S. (1970). A pharmacological model of paradoxical sleep: the role of cholinergic and monoamine systems. *Physiol. Behav.* **5**, 175–82.

Kayama, Y., Ohta, M. & Jodo, E. (1992). Firing of 'possibly' cholinergic neurons in the rat laterodorsal tegmental nucleus during sleep and wakefulness. *Brain Res.* **569**, 210–20.

Keifer, J. C., Baghdoyan, H. A. & Lydic, R. (1992). Sleep disruption and increased apneas after pontine microinjection of morphine. *Anesthesiology* **77**, 973–82.

Keifer, J. C., Baghdoyan, H. A., Becker, L. & Lydic, R. (1994). Halothane decreases pontine acetylcholine release and increases EEG spindles. *Neuroreport* **5**, 577–80.

Kitt, C. A., Höhmann, C., Coyle, J. T. & Price, D. L. (1994). Cholinergic innervation of mouse forebrain structures. *J. Comp. Neurol.* **341**, 117–29.

Kodama, T., Takahashi, Y. & Honda, Y. (1990). Enhancement of acetylcholine release during paradoxical sleep in the dorsal tegmental field of the cat brain stem. *Neurosci. Lett.* **114**, 277–82.

Krnjevic, K. (1967). Chemical transmission and cortical arousal. *Anesthesiology* **28**, 100–5.

Kshatri, A. M., Baghdoyan, H. A. & Lydic, R. (1998). Cholinomimetics, but not morphine, increase antinociceptive behavior from pontine reticular regions regulating rapid eye movement sleep. *Sleep* **21**, 677–85.

Kubin, L. (2001). Carbachol models of REM sleep: recent developments and new directions. *Arch. Ital. Biol.* **139**, 147–68.

Kumar, P. & Raju, T. R. (2001). Seizure susceptibility decreases with enhancement of rapid eye movement sleep. *Brain Res.* **922**, 299–304.

Lawrence, N. S., Ross, T. J. & Stein, E. A. (2002). Cognitive mechanisms of nicotine on visual attention. *Neuron* **36**, 539–48.

Le Novère, N. & Changeux, J.-P. (2001). LDICdb: the ligand-gated ion channel database. *Nucleic Acids Res.* **29**, 294–5.

Lee, L. H., Friedman, D. B. & Lydic, R. (1995). Respiratory nuclei share synaptic connectivity with pontine reticular regions regulating REM sleep. *Am. J. Physiol.* **268**, L251–62.

Léna, C., Popa, D., Grailhe, R. *et al.* (2004). β2-Containing nicotinic receptors contribute to the organization of sleep and regulate putative micro-arousals in mice. *J. Neurosci.* **24**, 5711–18.

Leonard, T. O. & Lydic, R. (1995). Nitric oxide synthase inhibition decreases pontine acetylcholine release. *Neuroreport* **6**, 1525–9.

Leonard, T. O. & Lydic, R. (1997). Pontine nitric oxide modulates acetylcholine release, rapid eye movement sleep generation, and respiratory rate. *J. Neurosci.* **17**, 774–85.

Loewi, O. (1936). *Nobel Prize Lecture.* http://nobelprize.org/nobel_prizes/medicine/laureates/1936/loewi-lecture.html.

Longo, V. G. & Silvestrini, B. (1957). Action of eserine and amphetamine on the electrical activity of the rabbit brain. *J. Pharmacol. Exp. Ther.* **120**, 160–70.

Lydic, R. (2001). Pain: a bridge linking anesthesiology and sleep research. *Sleep* **24**, 10–12.

Lydic, R. & Baghdoyan, H. A. (1993). Pedunculopontine stimulation alters respiration and increases ACh release in the pontine reticular formation. *Am. J. Physiol.* **264**, R544–54.

Lydic, R. & Baghdoyan, H. A. (2005). Sleep, anesthesiology, and the neurobiology of arousal state control. *Anesthesiology* **103**, 1268–95.

Lydic, R., Baghdoyan, H. A. & Lorinc, Z. (1991). Microdialysis of cat pons reveals enhanced acetylcholine release during state-dependent respiratory depression. *Am. J. Physiol.* **261**, R766–70.

Lydic, R., Keifer, J. C., Baghdoyan, H. A. & Becker, L. (1993). Microdialysis of the pontine reticular formation reveals inhibition of acetylcholine release by morphine. *Anesthesiology* **79**, 1003–12.

Lydic, R., Douglas, C. L. & Baghdoyan, H. A. (2002). Microinjection of neostigmine into the pontine reticular formation of C57BL/6J mouse enhances rapid eye movement sleep and depresses breathing. *Sleep* **25**, 835–41.

Lydic, R., Garza-Grande, R., Struthers, R. & Baghdoyan, H. A. (2006). Nitric oxide in B6 mouse and nitric oxide-sensitive soluble guanylate cyclase in cat modulate acetylcholine release in pontine reticular formation. *J. Appl. Physiol.* **100**, 1666–73.

Maquet, P., Degueldre, C., Delfiore, G. *et al.* (1997). Functional neuroanatomy of human slow wave sleep. *J. Neurosci.* **17**, 2807–12.

Marks, G. A. & Birabil, C. G. (1998). Enhancement of rapid eye movement sleep in the rat by cholinergic and adenosinergic agonists infused into the pontine reticular formation. *Neuroscience* **86**, 29–37.

Marks, G. A. & Birabil, C. G. (2000). Infusion of adenylyl cyclase inhibitor SQ22,536 into the medial pontine reticular formation of rats enhances rapid eye movement sleep. *Neuroscience* **98**, 311–15.

Marks, G. A., Shaffery, J. P., Speciale, S. G. & Birabil, C. G. (2003). Enhancement of rapid eye movement sleep in the rat by actions at A1 and A2A adenosine receptor subtypes with a differential sensitivity to atropine. *Neuroscience* **116**, 913–20.

Marrosu, F., Portas, C., Mascia, M. S. *et al.* (1995). Microdialysis measurement of cortical and hippocampal acetylcholine release during sleep-wake cycle in freely moving cats. *Brain Res.* **671**, 329–32.

Mavanji, V. & Datta, S. (2003). Activation of the phasic pontine-wave generator enhances improvement of learning performance: a mechanism for sleep-dependent plasticity. *Eur. J. Neurosci.* **17**, 359–70.

McCarley, R. W. & Hobson, J. A. (1975). Neuronal excitability modulation over the sleep cycle: a structural and mathematical model. *Science* **189**, 58–60.

Meuret, P., Backman, S. B., Bonhomme, V., Plourde, G. & Fiset, P. *et al.* (2000). Physostigmine reverses propofol-induced unconsciousness and attenuation of the auditory steady state response and bispectral index in human volunteers. *Anesthesiology* **93**, 708–17.

Mihailescu, S., Guzman-Marin, R. & Drucker-Colin, R. (2001). Nicotine stimulation of dorsal raphe neurons: effects on laterodorsal and pedunculopontine neurons. *Eur. Neuropsychopharmacol.* **11**, 359–66.

Mitani, A., Ito, K., Hallanger, A. E. *et al.* (1988). Cholinergic projections from the laterodorsal and pedunculopontine tegmental nuclei to the pontine gigantocellular tegmental field in the cat. *Brain Res.* **451**, 397–402.

Mitchell, J. F. (1963). The spontaneous and evoked release of acetylcholine from the cerebral cortex. *J. Physiol. Lond.* **163**, 98–116.

Mitler, M. M. & Dement, W. C. (1974). Cataplectic-like behavior in cats after microinjections of carbachol in pontine reticular formation. *Brain Res.* **68**, 335–43.

Mortazavi, S., Thompson, J., Baghdoyan, H. A. & Lydic, R. (1999). Fentanyl and morphine, but not remifentanil, inhibit acetylcholine release in pontine regions modulating arousal. *Anesthesiology* **90**, 1070–7.

Moruzzi, G. & Magoun, H. W. (1949). Brain stem reticular formation and activation of the EEG. *Electroencephalogr. Clin. Neurophysiol.* **1**, 455–73.

Muzur, A., Pace-Schott, E. F. & Hobson, J. A. (2002). The prefrontal cortex in sleep. *Trends Cogn. Sci.* **6**, 475–81.

Nofzinger, E. A., Mintun, M. A., Wiseman, M. B., Kupfer, D. J. & Moore, R. Y. (1997). Forebrain activation in REM sleep: an FDG PET study. *Brain Res.* **770**, 192–201.

Osman, N. I., Baghdoyan, H. A. & Lydic, R. (2005). Morphine inhibits acetylcholine release in rat prefrontal cortex when delivered systemically or by microdialysis to basal forebrain. *Anesthesiology* **103**, 779–87.

Parsons, S. M., Bahr, B. A., Rogers, G. A. *et al.* (1993a). Acetylcholine transporter-vesamicol receptor pharmacology and structure. *Prog. Brain Res.* **98**, 175–81.

Parsons, S. M., Prior, C. & Marshall, I. G. (1993b). Acetylcholine transport, storage, and release. *Int. Rev. Neurobiol* **35**, 279–390.

Paxinos, G. and Franklin, K. B. J. (2001). *The Mouse Brain in Stereotaxic Coordinates*. San Diego, CA: Academic Press.

Paxinos, G. & Watson, C. (1998). *The Rat Brain in Stereotaxic Coordinates*, 4th edn. New York, NY: Academic Press.

Prior, C., Marshall, I. G. & Parsons, S. M. (1992). The pharmacology of vesamicol: an inhibitor of the vesicular acetylcholine transporter. *Gen. Pharmacol.* **23**, 1017–22.

Reinoso-Suárez F,, de Andrés, I., Rodrigo-Angulo, M. L. & Garzón, M. (2001). Brain structures and mechanisms involved in the generation of REM sleep. *Sleep Med. Rev.* **5**, 63–77.

Reymond Shaw, I., Lavigne, G., Mayer, P. & Choinière, M. (2005). Acute intravenous administration of morphine perturbs sleep architecture in healthy pain-free young adults: a preliminary study. *Sleep* **28**, 677–82.

Richter, D. & Crossland, J. (1949). Variation in acetylcholine content of the brain with physiological state. *Am. J. Physiol.* **159**, 247–55.

Roehrs, T. & Roth, T. (2005). Sleep and pain: interaction of two vital functions. *Semin. Neurol.* **25**, 106–16.

Roth, M. T., Fleegal, M. A., Lydic, R. & Baghdoyan, H. A. (1996). Pontine acetylcholine release is regulated by muscarinic autoreceptors. *Neuroreport* **7**, 3069–72.

Saint-Mleux, B., Eggermann, E., Bisetti, A. *et al.* (2004). Nicotinic enhancement of the noradrenergic inhibition of sleep-promoting neurons in the ventrolateral preoptic area. *J. Neurosci.* **24**, 63–7.

Sakai, K. & Onoe, H. (1997). Critical role for M3 muscarinic receptors in paradoxical sleep generation in the cat. *Eur. J. Neurosci.* **9**, 415–23.

Salin-Pascual, R. J. & Jimenez-Anguiano, A. (1995). Vesamicol, an acetylcholine uptake blocker in presynaptic vesicles, suppresses rapid eye movement (REM) sleep in the rat. *Psychopharmacology, Berl.* **121**, 485–7.

Salin-Pascual, R. J., Moro-Lopez, M. L., Gonzalez-Sanchez, H. & Blanco-Centurion, C. (1999). Changes in sleep after acute and repeated administration of nicotine in the rat. *Psychopharmacology, Berl.* **145**, 133–8.

Saper, C. B., Chou, T. C. & Scammell, T. E. (2001). The sleep switch: hypothalamic control of sleep and wakefulness. *Trends Neurosci.* **24**, 726–31.

Sarter, M. & Bruno, J. P. (1997). Cognitive functions of cortical acetylcholine: toward a unifying hypothesis. *Brain Res. Rev.* **23**, 28–46.

Sarter, M. & Bruno, J. P. (2000). Cortical cholinergic inputs mediating arousal, attentional processing and dreaming: differential afferent regulation of the basal forebrain by telencephalic and brainstem afferents. *Neuroscience* **95**, 933–52.

Semba, K. (1991). The cholinergic basal forebrain: a critical role in cortical arousal. *Adv. Exp. Med. Biol.* **295**, 197–218.

Semba, K. (2000). Multiple output pathways of the basal forebrain: organization, chemical heterogeneity, and roles in vigilance. *Behav. Brain Res.* **115**, 117–41.

Shaw, I. R., Lavigne, G., Mayer, P. & Choinière, M. (2005). Acute intravenous administration of morphine perturbs sleep architecture in healthy pain-free young adults: a preliminary study. *Sleep* **28**, 677–82.

Shiromani, P. J. & Fishbein, W. (1986). Continuous pontine cholinergic microinfusion via mini-pump induces sustained alterations in rapid eye movement (REM) sleep. *Pharmacol. Biochem. Behav.* **25**, 1253–61.

Shiromani, P. J., Armstrong, D. M. & Gillin, J. C. (1988). Cholinergic neurons from the dorsolateral pons project to the medial pons: a WGA-HRP and choline acetyltransferase immunohistochemical study. *Neurosci. Lett.* **95**, 19–23.

Shuman, S. L., Capece, M. L., Baghdoyan, H. A. & Lydic, R. (1995). Pertussis toxin-sensitive G proteins mediate carbachol-induced REM sleep and respiratory depression. *Am. J. Physiol.* **269**, R308–17.

Sitaram, N., Wyatt, R. J., Dawson, S. & Gillin, J. C. (1976). REM sleep induction by physostigmine infusion during sleep. *Science* **191**, 1281–3.

Sitaram, N., Moore, A. M. & Gillin, J. C. (1978). Induction and resetting of REM sleep rhythm in normal man by arecholine: blockade by scopolamine. *Sleep* **1**, 83–90.

Soldatos, C. R., Kales, J. D., Scharf, M. B., Bixler, E. O. & Kales, A. (1980). Cigarette smoking associated with sleep difficulty. *Science* **207**, 551–3.

Steriade, M. (1999). Cellular substrates of oscillations in corticothalamic systems during states of vigilance. In *Handbook of Behavioral State Control, Cellular and Molecular Mechanisms*, ed. R. Lydic & H. A. Baghdoyan, pp. 327–48. New York, NY: CRC Press.

Steriade, M. & McCarley, R. W. (2005). *Brainstem Control of Wakefulness and Sleep.* New York, NY: Kluwer Academic/Plenum Publishers.

Stevens, D. R., Birnstiel, S., Gerber, U., McCarley, R. W. & Greene, R. W. (1993). Nicotinic depolarizations of rat medial pontine reticular formation neurons studied in vitro. *Neuroscience* **57**, 419–24.

Stickgold, R., Hobson, J. A., Fosse, R. & Fosse, M. (2001). Sleep, learning, and dreams: off-line memory reprocessing. *Science* **294**, 1052–57.

Thakkar, M., Portas, C. & McCarley, R. W. (1996). Chronic low-amplitude electrical stimulation of the laterodorsal tegmental nucleus of freely moving cats increases REM sleep. *Brain Res.* **723**, 223–7.

Tononi, G. & Pompeiano, O. (1996). Pharmacology of the cholinergic system. In *The Pharmacology of Sleep*, ed. A. Kales, pp. 143–210. Berlin: Springer.

Vanni-Mercier, G., Sakai, K., Lin, J. S. & Jouvet, M. (1989). Mapping of cholinoceptive brainstem structures responsible for the generation of paradoxical sleep in the cat. *Arch. Ital. Biol.* **127**, 133–64.

Vazquez, J., Guzman-Marin, R., Salin-Pascual, R. J. & Drucker-Colin, R. (1996). Transdermal nicotine on sleep and PGO spikes. *Brain Res.* **737**, 317–20.

Velazquez-Moctezuma, J., Shalauta, M. D., Gillin, J. C. & Shiromani, P. J. (1990a). Microinjections of nicotine in the medial pontine reticular formation elicits REM sleep. *Neurosci. Lett.* **115**, 265–8.

Velazquez-Moctezuma, J., Shiromani, P. J. & Gillin, J. C. (1990b). Acetylcholine and acetylcholine receptor subtypes in REM sleep generation. *Prog. Brain Res.* **84**, 407–13.

Verret, L., Leger, L., Fort, P. & Luppi, P.-H. (2005). Cholinergic and noncholinergic brainstem neurons expressing Fos after paradoxical (REM) sleep deprivation and recovery. *Eur. J. Neurosci.* **21**, 2488–504.

Vincent, S. R., Satoh, K., Armstrong, D. M. & Fibiger, H. C. (1983). NADPH-diaphorase: a selective histochemical marker for the cholinergic neurons of the pontine reticular formation. *Neurosci. Lett.* **43**, 31–6.

Walder, B., Tramèr, M. R. & Blois, R. (2001). The effects of two single doses of tramadol on sleep: a randomized, cross-over trial in healthy volunteers. *Eur. J. Anaesthesiol.* **18**, 36–42.

Webster, H. H. & Jones, B. E. (1988). Neurotoxic lesions of the dorsolateral pontomesencephalic tegmentum-cholinergic cell area in the cat. II. Effects upon sleep-waking states. *Brain Res.* **458**, 285–302.

Wetzel, W., Wagner, T. & Balschun, D. (2003). REM sleep enhancement induced by different procedures improves memory retention in rats. *Eur. J. Neurosci.* **18**, 2611–17.

Whitehouse, P. J. (2004). Paying attention to acetylcholine: the key to wisdom and quality of life? *Prog. Brain Res.* **145**, 311–17.

Xi, M. C., Liu, R. H., Yamuy, J., Morales, F. R. & Chase, M. H. (1997). Electrophysiological properties of lumbar motoneurons in the alpha-chloralose-anesthetized cat during carbachol-induced motor inhibition. *J. Neurophysiol.* **78**, 129–36.

Yamamoto, K., Mamelak, A. N., Quattrochi, J. J. & Hobson, J. A. (1990). A cholinoceptive desynchronized sleep induction zone in the anterodorsal pontine tegmentum: locus of the sensitive region. *Neuroscience* **39**, 279–93.

Zhang, W., Basile, A. S., Gomeza, J. et al. (2002). Characterization of central inhibitory muscarinic autoreceptors by the use of muscarinic acetylcholine receptor knock-out mice. *J. Neurosci* **22**, 1709–17.

6

Histamine in the control of sleep–wakefulness

MAHESH M. THAKKAR AND ROBERT W. McCARLEY

Summary

Wakefulness is a prerequisite for survival and is accompanied by an ensemble of other behaviors. Thus, the brain contains multiple and grossly redundant systems controlling wakefulness: the histaminergic system is one of them. The histaminergic system in the central nervous system (CNS) is exclusively localized within the tuberomammillary nucleus (TMN). It consists of histamine-containing neurons that innervate almost all the major regions of the CNS, including the spinal cord. Within the CNS, histamine mediates its effects via three G-protein coupled metabotropic receptors: the H_1, H_2, and H_3 receptors. Of these three receptors, the H_3 receptor functions as an autoreceptor and regulates the synthesis and release of histamine. The histaminergic system, like other monoaminergic systems, is implicated in the regulation of sleep–wakefulness. It has been suggested that TMN neurons are under inhibitory control of the sleep-inducing ventrolateral preoptic GABAergic neurons and induce wakefulness by activating the wakefulness-promoting cholinergic neurons of the basal forebrain via the H_1 receptor. Although the bulk of evidence is derived from pharmacological studies, numerous electrophysiological and biochemical studies also support the role of histamine in wakefulness.

Electrophysiological evidence suggests that the histaminergic neurons, like other monoaminergic neurons, have their highest discharge during wakefulness. Biochemical evidence also suggests that histamine release in the TMN and other target regions is highest during wakefulness. There is a high correlation between the amount of c-*fos* activation in the TMN and the amount of wakefulness.

Neurochemistry of Sleep and Wakefulness, ed. J. M. Monti *et al.* Published by Cambridge University Press.
© Cambridge University Press 2008.

Histamine decarboxylase knockout mice are unable to produce histamine and these animals are unable to maintain wakefulness in a novel environment. Systemic or intraventricular administration of histamine or H_1 receptor agonists induces wakefulness whereas systemic or intraventricular administration of H_1 receptor antagonists induces sleep. Local administration of an H_3 receptor agonist in the TMN induces sleep whereas local administration of an H_3 receptor antagonist into the TMN induces wakefulness.

Introduction

Wakefulness is a behavioral manifestation of cortical activation that is characterized by the presence of high-frequency gamma and low-frequency theta activity in the electroencephalogram (EEG). This cortical activation (or desynchronization) is a result of a concerted increase in activity of multiple neuronal aggregates, utilizing multiple neurotransmitters and localized in various regions of the brain. These include the cholinergic neurons of the ponto-mesencephalic tegmentum and basal forebrain, the monoaminergic neurons localized in the brainstem and the posterior hypothalamus, and the recently discovered orexinergic neurons found in the perifornical lateral hypothalamus. While the cholinergic neurons increase their activity during both wakefulness and rapid eye movement (REM) sleep and are responsible for promoting cortical activation during wakefulness and REM sleep, the monoaminergic systems, namely the norepinephrine (NE)-containing neurons of the locus coeruleus (LC), the serotonin (5-HT)-containing neurons of the raphe nuclei (RN), and the histamine (HA)-containing neurons of the tuberomammillary nucleus (TMN), are unique in the sense that these groups of neurons increase their discharge during wakefulness and completely cease firing during REM sleep. It is believed that the monoaminergic systems act in concert to promote wakefulness and inhibit REM sleep (Steriade & McCarley, 1990, 2005; Jones, 2003). Out of these three monoaminergic groups, the histaminergic neurons of the TMN have been the least studied and are the focus of this review. The interested reader is encouraged to consult more detailed reviews on the other monoaminergic neurons and their role in sleep–wakefulness (Steriade & McCarley, 2005; Jones, 2003).

History

Histamine, or 2(4-imidazolylethylamine, was first identified in the CNS during the early years of the twentieth century. However, HA was first given the status of a "neurotransmitter" in the 1970s, after biochemical studies revealed the presence of the HA-synthesizing enzyme L-histidine decarboxylase (HDC) in the brain and electrophysiological studies demonstrated that HA could be released by depolarization (Schwartz *et al.*, 1991). The development of antibodies against HA and HDC revealed the presence of histaminergic neurons in mammalian brain. Subsequent electrophysiological and biochemical studies demonstrated the presence of four subclasses of HA receptor. During the past decade, the availability of numerous biochemical, pharmacological, and molecular tools to manipulate histaminergic transmission selectively has led to a significant advance in our understanding of the function of HA as a neurotransmitter. It is now believed that HA may be a critical regulator of various functions, including wakefulness and sleep.

Synthesis and metabolism in the CNS

There are two distinct pools of HA in the brain: (1) the neuronal pool and (2) the non-neuronal pool, mainly contributed by the mast cells. The turnover of HA in mast cells is slower than in neurons; it is believed that the HA contribution from the mast cells is limited and that almost all brain histaminergic actions are the result of HA released by neurons (Haas & Panula, 2003). The blood–brain barrier is impermeable to HA. HA in the brain is formed from L-histidine, an essential amino acid. HA synthesis occurs in two steps: (1) neuronal uptake of L-histidine by L-amino acid transporters; and (2) subsequent decarboxylation of L-histidine by a specific enzyme, L-histidine decarboxylase (E.C. 4.1.1.22). It appears that the availability of L-histidine is the rate-limiting step for the synthesis of HA. The enzyme HDC is selective for L-histidine and its activity displays circadian fluctuations (Orr & Quay, 1975). HA synthesis can be reduced by inhibition of the enzyme HDC. α-Fluoromethylhistidine (α-FMH) is an irreversible and a highly selective inhibitor of HDC; a single systemic injection of α-FMH (10–50 mg/kg) can produce up to 90% inhibition of HDC activity within 60–120 min (Monti, 1993). Once synthesized, HA is taken up into vesicles by the vesicular monoamine transporter and is stored until released.

HA turnover is rapid in the brain, with a half-life of about 30 min. This can change very quickly depending on neuronal activity. There is no high-affinity uptake system for HA; once released, HA is inactivated by catabolism. In the brain, released HA is methylated almost exclusively by the enzyme histamine-N-methyltransferase (E.C. 2.1.1.8). The *tele*-methyl-HA is subsequently degraded by monoamine oxidase-B (MAO-B) and aldehyde dehydrogenase to produce *tele*-methylimidazoleacetic acid (Brown *et al.*, 2001).

When compared with other monoamines, HA levels are low, with the highest levels seen in the hypothalamus and the lowest in the cerebellum. In addition, synthesis and release of HA is under circadian control. In rats, the average HA

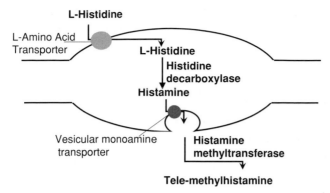

Figure 6.1 Histamine synthesis and metabolism in neurons. L-histidine is transported into neurons by the L-amino acid transporter. Once inside the neuron, L-histidine is converted into histamine by the specific enzyme histidine decarboxylase. Subsequently, histamine is taken up into vesicles by the vesicular monoamine transporter and stored there until released. In the absence of a high-affinity uptake mechanism in the brain, released histamine is rapidly degraded by histamine methyltransferase, which is located postsynaptically and in glia, to telemethylhistamine, a metabolite that does not show any histamine-like activity.

release during the dark period, when the animals are awake, is significantly higher than during the light period when the animals are inactive and sleeping (Mochizuki *et al.*, 1992; Monti, 1993; Orr & Quay, 1975).

Anatomical localization

HA research received a major boost after the development of antibodies against HA and HDC and the subsequent discovery of HA-containing neurons in the brain. The antibody against HA was developed by Panula and colleagues (Panula *et al.*, 1984). At about the same time, Watanabe and co-workers developed the antibody against HDC (Watanabe *et al.*, 1984). These studies showed that, in vertebrates, the HA-containing neurons are a restricted population of neurons localized within the TMN, which is a part of the posterior hypothalamus. The TMN (the name is derived from *tuber cinereum*, meaning a pale swelling) was named by Malone (Kohler *et al.*, 1985) and consists of several dense clusters of large, characteristic neurons, as well as scattered neurons with the same morphology and staining properties in the surrounding, more heterogenous regions. The TMN is located rostral to the mammillary bodies and caudal to the optic chiasm, forming the floor of the third ventricle in the posterior hypothalamus (Brown *et al.*, 2001).

The majority of TMN cells are large neurons (25–30 µm); small and medium-sized neurons are also present. Based on this morphological difference, Ericson and colleagues (Ericson *et al.*, 1987) divided the TMN nucleus into various subdivisions.

(1) the medial subgroup, situated on each side of the mammillary recess contains approximately 600 neurons.

(2) The ventral subgroup, situated at the ventral surface of the brain, rostral and caudal to the mammillary bodies, is the largest subgroup, containing approximately 2500 neurons (Kohler *et al.*, 1985). The ventral subgroup has fewer parvicellular neurons than the medial subgroup.

(3) The diffuse part of the TMN consists of a small group of neurons scattered within the lateral hypothalamic area, the posterior hypothalamic region, the perifornical area, the supramammillary nucleus, and the dorsomedial hypothalamic nucleus.

There is no evidence suggesting that these different subgroups have different projections and, therefore, the TMN is considered as a single functional unit of HA-containing neurons. Recently, however, HA-containing TMN neurons were shown to be functionally heterogeneous based on differential activation of c-*fos* gene expression following various acute stress stimuli (Miklos & Kovacs, 2003).

In addition to HA and its synthesizing machinery, some TMN neurons also contain GABA, glutamate decarboxylase (GAD, GABA-synthesizing enzyme), galanin, substance P, proenkephalin-derived peptides, and adenosine deaminase (i.e. the enzyme involved in the degradation of adenosine) (Yamamoto *et al.*, 1990; Kohler *et al.*, 1985; Patel *et al.*, 1986). While the functional significance of some of these co-localized neuroactive substances is unclear, the histaminergic neurons of the TMN, along with its projections, constitute a very extensive, far-reaching heterogenous system that could control and regulate several brain functions.

Projections of the TMN neurons

Although there are minor variations across different species with regard to target regions, TMN neurons target almost all the major regions of the CNS, including the spinal cord (Haas & Panula, 2003; Monti, 1993; Hough, 1988). The TMN efferent projections to the hypothalamus, diagonal band, septum, and olfactory bulb form the ventral ascending pathway, whereas TMN efferent projections innervating the thalamus, hippocampus, amygdala, and rostral forebrain form the dorsal ascending pathway. The descending TMN efferent projections are associated with the medial longitudinal fasciculus and innervate the brainstem and the spinal cord. Within the TMN there is no preferential localization of neuronal groups for any particular projections; in fact some neurons are known

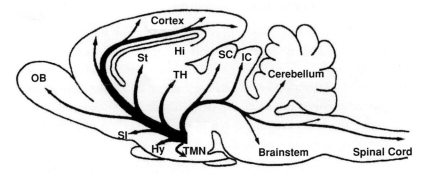

Figure 6.2 The location and distribution of the histamine-containing neurons in the brain. These neurons are localized in the tuberomammillary nucleus within the posterior hypothalamus and send projections throughout the brain. Abbreviations: Hi, hippocampus; Hy, hypothalamus; IC, inferior colliculus; OB, olfactory bulb; SC, superior colliculus; SI, substantia innominata; St, striatum; TH, thalamus; TMN, tuberomammillary nucleus. Adapted from Watanabe & Yanai (2001).

to send projections innervating both ascending and descending regions (Kohler *et al.*, 1985; Watanabe *et al.*, 1984; Wada *et al.*, 1991).

In all mammals, the highest density of histaminergic fibers is found in the hypothalamus, cerebral cortex, amygdala, and substantia nigra. The striatum, olfactory tubercle, and diagonal band receive moderate to dense histaminergic projections from the TMN (Kitahama *et al.*, 1984; Tago *et al.*, 1984; Panula *et al.*, 1993; Takagi *et al.*, 1986; Takeda *et al.*, 1984). The density of TMN projections to the hippocampus varies: the subiculum and dentate gyrus receive moderate to dense fibers, but the CA3 and CA1 regions are sparsely innervated. Similarly, TMN innervation to the thalamus is also variable, with the periventricular nuclei receiving moderate fiber innervation from the TMN. Within the brainstem, the TMN has moderate to dense projections to all the monoaminergic neuronal groups, the substantia nigra, superior colliculi, periaqueductal gray, nucleus of the trigeminal nerve, and nucleus tractus solitarius.

The histaminergic neurons have several well-developed primary and secondary dendrites that overlap with each other. Furthermore, long dendrites from histaminergic neurons located close to the mammillary recess or to the basal surface of the mammillary body appear to penetrate into the ependymal layer and make contact with cerebrospinal fluid. Thus, it is likely that neuroactive substances such as cytokines, present in the cerebrospinal fluid, may influence the discharge activity of TMN neurons (Wada *et al.*, 1991). Unlike the dopaminergic neurons, which are known to release dopamine from their dendrites, there is no evidence that these histaminergic dendrites store and/or release HA.

Afferents to histaminergic neurons

The histaminergic neurons of the TMN receive inputs from many different regions of the brain. The most prominent input sources to the TMN neurons are from the infralimbic cortex, lateral septum, and preoptic nucleus (Ericson *et al.*, 1991). The TMN also receives strong galanin and GABAergic inputs from the ventrolateral preoptic region (VLPO) (Sherin *et al.*, 1998). Galanin and GABAergic inputs from the VLPO are implicated in the suppression of TMN discharge during slow wave sleep, also termed non-REM (i.e. NREM) sleep. Other GABAergic inputs to the TMN also arise from the diagonal band of Broca and the lateral hypothalamus.

The perifornical lateral hypothalamus orexinergic neurons have reciprocal connections with TMN neurons (Peyron *et al.*, 1998). This is particularly important since orexin neurons are critical for behavioral state regulation (Mignot, 2004; Kilduff, 2001; Thakkar *et al.*, 2001) and disturbed orexin signaling causes narcolepsy (Lin *et al.*, 1999; Chemelli *et al.*, 1999; Thakkar *et al.*, 1999). Orexin neurons are known to innervate the entire brain and send dense projections to the monoaminergic neurons, including the TMN. A recent study suggests that the TMN histaminergic neurons are responsible for mediating the orexigenic effect of orexins (Jørgensen *et al.*, 2005).

Dopaminergic neurons of the ventral tegmental nucleus and the substantia nigra send scarce inputs to the TMN, and the major monoaminergic inputs to the TMN originate mainly from the epinephrinergic cell groups (C1–C3) (see Dahlstrom & Fuxe, 1964), norepinephrinergic cell groups (A1–A2) and serotoninergic cell groups (B5–B9) (Ericson *et al.*, 1989).

Physiology of histaminergic neurons

The electrophysiological properties of histaminergic neurons are very similar to those of other monoaminergic neurons. The discharge activity is spontaneous and regular. However, the discharge activity can change rapidly, depending on the behavioral state of the animal. Direct extracellular recordings of presumed histaminergic neurons in freely behaving cats and rats indicated a slow tonic and regular discharge during wakefulness that showed a gradual but significant decrease as the animal went from wakefulness to NREM sleep and a complete cessation of discharge during REM sleep (Vanni-Mercier *et al.*, 1984; Steininger *et al.*, 1999). Antidromic activation from the cerebral cortex displayed relatively slow conduction velocities, suggesting that the TMN neurons have unmyelinated axons. In urethane-anesthetized rats, spontaneous activity was slow and regular (2 Hz), with broad (4 ms) action potentials (Reiner et al., 1987).

In vitro electrophysiological studies also suggest that HA-containing TMN neurons are spontaneously active at the resting potential (−50 mV) with a broad-shouldered spike (mid-amplitude duration is c. 2 ms), primarily due to fast Na^+ and Ca^{2+} conductances and a deep (c. 15 mV) and long-lasting Ca^{2+}-independent afterhyperpolarization (AHP) (c. 450 ms duration). The latter returns the membrane potential to −80 mV (Haas & Reiner, 1988). The onset of an action potential is the result of a slow depolarizing potential mediated by a voltage-dependent Ca^{2+} current and a slow tetrodotoxin (TTX)-sensitive Na^+ current. The Ca^{2+} current is activated by the return to threshold following the afterhyperpolarization, whereas the Na^+ current appears to be persistent (Stevens et al., 2001). The spontaneous action potential is followed by an AHP, which is responsible for limiting the discharge activity. A fast transient K^+ outward current (A-type) with two components may be critical for membrane repolarization and, together with a hyperpolarization-activated current (I_h), provides the strong inward and outward rectifications, similar to those observed in other monoaminergic neurons (Greene et al., 1990; Haas & Panula, 2003).

Action of HA on TMN neurons

HA is known to inhibit HA-containing TMN neurons. This inhibition is mediated by the H_3 autoreceptors (Arrang et al., 1983) that are located on TMN cell somata, dendrites, and axonal varicosities. Originally discovered in 1983 (Arrang et al., 1983), the H_3 receptor is also known to regulate the release of other significant neurotransmitters, including acetylcholine, dopamine, glutamate, NE, and 5-HT (Brown et al., 1995; Schlicker et al., 1988, 1989, 1993; Clapham & Kilpatrick, 1992). Negatively coupled with cAMP, the H_3 autoreceptor inhibits Ca^{2+} current and provides the negative feedback controlling HA synthesis and release (Morisset et al., 2000; Drutel et al., 2001).

Action of other neurotransmitters and neuromodulators on TMN neurons

The TMN receives strong GABAergic input from the VLPO, DBB, and LH (Sherin et al., 1998; Yang & Hatton, 1997). Thus, it is not surprising that both $GABA_A$ and $GABA_B$ receptors are found on TMN neurons and that either one or both of these receptors together may be responsible for the GABA-mediated inhibition of TMN neurons (Stevens et al., 1999; Yang & Hatton, 1997). Furthermore, the VLPO galanin-containing neurons also send projections that inhibit TMN neurons (Sherin *et al.*, 1998; Schonrock *et al.*, 1991). Glycine is another important inhibitory neurotransmitter in the brain. Although glycine fibers are known to target TMN neurons (Rampon *et al.*, 1996) and glycine receptors are present on TMN neurons (Tamiya, 1991; Sato *et al.*, 1991; Araki *et al.*, 1988), in vitro studies indicate only a modest response of TMN neurons to glycine (Sergeeva *et al.*, 2001).

Glutamatergic AMPA (α-amino-3-hydroxy-5-methyl-4-isoxazolpropionic acid) and NMDA (*N*-methyl-D-aspartate) receptors are also found together with glutamatergic inputs from the LH (Yang & Hatton, 1997), although the physiological role of this excitation remains unclear (Haas & Panula, 2003).

There is clear evidence to indicate the presence of orexinergic projections to the TMN neurons; however, there is some controversy about the orexin receptor subtype present on TMN neurons. Although immunohistochemical techniques have suggested the presence of the orexin type I receptor on HA neurons (Backberg *et al.*, 2002), in situ hybridization studies indicated the presence of orexin type II receptors on histaminergic TMN neurons (Marcus *et al.*, 2001). However, irrespective of which subtype of orexin receptor is present on histaminergic TMN neurons, considerable evidence, from both in vivo and in vitro studies, suggests that orexins excite TMN neurons (Bayer *et al.*, 2001; Yamanaka *et al.*, 2002; Ishizuka *et al.*, 2002; Hong *et al.*, 2005; Eriksson *et al.*, 2001a). Dynorphin, which is co-localized with orexins in orexin neurons and may be co-released with orexins, has been suggested to suppress GABAergic inputs to the TMN, thus acting in concert with orexins to increase the excitability of TMN neurons (Eriksson *et al.*, 2004).

Although dopamine D_2 receptors are present on TMN neurons (Gurevich & Joyce, 1999), the role of dopamine in the TMN remains unknown. In contrast, 5-HT excites TMN neurons mainly by activation of Na^+/Ca^+ exchange mediated via the 5-HT$_{2C}$ receptor (Sergeeva *et al.*, 2003; Eriksson *et al.*, 2001b). Although NE has no direct effect on the membrane properties of TMN neurons, NE is shown to inhibit indirectly the GABA input onto TMN neurons via α_2 receptors, thereby exciting, or disinhibiting, TMN neurons (Stevens *et al.*, 2004).

TMN neurons are known to express α-bungartoxin-sensitive nicotinic receptors, predominantly of the α7 subtype. Although the origin of cholinergic innervation to the TMN is unclear (Uteshev *et al.*, 1996; Haas & Panula, 2003), cholinergic neurons of the mesopontine tegmentum are the most likely candidates for this innervation of the TMN. Similarly, although there is no evidence of purinergic transmission, ATP excites TMN neurons, mainly through the non-selective P_{2X} receptor (Vorobjev *et al.*, 2003; Furukawa *et al.*, 1994).

One of the distinctive features of TMN neurons is that they contain high levels of adenosine deaminase, a key enzyme involved in deamination of adenosine, a mediator of homeostatic sleep regulation (Thakkar *et al.*, 2003a, b).

Adenosine has no direct effect on TMN neurons (Haas & Panula, 2003); however, indirectly, adenosine, acting via adenosine A1 receptors, presynaptically inhibits the GABAergic input to TMN neurons.

HA receptors

HA receptors are classified into 4 subtypes: H_1, H_2, H_3, and H_4 (Hill et al., 1997). All four HA receptor types are metabotropic receptors and belong to the superfamily of G-protein coupled receptors. Ionotropic HA receptors are found in invertebrates (Hardie, 1989; Gisselmann et al., 2002) but are absent from vertebrates (Haas & Panula, 2003). Of the four HA receptors, only the H_1, H_2, and H_3 receptors are found in brain. The recently discovered H_4 receptor is predominantly present on leukocytes and may have a critical role in the immune system (Nguyen et al., 2001; Bakker, 2004; Haas & Panula, 2003).

The H_1 receptor

The H_1 receptor is a typical G protein-coupled metabotropic receptor (c. 490 amino acids) with seven putative transmembrane domains (Yamashita et al., 1991). Encoded from the intronless region on human chromosome 3, the H_1 receptor is coupled to phospholipase C through a pertussis-toxin-insensitive ($G_{q/11}$) G protein (Leurs et al., 2002). Stimulation of the H_1 receptor primarily leads to the activation of a second messenger signal cascade involving phospolipase C-mediated hydrolysis of phosphatidylinositol-4,5-bisphosphate into two different second messengers: (1) inositol-1,4,5-trisphosphate that mobilizes Ca^{2+} from intracellular stores; and (2) diacylglycerol, which activates protein kinase C. In addition, H_1 receptor activation leads to the formation of cGMP and two retrograde messengers, including nitric oxide and arachidonic acid (Richelson, 1978; Leurs et al., 1994). However, H_1 receptor-mediated presynaptic modulation is yet to be demonstrated. The H_1 receptor is known to potentiate the actions of G_s-coupled receptors, including adenosine A_2 and HA H_2 receptors (Daum et al., 1982; Leurs et al., 1994). Recent evidence suggests that brief exposure to HA may lead to internalization of the H_1 receptor, thereby attenuating the excitatory effects (Self et al., 2005).

The H_1 receptor is widely distributed throughout the brain. Receptor binding with the H_1 receptor antagonist [^{3}H] mepyramine in rat brain revealed that the highest levels of H_1 receptors are present in the hypothalamus (Tran et al., 1978; Palacios et al., 1981). High to moderate levels are seen in the cortex, cholinergic zones of the BF, bed nucleus of the stria terminalis, amygdala, thalamus, midbrain, and brainstem, especially in the cholinergic zone of the mesopontine tegmentum. Within the hippocampus, a high to moderate concentration of H_1

receptors is seen in several areas including the molecular layer of CA3, the hilus of the dentate gyrus, and the subiculum (Palacios et al., 1981). Moderate to low levels are observed in the LC, RN, and nucleus pontis oralis (Palacios et al., 1981).

In most cases, stimulation of the H_1 receptor leads to excitation, caused by depolarization or an increase in discharge frequency. However, several mechanisms are responsible for H_1-mediated excitation. In many neurons, activation of the H_1 leads to a reduction of a background voltage-independent "leakage" potassium current that is responsible for maintaining resting membrane potential (McCormick & Williamson, 1991; Reiner & Kamondi, 1994; Munakata & Akaike, 1994). Other mechanisms include activation of TTX-insensitive Na^+ channels (Gorelova & Reiner, 1996) in septal neurons, and activation of mixed cation channels in raphe neurons. Activation of the H_1 receptor is also reported to increase the number of gap junctions and increase c-fos expression in supraoptic neurons (Hatton & Yang, 1996; Vizuete et al., 1995).

The H₂ receptor

The H_2 receptor is the second class of HA receptors. This is another G-protein-coupled receptor but, unlike the H_1 receptor, the H_2 receptor is coupled to adenylyl cyclase via the GTP-binding G_s protein (Hill et al., 1997). Encoded by an intronless gene and located on human chromosome 5, the H_2 receptor is made up of c. 358 amino acids (Gantz et al., 1991; Traiffort et al., 1995). Activation of the H_2 receptor causes an accumulation of cAMP and activation of protein kinase A that eventually leads to the activation of cyclic-AMP-response element (CRE)-binding protein (CREB) (Hill et al., 1997). In neurons, the H_2 receptor mediates its excitatory effects by blocking the Ca^{2+}-dependent K^+ channel (Haas & Konnerth, 1983).

The localization of the H_2 receptor protein and its messenger RNAs was based on autoradiography using [^{125}I]iodoaminopotentidine, a selective H_2 receptor antagonist, for radioligand binding and a ^{33}P-labeled complementary RNA probe for in situ hybridization (Traiffort et al., 1992; Vizuete et al., 1997). Like that of the H_1 receptor, the distribution of the H_2 receptor in the brain is widespread. High to medium receptor densities are observed in the cerebral cortex, hippocampus, basal ganglia, amygdala, bed nucleus of stria terminalis, substantia nigra, superior colliculus, ventral tegmental area, and inferior olive (Vizuete et al., 1997). Medium to low densities are observed in the thalamus, substantia innominata, posterior hypothalamus, LC, RN, TMN, inferior colliculus, pontine nuclei, and solitary tract nucleus.

Stimulation of the H_2 receptor leads to blockade of a Ca^{2+}-dependent K^+ current through the small K^+ channel, thus causing a spike frequency adaptation (i.e. an accommodation of firing) and slow afterhyperpolarization

(Haas & Konnerth, 1983; Haas, 1984; Haas & Greene, 1986; Greene & Haas, 1990). Inhibition of protein kinase A prevents the effects of H_2-mediated HA on accommodation of firing and long-lasting afterhyperpolarization (Pedarzani & Storm, 1993). Other actions mediated by the H_2 receptor include (1) presynaptic facilitation of NE release in cortical neurons (Timm *et al.*, 1998), (2) depolarization via a direct action of cAMP, independent of protein kinase A, on a cation current (I_q or I_h) in hippocampal pyramidal cells (Pedarzani & Storm, 1995), (3) depolarization by acting in synergy with the H_1 receptor and reducing K^+ conductance (Munakata & Akaike, 1994), (4) excitation of local GABAergic interneurons (Haas & Greene, 1986; Greene & Haas, 1990), and (5) excitation of LC neurons by acting synergistically with H_1 receptors, although the exact mechanism has yet to be elucidated (Korotkova *et al.*, 2005).

The H_3 receptor

The third HA receptor functions as an autoreceptor and regulates the synthesis and release of HA. Identified initially in 1983 (Arrang *et al.*, 1983), this receptor is linked to pertussis toxin-sensitive $G_{i/o}$ protein and high-threshold Ca^+ channels. The H_3 receptor is encoded from a single gene on chromosome 20 in humans. However, unlike most G-protein-coupled receptors that are encoded from one exon, the human H_3 receptor gene consists of four exons and three introns (Tardivel-Lacombe *et al.*, 2000). Thus, occurrence of alternative splicing at various exon–intron junctions in the H_3 receptor gene leads to the existence of various functional and non-functional isoforms, of which three functional isoforms are known, each with distinct CNS expression profiles and each coupled differentially to adenylate cyclase and the mitogen-activated protein kinase signaling pathway (Drutel *et al.*, 2001). Analysis of the protein sequence revealed that the H_3 receptor consists of *c.* 450 amino acids with minor, yet significant, species differences that produce significant pharmacological heterogeneity (Hancock *et al.*, 2003). The H_3 receptor has low sequence homology with other G-protein-coupled receptors, including the H_1 and H_2 receptors (Lovenberg *et al.*, 1999). Although all HA receptors show constitutive signaling in heterologous expression systems (Lefkowitz *et al.*, 1993; Bakker *et al.*, 2000; Smit *et al.*, 1996), the H_3 receptor is unique because a high constitutive signaling activity is also observed in animals expressing normal levels of receptors (Rouleau *et al.*, 2002; Morisset *et al.*, 2000).

Autoradiographic studies with $[^3H]R$-(α)-methylhistamine have demonstrated the presence of high to moderate levels of H_3 receptor binding in almost all layers of the cerebral cortex, striatum, bed nuclei of the stria terminalis, substantia nigra, amygdala, olfactory nucleus, hippocampus, and hypothalamus, especially on the cell somata, dendrites, and axonal varicosities of HA-containing TMN neurons (Pollard *et al.*, 1993; Arrang *et al.*, 1987a, b). In situ hybridization studies with selective oligonucleotide probes targeted to recognize specifically different H_3 receptor isoform mRNAs revealed that all three isoforms were expressed in TMN neurons. However, other brain regions had differential expression of H_3 receptor isoforms. The functional relevance of this differential distribution remains unknown.

The activation of H_3 receptors not only controls the release of HA but also suppresses multiple Ca^{2+} channels including the high-voltage-activated N- and P-types that lead to a reduction in the discharge activity of TMN neurons (Takeshita *et al.*, 1998). In addition, stimulation of the H_3 receptor inhibits the release of various other neurotransmitters, including glutamate, 5-HT, NE, ACh, and dopamine (Schlicker *et al.*, 1988, 1989, 1993; Brown & Haas, 1999; Clapham & Kilpatrick, 1992), most likely by a $G_{i/o}$-mediated inhibition of high-voltage Ca^{2+} channels (Brown & Haas, 1999; Brown *et al.*, 2001).

HA and behavior

We have focused this chapter on the role of HA in the control of sleep–wakefulness. However, the CNS histaminergic system has been implicated in the regulation of a wide range of behavioral and physiological functions, including sleep–wakefulness, entrainment of circadian rhythms, motor activity, thermoregulation, learning and memory, stress, aggression, pain perception, self-stimulation, reinforcement, aversion, and regulation of blood pressure. There are excellent reviews, to which an interested reader is referred (White & Rumbold, 1988; Timmerman, 1989; Monti, 1993; Schwartz *et al.*, 1991; Brown *et al.*, 2001; Haas & Panula, 2003; Ohtsu & Watanabe, 2003; Fukui, 2005).

HA and sleep–wakefulness

The hypothesis of the role of HA in wakefulness stems from the observation that administration of the classical antihistamines (i.e. H_1 receptor antagonists) induced sedation. These first-generation antihistamines, used to treat inflammatory reactions, could cross the blood–brain barrier and block the central H_1 receptor (White & Rumbold, 1988). The first study examining the effect of antihistamines on sleep–wakefulness in cats reported an increase in NREM sleep and a decrease in REM sleep (Jewett, 1968). Similar results were also obtained in dogs (Wauquier *et al.*, 1981) and humans (Risberg *et al.*, 1975; Bassano & Caille, 1979; Nicholson *et al.*, 1985; Adam & Oswald, 1986). Intraventricular application of HA in the anesthetized rat caused a dose-dependent decrease in the duration of narcosis, whereas intraventricular application of HA in conscious animals produced classical signs of wakefulness, including EEG desynchronization, increased grooming, and exploratory behavior (Monnier et al., 1967; Kalivas, 1982; Monnier & Hatt, 1969; Wolf & Monnier, 1973). Pretreatment with H_1 receptor antagonists blocked these effects of HA, whereas H_2 antagonists had no effect (Kalivas, 1982). In addition, HA synthesis, release, and degradation were found to peak and ebb in a circadian fashion (Friedman & Walker, 1969; Orr & Quay, 1975) with high correlation with the behavioral state of the animals. These initial findings implicated HA, mediated via the central H_1 receptor, in the modulation of behavioral and cortical arousal.

Parallel research implicated the posterior hypothalamus, the region where histaminergic neurons were subsequently found, in the generation of arousal (Monti, 1993; Brown et al., 2001; Saper et al., 2001). Von Economo first observed that lesion of the posterior hypothalamus produced sleep (Von Economo, 1930, cited in Saper et al., 2001). Subsequently, numerous studies have demonstrated that experimental lesion of the posterior hypothalamus produces a state of somnolence and hypersomnia in rats, cats, and monkeys. Thus, bilateral lesions in the area of the mammillary bodies induced somnolence in monkeys (Ranson, 1939, cited in Monti, 1993). Bilateral transections of the posterior hypothalamus reduced wakefulness in rats (Nauta, 1946, cited in Monti, 1993). Localized and reversible inactivation by cooling the posterior hypothalamus induced behavioral sleep in rats (Naquet et al., 1966). Bilateral electrolytic lesions of the posterior hypothalamus and subthalamic region produced a continuous sleep-like state for more than one day in rats (McGinty, 1969). Similar results were also obtained when the posterior hypothalamus was lesioned in cats (Swett & Hobson, 1968).

These initial studies suggested that the posterior hypothalamus may contain a "wakefulness center" and provided the initial impetus to pursue further research to understand the role of HA and the posterior hypothalamus in sleep–wakefulness. The next cycle of research substantiating the role of HA in sleep–wakefulness consisted mainly of electrophysiological, biochemical/molecular, and pharmacological studies.

Electrophysiological studies

Several studies have examined the discharge activity of neurons in the posterior hypothalamus across sleep–wakefulness. Extracellular single-unit recordings of presumed histaminergic neurons performed in naturally sleeping, freely behaving cats (Vanni-Mercier et al., 1984; Sakai et al., 1990) revealed that these neurons displayed a typical discharge pattern that was characteristic of the monoaminergic LC and RN neurons: slow tonic discharge during wakefulness, reduced discharge during NREM sleep, and complete cessation during REM sleep, with resumption of firing in anticipation of wakefulness. These neurons were referred to as REM-off neurons. In addition, these REM-off neurons displayed long-duration action potentials and a slow conduction velocity, suggesting that they had unmyelinated axons, another characteristic of histaminergic neurons. Similar results were also obtained in urethane-anesthetized (Reiner & McGeer, 1987), and freely behaving rats (Steininger et al., 1999).

Biochemical and molecular studies

These studies could be categorized into three types: (1) Measurement of HA release and turnover, (2) measurement of c-Fos protein as a marker of neuronal activation, and (3) measurement of sleep–wakefulness in HDC knockout mice that cannot synthesize HA.

Measurement of HA release and turnover

The histaminergic system appears to be under strong circadian control. Thus, HA turnover undergoes circadian changes with peaks in the brain coinciding with the period of arousal. Indirect measurements of HA have been performed by measuring tissue levels of HA metabolites including tele-N-methylhistamine and tele-methylimidazoleacetic acid, but direct measurements of HA release have also been obtained in vivo by using techniques that include microdialysis sampling and push–pull cannula.

Using in vivo microdialysis sampling, Mochizuki and colleagues (Mochizuki et al., 1992) measured HA release from the anterior hypothalamic area, a region with a high concentration of histaminergic fibers, in freely behaving rats under a normal 12:12 h light:dark cycle. They found that HA release increased during the second half of the light period, in anticipation of wakefulness, and peaked during the dark period when the rats were generally awake and active (Mochizuki et al., 1992). The push–pull cannula technique was used by Prast et al. (1992) to measure HA release from the posterior hypothalamus in freely moving rats. They also found HA release to peak during the dark period (Prast et al., 1992). Diurnal variations in the levels of HA metabolites, with the peak appearing during the daytime, were also observed in the cerebrospinal fluid of rhesus monkeys (Prell et al., 1989) and human children (Kiviranta et al., 1994).

Microdialysis sampling coupled with radioenzymatic assay was used by Strecker and colleagues (Strecker et al., 2002) to measure extracellular HA release from the preoptic/anterior hypothalamus area of cats across the sleep–wakefulness cycle, sleep deprivation, and recovery sleep. There was a significant fluctuation of HA release across sleep–wakefulness, with highest levels during wakefulness followed by NREM sleep and the lowest level during REM sleep. However, HA release during 6 h of sleep deprivation was comparable to that during

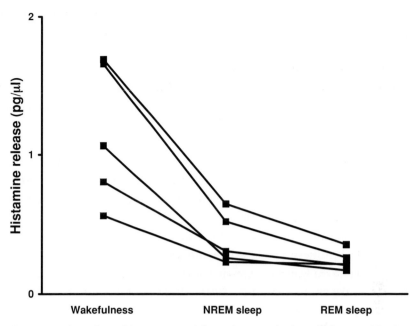

Figure 6.3 Histamine release measured from the posterior hypothalamus of freely behaving cats across the sleep–wakefulness cycle. The histamine release was higher during wakefulness compared with non-REM and REM sleep in each experiment, producing a highly significant group effect. Each experiment is represented by a single line ($n = 5$). Adapted from Strecker *et al.* (2002), to which the reader is referred for more details.

wakefulness and did not show any significant changes. These results suggested that HA may not relay information about sleep drive to the sleep-promoting neurons of the VLPO.

Measurement of c-Fos protein as a marker of neuronal activation

Since its discovery in the 1980s, expression of immediate-early gene c-*fos* and subsequent accumulation of c-Fos protein have often been used as evidence for neuronal activation (Morgan *et al.*, 1987; Hughes & Dragunow, 1995; Sagar *et al.*, 1988). Although the link between c-Fos accumulation and neuronal activation is indirect, c-*fos* expression is known to vary in different brain regions across spontaneous sleep–wakefulness (Pompeiano *et al.*, 1995; Cirelli & Tononi, 2000) and these changes are taken as surrogate markers for neuronal activity. Numerous recent studies have reported a high correlation between c-*fos* expression in the TMN and the amount of wakefulness.

Systemic administration of an H_3 receptor antagonist, ciproxifan (1 mg/kg in 0.2 ml, i.m.), induced c-*fos* expression in the vast majority of HA-immunoreactive neurons in the TMN (Vanni-Mercier *et al.*, 2003). Systemic administration of the anesthetics pentobarbital (100 mg/kg) and propofol (140 mg/kg) reduced c-Fos protein in the TMN when compared with saline controls. Similar results were also obtained with systemic administration of muscimol (10 mg/kg), a $GABA_A$ receptor agonist, and dexmedetomidine (500 μg/kg), an α_2 receptor agonist (Nelson *et al.*, 2002, 2003). However, it is important to note that neither sleep–wakefulness nor EEG was measured in these studies.

Infusion of prostaglandin D_2 (200 pmol/min) or the adenosine A_{2a} receptor agonist CGS21680 (20 pmol/min) for 2 h into the subarachnoid space under the BF, during the dark period, increased NREM sleep and reduced c-Fos protein in the TMN of rats when compared with saline-treated controls (Scammell *et al.*, 1998, 2001). In contrast, infusion of the adenosine A_1 receptor agonist N6-cyclopentyl-adenosine (2 pmol/min) in the same area did not have any effect on sleep–wakefulness or c-*fos* expression in the TMN.

In a recent study, c-*fos* expression was examined in TMN neurons in spontaneously awake animals (Ko *et al.*, 2003). These authors reported a strong correlation between c-*fos* expression in the TMN and the amount of wakefulness independent of the circadian cycle. In rats maintained on a normal 12:12 light:dark cycle, wakefulness was increased and c-*fos* expression was also increased in the TMN during the dark period relative to the light period. In rats maintained in constant darkness, increased wakefulness and increased c-Fos protein in the TMN were observed during the subjective night, irrespective of the lighting condition.

Measurement of sleep–wakefulness in HDC knockout mice

To evaluate the role of HA in the CNS, Ohtsu *et al.*, (2001) developed mice lacking the HA-synthesizing enzyme HDC. These HDC knockout (HDC$^{-/-}$) mice showed an absence of HA synthesis and were deficient in HA (Watanabe & Yanai, 2001). The HDC$^{-/-}$ mice appeared less reactive when handled, and had increased body mass. However, their general morphology and circadian sleep–wakefulness rhythm appeared normal. Spontaneous wakefulness or NREM sleep was not changed in HDC$^{-/-}$ mice, although REM sleep showed a significant increase, especially during the light period. The increase is REM sleep was primarily due to an increased number of REM episodes; mean REM sleep episode duration and latency to REM sleep were not changed in HDC$^{-/-}$ mice. The HDC$^{-/-}$ mice also exhibited increased delta and reduced theta power during wakefulness, an attenuated ability to anticipate darkness, as manifested by shorter bouts of wakefulness during the dark period, and an attenuated response to new environments, as manifested by indifference and unresponsiveness when placed in novel surroundings (Parmentier *et al.*, 2002).

Pharmacological studies

Most of the evidence supporting a role for HA in the control of wakefulness is derived from pharmacological studies. For ease of reference, these studies are divided into subgroups and detailed below.

Pharmacological manipulation of HA synthesis and degradation and its effects on sleep–wakefulness

Blockade of HA synthesis by intraperitoneal (i.p.) administration of α-FMH (100 mg/kg) during the light or inactive period in the rat resulted in decreased wakefulness during this period and increased NREM sleep during the dark or active period (Kiyono *et al.*, 1985). Monti and colleagues (Monti *et al.*, 1988) found similar results with systemic administration of a lower dose of α-FMH (50 mg/kg) in rats. They reported a significant reduction in wakefulness and increases in both NREM and REM sleep during the light period when the rats were housed under normal 12:12 h light:dark conditions. However, when the rats were housed under 16:8 h light:dark conditions, enhanced wakefulness was observed during the dark period (Monti *et al.*, 1988).

A significant decrease in wakefulness with a concomitant increase in NREM sleep was also seen with systemic (20 mg/kg) or local application of α-FMH (50 μg in 1 μl) in the TMN region of cats. Although the sleep-inducing effect of α-FMH began 8 h after systemic administration and lasted for one day (Lin *et al.*, 1988), the sleep-inducing effect appeared within 2 h of local application and its most prominent effect lasted for 9 h. In contrast, local microinjections of SKF-91488 (50 μg in 1 μl), a specific inhibitor of the catabolic enzyme HMT, produced an immediate increase in wakefulness, with a concomitant decrease in NREM and REM sleep that lasted for 6 h (Lin *et al.*, 1986).

Administration of HA and its effect on sleep–wakefulness

Local application of HA (5, 30 and 60 pg) in the TMN region of cats increased the latency to sleep, increased arousal, and reduced NREM sleep in a site-specific, dose-dependent manner. The highest dose produced the maximal effect, which lasted for 6 h. The HA-induced arousal was completely blocked when the cats were pretreated intraperitoneally with the H_1 receptor antagonist mepyramine (Lin *et al.*, 1986, 1988). In rats, intraventricular administration of HA blocked the increase in delta and theta activity (0–6 Hz) in the EEG induced by repeated low-frequency stimulation of the midbrain reticular formation. This effect was blocked if specific thalamic nuclei were lesioned (Tasaka *et al.*, 1993) or by simultaneous administration of an H_1 receptor antagonist, but not by an H2 receptor antagonist (Tasaka *et al.*, 1989). Application of HA

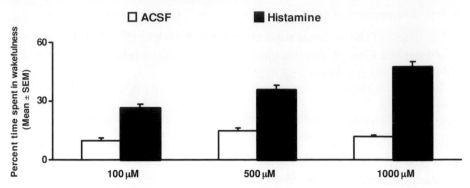

Figure 6.4 Microdialysis perfusion of histamine into the cholinergic zone of the basal forebrain increases wakefulness in a dose-dependent fashion. The animals spent almost half of their time in wakefulness during the 2 h period of perfusion of the highest dose (1,000 μM). In contrast, approximately 12% of the time was spent in wakefulness during the 2 h perfusion period of artificial CSF (i.e. the control day). Adapted from Ramesh *et al.* (2004).

in other regions also produced similar results. Local application of HA, either by microinjection or by reverse microdialysis, into the pontine tegmentum of cats induced a dose-dependent increase in wakefulness (Lin *et al.*, 1996). Similar results were also obtained when HA was applied locally in the preoptic region of cats (Lin *et al.*, 1994). In both the above studies, the HA-induced wakefulness was attenuated if the animals were pretreated with the H_1 receptor antagonist mepyramine.

In a recent study, Ramesh *et al.* (2004) applied different concentrations of HA (100, 500, and 1000 μM) by reverse microdialysis to the cholinergic zone of the basal forebrain of rats. They found that HA produced a site-specific, dose-dependent increase in wakefulness and a concomitant decrease in NREM sleep. REM sleep did not change. The increase in wakefulness was so marked that during administration of the highest dose of HA (1000 μM) the animals spent almost half the time in wakefulness. In contrast, during control (ACSF) perfusion, only 12% of the time was spent in wakefulness. These data suggest that cholinergic neurons of the basal forebrain are important in the histaminergic induction of wakefulness and cortical arousal.

Administration of H_1 receptor agonists or antagonists and their effect on sleep–wakefulness

Systemic administration of the H_1 receptor antagonists pyrilamine and diphenhydramine decreased wakefulness and increased NREM sleep in rats (Monti *et al.*, 1986); conversely, intracerebroventricular application of the

H_1-receptor agonist 2-thiazolylethylamine dose-dependently increased wakefulness and decreased both NREM sleep and REM sleep. Furthermore, the H_1 receptor antagonist pyrilamine blocked the wakefulness-inducing effects of the H_1-receptor agonist 2-thiazolylethylamine (Monti et al., 1986).

Similar results were obtained in cats. Intraperitoneal injections of the H_1 receptor antagonist mepyramine (1 and 5 mg/kg) dose-dependently increased NREM sleep and decreased wakefulness, REM sleep, and the latency to sleep within 1 h of injection (Lin et al., 1988). Similarly, local application of mepyramine (120 μg in 1 μl) into the TMN region increased NREM sleep, with a concomitant decrease in wakefulness within 1 h of injection. However, unlike the systemic injection, the latency to sleep remained unchanged and REM sleep was significantly increased following local injection of mepyramine in the TMN region (Lin et al., 1988).

A single oral dose of diphenhydramine (50 or 75 mg), an H_1 receptor antagonist, given at bedtime to normal human subjects did not have any effect on subjective sleep parameters, although motor activity tended to increase during the drug nights (Borbely & Youmbi-Balderer, 1988). However, diphenhydramine, an H_1 receptor antagonist, dose-dependently improved various sleep parameters in insomniac patients (Rickels et al., 1983; Kudo & Kurihara, 1990).

Local administration of the H_1 agonist 2-thiazolylethylamine (50 μg in 0.5 μl) into the pontine tegmentum increased wakefulness and reduced NREM sleep during the first 3 h after injection. In contrast, local application of mepyramine (5 μg in 0.25 μl) caused a decrease in wakefulness and an increase in NREM sleep.

Administration of H_2 receptor agonists or antagonists and their effects on sleep–wakefulness

Administration of H_2-receptor agonists and antagonists in rats had no effect on sleep–wakefulness (Monti et al., 1986, 1990). Although local application of impromidine (1 μg in 1 μl), an H_2 receptor agonist, into the preoptic region of the cat mimicked the effects of HA in inducing wakefulness, local application of impromidine (0.2 μg in 0.25 μl) in the pontine tegmentum had little effect.

Administration of H_3 receptor agonists or antagonists and their effects on sleep-wakefulness

The H_3 receptor functions as an autoreceptor, and its activation leads to a reduction in HA release. Lin and colleagues (1990) studied the effects of H_3 receptor ligands on sleep–wakefulness in cats and found that blockade of the H_3 receptor by oral administration of thioperamide produced a dose-dependent and long-lasting increase in wakefulness. The highest dose (10 mg/kg) produced a

60% increase in wakefulness for almost 10 h (Lin *et al.*, 1990). The arousing effects of thioperamide were prevented by pretreatment with (R)α-methylhistamine (20 mg/kg) or mepyramine (1 mg/kg). In contrast, oral administration of (R)α-methylhistamine to cats enhanced NREM sleep in a dose dependent manner. The highest dose of (R)α-methylhistamine (20 mg/kg) produced a 58% increase in NREM sleep that lasted for 6 h (Lin *et al.*, 1990).

Although systemic administration of thioperamide in rats induced a dose-dependent increase in wakefulness with a concomitant reduction in NREM and REM sleep, systemic administration of (R)α-methylhistamine had no effect (Monti *et al.*, 1991). In contrast, bilateral application of (R)α-methylhistamine into the TMN region of rats increased NREM sleep with a concomitant decrease in wakefulness and REM sleep. The NREM-sleep-inducing effect of (R)α-methylhistamine was attenuated if the rats were pretreated with thioperamide (4.0 mg/kg) (Monti *et al.*, 1991).

Oral administration of the H_3 receptor agonist BP 2.94 (20–30 mg/kg) to rats produced a dose-dependent increase in NREM sleep without a significant change in wakefulness or REM sleep. With the highest dose of BP 2.94 (30 mg/kg), the increase in NREM sleep was observed during the second hour and the effect lasted for 6 h. Pretreatment with the H_3 receptor antagonist carboperamide (30 mg/kg) prevented the sleep-inducing effects of BP 2.94. In contrast, oral administration of carboperamide (20–30 mg/kg) produced a dose-dependent increase in wakefulness with a concomitant decrease in NREM and REM sleep (Monti *et al.*, 1996).

In guinea pigs, oral administration (10 mg/kg) of SCH50971, a novel H_3 receptor agonist, depressed locomotor activity and increased total sleep time (McLeod *et al.*, 1998). Similar results were also obtained after oral administration of the H_3 receptor agonist BP 2.94 in the cat (Lin, 2000). In contrast, oral administration of ciproxifan (0.15–2 mg/kg), an H_3 receptor antagonist, induced wakefulness in cats (Ligneau *et al.*, 1998). However, in another study (Lamberty *et al.*, 2003) no major change in sleep–wakefulness was reported following intraperitoneal injections of immepip (5 or 10 mg/kg), also an H_3 receptor agonist, in rats, although cortical HA release was significantly reduced.

In order to explore the importance of the H_3 receptor in sleep–wakefulness, Toyota *et al.* (2002) compared the wake-promoting effects of the H_3 receptor antagonist thioperamide in wild-type and H_3 receptor KO mice. In wild-type mice, subcutaneous administration of thioperamide (10 mg/kg) increased wakefulness with a concomitant decrease in NREM sleep during the first 2 h after administration at lights-on. REM sleep was unaffected. In contrast, thioperamide had no effect on sleep–wakefulness in H_3 receptor KO mice (Toyota *et al.*, 2002).

Vanni-Mercier and colleagues (Vanni-Mercier *et al.*, 2003) investigated the pharmacological effects of H_3 receptor ligands on the discharge activity of presumed

TMN histaminergic neurons recorded in freely behaving cats. These wakefulness-on neurons had broad action potentials and exhibited a slow, regular tonic discharge activity. The firing rate peaked during active wakefulness, showed a significant decrease as the cats went from wakefulness to sleep, and was almost zero during REM sleep. Intramuscular injection of ciproxifan (1 mg/kg) induced a significant increase in the discharge activity of these wakefulness-selective neurons, although the neurons maintained their tonic, regular discharge. This effect was observed within 15 min of the injection of ciproxifan and lasted for 2 h. The EEG displayed all the signs of wakefulness including cortical activation and suppression of spindles and slow wave activity. Local application of α-MHA ((R)α-methylhistamine), an H_3 receptor agonist, into the TMN reversed the action of ciproxifan. In contrast, systemic injection of imetit (S-[2–4-(imidazolyl)ethyl]isothiourea), an H_3 receptor agonist (1 mg/kg, i.m.) produced a significant decrease in the discharge activity of the TMN wakefulness-active neurons. This effect was observed within 30 min of the injection and lasted for 3 h. Behaviorally, the animals appeared drowsy and the EEG showed an increase in cortical spindles and slow waves. The imetit-induced reduction in discharge activity was reversed by intramuscular injection of ciproxifan. Local administration of α-MHA (0.025–0.1 μg in 0.2 μl) into the TMN produced a dose-dependent decrease in the discharge activity of the TMN wakefulness-active neurons without affecting the behavior of the animal. The highest dose (0.1 μg in 0.2 μl) produced a complete cessation of discharge within 30 min of the injection (Vanni-Mercier et al., 2003).

Barbier et al. (2004) investigated the effects of a highly selective and novel non-imidazole H_3 receptor antagonist, 1, 1-[4-(3-piperidin-1-yl-propoxy)-benzyl]-piperidine (JNJ-5207852), on sleep and wakefulness in mice and rats. Systemic injections of JNJ-5207852 (1–10 mg/kg, s.c.) increased the time spent in wakefulness with a concomitant decrease in NREM and REM sleep in both mice and rats. The overall increase in wakefulness was due to an increase in the number of wakefulness bouts. Spectral analysis of the EEG also revealed a reduction in total delta power following systemic injections of this compound (Barbier et al., 2004).

Inactivation or lesion of the TMN and its effect on sleep–wakefulness

Inactivation of the ventrolateral posterior hypothalamus, which lies in and around the TMN, by local application of muscimol (0.1–1.0 μg in 0.5 μl), a potent GABA agonist, induced prolonged behavioral and EEG signs of NREM sleep, followed by a significant increase in REM sleep. Systemic administration of p-chlorophenylalanine (PCPA), a potent serotonin synthesis inhibitor, produces a long-lasting insomnia; local administration of muscimol in this region to cats rendered insomniac in this way induced both NREM and REM sleep with a short latency (Lin *et al.*, 1989).

Tuberomammillary nucleus neurons are known to express orexin type II receptors. Taking advantage of this, Gerashchenko *et al.* (2004) administered the neurotoxin saporin conjugated to orexin B (i.e. hypocretin 2, 50 ng in 0.25 μl) in the TMN and destroyed up to 83% of TMN histamine-containing neurons, together with most of the other neurons in adjacent cell groups in the posterior hypothalamus. However, even after destruction of more than 80% of histaminergic neurons, there was no effect on sleep–wakefulness, suggesting that the histaminergic TMN by itself may not be critical for wakefulness. This is true for other wakefulness-promoting regions and systems (Steriade & McCarley, 2005). Wakefulness is strongly buffered; downregulation of one particular system, such as the histaminergic system, is unlikely to affect it significantly. In addition, as Gerashchenko *et al.* (2004) noted, compensatory effects following the TMN lesion cannot be ruled out because the TMN neurons take several days to be destroyed following the administration of the neurotoxin.

Conclusion

Does the histaminergic system regulate wakefulness? The histaminergic system is localized within the TMN, which is a part of the posterior hypothalamus. Since the early part of the twentieth century, the posterior hypothalamus has been implicated in the regulation of wakefulness. Histaminergic neurons send widespread projections to wakefulness-promoting regions, including the orexin-rich perifornical hypothalamus and the cholinergic-rich basal forebrain. The histaminergic system also receives strong GABAergic and galaninergic inputs from the sleep-inducing VLPO region. The discharge activity of histaminergic neurons peaks during wakefulness and is almost silent during REM sleep. HA release parallels histaminergic discharge, and is at its highest level during wakefulness and lowest during REM sleep. Considerable pharmacological evidence suggests that the H_1 and the H_3 receptor, but not the H_2 receptor, are the key mediators of histaminergic action on wakefulness. HDC knockout mice that are unable to produce neuronal HA have difficulty in maintaining wakefulness in novel environments and are unable to exhibit normal wakefulness during the early part of the dark period. Thus, there is considerable evidence implicating the histaminergic system as a crucial player in the regulation of wakefulness. The challenge for future research is to identify the precise cellular and the molecular mechanisms by which HA acts to regulate wakefulness, the anatomical locations at which HA acts to control wakefulness, and what aspect of wakefulness is controlled by HA.

Acknowledgement

Supported by Veterans Affairs Medical Research Service, NIMH awards R01 MH62522 and R37 MH39683 and the NARSAD award.

References

Adam, K. & Oswald, I. (1986). The hypnotic effects of an antihistamine: promethazine. *Br. J. Clin. Pharmacol.* **22**, 715–17.

Araki, T., Yamano, M., Murakami, T. *et al.* (1988). Localization of glycine receptors in the rat central nervous system: an immunocytochemical analysis using monoclonal antibody. *Neuroscience* **25**, 613–24.

Arrang, J. M., Garbarg, M. & Schwartz, J. C. (1983). Auto-inhibition of brain histamine release mediated by a novel class (H3) of histamine receptor. *Nature* **302**, 832–7.

Arrang, J. M., Garbarg, M., Lancelot, J. C. *et al.* (1987a). Highly potent and selective ligands for histamine H3-receptors. *Nature* **327**, 117–23.

Arrang, J. M., Garbarg, M. & Schwartz, J. C. (1987b). Autoinhibition of histamine synthesis mediated by presynaptic H3-receptors. *Neuroscience* **23**, 149–57.

Backberg, M., Hervieu, G., Wilson, S. & Meister, B. (2002). Orexin receptor-1 (OX-R1) immunoreactivity in chemically identified neurons of the hypothalamus: focus on orexin targets involved in control of food and water intake. *Eur. J. Neurosci.* **15**, 315–28.

Bakker, R. A. (2004). Histamine H3-receptor isoforms. *Inflamm. Res.* **53**, 509–16.

Bakker, R. A., Wieland, K., Timmerman, H. & Leurs, R. (2000). Constitutive activity of the histamine H(1) receptor reveals inverse agonism of histamine H(1) receptor antagonists. *Eur. J. Pharmacol.* **387**, R5–7.

Barbier, A. J., Berridge, C., Dugovic, C. *et al.* (2004). Acute wake-promoting actions of JNJ-5207852, a novel, diamine-based H3 antagonist. *Br. J. Pharmacol.* **143**, 649–61.

Bassano, J. L. & Caille, E. J. (1979). Effects of two antihistaminic compounds (mequitazine, dexchlorpheniramine) on sleep. Sleep distortion by antihistaminics. *Waking Sleeping* **3**, 57–61.

Bayer, L., Eggermann, E., Serafin, M. *et al.* (2001). Orexins (hypocretins) directly excite tuberomammillary neurons. *Eur. J. Neurosci.* **14**, 1571–5.

Borbely, A. A. & Youmbi-Balderer, G. (1988). Effect of diphenhydramine on subjective sleep parameters and on motor activity during bedtime. *Int J. Clin. Pharmacol. Ther. Toxicol.* **26**, 392–6.

Brown, R. E. & Haas, H. L. (1999). On the mechanism of histaminergic inhibition of glutamate release in the rat dentate gyrus. *J. Physiol.* **515**, 777–86.

Brown, R. E., Fedorov, N. B., Haas, H. L. & Reymann, K. G. (1995). Histaminergic modulation of synaptic plasticity in area CA1 of rat hippocampal slices. *Neuropharmacology* **34**, 181–90.

Brown, R. E., Stevens, D. R. & Haas, H. L. (2001). The physiology of brain histamine. *Prog. Neurobiol.* **63**, 637–72.

Chemelli, R. M., Willie, J. T., Sinton, C. M. *et al.* (1999). Narcolepsy in orexin knockout mice: molecular genetics of sleep regulation. *Cell* **98**, 437–51.

Cirelli, C. & Tononi, G. (2000). On the functional significance of c-fos induction during the sleep-waking cycle. *Sleep* **23**, 453–69.

Clapham, J. & Kilpatrick, G. J. (1992). Histamine H3 receptors modulate the release of [3H]-acetylcholine from slices of rat entorhinal cortex: evidence for the possible existence of H3 receptor subtypes. *Br. J. Pharmacol.* **107**, 919–23.

Dahlstrom, A. & Fuxe, K. (1964). Evidence for the existence of monoamine in the cell bodies of brain stem neurons. *Acta Physiol.* **62**, 1–55.

Daum, P. R., Hill, S. J. & Young, J. M. (1982). Histamine H1-agonist potentiation of adenosine-stimulated cyclic AMP accumulation in slices of guinea-pig cerebral cortex: comparison of response and binding parameters. *Br. J. Pharmacol.* **77**, 347–57.

Drutel, G., Peitsaro, N., Karlstedt, K. *et al.* (2001). Identification of rat H3 receptor isoforms with different brain expression and signaling properties. *Mol. Pharmacol.* **59**, 1–8.

Ericson, H., Watanabe, T. & Kohler, C. (1987). Morphological analysis of the tuberomammillary nucleus in the rat brain: delineation of subgroups with antibody against L-histidine decarboxylase as a marker. *J. Comp. Neurol.* **263**, 1–24.

Ericson, H., Blomqvist, A. & Kohler, C. (1989). Brainstem afferents to the tuberomammillary nucleus in the rat brain with special reference to monoaminergic innervation. *J. Comp. Neurol.* **281**, 169–92.

Ericson, H., Blomqvist, A. & Kohler, C. (1991). Origin of neuronal inputs to the region of the tuberomammillary nucleus of the rat brain. *J. Comp. Neurol.* **311**, 45–64.

Eriksson, K. S., Sergeeva, O., Brown, R. E. & Haas, H. L. (2001a). Orexin/hypocretin excites the histaminergic neurons of the tuberomammillary nucleus. *J. Neurosci.* **21**, 9273–9.

Eriksson, K. S., Stevens, D. R. & Haas, H. L. (2001b). Serotonin excites tuberomammillary neurons by activation of Na(+)/Ca(2+)-exchange. *Neuropharmacology* **40**, 345–51.

Eriksson, K. S., Sergeeva, O. A., Selbach, O. & Haas, H. L. (2004). Orexin (hypocretin)/ dynorphin neurons control GABAergic inputs to tuberomammillary neurons. *Eur. J. Neurosci.* **19**, 1278–84.

Friedman, A. H. & Walker, C. A. (1969). Rat brain amines, blood histamine and glucose levels in relationship to circadian changes in sleep induced by pentobarbitone sodium. *J. Physiol.* **202**, 133–46.

Fukui, H. (2005). Review of some molecular and physiological studies of histamine H1 receptor function (Hiroshi Wada Symposium). *Inflamm. Res.* **54** (suppl. 1), S52–3.

Furukawa, K., Ishibashi, H. & Akaike, N. (1994). ATP-induced inward current in neurons freshly dissociated from the tuberomammillary nucleus. *J. Neurophysiol.* **71**, 868–73.

Gantz, I., Schaffer, M., DelValle, J. *et al.* (1991). Molecular cloning of a gene encoding the histamine H2 receptor. *Proc. Natl. Acad. Sci. USA* **88**, 429–33.

Gerashchenko, D., Chou, T. C., Blanco-Centurion, C. A., Saper, C. B. & Shiromani, P. J. (2004). Effects of lesions of the histaminergic tuberomammillary nucleus on spontaneous sleep in rats. *Sleep* **27**, 1275–81.

Gisselmann, G., Pusch, H., Hovemann, B. T. & Hatt, H. (2002). Two cDNAs coding for histamine-gated ion channels in *D. melanogaster*. *Nat. Neurosci.* **5**, 11–12.

Gorelova, N. & Reiner, P. B. (1996). Histamine depolarizes cholinergic septal neurons. *J. Neurophysiol.* **75**, 707–14.

Greene, R. W. & Haas, H. L. (1990). Effects of histamine on dentate granule cells in vitro. *Neuroscience* **34**, 299–303.

Greene, R. W., Haas, H. L. & Reiner, P. B. (1990). Two transient outward currents in histamine neurones of the rat hypothalamus in vitro. *J. Physiol.* **420**, 149–63.

Gurevich, E. V. & Joyce, J. N. (1999). Distribution of dopamine D3 receptor expressing neurons in the human forebrain: comparison with D2 receptor expressing neurons. *Neuropsychopharmacology* **20**, 60–80.

Haas, H. & Panula, P. (2003). The role of histamine and the tuberomamillary nucleus in the nervous system. *Nat. Rev. Neurosci.* **4**, 121–30.

Haas, H. L. (1984). Histamine potentiates neuronal excitation by blocking a calcium-dependent potassium conductance. *Agents Actions* **14**, 534–7.

Haas, H. L. & Greene, R. W. (1986). Effects of histamine on hippocampal pyramidal cells of the rat in vitro. *Exp. Brain Res.* **62**, 123–30.

Haas, H. L. & Konnerth, A. (1983). Histamine and noradrenaline decrease calcium-activated potassium conductance in hippocampal pyramidal cells. *Nature* **302**, 432–4.

Haas, H. L. & Reiner, P. B. (1988). Membrane properties of histaminergic tuberomammillary neurones of the rat hypothalamus in vitro. *J. Physiol.* **399**, 633–46.

Hancock, A. A., Esbenshade, T. A., Krueger, K. M. & Yao, B. B. (2003). Genetic and pharmacological aspects of histamine H3 receptor heterogeneity. *Life Sci.* **73**, 3043–72.

Hardie, R. C. (1989). A histamine-activated chloride channel involved in neurotransmission at a photoreceptor synapse. *Nature* **339**, 704–6.

Hatton, G. I. & Yang, Q. Z. (1996). Synaptically released histamine increases dye coupling among vasopressinergic neurons of the supraoptic nucleus: mediation by H1 receptors and cyclic nucleotides. *J. Neurosci.* **16**, 123–9.

Hill, S. J., Ganellin, C. R., Timmerman, H. *et al.* (1997). International Union of Pharmacology. XIII. Classification of histamine receptors. *Pharmacol. Rev.* **49**, 253–78.

Hong, Z. Y., Huang, Z. L., Qu, W. M. & Eguchi, N. (2005). Orexin A promotes histamine, but not norepinephrine or serotonin, release in frontal cortex of mice. *Acta Pharmacol. Sin.* **26**, 155–9.

Hough, L. B. (1988). Cellular localization and possible functions for brain histamine: recent progress. *Prog. Neurobiol.* **30**, 469–505.

Hughes, P. & Dragunow, M. (1995). Induction of immediate-early genes and the control of neurotransmitter-regulated gene expression within the nervous system. *Pharmacol. Rev.* **47**, 133–78.

Ishizuka, T., Yamamoto, Y. & Yamatodani, A. (2002). The effect of orexin-A and -B on the histamine release in the anterior hypothalamus in rats. *Neurosci. Lett.* **323**, 93–6.

Jewett, R. E. (1968). Effects of promethazine on sleep stages in the cat. *Exp. Neurol.* **21**, 368–82.

Jones, B. E. (2003). Arousal systems. *Front Biosci.* **8**, s438–51.

Jørgensen, E. A., Knigge, U., Watanabe, T., Warberg, J. & Kjaer, A. (2005). Histaminergic neurons are involved in the orexigenic effect of orexin-A. *Neuroendocrinology* **82**, 70–7.

Kalivas, P. W. (1982). Histamine-induced arousal in the conscious and pentobarbital-pretreated rat. *J. Pharmacol. Exp. Ther.* **222**, 37–42.

Kilduff, T. S. (2001). Sleepy dogs don't lie: a genetic disorder informative about sleep. *Genome Res.* **11**, 509–11.

Kitahama, K., Sakai, K., Tago, H. *et al.* (1984). Monoamine oxidase-containing neurons in the cat hypothalamus: distribution and ascending projection to the cerebral cortex. *Brain Res.* **324**, 155–9.

Kiviranta, T., Tuomisto, L. & Airaksinen, E. M. (1994). Diurnal and age-related changes in cerebrospinal fluid tele-methylhistamine levels during infancy and childhood. *Pharmacol. Biochem. Behav.* **49**, 997–1000.

Kiyono, S., Seo, M. L., Shibagaki, M. *et al.* (1985). Effects of alpha-fluoromethyl-histidine on sleep-waking parameters in rats. *Physiol. Behav.* **34**, 615–17.

Ko, E. M., Estabrooke, I. V., McCarthy, M. & Scammell, T. E. (2003). Wake-related activity of tuberomammillary neurons in rats. *Brain Res.* **992**, 220–6.

Kohler, C., Swanson, L. W., Haglund, L. & Wu, J. Y. (1985). The cytoarchitecture, histochemistry and projections of the tuberomammillary nucleus in the rat. *Neuroscience* **16**, 85–110.

Korotkova, T. M., Sergeeva, O. A., Ponomarenko, A. A. & Haas, H. L. (2005). Histamine excites noradrenergic neurons in locus coeruleus in rats. *Neuropharmacology* **49**, 129–34.

Kudo, Y. & Kurihara, M. (1990). Clinical evaluation of diphenhydramine hydrochloride for the treatment of insomnia in psychiatric patients: a double-blind study. *J. Clin. Pharmacol.* **30**, 1041–8.

Lamberty, Y., Margineanu, D. G., Dassesse, D. & Klitgaard, H. (2003). H3 agonist immepip markedly reduces cortical histamine release, but only weakly promotes sleep in the rat. *Pharmacol. Res.* **48**, 193–8.

Lefkowitz, R. J., Cotecchia, S., Samama, P. & Costa, T. (1993). Constitutive activity of receptors coupled to guanine nucleotide regulatory proteins. *Trends Pharmacol. Sci.* **14**, 303–7.

Leurs, R., Traiffort, E., Arrang, J. M. *et al.* (1994). Guinea pig histamine H1 receptor. II. Stable expression in Chinese hamster ovary cells reveals the interaction with three major signal transduction pathways. *J. Neurochem.* **62**, 519–27.

Leurs, R., Church, M. K. & Taglialatela, M. (2002). H1-antihistamines: inverse agonism, anti-inflammatory actions and cardiac effects. *Clin. Exp. Allergy* **32**, 489–98.

Ligneau, X., Lin, J., Vanni-Mercier, G. *et al.* (1998). Neurochemical and behavioral effects of ciproxifan, a potent histamine H3-receptor antagonist. *J. Pharmacol. Exp. Ther.* **287**, 658–66.

Lin, J. S. (2000). Brain structures and mechanisms involved in the control of cortical activation and wakefulness, with emphasis on the posterior hypothalamus and histaminergic neurons. *Sleep Med. Rev.* **4**, 471–503.

Lin, J. S., Sakai, K. & Jouvet, M. (1986). [Role of hypothalamic histaminergic systems in the regulation of vigilance states in cats.] *C. R. Acad. Sci. III* **303**, 469–74.

Lin, J. S., Sakai, K. & Jouvet, M. (1988). Evidence for histaminergic arousal mechanisms in the hypothalamus of cat. *Neuropharmacology* **27**, 111–22.

Lin, J. S., Sakai, K., Vanni-Mercier, G. & Jouvet, M. (1989). A critical role of the posterior hypothalamus in the mechanisms of wakefulness determined by microinjection of muscimol in freely moving cats. *Brain Res.* **479**, 225–40.

Lin, J. S., Sakai, K., Vanni-Mercier, G. *et al.* (1990). Involvement of histaminergic neurons in arousal mechanisms demonstrated with H3-receptor ligands in the cat. *Brain Res.* **523**, 325–30.

Lin, J. S., Sakai, K. & Jouvet, M. (1994). Hypothalamo-preoptic histaminergic projections in sleep-wake control in the cat. *Eur. J. Neurosci.* **6**, 618–25.

Lin, J. S., Hou, Y., Sakai, K. & Jouvet, M. (1996). Histaminergic descending inputs to the mesopontine tegmentum and their role in the control of cortical activation and wakefulness in the cat. *J. Neurosci.* **16**, 1523–37.

Lin, L., Faraco, J., Li, R. *et al.* (1999). The sleep disorder canine narcolepsy is caused by a mutation in the hypocretin (orexin) receptor 2 gene. *Cell* **98**, 365–76.

Lovenberg, T. W., Roland, B. L., Wilson, S. J. *et al.* (1999). Cloning and functional expression of the human histamine H3 receptor. *Mol. Pharmacol.* **55**, 1101–7.

Marcus, J. N., Aschkenasi, C. J., Lee, C. E. *et al.* (2001). Differential expression of orexin receptors 1 and 2 in the rat brain. *J. Comp. Neurol.* **435**, 6–25.

McCormick, D. A. & Williamson, A. (1991). Modulation of neuronal firing mode in cat and guinea pig LGNd by histamine: possible cellular mechanisms of histaminergic control of arousal. *J. Neurosci.* **11**, 3188–99.

McGinty, D. J. (1969). Somnolence, recovery and hyposomnia following ventro-medial diencephalic lesions in the rat. *Electroencephalogr. Clin. Neurophysiol.* **26**, 70–9.

McLeod, R. L., Aslanian, R., del Prado, M. *et al.* (1998). Sch 50971, an orally active histamine H3 receptor agonist, inhibits central neurogenic vascular inflammation and produces sedation in the guinea pig. *J. Pharmacol. Exp. Ther.* **287**, 43–50.

Mignot, E. (2004). Sleep, sleep disorders and hypocretin (orexin). *Sleep Med.* **5** (suppl. 1), S2–8.

Miklos, I. H. & Kovacs, K. J. (2003). Functional heterogeneity of the responses of histaminergic neuron subpopulations to various stress challenges. *Eur. J. Neurosci.* **18**, 3069–79.

Mochizuki, T., Yamatodani, A. & Okakura, K. (1992). Circadian rhythm of histamine release from the hypothalamus of freely moving rats. *Physiol. Behav.* **51**, 391–4.

Monnier, M. & Hatt, A. M. (1969). Afferent and central activating effects of histamine on the brain. *Experientia* **25**, 1297–8.

Monnier, M., Fallert, M. & Battacharya, I. C. (1967). The waking action of histamine. *Experientia* **23**, 21–2.

Monti, J. M. (1993). Involvement of histamine in the control of the waking state. *Life Sci.* **53**, 1331–8.

Monti, J. M., Pellejero, T. & Jantos, H. (1986). Effects of H1- and H2-histamine receptor agonists and antagonists on sleep and wakefulness in the rat. *J. Neural Transm.* **66**, 1–11.

Monti, J. M., D'Angelo, L., Jantos, H. & Pazos, S. (1988). Effects of a-fluoromethylhistidine on sleep and wakefulness in the rat. Short note. *J. Neural Transm.* **72**, 141–5.

Monti, J. M., Orellana, C., Boussard, M., Jantos, H. & Olivera, S. (1990). Sleep variables are unaltered by zolantidine in rats: are histamine H2-receptors not involved in sleep regulation? *Brain Res. Bull.* **25**, 229–31.

Monti, J. M., Jantos, H., Boussard, M. et al. (1991). Effects of selective activation or blockade of the histamine H3 receptor on sleep and wakefulness. *Eur. J. Pharmacol.* **205**, 283–7.

Monti, J. M., Jantos, H., Ponzoni, A. & Monti, D. (1996). Sleep and waking during acute histamine H3 agonist BP 2.94 or H3 antagonist carboperamide (MR 16155) administration in rats. *Neuropsychopharmacology* **15**, 31–5.

Morgan, J. I., Cohen, D. R., Hempstead, J. L. & Curran, T. et al. (1987). Mapping patterns of c-fos expression in the central nervous system after seizure. *Science* **237**, 192–7.

Morisset, S., Rouleau, A., Ligneau, X. et al. (2000). High constitutive activity of native H3 receptors regulates histamine neurons in brain. *Nature* **408**, 860–4.

Munakata, M. & Akaike, N. (1994). Regulation of K^+ conductance by histamine H1 and H2 receptors in neurones dissociated from rat neostriatum. *J. Physiol.* **480**, 233–45.

Naquet, R., Denavit, M. & be-Fessard, D. (1966). [Comparison between the role of the subthalamus and that of the different bulbomesencephalic structures in the maintenance of wakefulness.] *Electroencephalogr. Clin. Neurophysiol.* **20**, 149–64.

Nauta, W. (1946). Hypothalamic regulation of sleep in rats. An experimental study. *J. Neurophysiol.* **9**, 285–316.

Nelson, L. E., Guo, T. Z., Lu, J. et al. (2002). The sedative component of anesthesia is mediated by GABA(A) receptors in an endogenous sleep pathway. *Nat. Neurosci.* **5**, 979–84.

Nelson, L. E., Lu, J., Guo, T. et al. (2003). The alpha2-adrenoceptor agonist dexmedetomidine converges on an endogenous sleep-promoting pathway to exert its sedative effects. *Anesthesiology* **98**, 428–36.

Nguyen, T., Shapiro, D. A., George, S. R. et al. (2001). Discovery of a novel member of the histamine receptor family. *Mol. Pharmacol.* **59**, 427–33.

Nicholson, A. N., Pascoe, P. A. & Stone, B. M. (1985). Histaminergic systems and sleep. Studies in man with H1 and H2 antagonists. *Neuropharmacology* **24**, 245–50.

Ohtsu, H. & Watanabe, T. (2003). New functions of histamine found in histidine decarboxylase gene knockout mice. *Biochem. Biophys. Res. Commun.* **305**, 443–7.

Ohtsu, H. *et al.* (2001). Mice lacking histidine decarboxylase exhibit abnormal mast cells. *FEBS Lett.* **502**, 53–6.

Orr, E. & Quay, W. B. (1975). Hypothalamic 24-hour rhythms in histamine, histidine, decarboxylase and histamine-N-methyltransferase. *Endocrinology* **96**, 941–5.

Palacios, J. M., Wamsley, J. K. & Kuhar, M. J. (1981). The distribution of histamine H1-receptors in the rat brain: an autoradiographic study. *Neuroscience* **6**, 15–37.

Panula, P., Yang, H. Y. & Costa, E. (1984). Histamine-containing neurons in the rat hypothalamus. *Proc. Natl. Acad. Sci. USA* **81**, 2572–6.

Panula, P., Takagi, H., Inagaki, N. *et al.* (1993). Histamine-containing nerve fibers innervate human cerebellum. *Neurosci. Lett.* **160**, 53–6.

Parmentier, R., Ohtsu, H., Djebbara-Hannas, Z. *et al.* (2002). Anatomical, physiological, and pharmacological characteristics of histidine decarboxylase knock-out mice: evidence for the role of brain histamine in behavioral and sleep-wake control. *J. Neurosci.* **22**, 7695–711.

Patel, B. T., Tudball, N., Wada, H. & Watanabe T. (1986). Adenosine deaminase and histidine decarboxylase coexist in certain neurons of the rat brain. *Neurosci. Lett.* **63**, 185–9.

Pedarzani, P. & Storm, J. F. (1993). PKA mediates the effects of monoamine transmitters on the K+ current underlying the slow spike frequency adaptation in hippocampal neurons. *Neuron* **11**, 1023–35.

Pedarzani, P. & Storm, J. F. (1995). Protein kinase A-independent modulation of ion channels in the brain by cyclic AMP. *Proc. Natl. Acad. Sci. USA* **92**, 11716–20.

Peyron, C., Tighe, D. K., Van den Pol, A. N. *et al.* (1998). Neurons containing hypocretin (orexin) project to multiple neuronal systems. *J. Neurosci.* **18**, 9996–10015.

Pollard, H., Moreau, J., Arrang, J. M. & Schwartz, J. C. (1993). A detailed autoradiographic mapping of histamine H3 receptors in rat brain areas. *Neuroscience* **52**, 169–89.

Pompeiano, M., Cirelli, C., Arrighi, P. & Tononi, G. (1995). c-Fos expression during wakefulness and sleep. *Neurophysiol. Clin.* **25**, 329–41.

Prast, H., Dietl, H. & Philippu, A. (1992). Pulsatile release of histamine in the hypothalamus of conscious rats. *J. Auton. Nerv. Syst.* **39**, 105–10.

Prell, G. D., Khandelwal, J. K., Burns, R. S. & Green, J. P. (1989). Diurnal fluctuation in levels of histamine metabolites in cerebrospinal fluid of rhesus monkey. *Agents Actions* **26**, 279–86.

Ramesh, V., Thakkar, M. M., Strecker, R. E., Basheer, R. & McCarley, R. W. (2004). Wakefulness-inducing effects of histamine in the basal forebrain of freely moving rats. *Behav. Brain. Res.* **152**, 271–8.

Rampon, C., Luppi, P. H., Fort, P., Peyron, C. & Jouvet, M. (1996). Distribution of glycine-immunoreactive cell bodies and fibers in the rat brain. *Neuroscience* **75**, 737–55.

Ranson, S. W. (1939). Somnolence caused by hypothalamic lesions in the monkey. *Arch. Neurol. Psychiat.* **4**, 1–23.

Reiner, P. B. & Kamondi, A. (1994). Mechanisms of antihistamine-induced sedation in the human brain: H1 receptor activation reduces background leakage potassium current. *Neuroscience* **59**, 579–88.

Reiner, P. B. & McGeer, E. G. (1987). Electrophysiological properties of cortically projecting histamine neurons of the rat hypothalamus. *Neurosci. Lett.* **73**, 43–7.

Reiner, P. B., Semba, K., Fibiger, H. C. & McGeer, E. G. (1987). Physiological evidence for subpopulations of cortically projecting basal forebrain neurons in the anesthetized rat. *Neuroscience* **20**, 629–36.

Richelson, E. (1978). Histamine H1 receptor-mediated guanosine 3′,5′-monophosphate formation by cultured mouse neuroblastoma cells. *Science* **201**, 69–71.

Rickels, K., Morris, R. J., Newman, H. *et al.* (1983). Diphenhydramine in insomniac family practice patients: a double-blind study. *J. Clin. Pharmacol.* **23**, 234–42.

Risberg, A. M., Risberg, J. & Ingvar, D. H. (1975). Effects of promethazine on nocturnal sleep in normal man. *Psychopharmacologia* **43**, 279–84.

Rouleau, A., Ligneau, X., Tardivel-Lacombe, J. *et al.* (2002). Histamine H3-receptor-mediated [35S]GTP gamma[S] binding: evidence for constitutive activity of the recombinant and native rat and human H3 receptors. *Br. J. Pharmacol.* **135**, 383–92.

Sagar, S. M., Sharp, F. R. & Curran, T. (1988). Expression of c-fos protein in brain: metabolic mapping at the cellular level. *Science* **240**, 1328–31.

Sakai, K., el Mansari, M., Lin, J. S., Zhang, J. G. & Vanni-Mercier, G. (1990). The posterior hypothalamus in the regulation of wakefulness and paradoxical sleep. In *The Diencephalon and Sleep*, ed. M. Mancia & G. Marini, pp. 171–98. New York, NY: Raven Press.

Saper, C. B., Chou, T. C. & Scammell, T. E. (2001). The sleep switch: hypothalamic control of sleep and wakefulness. *Trends Neurosci.* **24**, 726–31.

Sato, K., Zhang, J. H., Saika, T. *et al.* (1991). Localization of glycine receptor alpha 1 subunit mRNA-containing neurons in the rat brain: an analysis using in situ hybridization histochemistry. *Neuroscience* **43**, 381–95.

Scammell, T., Gerashchenko, D., Urade, Y. *et al.* (1998). Activation of ventrolateral preoptic neurons by the somnogen prostaglandin D2. *Proc. Natl. Acad. Sci. USA* **95**, 7754–59.

Scammell, T. E., Gerashchenko, D. Y., Mochizuki, T. *et al.* (2001). An adenosine A2a agonist increases sleep and induces Fos in ventrolateral preoptic neurons. *Neuroscience* **107**, 653–63.

Schlicker, E., Betz, R. & Gothert, M. (1988). Histamine H3 receptor-mediated inhibition of serotonin release in the rat brain cortex. *Naunyn Schmiedebergs Arch. Pharmacol.* **337**, 588–90.

Schlicker, E., Fink, K., Hinterthaner, M. & Gothert, M. (1989). Inhibition of noradrenaline release in the rat brain cortex via presynaptic H3 receptors. *Naunyn Schmiedebergs Arch. Pharmacol.* **340**, 633–8.

Schlicker, E., Fink, K., Detzner, M. & Gothert, M. (1993). Histamine inhibits dopamine release in the mouse striatum via presynaptic H3 receptors. *J. Neural Transm. Gen. Sect.* **93**, 1–10.

Schonrock, B., Busselberg, D. & Haas, H. L. (1991). Properties of tuberomammillary histamine neurones and their response to galanin. *Agents Actions* **33**, 135–7.

Schwartz, J. C., Arrang, J. M., Garbarg, M., Pollard, H. & Ruat, M. (1991). Histaminergic transmission in the mammalian brain. *Physiol. Rev.* **71**, 1–51.

Self, T. J., Oakley, S. M. & Hill, S. J. (2005). Clathrin-independent internalization of the human histamine H1-receptor in CHO-K1 cells. *Br. J. Pharmacol.* **146**, 612–24.

Sergeeva, O. A., Eriksson, K. S. & Haas, H. L. (2001). Glycine receptor mediated responses in rat histaminergic neurons. *Neurosci. Lett.* **300**, 5–8.

Sergeeva, O. A., Amberger, B. T., Eriksson, K. S., Scherer, A. & Haas, H. L. (2003). Co-ordinated expression of 5-HT2C receptors with the NCX1 Na^+/Ca^{2+} exchanger in histaminergic neurones. *J. Neurochem.* **87**, 657–64.

Sherin, J. E., Elmquist, J. K., Torrealba, F. & Saper, C. B. (1998). Innervation of histaminergic tuberomammillary neurons by GABAergic and galaninergic neurons in the ventrolateral preoptic nucleus of the rat. *J. Neurosci.* **18**, 4705–21.

Smit, M. J., Leurs, R., Alewijnse, A. E. *et al.* (1996). Inverse agonism of histamine H2 antagonist accounts for upregulation of spontaneously active histamine H2 receptors. *Proc. Natl. Acad. Sci. USA* **93**, 6802–7.

Steininger, T. L., Alam, M. N., Gong, H., Szymusiak, R. & McGinty, D. (1999). Sleep-waking discharge of neurons in the posterior lateral hypothalamus of the albino rat. *Brain Res.* **840**, 138–47.

Steriade, M. & McCarley, R. W. (1990). *Brainstem Control of Wakefulness and Sleep.* New York, NY: Plenum Press.

Steriade, M. & McCarley, R. W. (2005). *Brain Control of Sleep and Wakefulness.* New York, NY: Kluwer-Elsevier.

Stevens, D. R., Kuramasu, A. & Haas, H. L. (1999). GABAB-receptor-mediated control of GABAergic inhibition in rat histaminergic neurons in vitro. *Eur. J. Neurosci.* **11**, 1148–54.

Stevens, D. R., Eriksson, K. S., Brown, R. E. & Haas, H. L. (2001). The mechanism of spontaneous firing in histamine neurons. *Behav. Brain Res.* **124**, 105–12.

Stevens, D. R., Kuramasu, A., Eriksson, K. S., Selbach, O. & Haas, H. L. (2004). Alpha 2-adrenergic receptor-mediated presynaptic inhibition of GABAergic IPSPs in rat histaminergic neurons. *Neuropharmacology* **46**, 1018–22.

Strecker, R. E., Nalwalk, J., Dauphin, L. J. *et al.* (2002). Extracellular histamine levels in the feline preoptic/anterior hypothalamic area during natural sleep-wakefulness and prolonged wakefulness: an in vivo microdialysis study. *Neuroscience* **113**, 663–70.

Swett, C. P. & Hobson, J. A. (1968). The effects of posterior hypothalamic lesions on behavioral and electrographic manifestations of sleep and waking in cats. *Arch. Ital. Biol.* **106**, 283–93.

Tago, H., Kimura, H., Kitahama, K. *et al.* (1984). Cortical projections of monoamine oxidase-containing neurons from the posterior hypothalamus in the rat. *Neurosci. Lett.* **52**, 281–6.

Takagi, H., Morishima, Y., Matsuyama, T. *et al.* (1986). Histaminergic axons in the neostriatum and cerebral cortex of the rat: a correlated light and electron microscopic immunocytochemical study using histidine decarboxylase as a marker. *Brain Res.* **364**, 114–23.

Takeda, N., Inagaki, S., Taguchi, Y. *et al.* (1984). Origins of histamine-containing fibers in the cerebral cortex of rats studied by immunohistochemistry with histidine decarboxylase as a marker and transection. *Brain Res.* **323**, 55–63.

Takeshita, Y., Watanabe, T., Sakata, T. *et al.* (1998). Histamine modulates high-voltage-activated calcium channels in neurons dissociated from the rat tuberomammillary nucleus. *Neuroscience* **87**, 797–805.

Tamiya, R. (1991). Synaptic inputs to histaminergic neurons in the rat posterior hypothalamus. *Osaka City Med. J.* **37**, 107–22.

Tardivel-Lacombe, J., Rouleau, A., Heron, A. *et al.* (2000). Cloning and cerebral expression of the guinea pig histamine H3 receptor: evidence for two isoforms. *Neuroreport* **20**, 755–9.

Tasaka, K., Chung, Y. H. & Sawada, K. (1989). Excitatory effect of histamine on EEGs of the cortex and thalamus in rats. *Agents Actions* **27**, 127–30.

Tasaka, K., Chung, Y. H., Mio, M. & Kamei, C. (1993). The pathway responsible for EEG synchronization and effect of histamine on this system. *Brain Res. Bull.* **32**, 365–71.

Thakkar, M. M., Ramesh, V., Cape, E. G. *et al.* (1999). REM sleep enhancement and behavioral cataplexy following orexin (hypocretin)-II receptor antisense perfusion in the pontine reticular formation. *Sleep Res. Online* **2**, 112–20.

Thakkar, M. M., Ramesh, V., Strecker, R. E. & McCarley, R. W. (2001). Microdialysis perfusion of orexin-A in the basal forebrain increases wakefulness in freely behaving rats. *Arch. Ital. Biol.* **139**, 313–28.

Thakkar, M. M., Delgiacco, R. A., Strecker, R. E. & McCarley, R. W. (2003a). Adenosinergic inhibition of basal forebrain wakefulness – active neurons: a simultaneous unit recording and microdialysis study in freely behaving cats. *Neuroscience* **122**, 1107–13.

Thakkar, M. M., Winston, S. & McCarley, R. W. (2003b). A1 receptor and adenosinergic homeostatic regulation of sleep-wakefulness: effects of antisense to the A1 receptor in the cholinergic basal forebrain. *J. Neurosci.* **23**, 4278–87.

Timm, J., Marr, I., Werthwein, S. *et al.* (1998). H2 receptor-mediated facilitation and H3 receptor-mediated inhibition of noradrenaline release in the guinea-pig brain. *Naunyn Schmiedebergs Arch. Pharmacol.* **357**, 232–9.

Timmerman, H. (1989). Histamine receptors in the central nervous system. *Pharm. Weekbl. Sci.* **20**(11), 146–50.

Toyota, H., Dugovic, C., Koehl, M. *et al.* (2002). Behavioral characterization of mice lacking histamine H3 receptors. *Mol. Pharmacol.* **62**, 389–97.

Traiffort, E., Pollard, H., Moreau, J. *et al.* (1992). Pharmacological characterization and autoradiographic localization of histamine H2 receptors in human brain identified with [125I]iodoaminopotentidine. *J. Neurochem.* **59**, 290–9.

Traiffort, E., Vizuete, M. L., Tardivel-Lacombe, J. et al. (1995). The guinea pig histamine H2 receptor: gene cloning, tissue expression and chromosomal localization of its human counterpart. *Biochem. Biophys. Res. Commun.* **211**, 570–7.

Tran, V. T., Chang, R. S. & Snyder, S. H. (1978). Histamine H1 receptors identified in mammalian brain membranes with [3H]mepyramine. *Proc. Natl. Acad. Sci. USA* **75**, 6290–4.

Uteshev, V. V., Stevens, D. R. & Haas, H. L. (1996). Alpha-bungarotoxin-sensitive nicotinic responses in rat tuberomammillary neurons. *Pflugers Arch. Eur. J. Physiol.* **432**, 607–13.

Vanni-Mercier, G., Sakai, K. & Jouvet, M. (1984). [Specific neurons for wakefulness in the posterior hypothalamus in the cat.] *C. R. Acad. Sci.* ser. Iii **298**, 195–200.

Vanni-Mercier, G., Gigout, S., Debilly, G. & Lin, J. S. (2003). Waking selective neurons in the posterior hypothalamus and their response to histamine H3-receptor ligands: an electrophysiological study in freely moving cats. *Behav. Brain. Res.* **144**, 227–41.

Vizuete, M. L., Dimitriadou, V., Traiffort, E. et al. (1995). Endogenous histamine induces c-fos expression within paraventricular and supraoptic nuclei. *Neuroreport* **6**, 1041–4.

Vizuete, M. L., Traiffort, E., Bouthenet, M. L. et al. (1997). Detailed mapping of the histamine H2 receptor and its gene transcripts in guinea-pig brain. *Neuroscience* **80**, 321–43.

Von Economo, C. (1930). Sleep as a problem of localization. *J. Nerv. Ment. Dis.* **71**, 249–59.

Vorobjev, V. S., Sharonova, I. N., Haas, H. L. & Sergeeva, O. A. (2003). Expression and function of P2X purinoceptors in rat histaminergic neurons. *Br. J. Pharmacol.* **138**, 1013–19.

Wada, H., Inagaki, N., Yamatodani, A. & Watanabe, T. (1991). Is the histaminergic neuron system a regulatory center for whole-brain activity? *Trends Neurosci.* **14**, 415–18.

Watanabe, T. & Yanai, K. (2001). Studies on functional roles of the histaminergic neuron system by using pharmacological agents, knockout mice and positron emission tomography. *Tohoku J. Exp. Med.* **195**(4), 197–217.

Watanabe, T., Taguchi, Y., Shiosaka, S. et al. (1984). Distribution of the histaminergic neuron system in the central nervous system of rats; a fluorescent immunohistochemical analysis with histidine decarboxylase as a marker. *Brain Res.* **295**, 13–25.

Wauquier, A., Van den Broeck, W. A., Awouters, F. & Janssen, P. A. (1981). A comparison between astemizole and other antihistamines on sleep-wakefulness cycles in dogs. *Neuropharmacology* **20**, 853–9.

White, J. & Rumbold, H. (1988). Behavioral effects of histamine and its antagonists: a review. *Psychopharmacology (Berl).* **95**, 1–14.

Wolf, P. & Monnier, M. (1973). Electroencephalographic, behavioural and visceral effects of intraventricular infusion of histamine in the rabbit. *Agents Actions* **3**, 196.

Yamamoto, T., Ochi, J., Daddona, P. E. & Nagy, J. I. (1990). Ultrastructural immunolocalization of adenosine deaminase in histaminergic neurons of the tuberomammillary nucleus of rat. *Brain Res.* **527**, 335–41.

Yamanaka, A., Tsujino, N., Funahashi, H. *et al.* (2002). Orexins activate histaminergic neurons via the orexin 2 receptor. *Biochem. Biophys. Res. Commun.* **290**, 1237–45.

Yamashita, M., Fukui, H., Sugama, K. *et al.* (1991). Expression cloning of a cDNA encoding the bovine histamine H1 receptor. *Proc. Natl. Acad. Sci. USA* **88**, 11515–19.

Yang, Q. Z. & Hatton, G. I. (1997). Electrophysiology of excitatory and inhibitory afferents to rat histaminergic tuberomammillary nucleus neurons from hypothalamic and forebrain sites. *Brain Res.* **773**, 162–72.

7

Dopamine in behavioral state control

DAVID B. RYE AND AMANDA A. H. FREEMAN

Dopamine is the most abundant of monoamines in the central nervous system (CNS). It modulates diverse behaviors including movement, motivation/reward, cognition, and feeding that share one notable attribute in common: they all play out on a backdrop of wakefulness (Bjorklund and Lindvall 1984; Marin *et al.* 1998; Durstewitz *et al.* 1999; Williams and Goldman-Rakic 1998). Dopamine's influence(s) upon normal and pathologic wake–sleep has unfortunately only recently begun to receive more widespread attention. The rebirth of interest in dopamine's participation in wake–sleep behaviors comes straight from the clinical arena. Here, sleepiness has been noted to be a common and disabling feature attending midbrain dopamine cell loss in Parkinson's disease (PD), as well as with dopamine agonist treatment of PD and additional disorders that interfere with normal sleep such as restless legs syndrome, and periodic leg movement and rapid eye movement sleep disorders (Rye 2004a,b; Rye and Jankovic 2002). Although this clinical experience argues that dopamine signaling is integral to maintaining wakefulness, a complete understanding is only beginning to emerge from recent scientific inquiries. What follows is a comprehensive account of the current state of knowledge of the brain's dopamine pathways as it pertains to their modulation of normal and pathologic wake–sleep state(s).

Synthesis and metabolism of dopamine

The family of catecholamines includes norepinephrine, epinephrine, and dopamine, of which dopamine is the most abundant in the CNS. It was

Neurochemistry of Sleep and Wakefulness, ed. J. M. Monti *et al.* Published by Cambridge University Press.
© Cambridge University Press 2008.

not until the 1950s that dopamine was recognized as a critical neurotransmitter, and not simply an intermediate in the single biosynthetic pathway it shares with norepinephrine and epinephrine. In the first and rate-limiting step of the pathway, L-tyrosine is hydroxylated via the enzyme tyrosine hydroxylase (TH) to form L-dihydroxyphenylalanine (L-DOPA) (Nagatsu *et al.* 1964). Removal of a carboxyl group from L-DOPA by DOPA decarboxylase then produces dopamine. In subsequent steps dopamine can then be further converted to norepinephrine and then to epinephrine by dopamine β-hydroxylase and phenylethanolamine-N-methyltransferase, respectively (Fig. 7.1).

Activation of TH is the rate-limiting step in the production of dopamine and it is under strict regulatory control by a variety of factors, including inhibitory feedback by the catecholamine products (e.g. dopamine). In order to convert tyrosine to L-DOPA, TH requires the binding of iron to the catalytic domain at the C-terminal. Catalytic activity of TH also requires (6R)-(1-erythro-1′,2′-dihydroxypropyl)-2-amino-4-hydroxy-5,6,7,8-tetrahydropteridine (6R-tetrahydrobiopterin; 6RBPH4; more commonly known as tetrahydrobiopterin (BH_4)), a naturally occurring pteridine cofactor, to reduce the iron to the ferrous form (Fe^{2+}). This allows the binding of the substrates (i.e., L-tyrosine and molecular oxygen) to the C-terminal (Nakashima *et al.* 1999). Following a catalytic cycle the molecular oxygen can oxidize a fraction of the iron to the ferric form, thus increasing the binding affinity for dopamine and L-DOPA. When either is bound to the regulatory domain of the N-terminus, the complex is inactivated by preventing the binding of BH_4. Biosynthesis of L-DOPA, and consequently dopamine, can be restored by phosphorylation of TH at serine 40 by cAMP-dependent protein kinase phosphorylation, thus decreasing the binding affinity for dopamine 300-fold and increasing the binding affinity for the pteridine cofactor (Ramsey and Fitzpatrick 1998; Ramsey *et al.* 1996). Endogenous levels of BH_4 are, in turn, regulated by guanosine triphosphate (GTP) cyclohydrolase activity, as its synthesis is downstream of the rate-limiting GTP enzyme (Nagatsu 1995). Mutations in the GTP cyclohydrolase I gene contribute to hereditary L-DOPA-responsive dystonia (Bandmann *et al.* 1998), the symptoms of which manifest in a circadian manner (i.e. worst in the evening and at night) and with greater penetrance in women (Nygaard 1993; Nygaard *et al.* 1993).

Following the release of dopamine, the primary mode of removal from the synapse is reuptake into the presynaptic neuron via the dopamine transporter (DAT). DAT is dependent upon the energy created by the Na^+/K^+ pump and is a member of the Na^+/Cl^--dependent plasma membrane transporter family, as are the norepinephrine and γ-aminobutyric acid (GABA) transporters. Imaging studies utilizing compounds with highly specific affinity for DAT

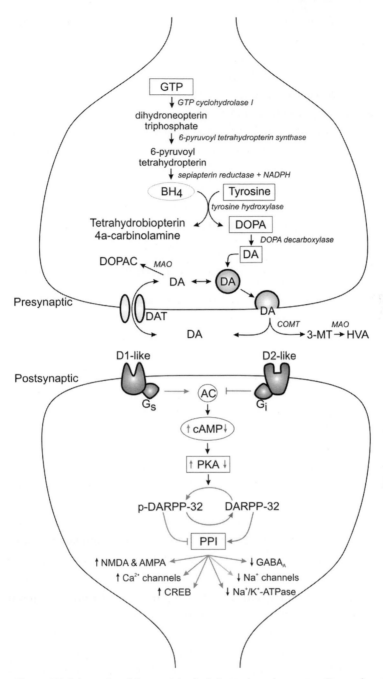

Figure 7.1 Schematic of the prototypical dopaminergic synapse. Pre- and post-synaptic components of a dopaminergic synapse summarizing molecular pathways for dopamine synthesis, metabolism, and second messenger effects following D1-like or D2-like receptor activation. (See also Plate 6.)

(i.e. 3β-(4-iodophenyl) tropane-2β-carboxylate, or β-CIT) permit visualization of the integrity of the dopamine system.

Once returned to the presynaptic terminal, dopamine is repackaged into synaptic vesicles via the vesicular monoamine transporter (VMAT) or metabolized to dihydroxyphenylacetic acid (DOPAC) by monoamine oxidase (MAO). Two alternative pathways are available for dopamine catabolism in the synapse, depending on whether the first step is catalyzed by MAO or catechol-O-methyltransferase (COMT). Thus, dopamine can be either deaminated to 3,4-dihydroxyphenylacetic acid (DOPAC) or methylated to 3-methoxytyramine (3-MT). In turn, deamination of 3-MT and methylation of DOPAC leads to homovanillic acid (HVA). In humans, cerebrospinal fluid levels of HVA have been used as a proxy for levels of dopaminergic activity within the brain (Stanley *et al.* 1985).

Physiological effects of dopamine at cellular and subcellular levels

The physiological effects of the dopaminergic system are best characterized as "neuromodulatory." Rather than eliciting excitatory (EPSPs) or inhibitory postsynaptic potentials (IPSPs) in a manner similar to glutamate and GABA, for example, dopamine allows the gating of inputs via alteration of membrane properties and specific ion conductances (Nicola *et al.* 2000). This enhanced or decreased response to other inputs affects the intensity, duration, and timing of output commensurate with environmental and homeostatic demands (Barbeau and Rossignol 1991; Kiehn and Kjaerulff 1996; Katz 1996). The multivariate control of dopamine is provided through five subtypes of seven transmembrane domain G-protein coupled receptors (D_1–D_5), which, based upon similarities in pharmacology, biochemistry, and amino acid homology, are divided into two classes, D_{1-like} (D_1, D_5) and D_{2-like} (D_2, D_3, D_4) (Missale *et al.* 1998). Ligand binding studies estimate the relative order of affinity for endogenous dopamine is $D_3 > D_4 > D_2 >> D_1$ obtained from references provided by a search of http://pdsp.med.unc.edu) (Sautel *et al.* 1995; Sokoloff *et al.* 1992). Furthermore, each receptor subtype has unique patterns of localization throughout the brain that increase the potential repertoire of the behavioral effects of dopamine.

$D1_{-like}$ receptors activate the G_s transduction pathway, stimulating the production of adenylyl cyclase, which increases the formation of cyclic adenosine monophosphate (cAMP) and ultimately increases the activity of cAMP-dependent protein kinase (PKA). PKA activates DARPP-32 (dopamine and cyclic adenosine 3′,5′-monophosphate-regulated phosphoprotein, 32 kDa) via phosphorylation, permitting phospho-DARPP-32 to then inhibit protein phosphatase-1 (PP-1). The downstream effect of decreased PP-1 activity is an increase in the phosphorylation states of assorted downstream effector proteins regulating neurotransmitter receptors and voltage-gated ion channels. Ultimately this results in increased activity of glutamate receptors (NMDA and AMPA), Ca^{2+} channels (L-, N-, and P-types), and CREB, as well as decreased activity of $GABA_A$ receptors, Na^+ channels, and Na^+/K^+-ATPase (Greengard et al. 1999). Alternatively, $D_{2\text{-like}}$ receptors stimulate the G_i transduction pathway, which is negatively coupled to the production of adenylylcyclase. Activation of $D_{2\text{-like}}$ receptors also leads to an increase in intracellular calcium concentrations. These two pathways can act independently, through decreased PKA and increased calcineurin, respectively, to return phospho-DARPP-32 to the inactive DARPP-32. In addition, calcineurin activity can be stimulated by the increase in intracellular calcium concentrations caused by glutamatergic activation of NMDA receptors. Other mechanisms of action mediated by $D_{2\text{-like}}$ receptors include increasing K^+ conductance and inhibiting Ca^{2+} entry via voltage-gated Ca^{2+} channels.

Both $D_{1\text{-like}}$ and $D_{2\text{-like}}$ receptors are found postsynaptically, exerting their effect on non-dopaminergic neurons targeted by dopaminergic projections. $D_{2\text{-like}}$ receptors can also be localized presynaptically on the dendrites, soma, and presynaptic terminals of dopaminergic cells. The presynaptic localization of the autoreceptors enables them to provide inhibitory feedback (Groves et al. 1975). The regulation in the somatodendritic region includes modulation of the firing rate of the dopaminergic cell, and in the nerve terminal autoreceptors control the synthesis and release of dopamine. In addition, dopamine acts upon receptors present on endothelial cells lining the brain's microvasculature, promoting vasoconstriction (Krimer et al. 1998). Although the exact mechanisms for the regulation of dopamine synthesis and for dopamine release remain to be elucidated, evidence does exist that these are distinct mechanisms (Cooper et al. 2002). For example, in the prefrontal and cingulate cortices, activation of autoreceptors regulates the release, but not the synthesis, of dopamine (Cooper et al. 2002). Low dose effects of dopaminomimetics are mediated by autoreceptor activation, as opposed to postsynaptic receptors, owing to their 10-fold higher affinity for dopamine.

Functional anatomy of central dopamine circuits

It has now been some 40 years since a group of Swedish scientists first described the nigrostriatal, mesocorticolimbic, and tuberoinfundibular dopamine neurons as giving rise to the three most conspicuous and behaviorally relevant dopamine circuits in the brain (Dahlstrom and Fuxe 1964). By using histofluorescence and subsequent immunohistochemical identification of TH (Hokfelt et al. 1984; Halasz et al. 1985) 16 unique monoaminergic cell groups were identified and given designations A1–A16, of which dopamine has been identified as a major transmitter in a portion of A2, located in the dorsal motor vagal complex, and groups A8–A16 (Lindvall and Bjorklund 1982). The chemoarchitecture, connectivity, and receptor distribution of the catecholamine system is comparable across vertebrate species with limited exceptions (Smeets and Gonzalez 2000). Operationally, these groups can be characterized as long projection, versus local circuit, neurons with unique functions (see Table 7.1).

The nigrostriatal pathway originates in the midbrain, from catecholamine cell groups A8 and A9, and projects to the caudate nucleus and putamen (collectively, often referred to as the dorsal striatum). This pathway is traditionally thought to modulate voluntary movement during waking; its destruction or degeneration, as seen in PD, results in impairments in the planning, initiation, and execution of movement and motor engrams (Kandel *et al.* 2000; Grillner *et al.* 2005; Albin *et al.* 1989; DeLong 1990). Heuristic models of this major dopaminergic circuit focus themselves upon the indirect actions of dopamine (i.e., via the dorsal striatum) upon the internal segment of the globus pallidus (GPi) and substantia nigra pars reticulata (SNr), and a series of parallel, segregated striato-pallidal-thalamocortical recurrent loops centered upon functionally distinct cortical regions (Alexander *et al.* 1986, 1990, 1997). The anatomy of the input and output connections of the A8–A9 neurons and associated behaviors are most often considered in isolation with the basal ganglia nuclei and the thalamus. Moreover, wakefulness has been the default "medium" through which the behavioral correlates of dopamine dysfunction are thought to play out in this major pathway. It is less well established or understood what relevance this dopaminergic system might have to modulation of normal and pathological sleep–wake states (see below).

The mesocorticolimbic pathway arises from the midbrain catecholamine cell group A10, within the ventral tegmental area, and targets the ventral striatum (nucleus accumbens), subcortical limbic nuclei such as the septum and amygdala, the hippocampus, and prefrontal cortex (4). Activation of this pathway is known to modulate various cognitive/emotive functions including reward, the psychomotor effects associated with drugs of abuse, and working memory (Tzschentke and Schmidt 2000; Fibiger and Phillips 1986; Goldman-Rakic 1995). Disruption of this pathway is thought to modify schizophrenia, attention deficit hyperactivity disorder, Tourette's syndrome, and major depression. Together, the nigrostriatal and mesocorticolimbic systems account for nearly 80% of the dopamine content in brain. Subsets of these midbrain dopaminergic neurons have unique phenotypes (e.g., co-release of glutamate and production of neuropeptides such as neurotensin), the functional significance of which is unclear (Seutin 2005).

The third major circuit, the tuberoinfundibular and tuberohypophyseal pathways, originate in the hypothalamic arcuate/periarcuate nuclei and periventricular hypothalamus (catecholamine cell groups A12 and A14, respectively). Activation of the A12 cluster modulates the release of numerous hormones in very complex ways; often in opposing ways at the cellular versus the presynaptic level. Dopamine in the tuberoinfundibular system/anterior pituitary tonically inhibits release of prolactin and luteinizing and thyroid stimulating hormones, and promotes growth hormone release, primarily via effects on releasing hormones (Krulich 1979; Behrends *et al.* 1998; Martin 1978; Benker *et al.* 1990; Muller 1973). The effects of dopamine upon the tuberohypophyseal system include generally inhibitory modulation of vasopressin release, and facilitation of oxytocin release (30).

The little studied A11 catecholamine cell group in the subparafascicular thalamus is the largest, likely sole, source of spinal dopamine (Bjorklund and Skagerberg 1979; Hokfelt *et al.* 1979; Skagerberg *et al.* 1982; Skagerberg and Lindvall 1985). Within the spinal cord, these axons target the intermediolateral column (IML) housing preganglionic sympathetic neurons, dorsal horn regions related to afferent nerve processing, and interneurons (e.g., Renshaw cells) (Skagerberg *et al.* 1982), where they likely dampen spinal nociceptive processing and sympathetic outflow, and enhance motor output predominantly via $D_{2\text{-like}}$ receptor mechanisms (Fleetwood-Walker *et al.* 1988; Gladwell and Coote 1999). Hypofunctioning of this circuit has been hypothesized to account for the sensorimotor disturbances encountered in restless legs syndrome/periodic leg movements of sleep (Clemens *et al.* 2006).

The axons of major projecting brain dopamine systems have a proclivity to collateralize extensively, i.e. individual axons branch and innervate two or more physically, and perhaps functionally, unique regions (Sanchez-Gonzalez *et al.* 2005; Freeman *et al.* 2001; Gaspar *et al.* 1992). In addition to innervating the striatum and frontal cortex, for example, A8–A9–A10 neurons also target the thalamus (principally the midline, intralaminar, and reticular nuclei that modulate thalamocortical excitability), the extended amygdala, the noradrenergic locus coeruleus, and the serotonergic raphe system. Axons of individual A11 cells branch extensively to all spinal cord levels along their course in the dorsolateral funiculi, as well as to the prefrontal cortex, amygdala, and nucleus of the solitary tract (Takada 1993). These arrangements are ideally suited to coordinate behaviors affected by disparate brain areas (e.g. environmental stimuli, cardiorespiratory homeostasis, and sleep–wake state) and bear remarkable semblance to other nuclei traditionally thought of as influencing the arousal state of the organism (i.e. those forming the Ascending Reticular Activating System) (cf. Brown and McCarley, this volume).

Circadian, homeostatic, and state influences on central dopamine signaling

Prior to embarking on a consideration of the role of dopamine in regulation of arousal state (see below), it is pertinent to preface this with a discussion of how this role, in turn, comes under the influence of circadian, homeostatic, and behavioral state factors. Such knowledge highlights the dynamic nature of dopamine signaling across the rest–activity cycle, thereby informing interpretations of how perturbations to central dopamine signaling affect arousal behaviors. Fluctuations in dopamine levels and receptor densities (and sensitivities), for example, may introduce variable effects on the 'state' of an organism in response to exogenous dopaminomimetic administration during high versus low levels of endogenous dopamine 'tone' across the activity–rest cycle. Indeed, it has long been appreciated that there are diurnal rhythms in content, turnover, release, and behavioral responsivity of most of the CNS dopamine systems outlined above, including those of the eye (Gaytan *et al.* 1998; O'Neill and Fillenz 1985; Doyle *et al.* 2002; Paulson and Robinson 1994; Megaw *et al.* 2006). Although we are far from a complete understanding, it is relatively safe to state that dopamine synthesis, release, and signaling in multiple mammalian species peaks early during the active period and nadirs early in the major inactive period (i.e., sleep). This rhythm is retained in cultures containing hypothalamic dopamine neurons that are in close proximity to the principal circadian pacemaker (i.e. the suprachiasmatic nucleus), and less evident, or absent, in cultures containing forebrain or midbrain dopamine neurons (Abe *et al.* 2002). Circadian influences upon brain dopamine systems are conveyed in part via melatonin, as a pinealectomy dampens rhythms in striatal dopamine content (Khaldy *et al.* 2002). There is increasing evidence of molecular control of dopaminergic transmission by genes involved in the circadian clock (McClung *et al.* 2005). Mice expressing an inactive protein of the circadian-associated gene *Clock* exhibit increased expression and phosphorylation of TH, and increased activity in A10 dopaminergic neurons and associated behaviors (McClung *et al.* 2005).

Diurnal variations in dopamine signaling

Insight into the state of dopaminergic "tone" is best obtained from measurements of extracellular dopamine in microdialysate samples collected from the behaving organism. Striatal (Paulson and Robinson 1994; Smith *et al.* 1992; Castaneda *et al.* 2004) and prefrontal cortical (Feenstra *et al.* 2000) dopamine levels rise in anticipation of, and are maintained throughout, the major wakefulness period in the rat, in concert with declines in dopamine metabolites (i.e., DOPAC, HVA, and 5-HIAA) (Smith *et al.* 1992; Whittaker *et al.* 1997). This pattern is mirrored by tissue contents of: (1) dopamine derived from whole brain (Lemmer and Berger 1978; Scheving *et al.* 1968), striatum, cerebellum, cortex (Matsumoto *et al.* 1981; Owasoyo *et al.* 1979), hippocampus, midbrain, and brainstem (Matsumoto *et al.* 1981); (2) TH (McGeer and McGeer 1973) and tetrahydrobiopterin (Mandell *et al.* 1980) (both necessary for dopamine synthesis); and (3) the dopamine transporter (DAT) (Whittaker *et al.* 1997), the principal determinant of dopamine signaling (Jaber *et al.* 1997). The greatest diurnal variations in dopamine content in the mouse, a nocturnal animal, occur within the hypothalamus (Matsumoto *et al.* 1981), peaking at midnight then dropping significantly by 4 a.m. It remains controversial whether rhythms of proteins involved in dopamine signaling in the rat striatum are mirrored by changes in dopamine receptor density (Bruinink *et al.* 1983; Watanabe and Seeman 1984; Naber *et al.* 1980), and whether they might be more pronounced in subcircuits traditionally considered to subserve "limbic" (O'Neill and Fillenz 1985) as opposed to "motor" (Paulson and Robinson 1994) behaviors. This being said, differential behavioral responsivity reflective of presumed ultradian variations in individual dopamine signaling pathways are well established following systemic apomorphine (Nagayama *et al.* 1978) and amphetamine (Gaytan *et al.* 1998; Evans *et al.* 1973) administration. While acknowledging that methamphetamine effects cannot be attributed solely to enhanced availability of synaptic dopamine, operant behaviors increase significantly only after administration during the active period while locomotor activity increases independent of time of administration (Evans *et al.* 1973). Pharmacokinetic investigations have further established that time of day also influences the kinetics of the metabolism of dopamine. L-DOPA, a precursor of dopamine (see above), has the highest plasma clearance rates in rats following administration at 2200 h, i.e., early in the major wake period (Naber *et al.* 1980). These diurnal variances in dopamine receptor activation and L-DOPA pharmacokinetics are evident in species as diverse as fruit flies (Andretic and Hirsh 2000) and humans (Garcia-Borreguero *et al.* 2001).

In non-human primates and humans, diurnal rhythms in the content and release of dopamine are evident in extracellular microdialysates from the putamen, amygdala, and cerebrospinal fluid (CSF), and in urine. These are generally concordant with those observed in rodents. The first studies to probe for diurnal variations in the monoamine content of human brain were those undertaken by Carlsson and colleagues on the hypothalamus in post mortem tissue (Carlsson *et al.* 1980). These studies confirm a daily peak in tissue dopamine content during the active period, 1500–1800 h, with a nadir in the early morning hours (Carlsson *et al.* 1980). Indirect measures of dopamine release in lumbar CSF (Hagan *et al.* 1999), urine (Kawano *et al.* 1990), and plasma (Sowers and Vlachakis 1984) reveal a maximum in the morning at around 0800 h with a nadir at

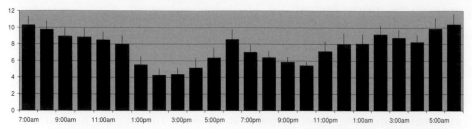

Figure 7.2 Diurnal variation of extracellular dopamine in the non-human primate putamen. Dopamine concentrations (nM) as determined by high-pressure liquid chromatography of microdialysates obtained from the putamen of two rhesus monkeys across their 12:12 h lights-on (waking 7:00 am–7:00 pm) and lights off (sleep; 7:00 pm–7:00 am) periods. Ten minute samples (2 μl/min sampling rate) were derived from nine individual 8 h sessions in each animal in which the sleep–wake state was monitored simultaneously by standard electrophysiological parameters.

approximately 0400 h. Ventricular CSF from rhesus monkeys is difficult to interpret secondary to analyses that utilize the dopamine metabolite HVA as a proxy for dopamine "turnover" and a sampling method unable to assess accurately the origin of this signal from the many potential sources of juxtaventricular dopamine (Perlow *et al.* 1977). To avoid these limitations, we have recently completed an assessment of the diurnal and state-related fluctuations of dopamine release in the putamen of two rhesus monkeys via *in vivo* microdialysis in combination with simultaneous electrophysiological monitoring of arousal state (Freeman 2006; Freeman *et al.* 2006). The 24 h rhythm of dopamine release describes two peaks, the more robust occurring immediately upon lights-on/awakening at 0700–0800 h, and a second, less pronounced inflection 12 h later in anticipation of the 1900 h lights-off (Fig. 7.2). Two troughs are observed: one during the mid-afternoon at 1400–1500 h, and a second at 2200 h at the beginning of the major sleep period. Elevations of dopamine across the major sleep period followed by decreases during successive hours of wakefulness are reminiscent of a homeostatic alerting signal; the secondary peak 1–3 h prior to the sleep period coincides with an interval of minimal sleep tendency reflective of the circadian alerting signal (Edgar *et al.* 1003; Strogatz *et al.* 1987). A second remarkable finding of this study is that the most conspicuous rise in extracellular dopamine occurs during the major sleep period, a state purported to be characterized by minimal discharge activity in motor-(Grace and Bunney 1980; Steinfels *et al.* 1983) and limbic-(Trulson and Preuseler 1984; Miller *et al.* 1983) related midbrain dopamine neurons. The observed rhythms across the wake–sleep cycle therefore reflect previously unappreciated state-related modulation of dopamine release by a burst firing mode, and/or modulation of nigrostriatal terminals by an afferent source yet to be defined, quite possibly the cerebrocortical mantle (see below and (Lena *et al.* 2005)). In humans, similar diurnal fluctuations of extracellular dopamine in the amygdala and adjacent limbic cortex occur (Zeitzer *et al.* 2001). Afternoon and end-of-day dips in extracellular dopamine appear to coincide with 10%–20% ultradian decreases in $D_{1\text{-like}}$ receptor density in the putamen and frontal cortex in humans (Karlsson *et al.* 2000). The functional significance of these diurnal rhythms across the wake–sleep cycle remains to be determined. More comprehensive analyses that include sleep deprivation and constant environmental conditions are needed in order to determine the relative contribution of striatal, limbic, and cortical dopamine to the homeostatic and circadian alerting signals.

Homeostatic influences upon dopamine signaling

The central dopamine systems also appear to be under homeostatic influences and this has been studied primarily in the nigrostriatal pathway. Among the central dopamine systems, plasticity in the nigrostriatal pathway in the setting of increased homeostatic demands upon sleep appears unique. Hypothalamic dopamine receptors, for example, are unaffected by sleep deprivation (Lal *et al.* 1981). Dopamine and its metabolites, as opposed to other monoamines, are increased in the striatum of REM sleep-deprived rats (Ghosh *et al.* 1976; Tufik *et al.* 1978; Farber *et al.* 1983; Asakura *et al.* 1999; Farooqui *et al.* 1996; Lara-Lemus *et al.* 1998). There is disagreement, on the other hand, concerning the precise receptor and regional changes that occur. Some investigators argue for no changes in the absolute receptor number (Farber *et al.* 1983; Hamdi *et al.* 1993); others describe increases in $D_{2\text{-like}}$ receptor binding (Zwicker and Calil 1986; Nunes *et al.* 1994; Brock *et al.* 1995). Still others argue for a $D_{1\text{-like}}$ receptor mediated increase in adenylate cyclase within mesocortical limbic pathways whose reversal with $D_{1\text{-like}}$, as opposed to $D_{2\text{-like}}$, antagonists facilitates rebound sleep (Fadda *et al.* 1992, 1993; Durán-Vázquez and Drucker-Colín 1997).

Dopamine availability in relation to behavioral state

There is a paucity of data concerning the release of dopamine during specific sleep stages or states compared with wakefulness. However, it would appear safe to conclude that striatal extracellular dopamine peaks during states of heightened thalamocortical arousal such as wakefulness (see above). These levels are generally maintained throughout the major wake period in rats compared with a more complex and dynamic rhythm evident in non-human primates (Fig. 7.2). Negative findings are more difficult to interpret given the temporal and spatial limitations of microdialysis (e.g. 'floor' or limit of detection effects in regions sparsely innervated by dopamine terminals). Moreover, there is the real possibility of species and regional brain differences in dopamine release. Despite the reported stability of dopamine neuronal firing rate across sleep–wake states, rates of dopamine release assessed in the cat by voltammetry (with a temporal resolution superior to that of microdialysis) fluctuate relative to sleep–wake state (Trulson 1985). One study of dopamine release in the amygdala and locus coeruleus in cats failed to detect variations in relation to sleep–wake state (Shouse et al. 2000). Dopamine release in the more densely innervated medial prefrontal cortex and nucleus accumbens of the rat is heightened in wakefulness and REM sleep compared with slow wave sleep (SWS) (Lena et al. 2005). In contrast, in the rhesus monkey putamen, discernable fluctuations in dopamine concentration in relation to specific sleep stages are not evident (Freeman et al. 2006). Nor does there seem to be a consistent sleep-stage-specific release of dopamine in limbic brain regions in humans (Zeitzer et al. 2001). The diurnal rhythm of dopamine originating and measured from systemic sources in humans also appears to be independent of sleep state (Sowers and Vlachakis 1984).

The modulation of wake–sleep state by dopamine

Psychomotor stimulants such as amphetamine exhibit a molecular structure remarkably similar to that of dopamine (Hardman et al. 2001) and, while promoting locomotion and stereotypic movements, coincidentally enhance wakefulness at the expense of SWS and REM sleep (Edgar and Seidel 1997). The wake-promoting effect of these agents (as distinct from their locomotor enhancing effects) is predicated upon their affinities for the DAT, and thereby, their abilities to enhance synaptic dopamine (Wisor et al. 2001). Increases in the availability of synaptic dopamine made possible by genetically based interference with DAT function in both mice (Wisor et al. 2001) and flies (Kume et al. 2005) promotes wakefulness. Additional compelling evidence that dopamine modulates the sleep–wake continuum comes from the human clinic. Clinicians have taken advantage of the wake-promoting effects of dopaminomimetics, but they are also becoming increasingly aware of their potential soporific effects. Conditions such as atypical depression, narcolepsy/cataplexy, and PD, for example, are characterized by variable degrees of sleepiness, inappropriate intrusion of sleep-onset REM sleep into daytime naps, alterations of proteins that govern dopamine transmission in targets of dopamine neurons, and hypoactivity that responds favorably to dopaminomimetics (Rye 2004a,b; Rye and Jankovic 2002). Heuristic models that once emphasized the monoamines serotonin, norepinephrine, histamine, and acetylcholine as important to wakefulness (Mignot et al. 2002) are therefore now being revised to incorporate an increasing number of compelling observations that point to dopamine as a critical modulator of wake–sleep state. The vast

Table 7.1 *Major dopaminergic modulatory systems of the brain.*

Abbreviations: MPO, medial preoptic area.

Origin		1° Projections	Function
Long projecting systems			
A8	Retrorubral field	Forebrain	Unknown
A9	Substantia nigra		
	Dorsal tier[a]	Striatal matrix	Motor behaviors
	Ventral tier[a]	Striatal patches	Limbic modulation
A10	Ventral tegmental area	Nucleus accumbens	Reward
		"Limbic" cortical and subcortical structures	Motivation, arousal, appetite
A11	Subparafascicular thalamus	Spinal cord	Sensorimotor modulation
Local circuits			
A12	Arcuate/periventricular hypothalamus	Median eminence/infundibular stalk	Modulate hormone release
		Intermediate and neural lobes of the hypophysis	
A13	Medial zona incerta	Local; anterior hypothalamus MPO	Unknown
A14	Periventricular hypothalamus	Local; anterior hypothalamus MPO	Unknown
A15	Olfactory tubercle	Local	Unknown
A16	Olfactory bulb Periglomerular cell		Increase dynamic range for odor detection[b]
A17	Retina inner nuclear layer Amacrine cells		Light adaptation – contrast sensitivity[c]

Adapted from Halasz *et al.* (1985) and (Kandel *et al.* (2000).

[a] (Gerfen *et al.* 1987).

[b] (Ennis *et al.* 2001).

[c] (Witkovsky 2004).

number of local circuit and long projecting dopamine systems in vertebrates (Table 7.1) precludes a complete accounting of how each might modulate normal and pathologic sleep-wake states. We will therefore focus our discussion on the largest contributor to dopamine content in the CNS, the mesotelencephalic system, for which the greatest and most relevant data exist. This being said, we will highlight other dopamine systems when appropriate, i.e., where converging lines of evidence present a compelling story that they affect arousal state (e.g. the hypothalamic A11 and retinal A17 cell groups). We recognize that hypothalamically mediated hormonal release by dopamine might also be relevant to this discussion, since many of these hormones are known to modulate behavioral state. Complex feedback loops include not only hypothalamic, but *also* mesotelencephalic dopamine neurons that express receptors for many of these molecules (Pi *et al.* 2002; Heuer *et al.* 2000; Lonstein and Blaustein 2004). These complex reciprocal interactions make it difficult to dissociate definitively the hormonal from the dopaminergic effects on state. The reader should be at least aware that these discussions are ongoing in neuroendocrinology, and that they may ultimately have relevance to an even more comprehensive account of the modulation of behavioral state by dopamine.

Exogenous dopaminomimetic effects on wake–sleep state

Notable effects on the proportion of time spent awake or asleep are consistently observed following the systemic administration of pharmacological agents that target any of the molecules involved in dopamine signaling (see above, Fig. 7.1). Because of differential regional expression in the peripheral nervous system and the CNS, and binding affinities of the different dopamine receptor subtypes, as well as their pre- versus postsynaptic localizations (reviewed in (Gillin *et al.* 1981; Rye and Bliwise 1997)), the effects of dopaminomimetics on sleep–wake state are complex and have been difficult to attribute to a specific receptor subtype, or to localize to a specific set of dopamine neurons or brain circuits. Strategies to comprehend this complexity have included systemic, intracerebroventricular, or focal brain delivery of pharmacological agents that activate or inactivate, more or less selectively, the pharmacologically and molecularly defined dopamine receptors. More recent paradigms have incorporated genetic engineering of some of the molecules involved in dopamine signaling such as DAT, and several of the molecularly defined dopamine receptor subtypes. Taken together, these studies show that dopamine is critical to arousal, as well as to normal rest and activity patterns. While providing some additional insights, however, many of the details remain a matter for scientific inquiry.

Pharmacological agents that interfere with the primary route of removal of dopamine, namely presynaptic reuptake via DAT, enhance wakefulness in proportion to their binding affinities for DAT (Cooper *et al.* 2002; Nishino *et al.* 1998). The most robust durations in the amount of time spent awake and alpha-power in the electroencephalogram, for example, are observed following administration of agents with the highest binding affinities for DAT. The wake-promoting effects are presumably due to an increased availability of synaptic dopamine resulting from blockade of the primary clearing mechanism. Genetically engineered mice lacking DAT exhibit increased activity levels and wake bout lengths during the second half of the active phase, and are immune to the wake-promoting effects of DAT blockers (Wisor *et al.* 2001). The regulation of arousal by dopamine through the DAT is also evident in invertebrates. A genetically engineered lesion rendering DAT inactive in *Drosophila melanogaster* (Porzgen *et al.* 2001) yields a hyperactive mutant appropriately named fumin, which literally translates from Japanese as 'sleepless' (Kume *et al.* 2005). These fruit flies spend an increased amount of time in the waking, active phase with a corresponding deficit in the inactive or sleep phase. Blockade of dopamine synthesis in wild-type flies either pharmacologically or via genetic manipulation renders them unresponsive to methamphetamine-induced increases in wake-like activity (Andretic *et al.* 2005).

The wake-promoting actions of dopamine signaling are further supported by consideration of the effects of a variety of dopaminomimetics on sleep–wake state. These effects are dose- and receptor-dependent and reveal that the effects of dopamine on behavioral state are best characterized as biphasic. This biphasic dose–response relation for systemically administered dopamine is manifest in several physiological and behavioral endpoints, including locomotion, pain sensitivity, blood pressure, prolactin secretion, oxytocin release, and heart rate (Calabrese 2001). It is therefore difficult to ascertain whether sleep–wake behaviors attributed to dopamine reflect direct, as opposed to indirect, actions on brain arousal circuits. In healthy, drug-naive humans, sleep is enhanced by low doses of the dopamine precursor L-dopa, an effect that habituates after one week of treatment (Andreu *et al.* 1999). This effect is thought to reflect activation of $D_{2\text{-like}}$ presynaptic autoreceptors; higher doses, usually sufficient to increase locomotor activity, enhance wakefulness and suppress SWS and REM sleep, likely reflecting actions at both $D_{1\text{-like}}$ and $D_{2\text{-like}}$ postsynaptic receptors (Logos *et al.* 1998; Isaac and Berridge 2003). Systemic (Trampus *et al.* 1991; Monti *et al.* 1990; Cianchetti *et al.* 1984) and intracerebroventricular delivery of $D_{1\text{-like}}$ agonists increase wakefulness at the expense of both SWS and REM sleep (Isaac and Berridge 2003). Conversely, $D_{1\text{-like}}$ antagonists promote sleep and increase the time spent in SWS and REM sleep (Trampus *et al.* 1991, 1993; Monti *et al.* 1990; Ongini *et al.* 1993). The actions of $D_{2\text{-like}}$ agonists are more clearly dose-related. Lower doses exhibit sedative effects believed to reflect their preferential activation of $D_{2\text{-like}}$ inhibitory autoreceptors; higher doses have the opposite effect (Lagos *et al.* 1998; Monti 1989; Mnti *et al.* 1988). Consistent with this observation, wakefulness follows administration of the dopamine autoreceptor antagonist (–)DS121 (Olive *et al.* 1998). The CNS site mediating the soporific effects of low doses of dopaminomimetics appears to be $D_{2\text{-like}}$ inhibitory autoreceptors on the cell bodies or terminal axonal fields of dopaminergic VTA neurons. Local applications of $D_{2\text{-like}}$ receptor antagonists in the VTA block sedation provoked by systemic agonists (Bagetta *et al.* 1988); amphetamine administration into the ventromedial forebrain targets of VTA neurons initiates and maintains alert waking (Berridge *et al.* 1999).

Investigations that take into account the molecular signatures of dopamine receptors provide further details. Dopamine signaling by way of the D_2 receptor has recently been shown to be necessary for light to disrupt circadian rest–activity rhythms (i.e. light 'masking' of endogenous circadian rhythms) (Doi *et al.* 2006). Converging lines of evidence suggest that this reflects dopamine and D_2 receptor modulation of non-visual photic responses in the retina (Steenhard and Besharse 2000, 2004; Ribelayga *et al.* 2004; Sakamoto *et al.* 2005), although contributions from central sites of action cannot be ruled out. Interest in the D_3 receptor is motivated by the fact that, with the lowest K_d for endogenous dopamine (55 nM), it is the receptor subtype most likely to be activated or inactivated by the physiological range of extracellular dopamine concentrations. Mice lacking a functional D_3 receptor exhibit marked increases in wakefulness (at the expense of both SWS and REM sleep) in both their light and their dark phases, suggesting that the actions of dopamine at this receptor are necessary for mediating normal sleep stages (Hue *et al.* 2003). These arousal state changes may be an epiphenomenon of heightened responses to novelty (Hue *et al.* 2003), or decrements in the gating of spinal sensorimotor excitability (Clemens *et al.* 2006; Clemens and Hochman 2004). However, consistent with a role for D_3 receptor activation in mediating normal sleep, systemic administration of low doses of the D_3-preferring agonists ropinirole in humans (Ferreira *et al.* 2002) and pramipexole in rats (Lagos *et al.* 1998) promote sleep at the expense of wakefulness. As wakefulness is a prerequisite for locomotion, dissociating dopamine and dopamine receptor effects on arousal as separate from those on locomotion will necessitate simultaneous recording of both behaviors and careful interpretation.

Wake–sleep-related physiology of mesotelencephalic dopamine neurons

Examination of the state-related discharge rates of individual motor (Grace and Bunney 1980; Steinfels *et al.* 1983; Miller *et al.* 1983) and limbic (Trulson and Preussler 1984; Miller *et al.* 1983) mesencephalic dopaminergic cells previously negated considerations of dopamine as a leading player in arousal state regulation. These interpretations were suspect, however, not only because of limitations in sampling and analysis, but also because of the observation that, at least in non-human primates, extracellular dopamine increases throughout sleep (see above, Fig. 7.2). In one study, neurons were recorded over only a single sleep–wake cycle and the interspike interval (ISI) analysis was limited to only three neurons across all behavioral states (Steinfels *et al.* 1983). Samples biased towards the medial substantia nigra pars compacta, owing to its high cell packing density, ignore the real potential for functional/anatomical differences between individual neurons. Miller *et al.* (Miller *et al.* 1983), in fact, reported that

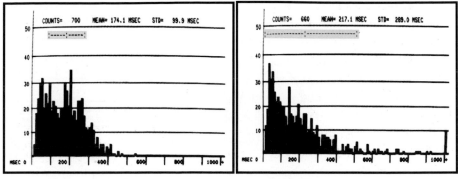

Slow-wave sleep   **Rapid eye movement (REM) sleep**

Figure 7.3 Interspike interval (ISI) histograms of midbrain dopamine neural firing in behaving rats (reproduced with permission from (Miller *et al.* 1983)). Note the nearly identical mean intervals, consistent with reported mean firing rate similarities between SWS and REM sleep, as opposed to the broader ISI range observed in REM sleep, reflective of the "burst" firing in a significant subpopulation of neurons (contrast the widths of the dashed bars above the histograms).

state-related changes in 6 of 17 pars compacta and 5 of 7 VTA dopaminergic neurons were "inconsistent," with the largest variance noted between SWS and REM sleep. Although the mean ISIs between SWS and REM sleep were no different, variance in interspike intervals (thought to represent burst firing) was significantly elevated in REM sleep (Fig. 7.3). Such "burst firing" drives synaptic release of dopamine more efficiently (Kitai *et al.* 1999; Chergui *et al.* 1994; Floresco *et al.* 2003) and is modulated by glutamatergic inputs from subthalamic (Urbain *et al.* 2000) and pedunculopontine tegmental neurons (PPN) (Steriade *et al.* 1990). The firing rates and patterns of the latter cell populations are themselves intimately related to behavioral state (particularly, to states of thalamocortical arousal). Thus, it is plausible that behavioral-state-specific alterations in dopamine neuron excitability do in fact, occur, and that they may account for differential release of dopamine across different stages of sleep or by time of night, as discussed above. Increases in extracellular release of dopamine across the night might alternatively point to synaptic mechanisms operating independently of neuronal firing. One possible mechanism, for example, is glutamatergic regulation of non-synaptic release of dopamine by way of reverse passage via DAT (Borland and Michael 2004; Mathe *et al.* 1999).

Wake–sleep-related functional anatomy of mesotelencephalic dopamine neurons

The mesocortical, mesolimbic, and mesostriatal systems are the most conspicuous of the brain circuits employing dopamine, and are traditionally taught to govern cognitive, emotive, and motor behaviors, respectively (see

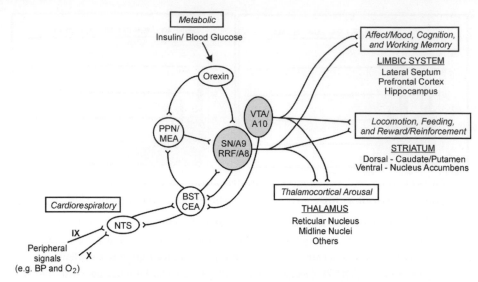

Figure 7.4 Summary of some of the wide array of afferent and efferent connections of midbrain dopaminergic neurons (SN/A9, RRF/A8, and VTA/A10 in center of figure). This emphasizes their potential involvement in coordination of seemingly disparate behaviors inclusive of the sleep–wake state of the organism. Abbreviations: BP, blood pressure; BST, bed nucleus of the stria terminalis; CEA, central nucleus of the amygdala; MEA, midbrain extrapyramidal area; NTS, nucleus of the solitary tract; O_2, oxygen tension; PPN, pedunculopontine tegmental nucleus; RRF, retrorubral field; SN, substantia nigra; VTA, ventral tegmental area.

above). Indeed, in terms of brain dopamine and its contributions to normal and pathologic behavior, these are the primary associations. It is noteworthy that this construct segregates behavioral correlates of dopamine function and dysfunction to individual subcircuits. The anatomy of the input and output connections of dopamine neurons and associated behaviors are considered in isolation, rather than as components of even more complex behavioral repertoires requiring coordination of physiological responses across larger regions of the brain, brainstem, and spinal cord. The default "medium" through which each of the behavioral correlates of dopamine function and dysfunction have traditionally been considered is the state of wakefulness. Thus, contemporary heuristic models of the principal CNS dopamine pathways are inadequate in accounting for the wake–sleep alterations observed with systemic dopaminomimetics and those accompanying the profound dopamine cell loss that occurs in PD. These shortcomings in contemporary models of central dopamine anatomy and physiology have led us and others to reconsider and reinvestigate the anatomical relations of midbrain dopamine neurons (Fig. 7.4). The rich diversity of their afferents and efferents, particularly with brain regions known to modulate states of thalamocortical arousal, is striking. Of particular interest are the dense inputs from the extended amygdala (bed nucleus of the stria terminalis and central nucleus of the amygdala) (Georges and Aston-Jones 2001), hypothalamic orexin (i.e. hypocretin) neurons (Nakamura *et al.* 2000; Korotkova *et al.* 2003; Uramura *et al.* 2001), glutamatergic and cholinergic pedunculopontine tegmental (PPN) neurons (Kitai *et al.* 1999; Rye 1997), medullary, noradrenergic A1 and A2 and pontine A4–A5 (locus coeruleus; LC) neurons (Jones and Moore 1977; Liprando *et al.* 2004; Mejias-Aponte *et al.* 2004), and serotonergic dorsal raphe cells (Lavoie and Parent 1990; Corvaja *et al.* 1993; Moukhles *et al.* 1997). The extended amygdala receives second-order chemo- and baroreceptor and other visceral information from the nucleus of the solitary tract, orexin neurons sensitive to circulating glucose and insulin (Griffond *et al.* 1999), and the PPN, LC, and dorsal raphe intimately involved in modulating thalamocortical arousal state (cf. Lydic & Baghdoyan, this volume; Brown & McCarley, this volume). Hence midbrain dopamine neurons are well positioned to integrate autonomic, metabolic, and sleep/wake homeostatic information relevant to survival. These considerations emphasize that many putative arousal systems might mediate their effects on behavioral state via midbrain dopamine neurons. Most of the aforementioned sources of input to midbrain dopaminergic neurons are excitatory and govern impulse-dependent terminal release of dopamine via multiple glutamate receptor subtypes (Kitai *et al.* 1999), orexin-2 (Nakamura *et al.* 2000; Korotkova *et al.* 2003; Uramura *et al.* 2001), muscarinic (Kitai *et al.* 1999; Gronier and Rasmussen 1998; Forster and Blaha 2000; Miller and Blaha 2004), nicotinic (Grenhoff *et al.* 1991), and α_1-adrenoreceptors (Grenhoff *et al.* 1995; Lategan *et al.* 1992; Tassin *et al.* 1979). The effects of serotonin on midbrain dopamine neurons are complex. In general, serotonin appears to exert tonic inhibitory control of midbrain dopamine neurons via the 2B/2C receptor subtypes, and predominates in the mesocorticolimbic, as opposed to nigrostriatal, pathways (Di Matteo *et al.* 2002; Cobb and Abercrombie 2003; Olijslagers *et al.* 2004; Balckburn *et al.* 2006). These inhibitory serotonergic influences are mediated indirectly via dampening of local somatodendritic dopamine efflux (Cobb and Abercrombie 2003), the latter being a regulator of terminal dopamine release through autoreceptor-mediated negative feedback (Cragg and Greenfield 1997). Synergistic inhibition of striatal dopamine release also occurs via presynaptic 5-HT2B/C receptors (Alex *et al.* 2005). Positive feedback circuits involving VTA dopaminergic neurons, the medial prefrontal cortex, and reciprocal corticofugal glutamatergic innervation of midbrain dopamine neurons, on the other hand, reinforce synaptic dopamine release through cortical 5-HT1A (Bortolozzi *et al.* 2005; Lejeune and Millan 1999) and α_1 adreno-receptors (Tzschentke and Schmidt 2000; Darracq *et al.* 1998; Ventura *et al.* 2003). Dopaminergic "tone" in midbrain neurons also comes under the influence of, and influences, local

GABA-ergic neurons that themselves have been implicated in the modulation of thalamocortical arousal states such as wakefulness and REM sleep (Lee *et al.* 2001).

Outputs from midbrain dopaminergic neurons are as diverse as their inputs, and this further underscores their defining a nexus for the integration and coordination of stress and environmental stimuli with sleep–wake states and cardiorespiratory homeostasis. The proclivity for their axons to branch extensively to two or more physically and functionally unique brain regions renders them ideally suited to coordinate behaviors affected by disparate brain areas; in this they resemble other constituents of the ascending reticular activating system (ARAS). It is unlikely that there exist individual dopaminergic neurons devoted solely to affecting striatal excitability and the corresponding behavioral engrams without coordination with thalamocortical arousal state. Midbrain dopaminergic neurons have the potential to modulate directly normal and pathological thalamocortical neuron excitability, and by inference sleep–wake state, by way of an extensive set of collaterals from the nigrostriatal and mesocorticolimbic pathways (Sanchez-Gonzalez *et al.* 2005; Freeman *et al.* 2001). Because most (at least 50% of) A8–A9–A10 neurons simultaneously target the thalamus and dorsal or ventral striatum, the broad spectrum of dopamine-mediated neuropsychiatric disorders should have a correlated disturbance of thalamocortical arousal (i.e. sleep–wake state), albeit not as well documented. Similarly, all the internal and external cues that modulate the expression of a dopamine phenotype in these neurons could also manifest disturbances in thalamocortical arousal. Although the physiological effects of dopamine on thalamic neurons and function have received limited study, dopamine is recognized as serving a modulatory role similar to the ascending cholinergic and noradrenergic pathways to the thalamus. Innervation of the thalamic reticular nucleus, as well as the thalamocortical relay nuclei, supports this role (Sherman and Guillery 2001). The excitatory or inhibitory effects attributable to this innervation are dependent on whether $D_{1\text{-like}}$ or $D_{2\text{-like}}$, pre- or postsynaptic receptors on relay cells or interneurons are activated. The effects of dopamine on thalamocortical relay cell excitability, and thereby the transfer of information to the cortex, have been most studied in the dorsal lateral geniculate nucleus, which subserves visual processing. In the anesthetized preparation, dopamine has been reported to suppress or enhance neural discharge via $D_{1\text{-like}}$ or $D_{2\text{-like}}$ receptors, respectively (Albrecht *et al.* 1996). The reverse is true in the thalamic slice preparation where $D_{1\text{-like}}$ excitatory effects have been described (Govindaiah and Cox 2005), and $D_{2\text{-like}}$ receptor mediated inhibition occurs via presynaptic mechanisms (Govindaiah and Cox 2006) and GABA-ergic interneurons (Munsch *et al.* 2005). In the mediodorsal thalamus, dopamine enhances membrane excitability and facilitates low-threshold spike (LTS) activity primarily via $D_{2\text{-like}}$ versus $D_{1\text{-like}}$ receptors (Lavin and Grace 1998). Endogenous dopamine may act at D_4 receptors in the thalamic reticular nucleus to inhibit GABA release, thereby modulating the gating of thalamocortical transmission and spindle generation (Floran *et al.* 2004).

Midbrain dopamine neurons might also modulate thalamocortical arousal state indirectly, by way of output pathways to, inter alia, the extended amygdala and ventral forebrain, perifornical orexin neurons, and the LC. The functional impact of these projections to areas known to modulate behavioral and cortical arousal state is, at best, limited. Pathways ascending from midbrain dopamine neurons interact with cholinergic magnocellular forebrain neurons, and thereby have the potential to modulate acetylcholine release in the entire cortical mantle (Napier and Potter 1989; Gaykema and Zaborszky 1996; Smiley *et al.* 1999). The physiological effects of this interaction are poorly defined and include putative direct (Maslowski and Napier 1991) and indirect (Momiyama and Sim 1996) (presynaptic) $D_{1\text{-like}}$ receptor-mediated excitatory effects, and $D_{2\text{-like}}$ receptor-mediated inhibition (Maslowski and Napier 1991) of cholinergic neuron excitability. The molecularly defined D_5 receptor, within the $D_{1\text{-like}}$ pharmacologically defined receptor subclass, may be particularly relevant in promoting acetylcholine release, because it is expressed by the majority of forebrain cholinergic neurons (Berlanga *et al.* 2005). Midbrain dopamine neurons may also affect thalamocortical arousal state via direct and indirect inhibition of perifornical orexin neurons (Li and van den Pol 2005; Bubser *et al.* 2005; Yamanaka *et al.* 2006). Dopaminergic innervation of the LC and surrounding area originates from the hypothalamic A11 and A13 (Luppi *et al.* 1995) and midbrain VTA-A10 cell groups (Ornstein *et al.* 1987) and has been implicated in inhibiting REM sleep and enhancing muscle tone in REM sleep (Crochet and Sakai 1999), as well as enhancing SWS and REM sleep via α_2 adrenoreceptors (Crochet and Sakai 2003). Although there is evidence both in the periphery (Hardman *et al.* 2001) and in the preoptic area of the brain (Cornil *et al.* 2002) that dopamine can indeed act when present in high concentrations via adrenoreceptors, placing these observations into a physiological perspective is difficult. The concentration of DA retrieved by microdialysis from the LC region in behaving cats, for example, is approximately 390 nM (Shouse *et al.* 2000), unlikely to be sufficient to activate adrenoreceptors (Keating and Rye 2003).

Some less obvious phenomena of catecholamine transport and biosynthesis further illustrate the complexities of deciphering how efferents from midbrain dopamine neurons contribute to sleep–wake regulation. The plasma membrane norepinephrine transporter (NET), which is responsible for the uptake of extracellular noradrenaline, can also readily transport dopamine, and does so *in vivo*. This "non-specific" uptake can be critical for the control of extracellular dopamine levels, particularly in areas of the brain that are rich in NET but poor in DAT, such as the prefrontal cortex (Carboni and Silvagni 2004). There is also evidence that noradrenergic neurons actually release dopamine. Norepinephrine synthesis is catalyzed from the conversion of dopamine by dopamine β-hydroxylase (DBH). This conversion is not always efficient, especially during sustained neuronal activity or genetic/pharmacological reduction in DBH activity, and this can result in increased dopamine synthesis and release from noradrenergic terminals (Carboni and Silvagni 2004; Devoto *et al.* 2005; Bourdelat-Parks *et al.* 2005).

Distinguishing the separate contributions of the midbrain dopamine neurons and dopaminoceptive structures to normal and pathological states of sleep and wakefulness will require additional anatomical, physiological, and pharmacological data. The findings to date are intriguing, although more data are needed before dopaminergic circuitry can be incorporated into current heuristic models of sleep and REM sleep regulation. However, some additional insights come from lesion studies, animal models, and clinical disorders, and these are discussed below.

Insights from the clinic, animal models, and lesion studies

Clinicians have long taken advantage of the wake-promoting effects of dopaminomimetics, inclusive of traditional psychostimulants, and are becoming increasingly aware of the potential somnogenic effects of dopamine agonists. Not as universally appreciated, however, are the dopaminomimetic effects on REM sleep in normal subjects, PD patients, and narcolepsy/cataplexy. For example, a common side effect of dopaminomimetics is exaggerated dream imagery. In PD patients, chronic L-dopa treatment promotes phasic REM sleep phenomena, such as heightened dream mentation, nightmares, and their daytime correlates: hallucinations and psychosis (Arnulf *et al.* 2000). In narcolepsy, although non-specific dopaminomimetics enhance wakefulness and mildly suppress cataplexy, D_2-D_3 receptor-specific agonists exacerbate cataplexy (Nishino *et al.* 1991). These findings are relevant to our understanding of the mechanisms underlying REM sleep, and of clinical disorders such as depression, PD, and narcolepsy/cataplexy, in which the electrophysiological measures of REM sleep are altered and for which dopaminomimetics are commonly prescribed. Studies in mice, rats, non-human primates, and humans point to dopaminergic neurons in the medial aspects of the midbrain (i.e. the VTA and periaqueductal midline regions) as critical for modulating states of thalamocortical arousal, i.e. in both wakefulness and REM sleep. Several reports have highlighted mesocorticolimbic dopaminergic circuits as being critical for modulating the quality, quantity, and timing of REM sleep

Control rat

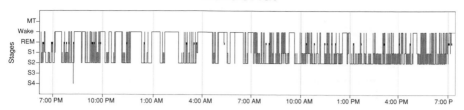

6-Hydroxydopamine lesioned rat

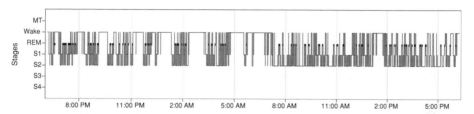

Figure 7.5 Histograms illustrating typical behavioral state changes observed following bilateral lesions of dopaminergic ventral tegmental pathways in rats receiving 6-hydroxydopamine into the nucleus accumbens (217). Notable amounts of REM sleep are evident during both the major wake (1900–0700) and major sleep (0700–1900) periods. Maintenance of the rest and activity periods to the 12:12 h light: dark schedule, respectively, demonstrates the relative preservation of circadian processes.

(Decker *et al.* 2002; Reid *et al.* 1996). Wakefulness is diminished and REM sleep is increased following destruction of dopaminergic VTA, medial substantia nigra, and periaqueductal grey neurons in rats (Decker *et al.* 2000, 2002; Sakata *et al.* 2002; Ulivelli *et al.* 2002; Lu *et al.* 2006) (Fig. 7.5). Furthermore, a narcolepsy-like phenotype (i.e. sleepiness and REM-sleep intrusion into daytime naps) occurs in methyl 4-phenyl-1,2,3,6-tetrahydropyridine-(MPTP) induced parkinsonism in non-human primates (Daley 2003; Daley *et al.* 1998, 1999), and in 30%–50% of patients with idiopathic PD (Arnulf *et al.* 2000, 2002; Rye *et al.* 1999, 2000). Decrements in alertness encountered with midbrain dopamine cell loss often appear as excessive sleep over a 24 h period (Ulivelli *et al.* 2002; Manni *et al.* 2004; Pacchetti *et al.* 2003), and are not readily attributable to medications or the quantity or quality of the prior night's sleep (Rye *et al.* 2000; Arnulf *et al.* 2002; Razmy *et al.* 2004; Baumann *et al.* 2005). Circadian body temperature, activity, and neuroendocrine rhythms are generally unaffected in the parkinsonism-like disorder induced by MPTP in mice and non-human primates (Almirall *et al.* 2001; Barcia *et al.* 2003; Leng *et al.* 2004). These findings emphasize that midbrain dopaminergic cell groups are critical to homeostatic sleep–wake mechanisms (e.g. process S) and are less integrated with circadian processes.

State-related dysfunction in PD

Sleep–wake state alterations in PD can be broadly classified into disturbances of: (1) thalamocortical arousal state; and (2) excessive nocturnal movement (Rye and Bliwise 2004; Rye and Iranzo 2005). The former includes the loss of sleep spindles and SWS, daytime sleepiness, and intrusion of REM sleep into daytime naps (i.e. sleep onset REM periods, or SOREMs), and the latter encompass periodic leg movements of sleep (PLMs) and REM sleep behavior disorder (RBD). The pathophysiological basis of sleepiness and SOREMs appears to be dopaminergic cell loss in PD, though excessive nocturnal movements are not as clearly related to dopaminergic deficits.

Sleepiness in PD is common, real, and increasingly recognized, and has attracted significant investigation, as recently reviewed (Rye 2006; Rye et al. 2003; Schapira 2004; Arnulf 2005). By self-report, 10%–75% of PD patients experience unintended sleep episodes or sleepiness that interferes with daily activities (Hobson et al. 2002; Tan et al. 2002; Brodsky et al. 2003). Nearly one half of these meet physiological criteria for narcolepsy (Arnulf et al. 2002). Employing the multiple sleep latency test (MSLT), which is a standardized measure of physiological sleep tendency across five daytime nap opportunities, pathological sleepiness has been documented in 20%–50% of PD patients, and a narcolepsy-like phenotype in 15%–50% of these (with a mean sleep latency [MSL] < 8 min, and more than two daytime naps with REM sleep) (Rye et al. 2000; Arnulf et al. 2002; Razmy et al. 2004; Baumann et al. 2005; Stevens et al. 2004; Roth et al. 2003). In all but one of these studies (Stevens et al. 2004), physiological impairments in arousal state bore little relationship to the primary motor manifestations of disease (e.g. treatment duration, disease duration, disability scales) or sleep architecture measures (e.g. total sleep time, stage percentage). The more recent of these studies has suggested that impaired arousal, or sleepiness, is associated with a greater dopaminergic drug load, in line with clinical experience (Razmy et al. 2004; Stevens et al. 2004; Kaynak et al. 2005). Contrary to what might be expected based upon the demands of sleep homeostatic mechanisms, poor nocturnal sleep in PD is typically associated with greater, rather than lesser, degrees of daytime alertness. Hence sleepiness in PD is unlikely to reflect inadequate sleep amounts or quality, but rather appears intrinsic to the disease and its treatment. Indeed, continuous electrophysiological recordings of sleepy PD subjects reveal a more naturalistic picture inclusive of "microsleeps," daytime napping, and excessive 24 h total sleep times (Ulivelli et al. 2002; Manni et al. 2004; Pacchetti et al. 2003).

In PD, the dissociation of arousal state from the motor manifestations of the disease and homeostatic sleep drives (i.e. sleep propensity should be inversely rather than directly related to the quantity and quality of the prior night's sleep) has several implications. First, it emphasizes that the integrity of dopamine pathways or exogenous dopaminomimetic drugs have significant interactions with homeostatic sleep mechanisms. Second, it suggests that the pathophysiological substrate of impaired thalamocortical arousal state is outside the nigrostriatal pathways that underlie the motor disabilities of PD. A threshold of 60%–90% of dopamine loss in the sensorimotor putamen is necessary for the emergence of the waking clinical symptoms of PD (Agid 1991). Cell loss then proceeds through associative (i.e. caudate) and eventually, limbic (i.e. nucleus accumbens) striatal subcircuits. Thus, it is loss of dopamine in these latter circuits, most characteristic of the advanced disease state, that is a potential factor in the narcolepsy-like phenotype discussed here.

Nocturnal motor dyscontrol in PD and atypical PD is also common and appears as PLMs (Bliwise et al. 1998; Wetter et al. 2000) and RBD (Comella et al. 1997; Gagnon et al. 2002). The recognition that RBD predates and is associated with neurodegenerative diseases which share waking symptoms with PD has attracted considerable attention. Histories consistent with RBD can be obtained from nearly 1 in 6 patients with idiopathic PD (Comella et al. 1997; Gagnon et al. 2002). Polysomnographic analysis reveals subclinical evidence of RBD in 50% of PD patients (Gagnon et al. 2002), and this electrophysiological correlate of RBD appears specific in distinguishing PD patients from age-matched controls and AD patients (Gagnon et al. 2002; Bliwise et al. 2003). The waking EEG in these patients also demonstrates subtle abnormalities that distinguish these patients from controls and PD patients without RBD (Lavia Fantini et al. 2003). RBD seems particularly high in patients presenting with L-dopa- or dopamine agonist-induced hallucinations (Comella et al. 1993). Nearly 65% of RBD cases presage the development of the waking motor symptoms of PD by several years (Schenck et al. 2003). Indeed, several investigators have suggested that RBD is almost predictive of a synucleinopathy (Turner et al. 2000; Boeve et al. 1998), and this has been confirmed in a recent neuropathological investigation of RBD plus dementia or parkinsonism (Boeve et al. 2003). The clinical and pathological associations are so strong that the criteria now include RBD as a core clinical feature strongly suggestive of a diagnosis of dementia with Lewy bodies (McKeith et al. 2000).

Substrates underlying impaired arousal in PD

The objective findings in a small number of newly diagnosed, unmedicated or young PD patients (Rye et al. 1999, 2000) emphasize that PD itself is a major factor in the expression of sleepiness and SOREMs. This is confirmed in animal models that control for potentially confounding variables such as age, co-morbidities, and medications. Rats spend less of their subjective day awake and exhibit inappropriate REM sleep intrusions following destruction of ascending dopamine pathways from the VTA (Decker *et al.* 2000; Sakata *et al.* 2002). In rats, lesions targeting presumptively wake-active dopaminergic neurons that extend dorsally from the VTA into the ventral periaqueductal gray have recently been shown to result in *c.* 20% reductions in wakefulness (Lu *et al.* 2006). Daytime sleepiness and SOREMs were reported in a non-human primate following systemic delivery of the dopamine neurotoxin MPTP (Daley *et al.* 1999), and this was subsequently confirmed in two additional animals (Daley 2003). These effects have been reversed with the dopamine precursor L-dopa and the dopamine reuptake blocker bupropion, but not with the $D_{2\text{-like}}$ agonist pergolide (Daley 2003; Daley *et al.* 1999). Presynaptic integrity of dopaminergic axons is necessary for the actions of L-dopa and bupropion. This suggests that their ability to reverse sleepiness and SOREMs reflects an action on surviving mesocorticolimbic dopaminergic circuits, which are less vulnerable to MPTP and lost only later in the course of idiopathic PD. Mice lacking DAT (Wisor *et al.* 2001) and PD patients with presumably extensive (>90%) loss of midbrain dopaminergic cells (Rye 2006; Rye *et al.* 2003) are immune to the wake-promoting effects of traditional psychostimulants, emphasizing the importance of midbrain dopamine neurons for the generation and maintenance of wakefulness. Enhancement of synaptic dopamine availability in mesocorticolimbic circuits may underlie the partial success of amphetamines in the treatment of PD that was first described nearly 30 years ago (Miller and Nieburg 1973; Parkes *et al.* 1975), providing beneficial alerting effects in sleepy patients.

The precise cellular and subcellular substrates underlying the lesion- and disease-related effects of dopaminergic cell loss on arousal remain unknown. These phenomena may reflect loss of the effects of dopamine on neural excitability in any one of the brain regions necessary for maintaining normal states of thalamocortical excitability. One plausible substrate, given the narcolepsy-like phenotype seen in nearly half of sleepy PD patients, is the orexin-containing neurons in the perifornical hypothalamus that are known to degenerate in primary narcolepsy/cataplexy (Silber and Rye 2001). Other plausible neural substrates that deserve future investigation as potential contributors to sleepiness and SOREMs when dopamine is depleted include the targets of VTA dopamine neurons such as the prefrontal cortex, the cholinergic magnocellular basal forebrain, and the midline thalamic nuclei. This is suggested by the finding that D_2 receptor antagonists microinjected into the VTA block the sedation seen with systemic dopamine agonists (Bagetta *et al.* 1988), and that infusions of amphetamine into the ventral forebrain targets of VTA neurons initiate and maintain alert wakefulness (Berridge *et al.* 1999). Alternatively, sleepiness and SOREMs may reflect extranigral pathology (Jellinger 1991), such as in the nuclei comprising the ascending reticular activating system, including the hypothalamic orexin system, the dorsal raphe, LC, and PPN region. This could also be extended to include the midline thalamic nuclei, which exhibit extensive pathology in idiopathic PD (Xuereb *et al.* 1991; Henderson *et al.* 2000a,b; Rub *et al.* 2002). Impairments in central release of orexins might also seem a parsimonious explanation for the narcolepsy-like phenotype seen in a subset of PD patients. However, in most of these cases cerebrospinal fluid orexin-1 levels are normal (Baumann *et al.* 2004; Overeem *et al.* 2002; Drouot *et al.* 2003). Alternatively, dysregulation of the brainstem PPN region, an area known to promote thalamocortical arousal and REM sleep, may also be an important factor given its position as the principal brainstem target of pathologic basal ganglionic outflow (Rye 1997).

Substrates underlying excessive nocturnal movement in PD

The extent to which PLMs and RBD-like phenomena are dopamine-related, disease-specific, or treatment-related phenomena, remains controversial (for extensive reviews see (Rye 2003, 2004b; Rye and Bliwise 2004; Rye and Iranzo 2005)). The precise substrates for a potential detrimental effect of midbrain dopamine cell loss on nocturnal movement remain ill-defined. Neuroimaging studies have revealed decreases in striatal DAT in patients with idiopathic RBD similar to those seen in early PD (Albin *et al* 2000; Eisensehr *et al.* 2000). These results suggest that dopamine might modulate brainstem circuits affecting PLMs and REM sleep atonia. This does not occur via direct dopaminergic innervation of the brainstem, however, but rather by indirect, multisynaptic routes linking the basal ganglia output nuclei with pontomedullary reticulospinal pathways via the dorsolateral pons, including the subcoeruleal region (Rye 1997). Increasingly, interest has focused on extranigral, non-dopaminergic pathology in sporadic PD, involving, for example, medullary and pontine regions containing multiple neuron types, which influence sleep–wake-related somatomotor activity (Braak *et al.* 2000). This pathology might occur before the extensive loss of midbrain dopaminergic neurons that underlies PD (Braak *et al.* 2002, 2003). This would account for the almost ubiquitous occurrence of sleep-related movement disorders in PD, as well as the fact that disturbed sleep, particularly RBD, can presage the development of the waking symptoms of PD. Indeed, these findings would also provide an explanation for the fact that RBD symptoms in PD patients do not respond in any consistent manner (as revealed by detailed electromyographic analysis) to dopamine agonists (Fantini *et al.* 2003), or to manipulations aimed at reversing the effects of dopamine loss on subcortical excitability (e.g. by deep brain subthalamic nucleus stimulation) (Iranzo *et al.* 2002).

Acknowledgments

The authors thank Drs Shawn Hochman and David Weinshenker for their insightful comments and expertise that contributed to this work. Special thanks to our close colleagues Drs Glenda Keating and Michael Decker, who contributed much to the body of this work. Dr Rye is supported by USPHS grants NS-36977, NS-40221, and NS-43374, and the Restless Legs Syndrome and Arthur L. Williams Jr. Foundations.

References

Abe M., Herzog E. D., Yamazaki S. *et al.* (2002). Circadian rhythms in isolated brain regions. *J. Neurosci.* **22**(1), 350–6.

Agid Y. (1991). Parkinson's disease: pathophysiology. *Lancet.* **337**, 1321–4.

Albin R., Koeppe R., Chervin R. *et al.* (2000). Decreased striatal dopaminergic innervation in REM sleep behavior disorder. *Neurology.* **55**, 1410–12.

Albin R., Young A., Penney J. (1989). The functional anatomy of basal ganglia disorders. *Trends Neurosci.* **12**, 366–75.

Albrecht D., Quäschling U., Zippel U., Davidowa H. (1996). Effects of dopamine on neurons of the lateral geniculate nucleus: an iontophoretic study. *Synapse.* **23**, 70–8.

Alex K., Yavanian G., McFarlane H., Pluto C., Pehek E. (2005). Modulation of dopamine release by striatal 5-HT2C receptors. *Synapse.* **55**, 242–51.

Alexander G. (1997). Anatomy of the basal ganglia and related motor structures. In: Watts R., Koller W., editors. *Movement Disorders: Neurologic Principles and Practice.* New York, NY: McGraw-Hill. pp. 73–86.

Alexander G. E., Crutcher M. D., DeLong M. R. (1990). Basal ganglia-thalamocortical circuits: parallel substrates for motor, oculomotor, "prefrontal" and "limbic" functions. *Prog. Brain Res.* **85**, 119–46.

Alexander G. E., DeLong M. R., Strick P. L. (1986). Parallel organization of functionally segregated circuits linking basal ganglia and cortex. *A. Rev. Neurosci.* **9**, 357–81.

Almirall H., Bautista V., Sanchez-Bahillo A., Trinidad-Herrero M. (2001). Ultradian and circadian body temperature and activity rhythms in chronic MPTP treated monkeys. *Neurophysiol. Clin.* **31**, 161–70.

Andreau N., Chale J., Senard J. *et al.* (1999). L-dopa induced sedation: a double-blind cross-over controlled study versus triazolam and placebo in healthy volunteers. *Clin. Neuropharmacol.* **22**, 15–23.

Andretic R., Hirsh J. (2000). Circadian modulation of dopamine receptor responsiveness in Drosophila melanogaster. *Proc. Natl. Acad. Sci. USA* **97**(4), 1873–8.

Andretic R., van Swinderen B., Greenspan R. J. (2003). Dopaminergic modulation of arousal in *Drosophila. Curr. Biol.* **15**(13), 1165–75.

Arnulf I., Bonnet A., Damier P. *et al.* (2000). Hallucinations, REM sleep, and Parkinson's disease: a medical hypothesis. *Neurology* **55**(2), 281–8.

Arnulf I., Konofal E., Merino-Andreu M. *et al.* (2002). Parkinson's disease and sleepiness: an integral part of PD. *Neurology*. **58**, 1019–24.

Arnulf I. (2005). Excessive daytime sleepiness in parkinsonism. *Sleep Med. Rev.* **9**, 185–200.

Asakura W., Matsumoto K., Ohta H., Watanabe H. (1992). REM sleep deprivation decreases apomorphine-induced stimulation of locomotor activity but not stereotyped behavior in mice. *Gen. Pharmacol.* **23**, 337–41.

Bagetta G., Sarro G. D., Priolo E., Nisticó G. (1988). Ventral tegmental area: site through which dopamine D_2-receptor agonists evoke behavioral and electrocortical sleep in rats. *Br. J. Pharmacol.* **95**, 860–6.

Bandmann O., Valente E., Holmans P. *et al.* (1998). Dopa-responsive dystonia: a clinical and molecular genetic study. *Ann. Neurol.* **44**, 649–56.

Barbeau H., Rossignol S. (1991). Initiation and modulation of the locomotor pattern in the adult chronic spinal cat by noradrenergic, serotonergic and dopaminergic drugs. *Brain Res.* **546**(2), 250–60.

Barcia C., Bautista V., Sanchez-Bahillo A. *et al.* (2003). Circadian determinations of cortisol, prolactin and melatonin in chronic methyl-phenyl-tetrahydropyridine-treated monkeys. *Neuroendocrinology* **78**, 118–28.

Baumann C., Dauvilliers Y., Mignot E., Bassetti C. (2004). Normal CSF hypocretin-1 (orexin A) levels in dementia with Lewy bodies associated with excessive daytime sleepiness. *Eur. Neurol.* **52**, 73–6.

Baumann C., Ferini-Strambi L., Waldvogel D., Werth E., Bassetti C. (2005). Parkinsonism with excessive daytime sleepiness – a narcolepsy like disorder? *J. Neurol.* **252**, 139–45.

Behrends J., Prank K., Dogu E., Brabant G. (1998). Central nervous system control of thyrotropin secretion during sleep and wakefulness. *Horm. Res.* **49**, 173–7.

Benker G., Jaspers C., Hausler G., Reinwein D. (1990). Control of prolactin secretion. *Klin. Wochenschr.* **68**, 1157–67.

Berlanga M., Simpson T., Alcantra A. (2005). Dopamine D5 receptor localization on cholinergic neurons of the rat forebrain and diencephalon: a potential neuroanatomical substrate involved in mediating dopaminergic influences on acetylcholine release. *J. Comp. Neurol.* **492**, 34–49.

Berridge C., O'Neil J., Wifler K. (1999). Amphetamine acts within the medial basal forebrain to initiate and maintain alert waking. *Neuroscience* **93**, 885–96.

Besharse J., Zhunag M., Freeman K., Fogerty J. (2004). Regulation of photoreceptor Per1 and Per2 by light, dopamine and a circadian clock. *Eur. J. Neurosci.* **20**, 167–4.

Bjorklund A, Lindvall O. (1984). Dopamine-containing systems in the CNS. In: Bjorklund A., Hokfelt T., editors. *Handbook of Chemical Neuroanatomy*. Amsterdam: Elsevier. pp. 55–122.

Bjorklund A., Skagerberg G. (1979). Evidence for a major spinal cord projection from the diencephalic A11 dopamine cell group in the rat using transmitter-specific fluorescent retrograde tracing. *Brain Res.* **177**(1), 170–5.

Blackburn T., Suzuki K., Ashby C., Jr. (2006). The acute and chronic administration of the 5-HT (2B/2C) receptor antagonist SB-200646A significantly alters the activity of spontaneously active midbrain dopamine neurons in the rat: an *in vivo* extracellular single cell study. *Synapse.* **59**, 502–12.

Bliwise D., Rye D., Dihenia B. *et al.* (1998). Periodic leg movements in elderly patients with Parkinsonism. *Sleep* **21**(Suppl.), 196.

Bliwise D., Rye D., He L., Ansari F. (2003). Influence of PLMs on scoring phasic leg muscle activity. *Sleep* **26**, A344.

Boeve B., Silber M., Ferman T. *et al.* (1998). REM sleep behavior disorder and degenerative dementia – An association likely reflecting Lewy body disease. *Neurology* **51**, 363–70.

Boeve B., Silber M., Pirisi J. *et al.* (2003). Synucleinopathy pathology and REM sleep behavior disorder plus dementia or parkinsonism. *Neurology* **61**, 40–5.

Borland L. M., Michael A. C. (2004). Voltammetric study of the control of striatal dopamine release by glutamate. *J. Neurochem.* **91**(1), 220–9.

Bortolozzi A., Diaz-Mataix L., Scorz M., Celada P., Artigas P. (2005). The activation of 5-HT receptors in prefrontal cortex enhances dopaminergic activity. *J. Neurochem.* **95**, 1597–607.

Bourdelat-Parks B., Anderson G., Donaldson Z. *et al.* (2005). Effects of dopamine beta-hydroxylase genotype and disulfiram inhibition on catecholamine homeostasis in mice. *Psychopharmacol. (Berl).* **183**, 72–80.

Braak H., Rub U., Sandmann-Keil D. *et al.* (2000). Parkinson's disease: affection of brain stem nuclei controlling premotor and motor neurons of the somatomotor system. *Acta Neuropathol. (Berl.)* **99**, 489–95.

Braak H., Tredici K., Bratzke H. *et al.* (2002). Staging of the intracerebral inclusion body pathology associated with idiopathic Parkinson's disease (preclinical and clinical stages). *J. Neurol.* **249**(Suppl. 3), III/1–IIII/5.

Braak H., Tredici K., Rub U. *et al.* (2003). Staging of brain pathology related to sporadic Parkinson's disease. *Neurobiol. Aging* **24**, 197–211.

Brock J. W., Hamdi A., Ross K., Payne S., Prasad C. (1995). REM sleep deprivation alters dopamine D2 receptor binding in the rat frontal cortex. *Pharmacol. Biochem. Behav.* **52**(1), 43–8.

Brodsky M., Godbold J., Roth T., Olanow C. (2003). Sleepiness in Parkinson's disease: a controlled study. *Mov. Disord.* **18**, 668–72.

Bruinink A., Lichtensteiger W., Schlumpf M. (1983). Ontogeny of diurnal rhythms of central dopamine, serotonin and spirodecanone binding sites and of motor activity in the rat. *Life Sci.* **33**(1), 31–8.

Bubser M., Fadel J., Jackson L. *et al.* (2005). Dopaminergic modulation of orexin neurons. *Eur. J. Neurosci.* **21**, 2993–3001.

Calabrese E. (2001). Dopamine: biphasic dose responses. *Crit. Rev. Toxicol.* **31**, 563–83.

Carboni E., Silvagni A. (2004). Dopamine reuptake by norepinephrine neurons: exception or rule? *Crit. Rev. Neurobiol.* **16**, 121–8.

Carlsson A., Svennerholm L., Winblad B. (1980). Seasonal and circadian monoamine variations in human brain examined post mortem. *Acta Pyschiatr. Scan. Suppl.* **280**, 275–5.

Castaneda T., de Prado B., Prieto D., Mora F. (2004). Circadian rhythms of dopamine, glutamate and GABA in the striatum and nucleus accumbens of the awake rat: modulation by light. *J. Pineal Res.* **36**, 177–85.

Chergui K., Suaud-Chagny M. F., Gonon F. (1994). Nonlinear relationship between impulse flow, dopamine release and dopamine elimination in the rat brain in vivo. *Neuroscience* **62**(3), 641–5.

Cianchetti C., Masala C., Olivari P., Giordano G. (1984). Sleep pattern alterations by naloxone. Partial prevention by haloperidol. *Psychopharmacology (Berl).* **83**(2), 179–82.

Clemens S., Hochman S. (2004). Conversion of the modulatory actions of dopamine on spinal reflexes from depression to facilitation in D3 receptor knock-out mice. *J. Neurosci.* **24**, 11337–45.

Clemens S., Rye D., Hochman S. (2006). Restless legs syndrome: revisiting the dopamine hypothesis from the spinal cord perspective. *Neurology* **67**, 125–30.

Cobb W., Abercrombie E. (2003). Differential regulation of somatodendritic and nerve terminal release by serotonergic innervation of substantia nigra. *J. Neurochem.* **84**, 576–84.

Comella C., Nardine T., Diederich N., Stebbins G. (1997). Sleep-related violence, injury, and REM sleep behavior disorder in Parkinson's disease. *Neurology* **48**(3), A539.

Comella C., Tanner C., Ristanovic R. (1993). Polysomnographic sleep measures in Parkinson's Disease patients with treatment-induced hallucinations. *Ann. Neurol.* **34**, 710–14.

Cooper J., Bloom F., Roth R. (2002). *The Biochemical Basis of Neuropharmacology.* 8th ed. New York: Oxford University Press.

Cornil C. A., Balthazart J., Motte P., Massotte L., Seutin V. (2002). Dopamine activates noradrenergic receptors in the preoptic area. *J. Neurosci.* **22**(21), 9320–30.

Corvaja N., Doucet G., Bolam J. (1993). Ultrastructure and synaptic targets of the raphe-nigral projection in the rat. *Neuroscience* **55**(2), 417–27.

Cragg S., Greenfield S. (1997). Differential autoreceptor control of somatodendritic and axon terminal dopamine release in substantia nigra, ventral tegmental area and striatum. *J. Neurosci.* **17**, 5738–46.

Crochet S., Sakai K. (2003). Dopaminergic modulation of behavioral states in mesopontine tegmentum: a reverse microdialysis study in freely moving cats. *Sleep* **26**, 801–6.

Crochet S., Sakai K. (1999). Effects of microdialysis application of monoamines on the EEG and behavioural states in the cat mesopontine tegmentum. *Eur. J. Neurosci.* **11**(10), 3738–52.

Dahlstrom A., Fuxe K. (1964). Evidence for the existence of monoamine-containing neurones in the central nervous system. I. Demonstration of monoamines in the cell bodies of brain stem neurones. *Acta Physiol. Scand.* (Suppl.) **232**, 1–55.

Daley J., Turner R., Becker D., Bliwise D., Rye D. (1998). Telemetric recording of sleep in macaca mulatta prior to systemic MPTP. *Sleep* **21**(Suppl.)(3), 6.

Daley J., Turner R., Bliwise D., Rye D. (1999). Nocturnal sleep and daytime alertness in the MPTP-treated primate. *Sleep* **22**(Suppl.), S218–19.

Daley J. (2003). *A Role for Dopamine in the Basal Ganglia in Sleep-Wake Regulation: Insights from the MPTP-Treated Primate*. Atlanta, GA: Emory University.

Darracq L., Blanc G., Glowinski J., Tassin J. (1998). Importance of the noradrenaline-dopamine coupling in the locomotor activating effects of D-amphetamine. *J. Neurosci.* **18**, 2729–39.

Decker M., Keating G., Freeman A., Rye D. (2000). Parkinsonian-like sleep-wake architecture in rats with bilateral striatal 6-OHDA lesions. *Soc. Neurosci. Abstr.* **26**, 1514.

Decker M. J., Keating G., Hue G. E., Freeman A., Rye D. B. (2002). Mesolimbic dopamine's modulation of REM Sleep. *J. Sleep. Res.* (suppl.) **51**, 51–2.

DeLong M. R. (1990). Primate models of movement disorders of basal ganglia origin. *Trends Neurosci.* **13**, 281–5.

Devoto P., Flore G., Saba P., Fa M., Gessa G. (2005). Stimulation of the locus coeruleus elicits noradrenaline and dopamine release in the medial prefrontal and parietal cortex. *J. Neurochem.* **92**, 368–74.

Di Matteo V., Cacchio M., Di Giulio C., Esposito E. (2002). Role of serotonin (2C) receptors in the control of brain dopaminergic function. *Pharmacol. Biochem. Behav.* **71**, 727–34.

Doi M., Yujnovsky I., Hirayama J. *et al.* (2006). Impaired light masking in dopamine receptor-null mice. *Nat. Neurosci.* **9**, 732–4.

Doyle S., Grace M., McIvor W. (2002). Menaker M. Circadian rhythms of dopamine in mouse retina: the role of melatonin. *Vis. Neurosci.* **19**, 593–601.

Drouot X., Moutereau S., Nguyen J. *et al.* (2003). Low levels of ventricular CSF orexin/hypocretin in advanced PD. *Neurology* **61**, 540–3.

Durán-Vázquez A., Drucker-Colín R. (1997). Differential role of dopamine receptors on motor asymmetries of nigro-stratal lesioned animals that are REM sleep deprived. *Brain Res.* **744**, 171–4.

Durstewitz D., Kroner S., Gunturkun O. (1999). The dopaminergic innervation of the avian telencephalon. *Prog. Neurobiol.* **59**(2), 161–95.

Edgar D. M., Dement W. C., Fuller C. A. (1993). Effect of SCN lesions on sleep in squirrel monkeys: evidence for opponent processes in sleep-wake regulation. *J. Neurosci.* **13**(3), 1065–79.

Edgar D. M., Seidel W. F. (1997). Modafinil induces wakefulness without intensifying motor activity or subsequent rebound hypersomnolence in the rat. *J. Pharmacol. Exp. Ther.* **283**(2), 757–69.

Eisensehr I., Linke R., Noachtar S. *et al.* (2000). Reduced striatal dopamine transporters in idiopathic rapid eye movement behaviour disorder. Comparison with Parkinson's disease and controls. *Brain* **123**(6), 1155–60.

Ennis M., Zhou F., Ciombor K. *et al.* (2001). Dopamine D2 receptor-mediated presynaptic inhibition of olfactory nerve terminals. *J. Neurophysiol.* **86**, 2986–97.

Evans H. L., Ghiselli W. B., Patton R. A. (1973). Diurnal rhythm in behavioral effects of methamphetamine, p-chloramethamphetamine and scopolamine. *J. Pharmacol. Exp. Ther.* **186**(1), 10–17.

Fadda P., Martellotta M. C., De Montis M. G., Gessa G. L., Fratta W. (1992). Dopamine D1 and opioid receptor binding changes in the limbic system of sleep deprived rats. *Neurochem. Int.* **20** (Suppl.), 153S–156S.

Fadda P., Martellotta M. C., Gessa G. L., Fratta W. (1993). Dopamine and opioids: interactions in sleep deprivation. *Prog. Neuropsychopharmacol. Biol. Psychiatry* **17**(2), 269–78.

Fantini M. L., Gagnon J. F., Filipini D., Montplaisir J. (2003). The effects of pramipexole in REM sleep behavior disorder. *Neurology* **61**(10), 1418–20.

Farber J., Miller J. D., Crawford K. A., McMillen B. A. (1983). Dopamine metabolism and receptor sensitivity in rat brain after REM sleep deprivation. *Pharmacol. Biochem. Behav.* **18**(4), 509–13.

Farooqui S. M., Brock J. W., Zhou J. (1996). Changes in monoamines and their metabolite concentrations in REM sleep-deprived rat forebrain nuclei. *Pharmacol. Biochem. Behav.* **54**(2), 385–91.

Feenstra M., Botterblom M., Mastenbrook S. (2000). Dopamine and noradrenaline efflux in the prefrontal cortex in the light and dark period: effects of novelty and handling and comparison to the nucleus accumbens. *Neuroscience* **100**, 741–8.

Ferreira J. J., Galitzky M., Thalamas C. *et al.* (2002). Effect of ropinirole on sleep onset: a randomized placebo controlled study in healthy volunteers. *Neurology* **58**(3), 460–2.

Fibiger H., Phillips A. (1986). Reward, motivation, cognition: Psychobiology of mesotelencephalic dopamine systems. In: *Handbook of Physiology,* Vol. 4. *Intrinsic regulatory systems of the brain.* Bethesda, MD: American Physiology Society; pp. 647–75.

Fleetwood-Walker S., Hope P., Mitchell R. (1988). Antinociceptive actions of descending dopaminergic tracts on cat and rat dorsal horn somatosensory neurones. *J. Physiol. Lond.* **399**, 335–48.

Floran B., Floran L., Erlij D., Aceves J. (2004). Activation of dopamine D4 receptors modulates [3H]GABA release in slices of the rat thalamic reticular nucleus. *Neuropharmacology* **46**, 497–503.

Floresco S. B., West A. R., Ash B., Moore H., Grace A. A. (2003). Afferent modulation of dopamine neuron firing differentially regulates tonic and phasic dopamine transmission. *Nat. Neurosci.* **6**(9), 968–73.

Forster G., Blaha C. (2000). Laterodorsal tegmental stimulation elicits dopamine efflux in the rat nucleus accumbens by activation of acetycholine and glutamate receptors in the ventral tegmental area. *Eur J Neurosci* **12**, 3596–604.

Freeman A., Ciliax B., Bakay R. *et al.* (2001). Nigrostriatal collaterals to thalamus degenerate in parkinsonian animal models. *Ann. Neurol.* **50**, 321–9.

Freeman A., Morales J., Beck J. *et al.* (2006). In vivo diurnal rhythm of dopamine measured in the putamen of non-human primates. *Sleep* **29**(Abstr. Suppl.), A69.

Freeman A. (2006). *Anatomy and Physiology of the Mesothalamic Dopamine System.* Atlanta, GA: Emory University.

Gagnon J., Bedard M-A., Fantini M. *et al.* (2002). REM sleep behavior disorder and REM sleep without atonia in Parkinson's disease. *Neurology* **59**, 585–9.

Garcia-Borreguero D., Larrosa O., Saiz T. *et al.* (2001). Circadian variation in neuroendocrine response to the administration of L-dopa in patients with restless legs syndrome: a pilot study. *Sleep* **24**(suppl.), (A16–A17).

Gaspar P., Stepniewska I., Kaas J. H. (1992). Topography and collateralization of the dopaminergic projections to motor and lateral prefrontal cortex in owl monkeys. *J. Comp. Neurol.* **325**(1), 1–21.

Gaykema R. P., Zaborszky L. (1996). Direct catecholaminergic-cholinergic interactions in the basal forebrain. II. Substantia nigra-ventral tegmental area projections to cholinergic neurons. *J. Comp. Neurol.* **374**(4), 555–77.

Gaytan O., Swann A., Dafny N. (1998). Diurnal differences in rat's motor response to amphetamine. *Eur. J. Pharmacol.* **345**(2), 119–28.

Georges F., Aston-Jones G. (2001). Potent regulation of midbrain dopamine neurons by the bed nucleus of the stria terminalis. *J. Neurosci.* **21**(16), RC160.

Gerfen C. R., Herkenham M., Thibault J. (1987). The neostriatal mosaic: II. Patch- and matrix-directed mesostriatal dopaminergic and non-dopaminergic systems. *J. Neurosci.* **7**, 3915–34.

Ghosh P. K., Hrdina P. D., Ling G. M. (1976). Effects of REMS deprivation on striatal dopamine and acetylcholine in rats. *Pharmacol. Biochem. Behav.* **4**(4), 401–5.

Gillin C., Kammen Dv., Post R. *et al.* (1981). What is the role of dopamine in the regulation of sleep-wake activity? In: Corsini G., Gessa G., editors. *Apomorphine and Other Dopaminomimetics.* New York: Raven Press, pp. 157–64.

Gladwell S., Coote J. (1999). Inhibitory and indirect excitatory effects of dopamine on sympathetic preganglionic neurones in the neonate rat spinal cord in vitro. *Brain Res.* **818**, 397–407.

Goldman-Rakic P. S. (1995). Cellular basis of working memory. *Neuron* **14**(3), 477–85.

Govindaiah G., Cox C. (2006). Depression of retinogeniculate synaptic transmission by presynaptic D(2)-like dopamine receptors in rat lateral geniculate nucleus. *Eur. J. Neurosci.* **23**, 423–34.

Govindaiah G., Cox C. (2005). Excitatory actions of dopamine via D1-like receptors in the rat lateral geniculate nucleus. *J. Neurophysiol.* **94**, 3708–18.

Grace A., Bunney B. (1980). Nigral dopamine neurons: intracellular recording and identification with L-dopa injection and histofluorescence. *Science Wash. DC* **210**, 654–6.

Greengard P., Allen P., Nairn A. (1999). Beyond the dopamine receptor: the DARPP-32/protein phosphatase-1 cascade. *Neuron* **23**, 435–7.

Grenhoff J., Janson A. M., Svensson T. H., Fuxe K. (1991). Chronic continuous nicotine treatment causes decreased burst firing of nigral dopamine neurons in rats partially hemitransected at the meso-diencephalic junction. *Brain Res.* **562**, 347–51.

Grenhoff J., North R., Johnson S. (1995). Alpha 1-adrenergic effects on dopamine neurons recorded intracellularly in the rat midbrain slice. *Eur. J. Neurosci.* **7**, 1707–13.

Griffond B., Risold P., Jacquemard C., Colard C., Fellmann D. (1999). Insulin-induced hypoglycemia increases preprohypocretin (orexin) mRNA in the rat lateral hypothalamic area. *Neurosci. Lett.* **262**(2), 77–80.

Grillner S., Hellgren J., Menard A., Saitoh K., Wikstrom M. (2005). Mechanisms for selection of basic motor programs – roles for the striatum and pallidum. *Trends Neurosci.* **28**, 364–70.

Gronier B., Rasmussen K. (1998). Activation of midbrain presumed dopaminergic neurons by muscarinic cholinergic receptors: an in vivo electrophysiological study in the rat. *Br. J. Pharmacol.* **124**, 455–64.

Groves P. M., Wilson C. J., Young S. J., Rebec G. V. (1975). Self-inhibition by dopaminergic neurons. *Science* **190**, 522–9.

Hagan M. M., Havel P. J., Seeley R. J. *et al.* (1999). Cerebrospinal fluid and plasma leptin measurements: covariability with dopamine and cortisol in fasting humans. *J. Clin. Endocrinol. Metab.* **84**(10), 3579–85.

Halasz B., Fuxe K., Agnati L. F. *et al.* editors. (1985). *The Dopaminergic System*. New York, NY: Springer Verlag.

Hamdi A., Brock J., Ross K., Prasad C. (1993). Effects of rapid eye movement sleep deprivation on the properties of striatal dopaminergic system. *Pharmacol. Biochem. Behav.* **46**, 863–6.

Hardman J., Limbird L., Goodman Gilman A. (2001). *Goodman and Gilman's The Pharmacological Basis of Therapeutics*. 10th ed. New York: McGraw-Hill Professional.

Henderson J., Carpenter K., Cartwright H., Halliday G. (2000a). Loss of thalamic intralaminar nuclei in progressive supranuclear palsy and Parkinson's disease: clinical and therapeutic implications. *Brain* **123**(7), 1410–21.

Henderson J., Carpenter K., Cartwright H., Halliday G. (2000b). Degeneration of the centre median-parafascicular complex in Parkinson's disease. *Ann. Neurol.* **47**(3), 345–52.

Heuer H., Schafer M., O'Donnell D., Walker P., Bauer K. (2000). Expression of thyrotropin-releasing hormone receptor 2 (TRH-R2) in the central nervous system of rats. *J. Comp. Neurol.* **428**, 319–26.

Hobson D. E., Lang A. E., Martin W. R. W., Razmy A., Rivest J., Fleming J. (2002). Excessive daytime sleepiness and sudden-onset sleep in Parkinson disease. *JAMA* **287**(4), 455–63.

Hokfelt T., Martensson R., Bjorklund A., Kleinau S., Goldstein M. (1984). Distributional maps of tyrosine-hydroxylase-immunoreactive neurons in the rat brain. In: Bjorklund A., Hokfelt T., editors. *Handbook of Chemical Neuroanatomy*. New York: Elsevier; pp. 277–379.

Hokfelt T., Phillipson O., Goldstein M. (1979). Evidence for a dopaminergic pathway in the rat descending from the A11 cell group to the spinal cord. *Acta Physiol. Scand.* **107**(4), 393–5.

Hue G., Decker M., Solomon I., Rye D. (2003). Increased wakefulness and hyper-responsivity to novel environments in mice lacking functional dopamine D3 receptors. In: *Society for Neuroscience*.

Iranzo A., Valldeoriola F., Santamaria J., Tolosa E., Rumia J. (2002). Sleep symptoms and polysomnographic architecture in advanced Parkinson's disease after chronic bilateral subthalamic stimulation. *J. Neurol. Neurosurg. Psychiatry* **72**, 661–4.

Isaac S. O., Berridge C. W. (2003). Wake-promoting actions of dopamine D1 and D2 receptor stimulation. *J. Pharmacol. Exp. Ther.* **307**(1), 386–94.

Jaber M., Jones S., Giros B., Caron M. G. (1997). The dopamine transporter: a crucial component regulating dopamine transmission. *Mov. Disord.* **12**(5), 629–33.

Jellinger K. (1991). Pathology of Parkinson's disease. Changes other than the nigrostriatal pathway. *Mol. Chem. Neuropathol.* **14**, 153–97.

Jones B., Moore R. (1977). Ascending projections of the locus coeruleus in the rat. II. Autoradiographic study. *Brain Res.* **127**, 23–53.

Kandel E. R., Schwartz J. H., Jessell T. M. (2000). *Principles of Neural Science*, 4th ed. New York, NY: McGraw-Hill

Karlsson P., Farde L., Halldin C. (2000). Circadian rhythm in central D1-like dopamine receptors examined by PET. In: *The 3rd International Symposium on functional Neuroreceptor Mapping*; 2000; New York, NY: *J. Neuroimaging*.

Katz P. (1996). Neurons, networks, and motor behavior. *Neuron*. **16**, 245–53.

Kawano Y., Kawasaki T., Kawazoe N. *et al.* (1990). Circadian variations of urinary dopamine, norepinephrine, epinephrine and sodium in normotensive and hypertensive subjects. *Nephron* **55**(3), 277–82.

Kaynak D., Kiziltan G., Kaynak H., Benbir G., Uysal O. (2005). Sleep and sleepiness in patients with Parkinson's disease before and after dopaminergic treatment. *Eur. J. Neurol.* **12**, 199–207.

Keating G., Rye D. (2003). Where you least expect it: dopamine in the pons aion of sleep and REM-sleep. *Sleep* **26**, 788–9.

Khaldy H., Leon J., Escames G. *et al.* (2002). Circadian rhythms of dopamine and dihydroxyphenyl acetic acid in the mouse striatum: effects of pinealectomy and of melatonin treatment. *Neuroendocrinology* **75**(3), 201–8.

Kiehn O., Kjaerulff O. (1996). Spatiotemporal characteristics of 5-HT and dopamine-induced rhythmic hindlimb activity in the in vitro neonatal rat. *J. Neurophysiol.* **75**(4), 1472–82.

Kitai S. T., Shepard P. D., Callaway J. C., Scroggs R. (1999). Afferent modulation of dopamine neuron firing patterns. *Curr. Opin. Neurobiol.* **9**(6), 690–7.

Korotkova T., Sergeeva O., Eriksson K., Haas H., Brown R. (2003). Excitation of ventral tegmental area dopaminergic and nondopaminergic neurons by orexins/hypocretins. *J. Neurosci.* **23**, 7–11.

Krimer L. S., Muly E. C. III, Williams G. V., Goldman-Rakic P. S. (1998). Dopaminergic regulation of cerebral cortical microcirculation. *Nat. Neurosci.* **1**(4), 286–9.

Krulich L. (1979). Central neurotransmitters and the secretion of prolactin, GH, LH and TSH. *A. Rev. Physiol.* **41**, 603–15.

Kume K., Kume S., Park S. K., Hirsh J., Jackson F. R. (2005). Dopamine is a regulator of arousal in the fruit fly. *J. Neurosci.* **25**(32), 7377–84.

Lagos P., Scorza C., Monti J. M. *et al.* (1998). Effects of the D3 preferring dopamine agonist pramipexole on sleep and waking, locomotor activity and striatal dopamine release in rats. *Eur. Neuropsychopharmacol.* **8**(2), 113–20.

Lal S., Thavundayil J., Nair N. P. *et al.* (1981). Effect of sleep deprivation on dopamine receptor function in normal subjects. *J. Neural Transm.* **50**(1), 39–45.

Lara-Lemus A., Drucker-Colin R., Mendez-Franco J., Palomero-Rivero M., Perez de la Mora M. (1998). Biochemical effects induced by REM sleep deprivation in naive and in D-amphetamine treated rats. *Neurobiology* **6**(1), 13–22.

Lategan A., Marien M., Colpaert F. (1992). Suppression of nigrostriatal and mesolimbic dopamine release in vivo following noradrenaline depletion by DSP-4: a microdialysis study. *Life Sci.* **50**, 995–9.

Lavia Fantini M., Gagnon J., Petit D. *et al.* (2003). Slowing of electroencephalogram in rapid eye movement sleep behavior disorder. *Ann. Neurol.* **53**, 774–80.

Lavin A., Grace A. A. (1998). Dopamine modulates the responsivity of mediodorsal thalamic cells recorded in vitro. *J. Neurosci.* **18**(24), 10566–78.

Lavoie B., Parent A. (1990). Immunohistochemical study of the serotoninergic innervation of the basal ganglia in the squirrel monkey. *J. Comp. Neurol.* **299**, 1–16.

Lee R. S., Steffensen S. C., Henriksen S. J. (2001). Discharge profiles of ventral tegmental area GABA neurons during movement, anesthesia, and the sleep-wake cycle. *J. Neurosci.* **21**(5), 1757–66.

Lejeune F., Millan M. (1999). Pindolol excites dopaminergic and adrenergic neurons, and inhibits serotonergic neurons, by activation of 5-HT1A receptors. *Eur. J. Neurosci.* **12**, 3265–75.

Lemmer B., Berger T. (1978). Diurnal rhythm in the central dopamine turnover in the rat. *Naunyn Schmiedebergs Arch. Pharmacol.* **303**(3), 257–61.

Lena I., Parrot S., Deschaux O. *et al.* (2005). Variations in the extracellular levels of dopamine, noradrenaline, glutamate, and aspartate across the sleep-wake cycle in the medial prefrontal cortex and nucleus accumbens of freely moving rats. *J. Neurosci. Res.* **81**, 891–9.

Leng A., Mura A., Hengerer B., Feldon J., Ferger B. (2004). Effects of blocking the dopamine biosynthesis and of neurotoxic dopamine depletion with 1-methyl-4-phenyl-1,2,3,6-tetrahydropyridine (MPTP) on voluntary wheel running in mice. *Behav. Brain Res.* **154**, 375–83.

Li Y., van den Pol A. (2005). Direct and indirect inhibition by catecholamines of hypocretin/orexin neurons. *J. Neurosci.* **25**, 173–83.

Lindvall O., Bjorklund A. (1982). Neuroanatomy of central dopamine pathways: review of recent progress. In: M Keal, editor. *Advances in Dopamine Research*. Oxford and New York: Pergamon Press; pp. 297–311.

Liprando L., Miner L., Blakely R., Lewis D., Sesack S. (2004). Ultrastructural interactions between terminals expressing the norepinephrine transporter and dopamine neurons in the rat and monkey ventral tegmental area. *Synapse* **52**, 233–44.

Lonstein J., Blaustein J. (2004). Immunoctyochemical investigation of nuclear progestin receptor expression within dopaminergic neurones of the female rat brain. *J. Neuroendocrinol.* **16**, 534–43.

Lu J., Jhou T. C., Saper C. B. (2006). Identification of wake-active dopaminergic neurons in the ventral periaqueductal gray matter. *J. Neurosci.* **26**(1), 193–202.

Luppi P. H., Aston-Jones G., Akaoka H., Chouvet G., Jouvet M. (1995). Afferent projections to the rat locus coeruleus demonstrated by retrograde and anterograde tracing with cholera-toxin B subunit and *Phaseolus vulgaris* leucoagglutinin. *Neuroscience* **65**(1), 119–60.

Mandell A. J., Bullard W. P., Yellin J. B., Russo P. V. (1980). The influence of D-amphetamine on rat brain striatal reduced biopterin concentration. *J. Pharmacol. Exp. Ther.* **213**(3), 569–74.

Manni R., Terzaghi M., Sartori I., Mancini F., Pacchetti C. (2004). Dopamine agonists and sleepiness in PD: a review of the literature and personal findings. *Sleep Med.* **5**, 189–93.

Marin O., Smeets W. J., Gonzalez A. (1998). Evolution of the basal ganglia in tetrapods: a new perspective based on recent studies in amphibians. *Trends Neurosci.* **21**(11), 487–94.

Martin J. (1978). Neural regulation of growth hormone secretion. *Med. Clin. N. Am.* **62**, 327–36.

Maslowski R. J., Napier T. C. (1991). Dopamine D1 and D2 receptor agonists induce opposite changes in the firing rate of ventral pallidal neurons. *Eur. J. Pharmacol.* **200**(1), 103–12.

Mathe J. M., Nomikos G. G., Blakeman K. H., Svensson T. H. (1999). Differential actions of dizocilpine (MK-801) on the mesolimbic and mesocortical dopamine systems: role of neuronal activity. *Neuropharmacology* **38**(1), 121–8.

Matsumoto M., Kimura K., Fujisawa A. *et al.* (1981). Diurnal variations in monoamine contents in discrete brain regions of the Mongolian gerbil (*Meriones unguiculatus*). *J. Neurochem.* **37**, 792–4.

McClung C., Sidiropoulou K., Vitaterna M. *et al.* (2005). Regulation of dopaminergic transmission and cocaine reward by the Clock gene. *Proc. Natl. Acad. Sci. USA* **102**, 9377–81.

McGeer E., McGeer P. (1973). Some characteristics of brain tyrosine hydroxylase. In: Mandel A., editor. *New Concepts in Neurotransmitter Regulation.* New York: Plenum Press; pp. 53–68.

McKeith I. G., Ballard C. G., Perry R. H. *et al.* (2000). Prospective validation of consensus criteria for the diagnosis of dementia with Lewy bodies [In Process Citation]. *Neurology* **54**(5), 1050–8.

Megaw P., Boelen M., Morgan I., Boelen M. (2006). Diurnal patterns of dopamine release in chicken retina. *Neurochem. Intl.* **48**, 17–23.

Mejias-Aponte C., Zhu Y., Aston-Jones G. S. (2004). Noradrenergic innervation of midbrain dopamine neurons: prominent inputs from A1 and A2 Cell groups. In: *Society for Neuroscience Annual Meeting*; Abstract No. 465.464.

Mignot E., Taheri S., Nishino S. (2002). Sleeping with the hypothalamus: emerging therapeutic targets for sleep disorders. *Nat. Neurosci.* **5** (Suppl), 1071–5.

Miller A., Blaha C. (2004). Nigrostriatal dopamine release modulated by mesopontine muscarinic receptors. *NeuroReport* **15**, 1805–8.

Miller E., Nieburg H. (1973). Amphetamines. Valuable adjunct in treatment of Parkinsonism. *NY State J. Med.* **73**, 2657–61.

Miller J., Farber J., Gatz P., Roffwarg H., German D. (1983). Activity of mesencephalic dopamine and non-dopamine neurons across stages of sleep and waking in the rat. *Brain Res.* **273**, 133–41.

Missale C., Nash S. R., Robinson S. W., Jaber M., Caron M. G. (1998). Dopamine receptors: from structure to function. *Physiol. Rev.* **78**(1), 189–225.

Momiyama T., Sim J. A. (1996). Modulation of inhibitory transmission by dopamine in rat basal forebrain nuclei: activation of presynaptic D1-like dopaminergic receptors. *J. Neurosci.* **16**(23), 7505–12.

Monti J., Hawkins M., Jantos H., D'Angelo L., Fernandez M. (1988). Biphasic effects of dopamine D-2 receptor agonists on sleep and wakefulness in the rat. *Psychopharmacology* **95**, 395–400.

Monti J. M., Fernandez M., Jantos H. (1990). Sleep during acute dopamine D1 agonist SKF 38393 or D1 antagonist SCH 23390 administration in rats. *Neuropsychopharmacology* **3**(3), 153–62.

Monti J. M. (1989). Effects of the selective dopamine D2 receptor agonist, quinpirole on sleep and wakefulness in the rat. *Eur. J. Pharmacol.* **169**, 61–6.

Moukhles H., Bosler O., Bolam J. *et al.* (1997). Quantitative and morphometric data indicate precise cellular interactions between serotonin terminals and postsynaptic targets in rat substantia nigra. *Neuroscience* **76**, 1159–71.

Muller E. (1973). Nervous control of growth hormone secretion. *Neuroendocrinology* **11**, 338–69.

Munsch T., Yanagawa Y., Obata K., Pape H. (2005). Dopaminergic control of local interneuron activity in the thalamus. *Eur. J. Neurosci.* **21**, 290–4.

Naber D., Wirz-Justice A., Kafka M. S., Wehr T. A. (1980). Dopamine receptor binding in rat striatum: ultradian rhythm and its modification by chronic imipramine. *Psychopharmacology (Berl).* **68**(1), 1–5.

Nagatsu I. (1995). Tyrosine hydroxylase: human isoforms, structure and regulation in physiology and pathology. *Essays Biochem.* **30**, 15–35.

Nagatsu T., Levitt M., Udenfriend S. (1964). Tyrosine hydroxylase, the initial step in norepinephrine synthesis. *J. Biol. Chem.* **239**, 2910–17.

Nagayama H., Takagi A., Nakamura E., Yoshida H., Takahashi R. (1978). Circadian susceptibility rhythm to apomorphine in the brain. *Commun. Psychopharmacol.* **2**(4), 301–10.

Nakamura T., Uramura K., Nambu T. *et al.* (2000). Orexin-induced hyperlocomotion and stereotypy are mediated by the dopaminergic system. *Brain Res.* **873**(1), 181–7.

Nakashima A., Mori K., Suzuki T. *et al.* (1999). Dopamine inhibition of human tyrosine hydroxylase type I is controlled by the specific portion in the N-terminus of the enzyme. *J. Neurochem.* **72**, 2145–53.

Napier T. C., Potter P. E. (1989). Dopamine in the rat ventral pallidum/substantia innominata: biochemical and electrophysiological studies. *Neuropharmacology* **28**(7), 757–60.

Nicola S., Surmeier J., Malenka R. (2000). Dopaminergic modulation of neuronal excitability in the striatum and nucleus accumbens. *A. Rev. Neurosci.* **23**, 185–215.

Nishino S., Arrigoni J., Valtier D. *et al.* (1991). Dopamine D2 mechanisms in canine narcolepsy. *J. Neurosci.* **11**, 2666–71.

Nishino S., Mao J., Sampathkumaran R., Shelton J., Mignot E. (1998). Increased dopaminergic transmission mediates the wake-promoting effects of CNS stimulants. *Sleep Res. Online* 1(1), 49–61.

Nunes G., Jr, Tufik S., Nobrega N. (1994). Autoradiographic analysis of D1 and D2 dopaminergic receptors in rat brain after paradoxical sleep deprivation. *Brain Res. Bull.* **34**(5), 453–6.

Nygaard T., Marsden C., Duvoisin R. (1988). Dopa-responsive dystonia. *Adv. Neurol.* **50**, 377–84.

Nygaard T. (1993). Dopa-responsive dystonia. Delineation of the clinical syndrome and clues to pathogenesis. *Adv. Neurol.* **1993**, 577–85.

O'Neill R. D., Fillenz M. (1985). Simultaneous monitoring of dopamine release in rat frontal cortex, nucleus accumbens and striatum: effect of drugs, circadian changes and correlations with motor activity. *Neuroscience* **16**(1), 49–55.

Olijslagers J., Werkman T., McReary A. *et al.* (2004). 5-HT2 receptors differentially modulate dopamine-mediated auto-inhibition in A9 and A10 midbrain areas of the rat. *Neuropharmacology* **46**, 504–10.

Olive M. F., Seidel W. F., Edgar D. M. (1998). Compensatory sleep responses to wakefulness induced by the dopamine autoreceptor antagonist (-)DS121. *J. Pharmacol. Exp. Ther.* **285**(3), 1073–83.

Ongini E., Bonizzoni E., Ferri N., Milani S., Trampus M. (1993). Differential effects of dopamine D1 and D2 receptor antagonist antipsychotics on sleep-wake patterns in the rat. *J. Pharmacol. Exp. Ther.*

Ornstein K., Milon H., McRae-Degueurce A. *et al.* (1987). Biochemical and radioautographic evidence for dopaminergic afferents of the locus coeruleus originating in the ventral tegmental area. *J. Neural Transm.* **70**(3–4), 183–91.

Overeem S., van Hilten J. J., Ripley B., Mignot E., Nishino S., Lammers G. J. (2002). Normal hypocretin-1 levels in Parkinson's disease patients with excessive daytime sleepiness. *Neurology* **58**(3), 465–8.

Owasoyo J. O., Walker C. A., Whitworth U. G. (1979). Diurnal variation in the dopamine level of rat brain areas: effect of sodium phenobarbital. *Life Sci.* **25**(2), 119–22.

Pacchetti C., Martignoni E., Terzaghi M. *et al.* (2003). Sleep attacks in Parkinson's disease: a clinical and polysomnographic study. *Neurol. Sci.* **24**, 195–6.

Parkes J. D., Tarsy D., Marsden C. D. *et al.* (1975). Amphetamines in the treatment of Parkinson's disease. *J. Neurol. Neurosurg. Psychiatry* **38**(3), 232–7.

Paulson P. E., Robinson T. E. (1994). Relationship between circadian changes in spontaneous motor activity and dorsal versus ventral striatal dopamine neurotransmission assessed with on-line microdialysis. *Behav. Neurosci.* **108**(3), 624–35.

Perlow M. J., Gordon E. K., Ebert M. E., Hoffman H. J., Chase T. N. (1977). The circadian variation in dopamine metabolism in the subhuman primate. *J. Neurochem.* **28**(6), 1381–3.

Pi X., Voogt J., Grattan D. (2002). Detection of prolactin receptor mRNA in the corpus striatum and substantia nigra of the rat. *J. Neurosci. Res.* **67**, 551–8.

Porzgen P., Park S. K., Hirsh J., Sonders M. S., Amara S. G. (2001). The antidepressant-sensitive dopamine transporter in *Drosophila melanogaster*: a primordial carrier for catecholamines. *Mol. Pharmacol.* **59**(1), 83–95.

Ramsey A., Fitzpatrick P. (1998). Effects of phosphorylation of serine 40 of tyrosine hydroxylase on binding of catecholamines: evidence for a novel regulatory mechanism. *Biochemistry* **37**, 8980–6.

Ramsey A., Hillas P., Fitzpatrick P. (1996). Characterization of the active site iron in tyrosine hydroxylase redox states of the iron. *J. Biol. Chem.* **271**, 24395–400.

Razmy A., Lang A., Shapiro C. (2004). Predictors of impaired daytime sleep and wakefulness in patients with Parkinsons disease treated with older (ergot) vs newer (nonergot) dopamine agonists. *Arch. Neurol.* **61**, 97–102.

Reid M., Tafti M., Nishino S. *et al.* (1996). Local administration of dopaminergic drugs into the ventral tegmental area modulates cataplexy in the narcoleptic canine. *Brain Res.* **133**, 83–100.

Ribelayga C., Wang Y., Mangel S. (2004). A circadian clock in the fish retina regulates dopamine release via activation of melatonin receptors. *J. Physiol.* **554**(2), 467–82.

Roth T., Rye D., Borchert L. *et al.* (2003). Assessment of sleepiness and unintended sleep in Parkinson's disease patients taking dopamine agonists. *Sleep Med.* **4**, 275–80.

Rub U., Del Tredici K., Schultz C. *et al.* (2002). Parkinson's disease: the thalamic components of the limbic loop are severely impaired by alpha-synuclein immunopositive inclusion body pathology. *Neurobiol. Aging* **23**, 245–54.

Rye D., Bliwise D. (2004). Movement disorders specific to sleep and the nocturnal manifestations of waking movement disorders. In: Watts R., Koller W., editors. *Movement Disorders: Neurologic Principles and Practice*, 2nd edn. New York, NY: McGraw-Hill. pp. 855–90.

Rye D., Bliwise D. (1997). Movement disorders specific to sleep and the nocturnal manifestations of waking movement disorders. In: Watts R., Koller W., editors. *Movement Disorders: Neurologic Principles and Practice*. New York: McGraw-Hill; pp. 687–713.

Rye D., Daley J., Freeman A., Bliwise D. (2003). Daytime sleepiness and sleep attacks in idiopathic parkinson's disease. In: Bedard M-A., Agid Y., Chouinard S. *et al.* editors. *Mental and Behavioral Dysfunction in Movement Disorders*. Totawa, NJ: Humana Press; pp. 527–38.

Rye D., Iranzo A. (2005). The nocturnal manifestations of waking movement disorders: focus on Parkinson's disease. In: Guilleminault C., editor. *Handbook of Clinical Neurophysiology: Clinical Neurophysiology of Sleep Disorders*. Philadelphia, PA: Elsevier BV; pp. 263–72.

Rye D., Johnston L., Watts R., Bliwise D. (1999). Juvenile Parkinson's disease with REM behavior disorder, sleepiness and daytime REM-onsets. *Neurology* **53**, 1868–70.

Rye D. (1997). Contributions of the pedunculopontine region to normal and altered REM sleep. *Sleep* **20**(9), 757–88.

Rye D. (2006). Excessive daytime sleepiness and unintended sleep in Parkinson's disease. *Curr. Neurol. Neurosci. Rep.* **6**, 169–76.

Rye D. (2003). Modulation of normal and pathologic motoneuron activity during sleep. In: Chokroverty S., Hening W., Walters A., editors. *Sleep and Movement Disorders*. Philadelphia, PA: Butterworth-Heinemann; pp. 94–119.

Rye D. (2004b). Parkinson's disease and RLS: the dopaminergic bridge. *Sleep Med.* **5**, 317–28.

Rye D. (2004a). The two faces of Eve: dopamine's modulation of wakefulness and sleep. *Neurology* **63** (suppl. 3), S2–S7.

Rye D. B., Bliwise D. L., Dihenia B., Gurecki P. (2000). FAST TRACK: daytime sleepiness in Parkinson's disease. *J. Sleep Res.* **9**(1), 63–9.

Rye D. B., Jankovic J. (2002). Emerging views of dopamine in modulating sleep/wake state from an unlikely source: PD. *Neurology* **58**(3), 341–6.

Sakamoto K., Liu C., Kasamatsu M. *et al.* (2005). Dopamine regulates melanopsin mRNA expression in intrinsically photoresponsive retinal ganglion cells. *Eur. J. Neurosci.* **22**, 3129–36.

Sakata M., Sei H., Toida K. *et al.* (2002). Mesolimbic dopaminergic system is involved in diurnal blood pressure regulation. *Brain Res.* **928**(1–2), 194–201.

Sanchez-Gonzalez M., Garcia-Cabezas M., Rico B., Cavada C. (2005). The primate thalamus is a key target for brain dopamine. *J. Neurosci.* **25**, 6076–83.

Sautel F., Griffon N., Levesque D. *et al.* (1995). A functional test identifies dopamine agonists selective for D3 versus D2 receptors. *Neuroreport* **6**, 329–32.

Schapira A. (2004). Excessive daytime sleepiness in Parkinson's disease. *Neurology* **63**(8 Suppl. 3), S24–7.

Schenck C., Bundlie S., Mahowald M. (2003). REM behavior disorder (RBD): delayed emergence of parkinsonism or dementia in 65% of older men initially diagnosed with idiopathic RBD, and an analysis of the minimum and maximum tonic and/or phasic electromyographic abnormalities found during REM sleep. *Sleep* **26**(Suppl.), A316.

Scheving L. E., Harrison W. H., Gordon P., Pauly J. E. (1968). Daily fluctuation (circadian and ultradian) in biogenic amines of the rat brain. *Am. J. Physiol.* **214**(1), 166–73.

Seutin V. (2005). Dopaminergic neurones: much more than dopamine? *Br. J. Pharmacol.* **146**, 167–9.

Sherman S. M., Guillery R. W. (2001). *Exploring the Thalamus*. San Diego, CA: Academic Press.

Shouse M. N., Staba R. J., Saquib S. F., Farber P. R. (2000). Monoamines and sleep: microdialysis findings in pons and amygdala. *Brain Res.* **860**(1–2), 181–9.

Silber M. H., Rye D. B. (2001). Solving the mysteries of narcolepsy. *Neurology* **56**, 1616–18.

Skagerberg G., Bjorklund A., Lindvall O., Schmidt R. H. (1982). Origin and termination of the diencephalo-spinal dopamine system in the rat. *Brain Res. Bull.* **9**(1–6), 237–44.

Skagerberg G., Lindvall O. (1985). Organization of diencephalic dopamine neurones projecting to the spinal cord in the rat. *Brain Res.* **342**(2), 340–51.

Smeets W., Gonzalez A. (2000). Catecholamine systems in the brain of vertebrates: new perspectives through a comparative approach. *Brain Res. Brain Res. Rev.* **33**, (308–79).

Smiley J., Subramanian M., Mesulam M-M. (1999). Monoaminergic-cholinergic interactions in the primate basal forebrain. *Neuroscience* **93**, 817–29.

Smith A. D., Olson R. J., Justice J. B., Jr. (1992). Quantitative microdialysis of dopamine in the striatum: effect of circadian variation. *J. Neurosci. Meth.* **44**(1), 33–41.

Sokoloff P., Andrieux M., Besancon R. *et al.* (1992). Pharmacology of human dopamine D3 receptor expressed in a mammalian cell line: comparison with D2 receptor. *Eur. J. Pharmacol.* **225**, 331–7.

Sowers J. R., Vlachakis N. (1984). Circadian variation in plasma dopamine levels in man. *J. Endocrinol. Invest.* **7**(4), 341–5.

Stanley M., Traskman-Bendz L., Dorovini-Zis K. (1985). Correlations between aminergic metabolites simultaneously obtained from human CSF and brain. *Life Sci.* **37**(14), 1279–86.

Steenhard B., Besharse J. (2000). Phase shifting the retinal circadian clock: xPer2 mRNS induction by light and dopamine. *J. Neurosci.* **20**, 8572–7.

Steinfels G., Heym J., Strecker R., Jacobs B. (1983). Behavioral correlates of dopaminergic unit activity in freely moving cats. *Brain Res.* **258**, 217–28.

Steriade M., Paré D., Datta S., Oakson G., Dossi R. C. (1990). Different cellular types in mesopontine cholinergic nuclei related to ponto-geniculo-occipital waves. *J. Neurosci.* **10**(8), 2560–79.

Stevens S., Comella C., Stepanski E. (2004). Daytime sleepiness and alertness in patients with Parkinson disease. *Sleep* **27**, 967–72.

Strogatz S. H., Kronauer R. E., Czeisler C. A. (1987). Circadian pacemaker interferes with sleep onset at specific times each day: role in insomnia. *Am. J. Physiol.* **253**(1), R172–8.

Takada M. (1993). Widespread dopaminergic projections of the subparafascicular thalamic nucleus in the rat. *Brain Res. Bull.* **32**, 301–9.

Tan E. K., Lum S. Y., Fook-Chong S. M. C. *et al.* (2002). Evaluation of somnolence in Parkinson's disease: comparison with age and sex matched controls. *Neurology* **58**(3), 465–8.

Tassin J., Lavielle S., Herve D. *et al.* (1979). Collateral sprouting and reduced activity of the rat mesocortical dopaminergic neurons after selective destruction of the ascending noradrenergic bundles. *Neuroscience* **4**, 1569–82.

Trampus M., Ferri N., Adami M., Ongini E. (1993). The dopamine D1 receptor agonists, A68930 and SKF 38393, induce arousal and suppress REM sleep in the rat. *Eur. J. Pharmacol.* **235**, 83–7.

Trampus M., Ferri N., Monopoli A., Ongini E. (1991). The dopamine D1 receptor is involved in the regulation of REM sleep in the rat. *Eur. J. Pharmacol.* **194**, 189–94.

Trulson M., Preussler D. (1984). Dopamine-containing ventral tegmental area neurons in freely moving cats: activity during the sleep-waking cycle and effects of stress. *Exp. Neurol.* **83**, 367–77.

Trulson M. E. (1985). Simultaneous recording of substantia nigra neurons and voltammetric release of dopamine in the caudate of behaving cats. *Brain Res. Bull.* **15**(2), 221–3.

Tufik S., Lindsey C. J., Carlini E. A. (1978). Does REM sleep deprivation induce a supersensitivity of dopaminergic receptors in the rat brain? *Pharmacology* **16**(2), 98–105.

Turner R., D'Amato C., Chervin R., (2000). Blaivas M. The pathology of REM-sleep behavior disorder with comorbid Lewy body dementia. *Neurology* **55**, 1730–2.

Tzschentke T., Schmidt W. (2000). Functional relationship among medial prefrontal cortex, nucleus accumbens, and ventral tegmental area in locomotion and reward. *Crit. Rev. Neurobiol.* **14**, 131–42.

Ulivelli M., Rossi S., Lombard C. *et al.* (2002). Polysomnographic characterization of pergolide-induced "sleep attacks" in an idiopathic PD patient. *Neurology* **58**(3), 462–5.

Uramura K., Funahashi H., Muroya S. *et al.* (2001). Orexin-a activates phospholipase C- and protein kinase C-mediated Ca^{2+} signaling in dopamine neurons of the ventral tegmental area. *NeuroReport* **12**, 1885–9.

Urbain N., Gervasoni D., Souliere F. *et al.* (2000). Unrelated course of subthalamic nucleus of globus pallidus neuronal activities across vigilance states in the rat. *Eur. J. Neurosci.* **12**, 3361–74.

Ventura R., Cabib S., Alcaro A., Orsini C., Puglisi-Allegra S. (2003). Norepinephrine in the prefrontal cortex is critical for amphetamine-induced reward and mesoaccumbens dopamine release. *J. Neurosci.* **23**, 1879–85.

Watanabe S., Seeman P. (1984). D2 dopamine receptor density in rat striatum over 24 hours: lack of detectable changes. *Biol. Psychiatry* **19**(8), 1249–53.

Wetter T., Collado-Seidel V., Pollmacher T., Yassouridis A., Trenkwalder C. (2000). Sleep and periodic leg movement patterns in drug-free patients with Parkinson's disease and multiple system atrophy. *Sleep* **23**(3), 361–7.

Whittaker J., Morcol T., Patrickson J. (1997). Circadian plasticity in dopaminergic parameters in the rat substantia nigra. *Soc. Neurosci. Abstr.* **23**(80.2), 190.

Williams S. M., Goldman-Rakic P. S. (1998). Widespread origin of the primate mesofrontal dopamine system. *Cereb. Cortex* **8**(4), 321–45.

Wisor J., Nishino S., Sora I. *et al.* (2001). Dopaminergic role in stimulant-induced wakefulness. *J. Neurosci.* **21**(5), 1787–94.

Witkovsky P. (2004). Dopamine and retinal function. *Doc. Ophthalmol.* **108**, 17–40.

Xuereb J. H., Perry R. H., Candy J. M. *et al.* (1991). Nerve cell loss in the thalamus in Alzheimer's disease and Parkinson's disease. *Brain* **114**, 1363–79.

Yamanaka A., Muraki Y., Ichiki K. *et al.* (2006). Orexin neurons are directly and indirectly regulated by catecholamines in a complex manner. *J. Neurophysiol.* Epub-ahead of print.

Zeitzer J., Lopez-Rodriguez F., Behnke E. *et al.* (2001). Serotonin and dopamine in the human cortex and limbic system during a 40h sleep deprivation challenge. *Sleep* **24**, A76.

Zwicker A., Calil H. (1986). The effects of REM sleep deprivation on striatal dopamine receptor sites. *Pharmacol. Biochem. Behav.* **24**, 809–12.

8

Glutamate neurotransmission and sleep

IRWIN FEINBERG AND IAN G. CAMPBELL

Glutamate (Glu) is the main excitatory neurotransmitter in vertebrate brain and GABA is the main inhibitory neurotransmitter. Brain excitability and arousal level therefore depend on the dynamic interplay between Glu and GABA activity: excitability can be lowered by increasing GABA or by decreasing Glu tone. Despite a vast literature on the reduction of arousal and the induction of sleep by GABAergic drugs, Glu has remained relatively neglected. The reason for this unequal treatment is obvious. Drugs that depress brain excitability by stimulating the GABA–benzodiazepine receptor have been extraordinarily useful as hypnotics and short-term anesthetics, and new ones are being constantly developed. However, diminishing returns have now begun to affect the hegemony of the GABAergic hypnotics. Their well recognized limitations include tachyphyllaxis, addiction, and withdrawal syndromes with life-threatening convulsions. Moreover, they induce a sleep pattern with a non-physiological electroencephalogram (EEG) that is typically experienced as non-refreshing. It may thus now be a propitious time to manipulate the other side of the excitation–inhibition equation and examine Glu in more detail. Altering brain excitability by enhancing or depressing Glu transmission could lead to the development of drugs with unique and perhaps more favorable clinical profiles. The discussion in this chapter illustrates the basic science and the clinical potential of this alternative approach.

In 30 years, Glu has progressed from a putative neurotransmitter to being recognized as the major excitatory neurotransmitter in the brain. As such, Glu plays a role in countless brain functions, and it is not surprising, therefore,

Neurochemistry of Sleep and Wakefulness, ed. J. M. Monti *et al.* Published by Cambridge University Press.
© Cambridge University Press 2008.

that Glu should be involved in wake–sleep relationships. We review here the evidence for Glu neurotransmission in areas of the brain that regulate vigilance and then describe a series of experiments in rats that point to potential therapeutic uses for Glu receptor agonists and antagonists in the treatment of sleep disorders.

Glutamate receptor types

Glu receptors can be divided into ionotropic and metabotropic receptors. The classification of ionic Glu receptor subtypes has been reviewed in several publications (Collingridge & Lester, 1989; Greenamyre & Porter, 1994; Monaghan et al., 1989) and the classification of mGluRs has been reviewed by others (Conn & Pin, 1997; Schoepp, 2001; Schoepp & Conn, 1993). The ionotropic receptors are divided into the three types according to agonist binding selectivity: AMPA, kainate, and NMDA. Glu binding to AMPA or kainate receptors induces a fast excitatory depolarization via sodium ion influx. NMDA receptor ionophores are also permeable to calcium, and the entry of calcium ions can induce prolonged changes within the neuron that are believed to be important for learning and synaptic plasticity. The metabotropic receptors can also induce prolonged changes to the intracellular environment, but do so via G-protein-coupled second messenger systems. Eight metabotropic Glu receptor (mGluR) subtypes have been identified to date, and they are grouped into three classes. Group I mGluRs are positively coupled to phospholipase C and inositol phosphate. Groups II and III mGluRs are negatively coupled to adenylate cyclase. In general, Glu binding at ionotropic receptors produces neuronal excitation, and Glu binding at metabotropic receptors negatively modulates this excitability.

Glutamate neurotransmission in areas of the brain important for sleep and arousal

Although sleep and wakefulness are global states, specific brain structures are known to be involved in their regulation. These sites include areas within the brainstem, hypothalamus, and the thalamus, and Glu plays an active role in the control of sleep and waking in these areas.

Many sites within the pons and medulla that contribute to the increased levels of arousal that characterize wakefulness and rapid eye movement (REM) sleep are under glutamatergic control. The pontine reticular formation, for example, is involved in phenomena related to REM sleep and to motor activity during wakefulness. Glutamatergic neurotransmission also mediates the responses of cells of the medial pontine reticular formation. These cells are depolarized and increase their firing rate in response to Glu or to agonists of the three classes of ionotropic Glu receptors (Stevens *et al.*, 1992), and specific ionotropic receptor antagonists can block this effect (Stevens *et al.*, 1992). The muscle atonia that characterizes REM sleep is produced in the medial medulla, and is also under glutamatergic control. Activity in the pontine inhibitory area causes release of Glu in the nucleus magnocellularis of the medulla and Glu levels in this nucleus increase during REM sleep (Kodama *et al.*, 1998). The pedunculopontine tegmentum (PPT) contains cholinergic neurons that project throughout the brainstem and forebrain and produce arousal during wakefulness and REM. In rats, low doses of Glu injected into the PPT increase REM sleep, and higher doses increase wakefulness (Datta *et al.*, 2001b). This effect is mediated through NMDA and kainate receptors (Datta 2002; Datta *et al.*, 2001a). The fact that lower levels of arousal induced by PPT injections of Glu stimulate REM sleep, but that higher doses produce wakefulness, can be understood in terms of the one-stimulus model of non-REM–REM (i.e. NREM–REM) sleep alternation (Feinberg & March, 1988, 1995). According to this model, NREM sleep is produced by a pulsatile inhibitory stimulus that decreases neuronal firing, reduces brain metabolic rate, causes functional deafferentation, and shuts down memory systems. When the strength of this stimulus wanes sufficiently, escape from inhibition occurs. This inhibitory escape *is* REM sleep, which is characterized by irregular firing of cells in many structures and a return of metabolic rate to near-waking levels. In normal sleep, the process then recurs with another inhibitory pulse until the sleep need has been met. This model explains the results from Datta and colleagues (Datta *et al.*, 2001b), as well as some other responses during REM sleep, e.g. that stimulation of brainstem arousal centers during NREM sleep first raises brain arousal to the intermediate level of REM sleep and further stimulation produces wakefulness.

The suprachiasmatic nucleus (SCN) of the hypothalamus contains neurons that generate the endogenous circadian rhythm. These rhythms are entrained to environmental light by projections from the retina via the retinohypothalamic tract (RHT). Multiple lines of evidence have established that the RHT neurons entrain the SCN via Glu neurotransmission (Ebling, 1996). Thus, gene expression studies demonstrate the presence of mRNA for NMDA, AMPA, and kainate receptor subunits in the SCN. Ionotropic Glu receptor antagonists injected into the SCN block the entraining effects of light. Glu injection within the SCN produces circadian phase shifts that can mimic the phase shifts produced by light exposure. The efferent pathways by which the SCN induces arousal are not yet clear, but they appear to have Glu as a primary transmitter. SCN neurons project to the hypocretin-(i.e. orexin-) and Glu-containing neurons of the lateral and posterior hypothalamus (Abrahamson *et al.*, 2001).

Hypocretin-(HCT-) containing cells of the lateral and dorsomedial hypothalamus are critical for the maintenance of wakefulness, and narcolepsy is characterized by a reduced number of these cells (Peyron *et al.*, 2000; Thannickal *et al.*, 2000). HCT-containing neurons project throughout the brain and produce excitation largely through Glu release. For example, HCT cells project to the locus coeruleus. Intraventricular injection of HCT or direct locus coeruleus injection of HCT causes a release of Glu in the locus coeruleus that occurs concurrently with increased wakefulness (Kodama & Kimura, 2002). HCT neurons also project to the paraventricular nucleus of the thalamus (PVT), yet another area implicated in the control of sleep–wakefulness. Cortically projecting glutamatergic neurons of the PVT are excited by HCT (Huang *et al.*, 2006). Not only does HCT cause a release of Glu, but Glu also excites HCT neurons. Thus, HCT neurons feed back positively on themselves via Glu release (Li *et al.*, 2002). HCT neurons are excited via AMPA and NMDA receptor-mediated neurotransmission, and this excitation is tonically inhibited by group III mGluRs (Acuna-Goycolea *et al.*, 2004).

The presence of sleep-active cells in the medial preoptic area (mPOA) of the hypothalamus suggests that this brain area plays an important role in sleep regulation. Patch clamp studies have shown that GABA receptors mediate inhibitory postsynaptic potentials (IPSPs) in the mPOA and Glu receptors mediate EPSPs (Hoffman *et al.*, 1994). Stimulation of afferents to the mPOA produces EPSPs that are blocked by AMPA and NMDA receptor antagonists. It also induces IPSPs that are blocked by GABAa receptor antagonists (Malinina *et al.*, 2005). Microdialysis studies in the mPOA show that Glu is elevated in wakefulness relative to NREM sleep (Azuma *et al.*, 1996). In addition, the wakefulness-promoting drug modafinil increases Glu levels in the mPOA by decreasing GABA levels (Ferraro *et al.*, 1999). Thus, as in other areas of the brain, Glu and GABA work in dynamic opposition to control activity in this sleep center.

The basal forebrain is an important way station in the activation of the cerebral cortex from the reticular activating system. AMPA and NMDA injections into the basal forebrain increase wakefulness and reduce sleep (Cape & Jones, 2000; Manfridi *et al.*, 1999), effects that are blocked by AMPA and NMDA receptor antagonists (Manfridi *et al.*, 1999). The excitatory cortical projections of the basal forebrain have long been considered purely cholinergic, but many basal forebrain neurons that project to the cortex are now known to contain Glu, which may function as a co-transmitter or even as the primary excitatory neurotransmitter (Manns *et al.*, 2001). The basal forebrain also affects vigilance via synapses to HCT cells in the lateral hypothalamus; some of these synapses are glutamatergic (Henny & Jones, 2006).

Vigilance state and the EEG are affected by both cortical and thalamic glutamatergic processes. Application of Glu receptor antagonists to the ventroposterolateral thalamus increases sleep and decreases wakefulness (Juhasz *et al.*, 1990). The burst duration of cortical cells during NREM sleep is increased by NMDA and decreased by an NMDA receptor antagonist (Armstrong-James & Fox, 1988). The slow-wave EEG and sleep spindles that characterize NREM sleep are generated via thalamocortical circuits. Slow-wave oscillations in the cortex are altered by the NMDA receptor antagonist ketamine (Amzica & Steriade, 1995). In brain slice recordings from thalamocortical cells, <1 Hz oscillations can be initiated with mGluR agonists (Hughes *et al.*, 2002). Stimulating corticothalamic fibers also induces <1 Hz oscillations in thalamocortical cells that can be blocked by metabotropic Glu receptor antagonists (Hughes *et al.*, 2002).

The effects of systemic glutamate receptor antagonists and agonists on sleep and EEG

In this section, we describe a series of experiments in rats on the effects on sleep and EEG of systemic administration of drugs that alter Glu neurotransmission. We began by studying the effects of non-competitive NMDA antagonists, which have an unusual, counterintuitive effect on limbic system metabolism. Despite blocking excitatory neurotransmission, these compounds induce limbic hypermetabolism. We used this drug-induced hypermetabolism to test a component of the homeostatic model of NREM sleep delta power (Feinberg, 1974), i.e. that the drive for delta power homeostasis is determined by the intensity of awake brain activity as well as by the duration of wakefulness. We then tested the sleep and EEG effects of a competitive NMDA receptor antagonist that did not alter limbic metabolism, and we also investigated the effects of an AMPA receptor antagonist. Because Glu is the main excitatory neurotransmitter in the brain, it is not surprising that the sleep effects of these drugs were accompanied by numerous side effects. The metabotropic Glu receptors are modulators of excitatory neurotransmission. As described below, mGluR agonists and antagonists affect sleep and the EEG without producing behavioral impairment: they hold promise as clinically useful compounds for altering sleep and wakefulness regulation.

Effects of NMDA channel blockade and increased limbic system metabolism on subsequent sleep

Our first studies with compounds that alter Glu neurotransmission were not targeted at decreasing brain excitability. Rather, as noted above, we used the limbic hypermetabolism induced by non-competitive NMDA receptor antagonists to test whether an increase in the metabolic rate of these limbic structures would increase the homeostatic drive, producing higher levels of EEG delta power in subsequent sleep. The intensity of neuronal activity, in this area as in any other, is proportional to metabolic rate. Thus, increasing the intensity of limbic metabolism should, according to our model, increase the drive for sleep homeostasis. This would be demonstrated by an increase in EEG delta power during NREM sleep. The later two-process homeostatic model (Borbely, 1982) did not include a component for waking intensity and differs from the original model of delta homeostasis in other major respects. In fact, the "intensity" component of the 1974 homeostatic model was introduced to account for the marked decline of NREM sleep delta power during adolescence. We proposed that this decline was due to a decreasing intensity in metabolic rate of awake brain activity across adolescence (Chugani et al., 1987; Kennedy & Sokoloff, 1957). This reduces the amount of homeostatic recovery needed during sleep.

We wanted to go beyond indirect and inferential evidence, however, and test experimentally the hypothesis that an increase in awake brain metabolic rate would increase NREM sleep delta power during subsequent sleep. However, brain metabolism during wakefulness is under tight homeostatic control and is not easily manipulated. We therefore used non-competitive NMDA antagonists to stimulate the metabolic rate of limbic brain structures. Deoxyglucose studies by others had demonstrated that NMDA channel blockade in rats, using ketamine, PCP, or MK-801, significantly increased glucose uptake in limbic structures, including the hippocampus, cingulate, and entorhinal cortex (Crosby et al., 1982; Hammer & Herkenham, 1983; Kurumaji et al., 1989; Nelson et al., 1980). However, these metabolic effects were not global. NMDA channel blockade produced a mosaic of metabolic changes, including, notably, a decrease in metabolic rate in sensory and motor systems.

While recognizing the complexities of NMDA channel blockade effects, we nevertheless decided to examine this question by administering ketamine to rats intraperitoneally (i.p.) at subanesthetic doses of 15, 25 and 50 mg/kg (Feinberg & Campbell, 1993). The drugs were first administered 6 h into the dark period. We administered the drug three times at each dose to produce a sustained change in the metabolic rate of affected brain structures. The second and third doses were given when the preceding motor effects had worn off. The motor effects of NMDA channel blockade are dramatic. Locomotion increases, stereotyped head swinging emerges, and finally the animals become ataxic. Ketamine injected during the dark period produced a sustained increase in EEG delta power in NREM sleep during the subsequent light period. We also showed that the ketamine stimulation of NREM sleep delta power is dose-dependent across the 25 and 50 mg/kg doses (Feinberg & Campbell, 1995).

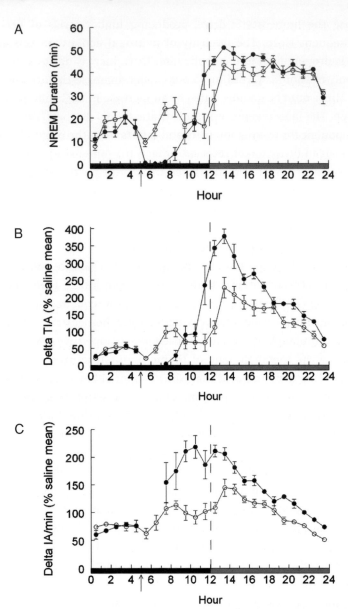

Figure 8.1 The duration of NREM sleep and delta activity during NREM sleep following saline (open circles) or 0.5 mg/kg MK-801 (filled circles), administered 6 h after the start of the dark period. MK-801 initially produced a period of wakefulness approximately 3 h long. In the subsequent light period, NREM sleep duration (A), total integrated amplitude (TIA, a period amplitude measure similar to power) of NREM sleep delta (B), and NREM sleep delta integrated amplitude per minute (IA/min) (C) were all significantly increased above control levels.

The question remained as to whether the effect on delta power was the result of NMDA channel blockade, since ketamine affects multiple receptor systems. We therefore repeated the experiment with MK-801 (Campbell & Feinberg, 1996a), a more specific NMDA antagonist than ketamine. MK-801 was administered i.p. at doses of 0.3 and 0.5 mg/kg. MK-801 injected during the dark period induced an extended period of stereotypical behavior similar to that produced by ketamine. Figure 8.1 shows that, during the subsequent light period, MK-801 increased NREM sleep duration and also increased EEG delta power in NREM sleep. It remained possible, however, that the average 3 h increase in dark-period wakefulness induced by this drug had some unique stimulatory effect on NREM sleep delta mechanisms, which in turn produced the experimental effects. To test this possibility, we performed 3 h of sleep deprivation during the dark period at a time that corresponded to the wakefulness induced by the drugs. The 11% increase in delta power produced by this manipulation approached significance but was far less than the 55% increase produced by 0.5 mg/kg MK-801.

Thus, we had strong evidence that NMDA channel blockade during wakefulness increases NREM sleep delta power during subsequent sleep, and this increase is greater than that produced by other pharmacological manipulations. However, at the time that these experiments were being performed, it was reported that MK-801 caused vacuolization in the same structures that responded with hypermetabolism (Olney et al., 1989). Moreover, these neurotoxic changes had a declining time course that resembled the physiological decline in delta power across sleep. Neurotoxicity could itself produce EEG slowing, raising the possibility that the delta power increase we were measuring was that of pathological slowing rather than changes in the physiological delta power of NREM sleep. We therefore designed an experiment to separate the time course of the vacuolization effect from that of delta power stimulation following MK-801. Reasoning that if our basic hypothesis was correct and that the hypermetabolism in limbic structures increased the homeostatic delta drive, we hypothesized that this drive would still be present after 12 h of sleep deprivation when the vacuolization effect was exhausted.

We therefore performed the following experiment. We administered 0.3 mg/kg of MK-801 at the onset of the 12 h dark period. In one group of rats, there was no further manipulation. In a second group of rats, the drug was followed by 12 h of total sleep deprivation. In the third group of rats, saline was administered at the onset of the dark period and this was followed by 12 h of sleep deprivation. The dependent variable was the total integrated delta amplitude over the 12 h light period that followed (Fig. 8.2). The stimulation of delta power by MK-801 alone was immediate and had largely dissipated by the start of the light period 12 h later. Twelve hours of sleep deprivation produced a marked

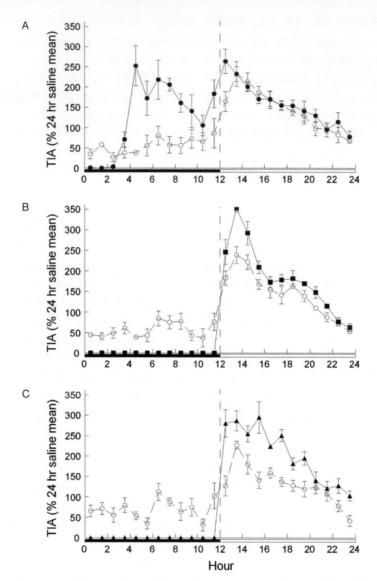

Figure 8.2 A comparison of the effects on standardized NREM sleep delta total integrated amplitude (TIA) produced by (A) MK-801, (B) 12 h total sleep deprivation (TSD), and (C) MK-801 + TSD shows that the delta increase produced by MK-801 persists across a 12 h period of sleep deprivation. MK-801 injected at the start of the dark period produced a large increase in TIA that returned to baseline levels by the second hour of the light period. TSD throughout the 12 h dark period produced a 28% increase in TIA in the subsequent light period. MK-801 followed by TSD for the remainder of the dark period produced a 60% increase in light period delta TIA that was significantly greater than the effect of MK-801 alone or TSD alone. This finding indicated that MK-801 increased the homeostatic drive for delta.

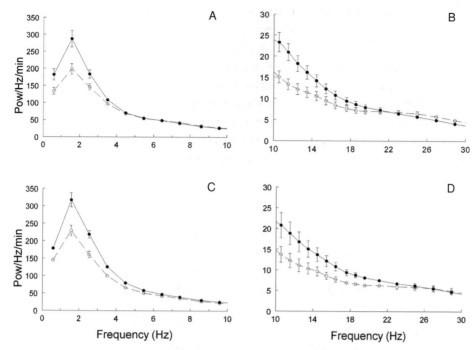

Figure 8.3 The similarity of the EEG effects of 12 h total sleep deprivation (TSD) and 0.5 mg/kg MK-801. Standardized power density functions for the 12 h light period are shown for the frequency ranges most affected by the two treatments. Both TSD and MK-801 increased power in the 1–4 Hz frequency band during NREM sleep and the 10–20 Hz frequency band during REM sleep. (A) MK-801 vs. saline, NREM; (B) MK-801 vs. saline, REM; (C) 12 h TSD vs. control, NREM; (D) 12 h TSD vs. control, REM.

increase in delta power. However, the 0.3 mg/kg dose of MK-801 followed by 12 h of sleep deprivation produced a larger and more sustained increase in light period delta power that significantly exceeded that produced by either of the other two manipulations (Campbell & Feinberg, 1996b). Thus, we had successfully separated the time course of the delta effect from that of neurotoxicity, adding confidence to our inference that NMDA channel blockade increased the drive for sleep homeostasis by increasing the metabolic rate of limbic brain structures while the animal was awake.

We also tested the hypothesis that the delta power increase produced by MK-801 was physiological by comparing the EEG spectral density function after MK-801 with that following 12 h of sleep deprivation (Campbell & Feinberg, 1999). We compared the spectra in NREM and REM sleep and waking, and noted that the EEG spectral functions after sleep deprivation and MK-801 were strikingly similar during all three vigilance states. Figure 8.3 displays some of the principal results. As noted above, both sleep deprivation and MK-801 markedly increased delta power in NREM sleep. Another striking similarity was the increase in power in the 10–20 Hz frequency band during REM sleep produced by both sleep deprivation and MK-801. These results add further support to our hypothesis that NMDA channel blockade induced brain changes during wakefulness that increased the drive for sleep homeostasis.

The experiments described above represented two methodological approaches that were innovative when introduced but are now coming into more widespread use. The first was the attempt to increase delta sleep by altering the metabolic state of the brain during waking; this manipulation followed from the intensity component of our 1974 homeostatic model. Apart from the theoretical basis of our model, modifying the awake state of the brain seems a logical test of sleep systems if one assumes that sleep performs some brain function that reverses changes induced by wakefulness. The second innovation was the imposition of a period of sleep deprivation after the experimental manipulation to determine whether a persistent need for sleep homeostasis had been induced; so far as we know, only one other group has adopted this technique to date (Meerlo *et al.*, 2001).

Ionotropic glutamate receptor antagonists that decrease brain excitability

Our research into the effects of Glu perturbations on sleep established that non-competitive NMDA channel blockade produced a notable increase in NREM sleep delta power and that this increase persisted after 12 h of sleep deprivation. But would a competitive NMDA receptor blocker that does not increase limbic metabolism also increase delta power? To investigate this possibility we administered CPPene, a competitive NMDA antagonist that does not produce limbic hypermetabolism (Kurumaji *et al.*, 1989). The results were different from those obtained after non-competitive NMDA channel blockade. CPPene increased NREM and REM sleep duration and decreased the duration of wakefulness. Unlike the non-competitive antagonists, MK-801 and ketamine, CPPene had an effect during the first 6 h after injection. The EEG effects were also very different from those produced by MK-801 and ketamine. Rather than being elevated, NREM sleep delta power was significantly decreased by the 1.25 mg/kg dose of CPPene. All three CPPene doses also significantly increased high-frequency (i.e. 20–50 Hz) EEG power during REM sleep. CPPene also increased food consumption in the first hour after injection. We hypothesized that the eating and sleep effects resulted from decreased excitatory neurotransmission in hypothalamic structures; as noted above, excitatory transmission is well represented in this brain structure and is crucial for sleep and other vegetative functions. The excitation–inhibition balance of the brain can be modified by altering excitatory as well as inhibitory tone, as has more commonly been done with the GABAergic hypnotics and anesthetics. The decreased wakefulness and increased sleep induced by CPPene may result from inhibition of excitatory neurotransmission at NMDA receptors.

We also tested the sleep and EEG effects of directly decreasing brain excitation by systemically injecting the competitive AMPA antagonist, NBQX (unpublished observations). These injections significantly increased NREM sleep duration during the 6 h after the injection but only at a high dose that also produced ataxia. This dose also decreased spectral power across a wide range of EEG frequencies (1–50 Hz). This indicates that the response was clearly not physiological.

Manipulations of the metabotropic Glu receptor

We then decided to alter the balance of brain excitation and inhibition by modifying the actions of mGlu receptors (mGluRs). Our reasoning was as follows. One of the salient features of sleep is that it is a protracted state of diminished brain arousal. Therefore, mGluR perturbations, which modify neuronal excitability over prolonged periods by inducing changes through G-protein coupled receptors, might produce more prolonged changes relevant to natural sleep than those induced through fast-acting excitatory receptor systems. In our first experiment, we used the mGlu2/3 (group II) receptor agonist to reduce excitatory tone, and measured the effects on sleep–wake states and the EEG.

In rats we injected the potent and selective mGlu2/3 agonist LY379268 subcutaneously (s.c.) at the midpoint of the dark period. As in our previous experiments, each animal received a saline injection that provided baseline values. The results were dramatic. In the 6 h post-injection (Fig. 8.4), 1 mg/kg LY379268 totally abolished REM sleep and reduced it by 80% in the next 6 h period. These effects, and the associated changes in EEG spectra described below, were significantly dose-dependent. LY379268 at the doses we gave had little effect on NREM sleep or wakefulness duration. However, the effects of LY379268 on the awake and NREM sleep EEG spectra were significant. During the 6 h post-injection period, power density in the fast NREM sleep frequencies (i.e. 10–50 Hz) was profoundly reduced. In the awake EEG, power density in fast EEG frequencies was also reduced, although less markedly than during NREM sleep. Of particular interest, in view of the important hippocampal information-processing role attributed to these frequencies, was the specific suppression of theta EEG power during wakefulness.

LY341495 is an antagonist that has been shown to block mGlu2/3 receptors in several preparations. We injected 1, 5, and 10 mg/kg of LY341495 s.c. to rats. This

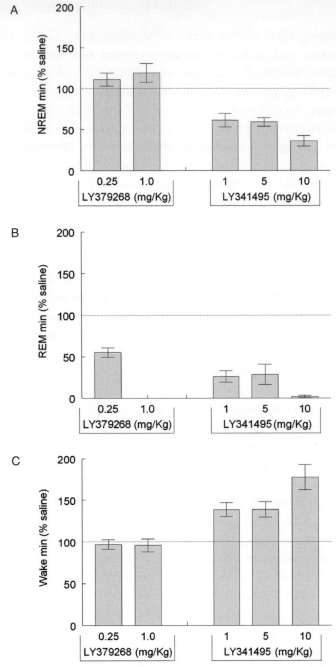

Figure 8.4 Vigilance state effects of the mGlu2/3 agonist LY379268 and antagonist LY341495. (A) NREM; (B) REM; (C) Wakefulness. During the 6 h following injection, LY379268 had little effect on NREM sleep or wakefulness duration, but at the higher dose the compound completely abolished REM sleep. Paradoxically, both LY379268 and LY341495 markedly decreased REM sleep. The mGlu2/3 antagonist, however, also decreased NREM sleep and increased wakefulness, demonstrating significant arousing effects.

experiment was designed to test the hypothesis that blocking mGlu2/3 receptors in normal animals would increase brain arousal levels, and that this increase would be correlated with increased wakefulness and increased fast EEG and theta activity.

Figure 8.4 shows the effects of LY341495 on vigilance states in the 6 h post-injection period. Both NREM and REM sleep were significantly reduced by all three doses, and waking was notably increased. Thus, antagonizing mGlu2/3 receptors increased behavioral arousal. Heightened arousal levels were also evident in the EEG spectral data. Figure 8.5 shows that, in NREM sleep, all three doses decreased low-frequency power to a similar extent; the lower the frequency, the greater the reduction in power. Spectral power returned to baseline levels in the 10–20 Hz frequency band, and then increased above baseline across the 20–50 Hz band with the greatest increase in the highest frequencies. This enhancement of power in the fast EEG frequencies was also significantly dose-dependent.

Figure 8.5 also displays the results of the mGlu2/3 antagonist on the awake spectral density function. Slow frequencies are normally minimal in the awake EEG and thus were not depressed as they were in NREM sleep. However, power in the high-frequency band (20–50 Hz) of the awake EEG spectrum was increased. As in NREM sleep, the higher the frequency, the greater the power enhancement, and this effect was also dose-dependent. Of particular interest was the notable increase in power in the theta frequency band (6–8 Hz) following both the 5 and 10 mg/kg doses. As noted above, this result, in conjunction with the theta suppression caused by LY379268, could provide a powerful tool for investigating the relationship between theta waves and memory and learning.

These data thus confirm our initial hypothesis that mGlu2/3 receptors are tonically active in lowering the level of brain arousal. Thus, antagonizing these receptors increases arousal as evidenced by the increase in waking and the stimulation of high-frequency EEG power. The striking increase in theta power was unexpected but is also consistent with increased arousal.

We also determined if the effects of LY341495 on sleep and the EEG were due to an action at the mGlu2/3 receptor, by testing whether LY341495 would specifically block the sleep and EEG effects of the highly selective mGlu2/3 agonist LY379268. In fact, LY341495 blocked and, with increasing doses, reversed the effects of 1 mg/kg LY379268 on wakefulness and EEG spectral power.

Hence an mGluR agonist and antagonist can both suppress REM sleep. This might seem incompatible with the opposing actions of these compounds on brain excitation that we have proposed. However, this apparent discrepancy can be explained by the one-stimulus model of NREM–REM sleep alternation described above. According to this model, REM sleep is a brain state of excitation or arousal that is intermediate between that of wakefulness and NREM

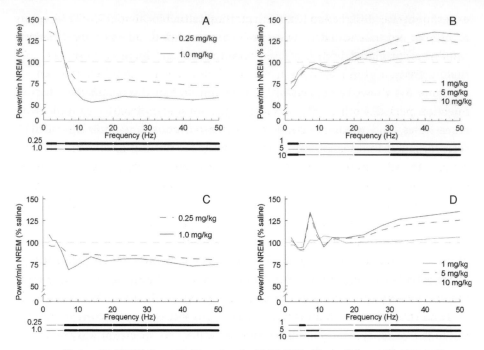

Figure 8.5 NREM sleep (A, B) and wake (C, D) EEG effects of the mGlu2/3 agonist LY379268 (A, C) and antagonist LY341495 (B, D). During the 6 h following injection, LY379268 increased NREM sleep low-frequency EEG power, decreased NREM sleep high-frequency EEG power (A), and decreased awake high-frequency EEG power (C). LY341495 produced the opposite effects on the EEG frequency spectrum during both NREM sleep (B) and wakefulness (D). The drugs also had pronounced effects on awake EEG theta power, with LY379268 producing a sharp decrease and LY341495 producing a sharp increase.

sleep. Thus, increasing excitation can reduce REM sleep by raising the arousal level to that of wakefulness, and conversely, decreasing excitation can change REM sleep to NREM sleep; for further discussion see (Feinberg *et al.*, 2005).

We interpreted the effects of LY379268 and LY341495 on vigilance states and the EEG as expressions of altered brain excitability or arousal level. mGlu2/3 receptors are located presynaptically outside the area of active synaptic transmission, indicating that their function might be to counteract the effects of excessive or extra-synaptic Glu release (Schoepp, 2001). However, our data, showing that mGLu2/3 antagonism with LY341495 affects the vigilance state and EEG spectral profile, demonstrated that these receptors maintain an excitatory tone even if an excess of Glu is not present. The notable suppression of REM sleep by LY379268 and by LY341495 are of clinical interest since their effect equals or exceeds that produced by MAO inhibitors, the most potent previously known drugs to suppress REM sleep. Thus, in addition to their potential clinical interest as sleep or psychiatric drugs, these findings suggest that LY379268 and LY341495 could provide a useful probe to test models that relate learning to specific EEG frequencies. For example, the suppression of EEG power in the theta frequencies during wakefulness by LY379268 could be used to test the putative relation of hippocampal theta to learning and memory. Such studies would be feasible since motor behavior, although somewhat diminished overall, is essentially normal in animals given 1 mg/kg LY379268 and even higher doses (Cartmell & Schoepp, 2000). Similarly, the presumptive role of REM sleep in learning could be tested by administering learning tasks prior to its total suppression by LY379268 injection. These REM-sleep-suppressing effects could be separated from the effects on theta power because both LY379268 and LY341495 suppress REM sleep but have opposite effects on theta. Finally, the opposite effects of these compounds on high frequencies in the awake EEG could be used to evaluate theories that relate activity in the gamma frequency band (i.e. 40–50 Hz) to learning and to the integration, or "binding", of neural processing.

Hence the powerful brain effects of mGlu2/3 receptor agonism and antagonism offer tools to investigate the effects of varying the levels of brain arousal on memory and behavior. The question remains as to whether they might also offer clinical potential. The available data suggest that mGlu2/3 receptor agonists and antagonists might eventually prove useful as sedative-hypnotic and analeptic agents. For example, they might be used to treat insomnia, a pervasive, troubling and unsolved pharmacological problem. Most insomniacs have essentially a normal sleep EEG; one of us (I.F.) has hypothesized that the memory systems of insomniacs do not shut down normally during sleep (Feinberg & Floyd, 1982). As a consequence of this failure, insomniacs believe they have been awake much of the night and experience their sleep as unrestorative. The failure of memory systems to shut down sufficiently during sleep could be due to hyperarousal that might be reversed by mGlu2/3 agonist-type drugs. Antagonists at mGlu2/3 receptors could also be used in conditions where sustained arousal is needed, for example to counteract the sleep attacks of narcolepsy, and possibly to treat attention-deficit hyperactivity disorder.

Whether or not manipulating glutamate transmission might lead to useful and novel sleep-inducing agents, the data discussed in this chapter show how such experiments could be applied in the investigation of important problems in basic neuroscience. Conceptually, excitation and inhibition in the CNS must be reciprocally interrelated rather than independent processes. Just as the contraction of a muscle involves coordinated relaxation of its antagonistic muscle, so increased central arousal should involve a precisely coordinated decrease in inhibition. Sleep, a state of generalized brain inhibition, offers a rich field for investigating these dynamically related processes, and it can be approached at all levels of integration. As noted in our introductory comments, most sleep research has understandably focused on the clinically useful inhibitory effects of increased GABAergic transmission. This near-exclusive focus has left relatively untouched an entire research area involving excitatory neurotransmission and sleep.

References

Abrahamson, E. E., Leak, R. K. & Moore, R. Y. (2001). The suprachiasmatic nucleus projects to posterior hypothalamic arousal systems. *Neuroreport* **12**, 435–40.

Acuna-Goycolea, C., Li, Y. & Van Den Pol, A. N. (2004). Group III metabotropic glutamate receptors maintain tonic inhibition of excitatory synaptic input to hypocretin/orexin neurons. *J. Neurosci.* **24**, 3013–22.

Amzica, F. & Steriade, M. (1995). Short- and long-range neuronal synchronization of the slow (<1 Hz) cortical oscillation. *J. Neurophysiol.* **73**, 20–38.

Armstrong-James, M. & Fox, K. (1988). Evidence for a specific role for cortical NMDA receptors in slow-wave sleep. *Brain Res.* **451**, 189–96.

Azuma, S., Kodama, T., Honda, K. & Inoue, S. (1996). State-dependent changes of extracellular glutamate in the medial preoptic area in freely behaving rats. *Neurosci. Lett.* **214**, 179–82.

Borbely, A. (1982). A two-process model of sleep regulation. *Hum. Neurobiol.* **1**, 195–204.

Campbell, I. G. & Feinberg, I. (1996a). Noncompetitive NMDA channel blockade during waking intensely stimulates NREM delta. *J. Pharmacol. Exp. Ther.* **276**, 737–42.

Campbell, I. G. & Feinberg, I. (1996b). NREM delta stimulation following MK-801 is a response of sleep systems. *J. Neurophysiol.* **76**, 3714–20.

Campbell, I. G. & Feinberg, I. (1999). Comparison of MK-801 and sleep deprivation effects on NREM, REM, and waking spectra in the rat. *Sleep* **22**(4), 423–32.

Cape, E. G. & Jones, B. E. (2000). Effects of glutamate agonist versus procaine microinjections into the basal forebrain cholinergic cell area upon gamma and theta EEG activity and sleep–wake state. *Eur. J. Neurosci.* **12**, 2166–84.

Cartmell, J. & Schoepp, D. D. (2000). Regulation of neurotransmitter release by metabotropic glutamate receptors. *J. Neurochem.* **75**, 889–907.

Chugani, H. T., Phelps, M. E. & Mazziotta, J. C. (1987). Positron emission tomography study of human brain functional development. *Ann. Neurol.* **22**, 487–97.

Collingridge, G. L. & Lester, R. A. (1989). Excitatory amino acid receptors in the vertebrate central nervous system. *Pharmacol. Rev.* **41**, 143–210.

Conn, P. J. & Pin, J. P. (1997). Pharmacology and functions of metabotropic glutamate receptors. *A. Rev. Pharmacol. Toxicol.* **37**, 205–37.

Crosby, G., Crane, A. M. & Sokoloff, L. (1982). Local changes in cerebral glucose utilization during ketamine anesthesia. *Anesthesiology* **56**, 437–43.

Datta, S. (2002). Evidence that REM sleep is controlled by the activation of brain stem pedunculopontine tegmental kainate receptor. *J. Neurophysiol.* **87**, 1790–8.

Datta, S., Patterson, E. H. & Spoley, E. E. (2001a). Excitation of the pedunculopontine tegmental NMDA receptors induces wakefulness and cortical activation in the rat. *J. Neurosci. Res.* **66**, 109–16.

Datta, S., Spoley, E. E. & Patterson, E. H. (2001b). Microinjection of glutamate into the pedunculopontine tegmentum induces REM sleep and wakefulness in the rat. *Am. J. Physiol. Regul. Integr. Comp. Physiol.* **280**, R752–9.

Ebling, F. J. (1996). The role of glutamate in the photic regulation of the suprachiasmatic nucleus. *Prog. Neurobiol.* **50**, 109–32.

Feinberg, I. (1974). Changes in sleep cycle patterns with age. *J. Psychiat. Res.* **10**, 283–306.

Feinberg, I. (1978). Efference copy and corollary discharge: implications for thinking and its disorders. *Schizophrenia Bull.* **4**, 636–40.

Feinberg, I. (1982). Schizophrenia: caused by a fault in programmed synaptic elimination during adolescence? *J. Psychiat. Res.* **17**, 319–34.

Feinberg, I. & Campbell, I. G. (1993). Ketamine administration during waking increases delta EEG intensity in rat sleep. *Neuropsychopharmacology* **9**, 41–8.

Feinberg, I. & Campbell, I. G. (1995). Stimulation of NREM delta EEG by ketamine administration during waking: demonstration of dose-dependence. *Neuropsychopharmacology* **12**(1), 89–90.

Feinberg, I. & Campbell, I. G. (1997). Coadministered pentobarbital anesthesia postpones but does not block the motor and sleep EEG responses to MK-801. *Life Sci.* **60**, PL217–22.

Feinberg, I. & Floyd, T. C. (1982). The regulation of human sleep. *Hum. Neurobiol.* **1**, 185–94.

Feinberg, I. & March, J. D. (1988). Cyclic delta peaks during sleep: result of a pulsatile endocrine process? [letter]. *Arch. Gen. Psychiat.* **45**, 1141–2.

Feinberg, I. & March, J. D. (1995). Observations on delta homeostasis, the one-stimulus model of NREM-REM alternation, and the neurobiologic implications of experimental dream studies. *Behav. Brain Res.* **69**, 97–108.

Feinberg, I., Schoepp, D. D., Hsieh, K. C., Darchia, N. & Campbell, I. G. (2005). The mGlu2/3 antagonist LY341495 stimulates waking and fast EEG power and blocks the effects of the mGlu2/3 agonist LY379268 in rats. *J. Pharmacol. Exp. Ther.* **312**, 826–33.

Ferraro, L., Antonelli, T., Tanganelli, S. *et al.* (1999). The vigilance promoting drug modafinil increases extracellular glutamate levels in the medial preoptic area and the posterior hypothalamus of the conscious rat: prevention by local GABAA receptor blockade. *Neuropsychopharmacology* **20**, 346–56.

Greenamyre, J. T. & Porter, R. H. P. (1994). Anatomy and physiology of glutamate in the CNS. *Neurology* **44**, S7–S13.

Hammer, R. P. & Herkenham, M. (1983). Altered metabolic activity in the cerebral cortex of rats exposed to ketamine. *J. Comp. Neurol.* **220**, 396–404.

Henny, P. & Jones, B. E. (2006). Vesicular glutamate (VGlut), GABA (VGAT), and acetylcholine (VACht) transporters in basal forebrain axon terminals innervating the lateral hypothalamus. *J. Comp. Neurol.* **496**, 453–67.

Hoffman, N. W., Wuarin, J. P. & Dudek, F. E. (1994). Whole-cell recordings of spontaneous synaptic currents in medial preoptic neurons from rat hypothalamic slices: mediation by amino acid neurotransmitters. *Brain Res.* **660**, 349–52.

Huang, H., Ghosh, P. & van den Pol, A. N. (2006). Prefrontal cortex-projecting glutamatergic thalamic paraventricular nucleus excited by hypocretin: a feedforward circuit that may enhance cognitive arousal. *J. Neurophysiol.* **95**, 1656–68.

Hughes, S. W., Cope, D. W., Blethyn, K. L. & Crunelli, V. (2002). Cellular mechanisms of the slow (<1 Hz) oscillation in thalamocortical neurons in vitro. *Neuron* **33**, 947–58.

Juhasz, G., Kekesi, K., Emri, Z., Soltesz, I. & Crunelli, V. (1990). Sleep-promoting action of excitatory amino acid antagonists: a different role for thalamic NMDA and non-NMDA receptors. *Neurosci. Lett.* **114**, 333–8.

Kennedy, C. & Sokoloff, L. (1957). An adaptation of the nitrous oxide method to the study of the cerebral circulation in children: normal values for cerebral blood flow and cerebral metabolic rate during childhood. *J. Clin. Invest.* **36**, 1130–7.

Kodama, T. & Kimura, M. (2002). Arousal effects of orexin-A correlate with GLU release from the locus coeruleus in rats. *Peptides* **23**, 1673–81.

Kodama, T., Lai, Y. Y. & Siegel, J. M. (1998). Enhanced glutamate release during REM sleep in the rostromedial medulla as measured by in vivo microdialysis. *Brain Res.* **780**, 178–81.

Kurumaji, A., Nehls, D. G., Park, C. K. & McCulloch, J. (1989). Effects of NMDA antagonists, MK-801 and CPP, upon local cerebral glucose use. *Brain Res.* **496**, 268–84.

Li, Y., Gao, X. B., Sakurai, T. & van den Pol, A. N. (2002). Hypocretin/orexin excites hypocretin neurons via a local glutamate neuron-A potential mechanism for orchestrating the hypothalamic arousal system. *Neuron* **36**, 1169–81.

Malinina, E., Druzin, M. & Johansson, S. (2005). Fast neurotransmission in the rat medial preoptic nucleus. *Brain Res.* **1040**, 157–68.

Manfridi, A., Brambilla, D. & Mancia, M. (1999). Stimulation of NMDA and AMPA receptors in the rat nucleus basalis of Meynert affects sleep. *Am. J. Physiol.* **277**, R1488–92.

Manns, I. D., Mainville, L. & Jones, B. E. (2001). Evidence for glutamate, in addition to acetylcholine and GABA, neurotransmitter synthesis in basal forebrain neurons projecting to the entorhinal cortex. *Neuroscience* **107**, 249–63.

Meerlo, P., de Bruin, E. A., Strijkstra, A. M. & Daan, S. (2001). A social conflict increases EEG slow-wave activity during subsequent sleep. *Physiol. Behav.* **73**, 331–5.

Monaghan, D. T., Bridges, R. J. & Cotman, C. W. (1989). The excitatory amino acid receptors: their classes, pharmacology and distinct properties in the function of the central nervous system. *A. Rev. Pharmacol. Toxicol.* **29**, 365–402.

Nelson, S. R., Howard, R. B., Cross, R. S. & Samson, F. (1980). Ketamine-induced changes in regional glucose utilization in the rat brain. *Anesthesiology* **52**, 330–4.

Olney, J. W. & Farber, N. B. (1995). Glutamate receptor dysfunction and schizophrenia. *Arch. Gen. Psychiat.* **52**, 998–1007.

Olney, J. W., Labruyere, J. & Price, M. T. (1989). Pathological changes induced in cerebrocortical neurons by phencyclidine and related drugs [see comments]. *Science* **244**, 1360–2.

Peyron, C., Faraco, J., Rogers, W. *et al.* (2000). A mutation in a case of early onset narcolepsy and a generalized absence of hypocretin peptides in human narcoleptic brains. *Nat. Med.* **6**, 991–7.

Schoepp, D. D. (2001). Unveiling the functions of presynaptic metabotropic glutamate receptors in the central nervous system. *J. Pharmacol. Exp. Ther.* **299**, 12–20.

Schoepp, D. D. & Conn, P. J. (1993). Metabotropic glutamate receptors in brain function and pathology. *Trends Pharmacol. Sci.* **14**, 13–20.

Stevens, D. R., McCarley, R. W. & Greene, R. W. (1992). Excitatory amino acid-mediated responses and synaptic potentials in medial pontine reticular formation neurons of the rat in vitro. *J. Neurosci.* **12**, 4188–94.

Thannickal, T. C., Moore, R. Y., Nienhuis, R. *et al.* (2000). Reduced number of hypocretin neurons in human narcolepsy. *Neuron* **27**, 469–74.

9

Serotonin and sleep–wake regulation

JAIME M. MONTI, HÉCTOR JANTOS, AND DANIEL MONTI

Although many questions remain about the complicated role of serotonin and its receptors in regulating sleep and waking, recent neurochemical, electrophysiological, and neuropharmacological studies have revealed much detailed information about this process.

Neural structures and neurotransmitters involved in the regulation of sleep and waking in laboratory animals

The neural structures involved in the promotion of the waking (W) state are located in the (1) brainstem [dorsal raphe nucleus (DRN), median raphe nucleus (MRN), locus coeruleus (LC), laterodorsal and pedunculopontine tegmental nuclei (LDT/PPT), and medial-pontine reticular formation (mPRF)]; (2) hypothalamus [tuberomammillary nucleus (TMN) and lateral hypothalamus (LH)]; (3) basal forebrain (BFB) (medial septal area, nucleus basalis of Meynert); and (4) midbrain ventral tegmental area (VTA) and substantia nigra pars compacta (SNc) (Pace-Schott & Hobson, 2002; Jones, 2003). The following neurotransmitters function to promote W: (1) acetylcholine (ACh: LDT/PPT, BFB); (2) noradrenaline (NA: LC); (3) serotonin (5-HT: DRN, MRN); (4) histamine (HA: TMN); (5) glutamate (GLU: mPRF, BFB, thalamus); (6) orexin (OX: LH); and (7) dopamine (DA: VTA, SNc) (Zoltoski et al., 1999; Monti, 2004).

The neural structures involved in the regulation of W give rise to mainly ascending projections. In this respect (1) NA-, 5-HT-, and HA-containing neurons send long ascending projections to the forebrain and cerebral cortex;

Neurochemistry of Sleep and Wakefulness, ed. J. M. Monti et al. Published by Cambridge University Press.
© Cambridge University Press 2008.

(2) DA-containing cells project into the basal ganglia and the frontal cortex; (3) cholinergic neurons from the midbrain tegmentum project to the thalamus (ventromedial, intralaminar, and midline nuclei) and the BFB, and cholinergic BFB neurons have widespread rostral projections to the cerebral cortex and the hippocampus; (4) orexin-containing neurons from the LH project to the entire forebrain and brainstem arousal systems; and (5) glutamatergic neurons make up the projection neurons of the mPRF and thalamus (Baghdoyan & Lydic, 2002; Jones, 2003). All these ascending projections into the forebrain follow a dorsal and a ventral route (Jones, 2003). The dorsal route terminates in non-specific thalamic nuclei, which in turn project to the cerebral cortex. Glutamate is involved in this step. The ventral route passes through the hypothalamus and continues into the BFB, where cells in turn project to the cerebral cortex and hippocampus. Acetylcholine participates in this step. In addition, a number of neural structures send descending projections to the spinal cord that modulate muscle tone.

Saper *et al.* (1997) have proposed that projections from the BFB (ACh-containing neurons) and LH (OX-containing cells) to the cerebral cortex are topographically organized and are involved in specific behaviors, whereas the ascending monoaminergic systems (NA, 5-HT, HA) that originate in the brainstem and the posterior hypothalamus play a more generalized role in cortical function.

Neurons in the BFB, preoptic area, and anterior hypothalamus constitute the sleep-inducing system. Electrical stimulation of the preoptic area and the horizontal limb of the diagonal band leads to sleep with electrocortical synchronization (Sterman & Clemente, 1962). In contrast, lesions involving the preoptic area and the horizontal limb of the diagonal band disrupt slow wave sleep (SWS) and REM sleep (REMS) (Lucas & Sterman, 1975). Recording of single-cell activity in the preoptic/anterior hypothalamic area of several species has enabled the identification of neurons that increase their discharge rates during SWS (Alam *et al.*, 1995, 1997; Szymusiak *et al.*, 2001). A majority of these neurons contain γ-aminobutyric acid (GABA) and galanin, two inhibitory neurotransmitters, and project to the basal forebrain and to brainstem and hypothalamic areas involved in the promotion of W. Thus, the GABA/galanin-containing cells in the preoptic/anterior hypothalamic area can in part promote sleep by inhibiting 5-HT, NA, HA, OX, and ACh neurons.

Adenosine has been proposed to induce sleep by inhibiting cholinergic neurons of the BFB and the brainstem. In this respect, adenosine and the adenosine transport inhibitor NBTI decrease the discharge rate of BFB neurons during W, whereas the adenosine A_1 receptor antagonist CPDX induces the opposite effects (Alam *et al.*, 1999; Strecker *et al.*, 2000). In addition, perfusion of adenosine into the LDT of the cat results in a significant decrease of W and the enhancement of sleep (Portas *et al.*, 1997).

Cholinergic neurons of the LDT/PPT act to promote REMS. The predominantly glutamatergic neurons of the REMS-induction region of the mPRF are in turn activated by cholinergic cells; this activation results in the occurrence of tonic and phasic components of REMS. All these neurons are inhibited by serotonergic (DRN), noradrenergic (LC), histaminergic (TMN), orexinergic (LH), and dopaminergic (VTA, SN) cells. Two types of neuron have been characterized in the LDT/PPT. One type of neuron has higher firing rates during W and REMS (wake-REM-on neurons) than during non-REM sleep (NREMS), whereas the other type increases its firing rate from W to NREMS and still more during REMS (REM-on neurons). The release of 5-HT, NA, HA, and ACh in areas relevant to REMS is abundant during W, whereas during REMS only ACh is released at a significant rate. The release of all neurotransmitters is reduced during SWS (Baghdoyan & Lydic, 2002; Saper *et al.*, 1997; Mallick *et al.*, 2002).

Changing concepts on the role of serotonin in the regulation of sleep and waking

In the 1970s, based on lesion studies and neuropharmacological analysis, 5-HT was hypothesized to be responsible for the initiation and maintenance of SWS (Jouvet, 1972). However, a series of findings from several laboratories seriously challenged the serotonergic hypothesis of sleep. Thus, the firing rate of 5-HT-containing DRN neurons decreases during SWS relative to W (Trulson & Jacobs, 1979); reduction of brain 5-HT levels by *p*-chlorophenylalanine (PCPA) fails to disrupt sleep in humans, and in some studies, also in the rat (Wyatt *et al.*, 1969; Rechtschaffen *et al.*, 1973); 5,7-dihydroxytryptamine, which produces a more selective and extensive depletion of brain 5-HT than do raphe lesions, does not significantly affect SWS (Ross *et al.*, 1976); and there is no significant difference between tryptophan-deficient and -replete rats in time spent in SWS (Clancy *et al.*, 1978). Concerning those studies showing that PCPA increases W in the rat (Mouret *et al.*, 1968; Laguzzi & Adrien, 1980), it should be taken into consideration that this 5-HT synthesis inhibitor also induces increased responsiveness to noxious or neutral environmental stimuli and enhances motor activity, aggressivity, and sexual activity (Tenen, 1967; Tagliamonte *et al.*, 1969; Sheard, 1969; Borbély *et al.*, 1973). Therefore, insomnia after PCPA in the rat and the cat could be related to a general hyper-responsiveness to stimuli rather than to impairment of sleep regulation itself. Even in the studies in which insomnia followed PCPA administration, the effect was a transitory one, and SWS returned while 5-HT levels remained depleted (Dement *et al.*, 1972). Moreover, in rats subjected to combined treatment with PCPA and sleep deprivation, delta activity reached the same high levels as after deprivation alone, which tends to indicate that SWS-regulating mechanisms are not disrupted in PCPA-treated rats (Tobler & Borbély, 1982).

With regard to an alternative hypothesis (Jouvet, 1984), there is no firm evidence to support the proposal that 5-HT released during W might act as a neurohormone and induce the synthesis and/or release of hypnogenic factors secondarily responsible for SWS and REMS occurrence. Therefore, based on neurochemical, electrophysiological, and neuropharmacological approaches, it is currently accepted that 5-HT functions to promote W and to inhibit REMS.

Efferent and afferent connections of the DRN and MRN in the rat

Serotonergic neurons of raphe regions of the brainstem are regarded as forming caudal and rostral cell groups. The most caudal nuclei project mainly to the medulla and the spinal cord, whereas the most rostral cell aggregates innervate the telencephalon, diencephalon, mesencephalon, and rhombencephalon (Cooper et al., 1996; Stanford, 2001). The two major midbrain nuclei contributing ascending serotonergic innervation are the DRN and the MRN. Vertes & Kocsis (1994) and Vertes et al. (1999) have proposed that the DRN and the MRN project to complementary neuroanatomical structures in the forebrain, and that their activity would be coordinated during certain behavioral states, such as W and REMS, in which the global release of 5-HT is dramatically enhanced and reduced, respectively.

Efferent connections

The main projections of the DRN and the MRN ascend through the forebrain within the median forebrain bundle. The basal ganglia, substantia nigra, and amygdala are mainly innervated by the DRN, whereas MRN axons project densely to the basal forebrain, septal nuclei, thalamus, posterior hypothalamus, LDT, and DRN. The hippocampus receives an overlapping innervation from the DRN and the MRN (Hensler et al., 1994; Vertes et al., 1999) (Table 9.1).

McQuade & Sharp (1997) tested whether electrical stimulation of the DRN or the MRN releases 5-HT in rat forebrain regions in a pattern that correlates with the distribution of 5-HT projections from the serotonergic nuclei. Stimulation of the DRN evoked the release of 5-HT in the frontal cortex, dorsal striatum, globus pallidus, and ventral hippocampus. Conversely, 5-HT release in dialysates collected from the dorsal and ventral hippocampus and the medial septum was increased in response to MRN stimulation. Thus, the functional mapping of DRN

Table 9.1 *Efferent connections of the dorsal raphe nucleus and the median raphe nucleus of the rat*

Dorsal raphe nucleus	Median raphe nucleus
Telencephalon	
Cerebral cortex	
frontal, piriform, insular, occipital, entorhinal, cingulate, and infralimbic cortices	cingulate, entorhinal, insular, parietal, occipital, piriform, and infralimbic cortices
Limbic system	
ventral hippocampus, lateral septal nucleus, amygdala (central, lateral and basolateral nuclei)	dorsal and ventral hippocampus, lateral and medial septal nuclei, amygdala (central, cortical, medial, lateral, and posterior nuclei)
Basal forebrain	
diagonal band (horizontal and vertical limb)	diagonal band (horizontal and vertical limb)
Neostriatum	
posteromedial regions of the striatum	
Diencephalon	
Thalamus	
midline, intralaminar, and anterior nuclei	anteromedial, anterodorsal, central, lateral habenular, mediodorsal, paracentral, parafascicular, and reuniens nuclei
Hypothalamus	
preoptic area, lateral hypothalamic area, supramammillary nucleus	preoptic area; anterior, lateral, dorsomedial, and posterior nuclei; mammillary nuclei
Mesencephalon	
interpeduncular nucleus, substantia nigra–pars compacta, ventral tegmental area, central gray, mesencephalic reticular formation, pedunculopontine tegmental nucleus, laterodorsal tegmental nucleus	interpeduncular nucleus, substantia nigra–pars compacta, ventral tegmental area, central gray, mesencephalic reticular formation, pedunculopontine tegmental nucleus, laterodorsal tegmental nucleus
Rhombencephalon	
pontine reticular formation, nucleus reticularis pontis oralis, nucleus reticularis pontis caudalis, nucleus reticularis gigantocellularis, locus coeruleus, median raphe nucleus, nucleus raphe pontis	nucleus reticularis pontis oralis, nucleus reticularis pontis caudalis, nucleus reticularis gigantocellularis, nucleus raphe dorsalis, nucleus raphe pontis, nucleus raphe magnus, central gray

From: Vertes (1991), Van Bockstaele *et al.* (1993), Losier & Semba (1993), Vertes & Kocsis (1994), Steiniger *et al.* (1997), Morin & Meyer-Bernstein (1999), and Vertes *et al.* (1999).

Table 9.2 *Afferent connections to the dorsal raphe nucleus and the median raphe nucleus of the rat*

Dorsal raphe nucleus	Median raphe nucleus
Telencephalon	
Cerebral cortex	
frontal, cingulate, orbital, and insular cortices	prefrontal and cingulate cortices
Limbic system	
amygdala (central, anterior, medial, and basolateral nuclei), medial and lateral septal nuclei	medial septal nucleus
Basal forebrain	
accumbens nuclei, ventral pallidum, bed nucleus of the stria terminalis, diagonal band	bed nucleus of the stria terminalis, diagonal band, ventral pallidum
Diencephalon	
Thalamus	
	lateral and medial habenular nuclei
Hypothalamus	
medial and lateral preoptic areas; anterior, lateral, and posterior hypothalamic areas; dorsomedial and ventromedial nuclei; tuberomammillary nucleus	medial and lateral preoptic areas, lateral hypothalamic area, dorsomedial nucleus, complex of mammillary bodies
Mesencephalon	
substantia nigra–pars reticulata, interpeduncular nucleus, central gray	ventral tegmental area, laterodorsal tegmental nucleus, interpeduncular nucleus
Rhombencephalon	
raphe nuclei, locus coeruleus, pontine reticular formation	dorsal raphe nucleus, central gray

From: Marcinkiewicz *et al.* (1989), Behzadi *et al.* (1990), Vertes (1991), Iwakiri *et al.* (1993), Baker *et al.* (1990), Vertes & Kocsis (1994), Gonzalo-Ruiz *et al.* (1995), Bunin *et al.* (1998), Hájos *et al.* (1998), and Peyron *et al.* (1998).

and MRN 5-HT pathways is correlated to a large extent with that obtained after anatomical studies.

Afferent connections

The DRN receives extensive projections from the cortex, amygdala, basal forebrain, and preoptic and hypothalamic areas (Peyron *et al.*, 1998) (Table 9.2). Neurons that project to the MRN are primarily from the cortex, basal forebrain, hypothalamus, and mesencephalic and rhombencephalic nuclei (Table 9.2). Thus, in summary 5-HT neurons of the DRN and the MRN innervate brain areas involved in sleep/wake regulation. These areas include the cholinergic nuclei of the mesencephalon and the basal forebrain, the dopaminergic neurons of the VTA and the SNc, the noradrenergic cells of the LC, the GABAergic, histaminergic, and orexinergic cell aggregates of the hypothalamus, and the glutamatergic neurons of the thalamus and the brainstem reticular formation. In turn, inputs to the 5-HT DRN and MRN cells have been found from the basal forebrain, the hypothalamus, and the cholinergic, dopaminergic, and noradrenergic nuclei of the brainstem. There is also a reciprocal interaction between the DRN and the MRN.

Chemoarchitecture of the DRN

The mechanism of action of neuroactive substances microinjected into the DRN on sleep variables will be discussed below. However, it is of interest to mention at this point the non-serotonergic interneurons and projection neurons that are present in the DRN in addition to the 5-HT-containing cells. In this respect, neurons producing DA, glutamate, GABA, and the tachykinin substance P (SP) have been characterized in the DRN of several species (Chan-Palay et al., 1978; Ochi & Shimizu, 1978; Nanopoulos et al., 1982; Clements et al., 1991; Charara & Parent, 1998; Li et al., 2001). Interestingly, a number of GABAergic neurons synapse with serotonergic perikarya and dendrites in the DRN, whereas others project to the midbrain reticular formation and the hypothalamus (Wang et al., 1992; Ford et al., 1995).

Rates of firing of aminergic, cholinergic, and orexinergic neurons involved in the regulation of sleep and waking

The activity of serotonergic DRN neurons is at its highest during W; it diminishes during SWS and is virtually suppressed when the animal starts REMS (Trulson & Jacobs, 1979). A similar pattern has been described with noradrenergic LC and histaminergic TMN neurons (Aston-Jones & Bloom, 1981; Sakai et al., 1990; Steininger et al., 1999). There is also evidence that orexinergic LH neurons discharge at their maximal rate during W, decrease firing during SWS, and cease firing during REMS (Lee et al., 2005). Moreover, studies assessing orexin release in the brain have shown that it is maximal during W (Zeitzer et al., 2003) (Table 9.3). Unlike 5-HT, NA, and HA cells, DA neurons in the VTA and the SNc show a change in the temporal pattern rather than the firing rate during W. It manifests

Table 9.3 *Rates of firing of aminergic, cholinergic, orexinergic, and GABAergic neurons involved in the regulation of sleep and waking*

Neurotransmitter system	W	SWS	REMS	Neurotransmitter release
Dorsal raphe nucleus (serotonin)	highest	lower	lowest	increased during W
Locus coeruleus (noradrenaline)	highest	lower	lowest	increased during W
Tuberomammillary nucleus (histamine)	highest	lower	lowest	increased during W
Ventral tegmental area and substantia nigra-pars compacta (dopamine)	no change of mean firing rate across the sleep–wake cycle; increase of burst firing during behavioral and EEG arousal		increased during W	
Pedunculopontine, pontine, and laterodorsal tegmental nuclei (acetylcholine)	highest (wake-REM-on neurons)	lowest	highest (REM-on neurons)	increased during W and REMS
Lateral hypothalamic area (orexin)	highest (active W)	lower	lowest	increased during W
Ventrolateral and medial preoptic area (GABA and galanin)	lower	higher	higher	?

as burst firing and is accompanied by a more efficient release of DA (Grace, 2002; Rye & Jankovic, 2002) (Table 9.3).

Takakusaki *et al.* (1997) characterized two types of neurons in the PPT according to their action potential duration: short-duration and long-duration neurons. The fast-firing neurons have higher firing rates during W and REMS than during SWS (wake-REM-on neurons). In contrast, the slow-firing cells increase their firing rates from W to SWS and still more during REMS (REM-on neurons). This finding is correlated with reports describing increased release of ACh in the brainstem during W and REMS (McCarley *et al.*, 1978; Kodama *et al.*, 1990) (Table 9.3). The discharge rate of many cells in the BFB is positively correlated with W and REMS. However, none has yet been identified as cholinergic (Marrosu *et al.*, 1995).

Sleep-active neurons have been identified in the ventrolateral and medial preoptic areas. These neurons exhibit increased discharge during SWS and REMS rather than W. Sleep-active neurons colocalize GABA and are excited by adenosine and prostaglandin D_2 (McGinty & Szymusiak, 2001) (Table 9.3).

Operational characteristics of the 5-HT receptors

The 5-HT receptors represent separate and distinct gene products. They can be classified into at least seven classes, designated 5-HT_{1-7}. The 5-HT_1, 5-HT_2, and 5-HT_5 classes consist of five ($5\text{-HT}_{1A\text{-}B\text{-}D\text{-}E\text{-}F}$), three ($5\text{-HT}_{2A\text{-}B\text{-}C}$), and two ($5\text{-HT}_{5A\text{-}B}$) subtypes, respectively, whereas the 5-HT_3, 5-HT_4, 5-HT_6, and 5-HT_7 classes have at present one subtype each (Hoyer *et al.*, 1994; Hoyer & Martin, 1996; Baez *et al.*, 1995). Except for the 5-HT_3 receptor, all other 5-HT receptors are structurally related to the superfamily of G-protein-coupled receptors.

Results obtained from studies of the administration of selective and relatively selective receptor agonists and antagonists have led to the proposal that 5-HT_{1A}, 5-HT_{1B}, 5-HT_{2A}, 5-HT_{2C}, 5-HT_3, and 5-HT_7 receptors are implicated in the regulation of sleep and waking. It should be emphasized that the density of a given 5-HT receptor subtype can be high at some central sites and low at some others. However, even the few receptors present at a given neuroanatomical location might be functionally important. Thus, CNS structures have been included in Tables 9.4 to 9.7 irrespective of the binding density or the level of receptor mRNA.

The 5-HT$_{1A}$ receptor

The 5-HT_{1A} receptor is located on the soma and the dendrites (somatodendritic autoreceptor) of 5-HT neurons, and at postsynaptic sites. Wang & Aghajanian (1977), and Aghajanian & Lakoski (1984) have shown that the somatodendritic autoreceptor mediates collateral inhibition, and that the ionic basis

Table 9.4 *Distribution of the 5-HT$_{1A}$ receptor in rat brain*

Telencephalon

Cerebral cortex
cingular, frontal, parietal, insular, piriform, and entorhinal cortices

Limbic system
medial and lateral septal nuclei, hippocampal formation (C$_1$–C$_3$ fields and dentate gyrus),
amygdala (cortical nucleus)

Diencephalon

Thalamus
medial habenular, centromedial, centrolateral, and reticular thalamic nuclei

Hypothalamus
ventromedial and supraoptic nuclei

Mesencephalon
superior colliculi, penduculopontine and laterodorsal tegmental nuclei

Rhombencephalon
dorsal raphe, median raphe, raphe pallidus, and raphe obscurus nuclei; locus coeruleus;
nucleus paragigantocellularis; nucleus reticularis magnocellularis

From: Luebke *et al.* (1992), Austin *et al.* (1994), Kia *et al.* (1996a,b), Thakkar *et al.* (1998), and
Tohyama & Takatsuji (1998).

for inhibition is the opening of K$^+$ channels and closing of Ca^{2+} channels to
produce hyperpolarization. The 5-HT$_{1A}$ receptor is coupled to adenylate cyclase.
Its activation inhibits the enzyme, which could be related to the coupling of the
5-HT$_{1A}$ receptor to a G$_i$ protein. Stimulation of the somatodendritic 5-HT$_{1A}$ receptor inhibits the firing rate of serotonergic neurons, whereas activation of the
postsynaptic receptor induces inhibitory responses on target structures. Brain
areas rich in 5-HT$_{1A}$ receptors include the cerebral cortex, the hippocampus,
the septal nuclei, the hypothalamus, and some amygdaloid and raphe nuclei,
particularly the DRN (Table 9.4).

The 5-HT$_{1B}$ receptor

Initially, it was proposed that the 5-HT$_{1B}$ receptor is located exclusively
in the brain of the rat and some other rodents, whereas the 5-HT$_{1D}$ receptor,
a close species homolog, is specific to the guinea pig and higher mammalian
species, including humans (Waeber *et al.*, 1989). However, recent studies have
characterized the 5-HT$_{1B}$ receptor also in the human brain (Bidmon *et al.*, 2001;
Varnäs *et al.*, 2005). The 5-HT$_{1B}$ receptor is linked to the inhibition of adenylate
cyclase, and is located at presynaptic (5-HT axon terminals) and postsynaptic

Table 9.5 *Distribution of the 5-HT$_{1B}$ receptor in rat brain*

Telencephalon

Cerebral cortex
frontal, parietal, cingulate, entorhinal, and olfactory cortices

Limbic system
amygdala (central, lateral, and basolateral nuclei), lateral septal nucleus, hippocampus (CA$_1$ field)

Basal ganglia
accumbens nucleus, caudate–putamen, subthalamic nucleus

Diencephalon

Thalamus
lateral habenular, paraventricular, anteromedial, anteroventral, paracentral, reuniens, and medial geniculate nuclei

Hypothalamus
lateral preoptic area; anterior, lateral, and dorsal hypothalamic areas; lateral mammillary nucleus; suprachiasmatic nucleus; arcuate nucleus

Mesencephalon
central gray, interpeduncular nucleus, substantia nigra–pars compacta

Rhombencephalon
locus coeruleus, dorsal raphe nucleus, raphe magnus nucleus, cerebellum (deep nuclei)

From: Lebel & Koe (1992), Bruinvels *et al.* (1994), Doucet *et al.* (1995), Sari *et al.* (1997, 1999), Riad *et al.* (2000), and Makarenko *et al.* (2002).

sites. It is involved in the regulation of the synaptic release of 5-HT and of other neurotransmitters, including ACh, NA, GABA, and glutamate, which is indicative of its role as auto- and heteroreceptor, respectively. The mapping of the 5-HT$_{1B}$ receptor mRNA and its visualization by autoradiography tends to indicate that its distribution is widespread in the CNS of several species, including man (Table 9.5).

The 5-HT$_{2A}$ and 5-HT$_{2C}$ receptors

The 5-HT$_{2A}$ and 5-HT$_{2C}$ receptors have striking amino acid homology, and their actions are mediated by the activation of phospholipase C, with a resulting depolarization of the host cell (Cooper *et al.*, 1996; Stanford, 2001). Receptors corresponding to the 5-HT$_2$ subfamily are located within postsynaptic structures, predominantly on proximal and distal dendritic shafts. Autoradiographic and immunohistochemical studies have demonstrated that each receptor subtype displays a particular regional distribution in the brain (Table 9.6).

Table 9.6 *Distribution of 5-HT$_{2A}$ and 5-HT$_{2C}$ receptors in rat brain*

5-HT$_{2A}$ receptor	5-HT$_{2C}$ receptor
Telencephalon	
Cerebral cortex	
frontal, piriform, cingulate and entorhinal cortices	frontal, parietal, occipital, piriform and cingulate cortices
Olfactory system	
olfactory bulb	olfactory bulb
Limbic system	
medial and lateral septal nuclei, hippocampal formation, amygdala (cortical, central, medial, lateral, basomedial, and basolateral nuclei)	lateral septal nucleus, hippocampal formation, amygdala (medial, lateral, and basolateral nuclei)
Basal forebrain	
nucleus of the diagonal band of Broca, ventral pallidum	nucleus of the diagonal band of Broca, ventral pallidum, bed nucleus of the stria terminalis
Basal ganglia	
nucleus accumbens, caudate–putamen, globus pallidus, subthalamic nucleus	nucleus accumbens, caudate–putamen, globus pallidus, subthalamic nucleus
Diencephalon	
Thalamus	
medial and lateral habenular, reticular, intralaminar, reuniens, anterior, lateral, and posterior nuclei	medial and lateral habenular, lateral, reuniens, and geniculate nuclei
Hypothalamus	
medial and lateral preoptic areas, anterior and lateral hypothalamic areas, ventromedial nucleus, mammillary nucleus	medial preoptic area, ventromedial nucleus, dorsomedial nucleus, mammillary nucleus
Mesencephalon	
central gray, substantia nigra–pars compacta, ventral tegmental area	central gray, substantia nigra–pars compacta
Rhombencephalon	
laterodorsal and pedunculopontine tegmental nuclei, dorsal raphe nucleus, median raphe nucleus, locus coeruleus, pontine reticular formation, gigantocellular reticular nucleus	laterodorsal and pedunculopontine tegmental nuclei, dorsal raphe nucleus, median raphe nucleus

From: Mengod *et al.* (1990), Pompeiano *et al.* (1994), Abramowski *et al.* (1995), Wolf & Schutz (1997), Duxon *et al.* (1997), Hamada *et al.* (1998), Cornea-Hébert *et al.* (1999), Vergé & Calas (2000), Clemett *et al.* (2000), and Nichols (2004).

Table 9.7 *Distribution of the 5-HT$_3$ receptor in rat brain*

Telencephalon

Cerebral cortex

piriform, entorhinal

Olfactory system

olfactory bulb, anterior olfactory nucleus

Limbic system

hippocampus (dentate gyrus, CA$_1$, CA$_2$, and CA$_3$ fields), amygdala (cortical, basomedial, basolateral, and lateral nuclei), lateral septal nucleus

Basal ganglia

nucleus accumbens, globus pallidus, caudate–putamen

Mesencephalon

Interpeduncular nucleus, central gray, mesencephalic reticular formation

Rhombencephalon

dorsal raphe nucleus, central gray, gigantocellular reticular nucleus

From: Kilpatrick *et al.* (1987, 1988), Waeber *et al.* (1990), Pratt *et al.* (1990), Gehlert *et al.* (1991), Laporte *et al.* (1992), and Morales *et al.* (1998).

The 5-HT$_3$ receptor

The 5-HT$_3$ receptor is not coupled to G proteins. It directly activates a 5-HT-gated cation channel, which leads to depolarization of a variety of cells. As a result, there is an increase in the release of DA, NA, GABA, ACh, and 5-HT at central sites (Stanford, 2001). The 5-HT$_3$ receptor is present in cortical and subcortical structures (Table 9.7).

The 5-HT$_7$ receptor

The 5-HT$_7$ receptor is part of the G-protein superfamily of receptors, which contains seven transmembrane regions, and its stimulation leads to an increase in cAMP production (Thomas & Hagan, 2004). The 5-HT$_7$ receptor is expressed in a number of telencephalic, diencephalic, mesencephalic, and rhombencephalic areas (Table 9.8).

Role of 5-HT receptors in the modulation of sleep and waking

Serotonin shares with other neurotransmitters the ability to promote W and to suppress REMS. However, 5-HT participates in a variety of functions in addition to regulation of the behavioral state. Thus, as depicted in Tables 9.4–9.8, 5-HT$_{1A}$, 5-HT$_{1B}$, 5-HT$_{2A/2C}$, 5-HT$_3$, and 5-HT$_7$ receptors are present in structures that

Table 9.8 *Distribution of the 5-HT$_7$ receptor in rat brain*

Telencephalon

Cerebral cortex
frontal, parietal, temporal, occipital, cingulate, entorhinal, and piriform cortices

Olfactory system
olfactory tubercle

Limbic system
hippocampus (dentate gyrus, CA$_1$, CA$_2$, and CA$_3$ fields), amygdala (cortical, central, medial, lateral, basomedial, and basolateral nuclei), medial and lateral septal nuclei

Basal forebrain
nucleus of the diagonal band of Broca

Basal ganglia
claustrum, ventral pallidum, globus pallidus, caudate–putamen, nucleus accumbens

Diencephalon

Thalamus
central, anterior, lateral, medial, posterior, paraventricular, mediodorsal, laterodorsal, habenular, reuniens, and geniculate nuclei

Hypothalamus
medial and lateral preoptic areas; anterior and lateral hypothalamic areas; ventromedial, dorsomedial, medial mammillary, and supramammillary nuclei

Mesencephalon
substantia nigra–pars reticulata, central gray, interpeduncular nucleus, superior and inferior colliculus

Rhombencephalon
Dorsal raphe nucleus, median raphe nucleus, locus coeruleus

From: To *et al.* (1995), Gustafson *et al.* (1996), and Neumaier *et al.* (2001).

are not relevant to the modulation of S and W. On the other hand, almost all these receptors are expressed on neurons with cell bodies located in the cerebral cortex, hippocampus, thalamus, LC, and DRN. In addition, 5-HT$_{1B}$, 5-HT$_{2A/2C}$, and 5-HT$_7$ receptors have been characterized in the preoptic area, anterior and lateral hypothalamic areas, and TMN, whereas 5-HT$_{1A}$ and 5-HT$_{2A/C}$ receptors have been found in the PPT/LDT and the mPRF.

The 5-HT$_{1A}$ receptor

Full agonists at pre- and postsynaptic 5-HT$_{1A}$ receptors
Currently, a number of ligands are available that show affinity for the 5-HT$_{1A}$-receptor binding site in rat and cat brain. They include 8-OH-DPAT

[8-hydroxy-2-(di-*n*-propylamino)tetralin] and flesinoxan, which are full agonists at pre- and postsynaptic sites, and the azapirones, buspirone, gepirone, and ipsapirone, which behave as full agonists at the somatodendritic autorecep-tor but only as partial agonists at the postsynaptic level. Until recently, 8-OH-DPAT was considered a selective 5-HT$_{1A}$ receptor agonist. However, it is now known that the compound is also a partial agonist for the 5-HT$_7$ receptor (Vanhoenacker *et al.*, 2000). All these compounds share the ability to inhibit the firing rate of DRN serotonergic neurons and to produce hyperpolariza-tion of intracellularly recorded cells (Sprouse & Aghajanian, 1987, 1988; Gobert *et al.*, 1995). Direct administration of 8-OH-DPAT into the DRN reduces the synthesis and release of 5-HT at postsynaptic sites; this effect is prevented by 5-HT$_{1A}$-receptor antagonists (Hillegaart, 1990). The mixed β-adrenoceptor and 5-HT$_{1A/B}$ receptor antagonist (−)pindolol acts at both pre- and postsynap-tic sites, as do WAY 100635 {*N*-[2-[4-(2-methoxyphenyl)-1-piperazinyl]ethyl]-*N*-(2-pyridinyl)cyclohexanecarboxamide} and p-MPPI {4-iodo-*N*-[2-[4-(methoxyphenyl)-1-piperazinyl]ethyl]-*N*-2-pyridinylbenzamide}, two selective high-affinity silent antagonists. WAY 100635 and p-MPPI produce dose-related increases of the basal firing rate of 5-HT neurons in the DRN of several species (Fornal *et al.*, 1996; Mundey *et al.*, 1996; Bjorvatn *et al.*, 1998). The effects are evident during W but not during sleep. In vitro and in vivo studies have shown that WAY 100635 and p-MPPI block the ability of 8-OH-DPAT to inhibit the firing of DRN neurons in the rat and the cat, respectively (Forster *et al.*, 1995; Fletcher *et al.*, 1996; Bjorvatn *et al.*, 1998).

Systemic injection of flesinoxan increases W and reduces SWS and REMS in the rat (Monti & Jantos, 2003). Similar effects have been observed following the administration of 8-OH-DPAT to vehicle-treated and serotonin-depleted animals (Dugovic & Wauquier, 1987; Monti & Jantos, 1992; Monti *et al.*, 1990, 1994). Pre-treatment with (−)pindolol or p-MPPI reverses the effect of 8-OH-DPAT on W and SWS (Monti & Jantos, 1992; Sorensen *et al.*, 2001). All these findings indicate that the postsynaptic 5-HT$_{1A}$ receptor has a role in the occurrence of arousal.

Reduction of REMS after flesinoxan or 8-OH-DPAT administration could be related to the activation of postsynaptic 5-HT$_{1A}$ receptors on REM-on neurons of the LDT/PPT, similar to the physiologic effect of 5-HT. Direct infusion of either 8-OH-DPAT or flesinoxan into the DRN significantly increased REMS in rats; this effect was prevented by local infusion of WAY 100635 (Monti *et al.*, 2002). In contrast, microinjection of (−)pindolol, WAY 100635, or p-MPPI into the DRN reduced REMS (Monti *et al.*, 2000, 2002; Sorensen *et al.*, 2001). Portas *et al.* (1996) provided direct evidence that suppression of DRN serotonergic activity increases REMS. In this study, extracellular 5-HT was measured in the DRN and, simulta-neously, behavioral state changes were determined from polygraphic recordings. Microdialysis perfusion of 8-OH-DPAT into the DRN decreased 5-HT levels by 50%

during W, and significantly increased REMS. In agreement with the reciprocal interaction model proposed by McCarley & Hobson (1975), inhibition of DRN activity following somatodendritic 5-HT$_{1A}$ receptor stimulation suppressed 5-HT inhibition of mesopontine cholinergic neurons, and increased REMS.

Microinjection of 8-OH-DPAT or flesinoxan into the LDT or the mPRF, where structures that act to promote and to induce REMS are located, selectively inhibited REMS in the cat and the rat (Sanford et al., 1994; Horner et al., 1997; Monti & Jantos, 2003). Furthermore, direct infusion of WAY 100635 into the LDT increased REMS (Monti & Jantos, 2004).

It can be concluded that direct administration of 5-HT$_{1A}$ receptor agonists into the DRN inhibits serotonin-containing neurons and enhances REMS. On the other hand, infusion of 5-HT$_{1A}$ agonists into areas in which the cholinergic or the glutamatergic REMS induction neurons are located results in the suppression of REMS. The inhibitory effect of postsynaptic 5-HT$_{1A}$ receptors on REMS occurrence is further supported by studies carried out in mutant mice that do not express this receptor subtype (Boutrel et al., 2002). Accordingly, REMS was significantly increased during both the light and the dark phase in 5-HT$_{1A}$ knockout mice compared with wild-type animals. Furthermore, systemic 8-OH-DPAT had no effect on sleep or W in these mutant mice.

Full agonists at 5-HT$_{1A}$ autoreceptors and partial agonists at postsynaptic 5-HT$_{1A}$ receptors

Buspirone, ipsapirone, and gepirone have been shown to increase time awake and to reduce SWS and REMS when given s.c. or i.p. to rats (Lerman et al., 1986; Monti et al., 1995a). Subcutaneous injection of the azapirones into 5,7-dihydroxytryptamine-pretreated rats led also to an increase of W and a reduction of sleep; this result further supports the dependence of these effects on postsynaptic 5-HT$_{1A}$ receptors (Monti et al., 1995a). Similar sleep-disrupting effects of buspirone and ipsapirone have been described in human subjects with normal sleep and in patients with insomnia. Thus, buspirone administration increased W, prolonged REMS latency, and decreased REMS time in insomniac patients (Seidel et al., 1985; Manfredi et al., 1991), whereas ipsapirone prolonged REMS latency and reduced REMS and SWS in healthy subjects (Gillin et al., 1994; Driver et al., 1995). The decrease of REMS after administration of buspirone, gepirone, or ipsapirone is compatible with the reciprocal interaction hypothesis of the regulation of desynchronized sleep. Accordingly, the azapirones would be acting on postsynaptic 5-HT$_{1A}$ receptors in the LDT/PPT nuclei to inhibit REM-on neurons.

Selective serotonin reuptake inhibitors

The effects of acute administration of selective serotonin reuptake inhibitors (SSRIs) on sleep have been studied in laboratory animals, healthy adults, and depressed patients (Armitage, 1996; Staner *et al.*, 1999; Oberndor-fer *et al.*, 2000). SSRIs are potent REMS suppressors, prolonging the latency to the first REM period. Direct infusion of fluoxetine into the DRN induced a significant increment of REMS in the rat. In contrast, microinjection of fluoxetine into the LDT or the mPRF produced the opposite effect; and pretreatment with WAY 100635 prevented the reduction of REMS induced by the microinjection of fluoxetine into the LDT (Monti & Jantos, 2004). The inhibitory effect of SSRIs on REMS has been proposed to result from enhancement of CNS serotonergic neurotransmission.

Monaca *et al.* (2003) examined the effect of the SSRI citalopram on REMS in 5-HT$_{1A}$ and 5-HT$_{1B}$ knockout mice. Citalopram suppressed REMS in wild-type and 5-HT$_{1B}^{-/-}$ mice but not in 5-HT$_{1A}^{-/-}$ mutants. The 5-HT$_{1A}$ receptor antagonist WAY 100635 prevented the citalopram-induced inhibition of REMS in wild-type and 5-HT$_{1B}$ knockout mice. However, pretreatment with the 5-HT$_{1B}$ receptor antagonist GR 127935 [2′-methyl-4′-(5-methyl-(1,2,4)oxadiazol-3-yl)-biphenyl-4-carboxylic acid ((4-methoxy-piperazine-1-yl)-phenyl)amide] was ineffective in this respect. It was concluded that the action of citalopram on REMS in the mouse depends exclusively on the activation of 5-HT$_{1A}$ receptors. Notwithstanding this, there is unequivocal evidence showing that administration of selective 5-HT$_{1B}$ receptor agonists suppresses REMS in the rat.

The 5-HT$_{1B}$ receptor

Full agonists at postsynaptic 5-HT$_{1B}$ receptors

Few studies have been published on the effect of 5-HT$_{1B}$ receptor ligands on sleep variables. Systemic administration of the selective 5-HT$_{1B}$ receptor agonists CGS 12066B [7-trifluoromethyl-4(4-methyl-1-piperazinyl)-pyrrolo(1,2-a)quinozaline] or CP-94,253 [3-(1,2,5,6-tetrahydro-4-pyridyl)-5-propoxypyrrolo(3,2-b)pyridine] significantly increased W and reduced SWS and REMS in the rat (Bjorvatn & Ursin, 1994; Monti *et al.*, 1995b). The mixed β-adrenoceptor/5-HT$_{1A/1B}$ receptor antagonist pindolol antagonized the increase of W and reduction of SWS induced by CP-94,253. However, pindolol failed to prevent the suppression of REMS (Monti *et al.*, 1995b).

The quantitation of spontaneous sleep–waking cycles in 5-HT$_{1B}$ receptor knockout mice has shown that REMS is increased whereas SWS is reduced during the light phase (Boutrel *et al.*, 1999). On the other hand, systemic administration of CP-94,253 to wild-type mice tends to suppress REM, whereas the 5-HT$_{1B}$ antagonist GR 127935 induces the opposite effect. Thus, the limited available evidence indicates that 5-HT$_{1B}$ receptor activation facilitates the occurrence of W and negatively influences REMS.

The 5-HT$_{2A/2B/2C}$ receptors

5-HT$_{2A}$ and 5-HT$_{2C}$ serotonin receptors have been detected in numerous rat brain regions involved in the regulation of sleep and W, including the
cerebral cortex, hippocampus, hypothalamus, mPRF, LC, LDT/PPT, and DRN (Pompeiano *et al.*, 1994; Abramowski *et al.*, 1995; Cornea-Hébert *et al.*, 1999; Clemett
et al., 2000; Fay & Kubin, 2000; López-Giménez *et al.*, 2001). In contrast, 5-HT$_{2B}$
receptors are expressed in discrete brain nuclei of the rat (Duxon *et al.*, 1997).
Serotonin-containing neurons of the DRN do not express 5-HT$_{2A}$ or 5-HT$_{2C}$ receptors. The 5-HT$_{2A}$ and 5-HT$_{2C}$ receptor-containing neurons are predominantly
GABAergic interneurons and projection neurons (Clemett *et al.*, 2000; López-
Giménez *et al.*, 2001; Mirkes & Bethea, 2001; Serrats *et al.*, 2005). The GABAergic regulation of cholinergic LDT/PPT nuclei arises both from local inhibitory
GABAergic interneurons that express 5-HT$_{2A/2C}$ receptors and from GABAergic
cells that contribute to the efferent projections of the DRN (Van Bockstaele
et al., 1993; Ford *et al.*, 1995; Clemett *et al.*, 2000; Janowski & Sesack, 2004).

5-HT$_2$ receptor agonists

Systemic administration of the 5-HT$_{2A/2C}$ receptor agonists DOI
[1-(2,5-dimethoxy-4-iodophenyl)-2-aminopropane] or DOM [1-(2,5-dimethoxy-4-
methylphenyl)-2-aminopropane] has been shown to reduce SWS and REMS and
to augment W in the rat (Dugovic & Wauquier, 1987; Dugovic *et al.*, 1989; Monti
et al., 1990). In addition, systemic or intrathalamic injection of DOI decreased
the neocortical high-voltage spindle activity that occurs during relaxed W in
the rat (Jäkälä *et al.*, 1995). The i.p. and p.o. administration of the selective
5-HT$_{2C}$ receptor agonists RO 60–0175/ORG 35030 [(S)-2-(chloro-5-fluoro-indol-1-yl)-
1-methylethylamine] or RO-60–0332/ORG 35035 {[S]-2-[4,4,7-trimethyl-1,4-dihydro-
indeno(1,2-b)pyrrol-1-yl]-1-methylethylamine} induced also an increase of W and
a reduction of REMS in the rat (Martin *et al.*, 1998).

5-HT$_2$ receptor antagonists

Injection of the 5-HT$_{2A/2C}$ receptor antagonists ritanserin, ketanserin,
ICI 170,809 [2(2-dimethylamino-2-methylpropylthio)-3-phenylquinoline], or sertin-
dole at the beginning of the light period induced a significant increase of SWS
and a reduction of REMS in the rat. Waking was also diminished in most studies
(Dugovic *et al.*, 1989; Tortella *et al.*, 1989; Monti *et al.*, 1990; Silhol *et al.*, 1991;
Coenen *et al.*, 1995; Kirov & Moyanova, 1998a,b) (Table 9.9).

More recently, the action of subtype-selective 5-HT$_2$ receptor antagonists on
sleep variables was assessed in the rat. Systemic administration of the 5-HT$_{2A}$

Table 9.9 *The effect of 5-HT$_{2A/2C}$ receptor antagonists on sleep and waking in the rat*
Symbols: +, increase; −, decrease; n.s., not significant.

Compound	W	SWS	REMS	Reference
Ritanserin (i.p.)	n.s.	+	−	Dugovic & Wauquier (1987)
Ritanserin (i.p.)	−	+	−	Dugovic et al. (1989)
Ritanserin (i.p.)	n.s.	+	−	Monti et al. (1990)
Ritanserin (i.p.)	−	+	−	Silhol et al. (1991)
Ritanserin (i.p.)	−	+	−	Kirov & Moyanova (1998b)
Ritanserin (i.p.)	−	+	−	Kantor et al. (2002)
		(increase of EEG power density in the low frequency range)		
Ketanserin (i.p.)	−	+	−	Kirov & Moyanova (1998a)
ICI 169,369 (p.o.)	+	n.s.	−	Tortella et al. (1989)
ICI 170,809 (p.o.)	+	delayed increase of non-REM sleep	−	
Sertindole (i.p.)	n.s.	+	−	Coenen et al. (1995)

antagonist EMD 281014 {7-[4-(2-(4-fluorophenyl)ethyl)-piperazine-1-carbonyl]-1H-indole-3-carbonitrile} significantly reduced REMS (Monti & Jantos, 2006b), whereas the 5-HT$_{2B}$ antagonist SB-215505 [6-chloro-5-methyl-1-(5-quinolylcarbamoyl)indoline] augmented W and suppressed SWS and REMS (Kantor et al., 2004). Moreover, oral administration of the 5-HT$_2$ antagonist SB-243213 in the rat {5-methyl-1-[[-2-[(-2-methyl-3-pyridyl)oxy]-5-pyridyl] carbamoyl]-6-trifluoromethylindoline} significantly increased SWS and reduced REMS during the light period (Smith et al., 2002). However, REMS suppression was the only noticeable effect when the compound was given by the subcutaneous route (Monti & Jantos, 2006b) (Table 9.10).

The contribution of the 5-HT$_{2C}$ receptor to sleep expression has been studied also in 5-HT$_{2C}$ receptor knockout mice. Compared with wild-type animals, mice lacking the 5-HT$_{2C}$ receptor have greater amounts and longer episodes of W, less non-REM sleep, and fewer non-REM to REMS transitions (Frank et al., 2002).

Effect of 5-HT$_2$ antagonists on the DOI-induced disruption of sleep and W
Pretreatment with ritanserin prevented the enhancement of W and the deficit of SWS induced by DOI and DOM, but not the REMS suppression (Dugovic et al., 1989; Monti et al., 1990). Ritanserin also antagonized the DOI-induced decrease of neocortical high-voltage spindle activity (Jäkälä et al., 1995). In order to gain further insight into the roles of 5-HT$_{2A}$ and 5-HT$_{2C}$ receptors in the

Table 9.10 *The effect of subtype-selective 5-HT$_2$ receptor antagonists on sleep and waking in the rat*

Symbols: +, increase; −, decrease; n.s., not significant.

Compound	W	SWS	REMS	Reference
EMD 281014 (s.c.) (5-HT$_{2A}$ antagonist)	n.s.	n.s.	−	Monti & Jantos (2006b)
SB-215505 (i.p.) (5-HT$_{2B}$ antagonist)	+ increase of motor activity	−	−	Kantor *et al.* (2004)
SB-243213 (p.o.) (5-HT$_{2C}$ antagonist)	n.s.	+	−	Smith *et al.* (2002)
SB-243213 (s.c.) (5-HT$_{2C}$ antagonist)	n.s.	n.s.	−	Monti & Jantos (2006b)
SB-242084 (i.p.) (5-HT$_{2C}$ antagonist)	+	−	n.s.	Kantor *et al.* (2004)

DOI-induced disruption of the sleep–wake cycle, animals were pretreated with either EMD 281014 or SB-243213, which selectively block the 5-HT$_{2A}$ or the 5-HT$_{2C}$ receptor, respectively. EMD 281014 prevented the increase of W and the reduction of SWS induced by DOI. However, REMS remained suppressed. In contrast, SB-243213 failed to reverse the DOI-induced disruption of sleep and W (Monti & Jantos, 2006b). Thus, on the basis of these results it appears that 5-HT$_{2A}$ receptor mechanisms predominate in the DOI-mediated effects on sleep and W. However, the role of the 5-HT$_{2C}$ receptor cannot be excluded, and further studies using additional 5-HT$_{2C}$ antagonists are warranted. The failure of EMD 281014 to prevent the suppression of REMS tends to indicate that the effect of DOI is not restricted to the 5-HT system. In this respect, it has been reported that systemic administration of DOI tends to increase the firing rate and burst firing of DA neurons and the release of DA in the ventral tegmental area of the rat (Pehec *et al.*, 2001; Bortolozzi *et al.*, 2005). Moreover, dopamine D$_1$ and D$_2$ receptor agonists have been shown to inhibit REMS in the rat (Monti *et al.*, 1988, 1990). Thus, the increased release of DA after DOI administration could be contributing to its REMS-suppressing effect. GABA has been considered also to be participating in the DOI-induced inhibition of REMS. In this respect, Amici *et al.* (2004) observed that DOI microinjected into the LDT decreased the number of sequential REMS episodes of the rat. Taking into account that GABAergic interneurons in the LDT/PPT express 5-HT$_{2A/2C}$ receptors, they proposed that the inhibitory effect of DOI on REMS could be related to the local release of GABA.

The 5-HT$_3$ receptor

5-HT$_3$ receptor agonists and antagonists

Not much is known about the role of the 5-HT$_3$ receptor in the regulation of sleep and waking. A limited number of selective agonists for the

5-HT$_3$ receptor are available. They include 2-methyl-5-HT, phenylbiguanide, and m-chlorophenylbiguanide (m-CPBG). However, because of their low lipophilicity, and hence poor brain penetration, currently available 5-HT$_3$ receptor agonists have to be administered directly into the brain (Kilpatrick & Tyers, 1992). In addition, highly selective and potent 5-HT$_3$ receptor antagonists that cross the blood–brain barrier are available. They include MDL 72222 (1aH,3a,5aH-tropan-3-yl-3,5-dichlorobenzoate), granisetron, ondansetron, and tropisetron. m-CPBG injected into the left lateral ventricle increased W and REMS latency, whereas SWS, REMS, and the number of REM periods were reduced in the rat (Ponzoni et al., 1993). In contrast, systemic administration of MDL 72222 or ondansetron significantly increased SWS and/or REMS, respectively (Tissier et al., 1990; Adrien et al., 1992; Ponzoni et al., 1993). Moreover, pretreatment with MDL 72222 prevented the increase of W and reduction of SWS and REMS induced by m-CPBG (Ponzoni et al., 1993). Concerning the mechanism underlying the m-CPBG-induced disruption of the sleep–wake cycle, it has been proposed that 5-HT$_3$ receptor agonists presumably act by increasing the release of several endogenous neurotransmitters (Kilpatrick & Tyers, 1992), which during a second step would augment W and diminish sleep. In this respect, it has been found that microinjection of m-CPBG into the nucleus accumbens increased W and reduced SWS in the rat. The effect of m-CPBG was markedly attenuated in 6-hydroxytryptamine-treated animals, and was antagonized by MDL 72222 and the DA D$_1$ or D$_2$ receptor antagonists SCH 23390 (7-chloro-8-hydroxy-3-methyl-1-phenyl-2,3,4,5-tetrahydro-1H-3-benzazepine), and YM-09151−2[cis-N-(1-benzyl-2-methylpyrrolidin-3-yl)-5-chloro-2-methoxy-4-methylaminobenzamide], respectively (Ponzoni et al., 1995; Monti et al., 1999). Thus, presently available evidence supports the proposal that the increase of W and reduction of SWS after 5-HT$_3$ receptor activation is related, at least in part, to the increased availability of DA at central sites.

The 5-HT$_7$ receptor

5-HT$_7$ receptor antagonists

Recently, SB-269970 (1-[3-hydroxy-phenyl-sulphonyl]-2-[2-(4-methyl-1-piperidinyl)-ethyl] pyrrolidine) and SB-656104 (6-((R)-2-{2-[4-(4-chloro-phenoxy)-piperidin-1-yl]-ethyl} pyrrolidine-1-sulphonyl)-1H-indole) have been reported to be potent 5-HT$_7$ receptor antagonists (Hagan et al., 2000; Forbes et al., 2002). Selective 5-HT$_7$ receptor agonists are not available at the present time. Systemic administration of SB-269970 or SB-656104 to rats at the beginning of the light period has been shown to reduce the total amount of REMS and to increase REMS latency. Values of W and SWS were not significantly modified (Hagan et al., 2000; Thomas et al., 2003). Hedlund et al. (2005) established that 5-HT$_7$

receptor knockout mice show a normal sleep pattern compared with their wild-type counterparts. However, during the light period, the 5-HT$_7^{-/-}$ mice spent less time in REMS. In contrast, there was no difference between the genotypes in time spent in W or SWS. Infusion of SB-269970 directly into the DRN also induced a suppression of REMS in the rat (Monti & Jantos, 2006a).

Glass *et al.* (2003) and Roberts *et al.* (2004) have proposed, on the basis of a series of functional studies, that 5-HT$_7$ receptors in the DRN are localized on GABAergic cells and terminals. Thus, it is conceivable that microinjection of SB-269970 into the DRN reduces GABAergic inhibition of 5-HT neurons and increases 5-HT release at postsynaptic sites, including the LDT/PPT and the mPRF, with the resultant suppression of REMS. To test this hypothesis, muscimol was microinjected into the DRN prior to the administration of the 5-HT$_7$ receptor antagonist. It was observed that the GABA$_A$ receptor agonist prevented the SB-269970-induced decrease of REMS (Monti & Jantos, 2006a). Thus, knockout mice strains that lack the 5-HT$_7$ receptor and rats given a 5-HT$_7$ receptor antagonist spend less time in REMS, which might be related to a reduction of the inhibitory effect of GABA on DRN 5-HT neurons.

Conclusions

Attempts to characterize the role of serotonin receptors on sleep variables have been limited to the 5-HT$_{1A}$, 5-HT$_{1B}$, 5-HT$_{2A}$, 5-HT$_{2C}$, 5-HT$_3$, and 5-HT$_7$ receptors. Most studies have examined the effect of systemic administration of selective and relatively selective agonists and antagonists on sleep and W in the rat. Recently, results from several studies have quantified the spontaneous sleep/waking cycles in serotonin 5-HT$_{1A}$, 5-HT$_{1B}$, or 5-HT$_7$ receptor knockout mice. Much less is known about the effect of local microinjection of serotonin receptor ligands into CNS structures relevant to the regulation of sleep and W, including the DRN, the LDT/PPT, and the mPRF.

All serotonin receptor agonists studied to date share the ability to promote W and to suppress REMS when given by the i.c.v., i.p., or s.c. route. Are all these receptors (tentatively including the 5-HT$_4$, 5-HT$_5$, and 5-HT$_6$ receptors) necessary to increase W and to reduce sleep? Are the behavioral changes qualitatively and the quantitatively similar, irrespective of the receptor involved? Is the response influenced by other neurotransmitters, via afferent inputs, including NA, ACh, HA, DA, or OX? Currently there are no answers to these questions. However, Steinbusch (1984) has shown that 5-HT cells in the rat DRN appear in topographically organized groups. These subpopulations of neurons differ in their morphological characteristics, cellular properties, and afferent and efferent connections (Abrams *et al.*, 2005). In addition, the subpopulations of 5-HT neurons co-express different neurotransmitters and neuromodulators, including DA, glutamate, GABA, SP, and corticotropin-releasing factor (Clements *et al.*, 1991; Charara & Parent, 1998; Li *et al.*, 2001; Commons *et al.*, 2003). Thus, the possibility exists that efferent projections from each subpopulation of 5-HT neurons form synapses with only one subtype of serotonin receptor. This would allow different 5-HT subsystems to influence specifically and separately the neurons involved in the regulation of W and REMS.

The characterization of subpopulations of 5-HT neurons adds to the appreciation that each 5-HT receptor family makes use of a particular signal transduction pathway. Accordingly, the 5-HT_1 family, like the 5-HT_5 receptor, are negatively coupled to adenylate cyclase. On the other hand, the 5-HT_2 family is coupled to phospholipase C whereas the 5-HT_4 and 5-HT_7 receptors are positively coupled to adenylate cyclase. As an exception, the 5-HT_3 receptor incorporates an ion channel that regulates ion flux in a G-protein-independent manner (Cooper *et al.*, 1996). Thus, activation of the postsynaptic 5-HT_{1A}, 5-HT_{1B}, and 5-HT_5 receptors induces the hyperpolarization of target neurons. In contrast, activation of the 5-HT_{2A}, 5-HT_{2C}, 5-HT_3, 5-HT_4, and 5-HT_7 receptors leads to the depolarization of a variety of postsynaptic cells. However, presently available evidence tends to indicate that REMS occurrence is not facilitated by the depolarization of postsynaptic neurons. This is partly related to the finding that 5-HT_{2A}, 5-HT_{2C}, and 5-HT_3 receptors are expressed also on GABAergic cells that innervate structures involved in the promotion and the induction of REMS.

Although the process by which activation of 5-HT_{1A} and 5-HT_{1B} receptors facilitates the state of wakefulness is still unknown, it should be mentioned that many of the GABAergic cells in the basal forebrain, hippocampus, and neocortex on which 5-HT_{1A} and 5-HT_{1B} receptors are expressed are hyperpolarized by serotonin released from the DRN (Parnavelas, 1990; Araneda & Andrade, 1991; Hesen & Joëls, 1996; Detari *et al.*, 1999; Newberry *et al.*, 1999). Thus, inhibition of GABAergic neurons following the activation of 5-HT_{1A} and 5-HT_{1B} receptors could account, at least in part, for their facilitatory effect on W. In other words, activation of the 5-HT_{1A} and 5-HT_{1B} receptors may attenuate GABAergic input and thereby indirectly increase the release of ACh and glutamate at cortical and subcortical sites. However, 5-HT_{1A} and 5-HT_{1B} receptor-dependent inhibition of cholinergic and glutamatergic neurons in the LDT/PPT and the mPRF, respectively, would be directly responsible for REMS suppression.

Activation of 5-HT_{2A} and 5-HT_{2C} receptors enhances the release of ACh in the mPFC and the hippocampus, and of DA in the mPFC and the VTA of the rat. Thus, the increased availability of DA and ACh at central sites after $5\text{-HT}_{2A/2C}$ receptor activation could be responsible, at least in part, for the increased incidence of W. Mesopontine cholinergic cells do not express $5\text{-HT}_{2A/2C}$ receptors. The LDT/PPT neurons that express these receptors correspond mainly to inhibitory GABAergic interneurons. Accordingly, the suppression of REMS after stimulation of 5-HT$_{2A/2C}$ receptors can be related to the activation of GABAergic interneurons located within and around the LDT/PPT that express these receptors.

Not much is known about the mechanisms subserving the increase of W and reduction of REMS after activation of 5-HT$_3$ receptor. This receptor is well known for stimulating the release of DA, ACh, NA, 5-HT, and GABA in the brainstem, the limbic system, the basal forebrain, and the cortex, which can tentatively explain its disruption of sleep variables. However, further studies are needed to resolve this issue.

In conclusion, based on neurochemical, electrophysiological, and neuropharmacological approaches, it is presently accepted that 5-HT functions to promote W and to inhibit REMS. Available evidence indicates that 5-HT$_{1A}$, 5-HT$_{1B}$, 5-HT$_{2A}$, 5-HT$_{2B}$, 5-HT$_{2C}$, 5-HT$_3$, and 5-HT$_7$ receptors are involved in these effects.

References

Abramowski, D., Rigo, M., Duc, D., Hoyer, D. & Staufenbiel, M. (1995). Localization of the 5-hydroxytryptamine$_{2C}$ receptor protein in human and rat brain using specific antisera. *Neuropharmacology* **34**, 1635–45.

Abrams, J. K., Johnson, P. L., Hay-Schmidt, A. *et al.* (2005). Serotonergic systems associated with arousal and vigilance behaviors following administration of anxiogenic drugs. *Neuroscience* **133**, 983–97.

Adrien, J., Tissier, M. H., Lanfumey, L. *et al.* (1992). Central action of 5-HT$_3$ receptor ligands in the regulation of sleep-wakefulness and raphe neuronal activity in the rat. *Neuropharmacology* **31**, 519–29.

Aghajanian, G. K. & Lakoski, J. M. (1984). Hyperpolarization of serotoninergic neurons by serotonin and LSD: studies in brain slices showing increased K$^+$ conductance. *Brain Res.* **305**, 181–5.

Alam, M. N., McGinty, D. & Szymusiak, R. (1995). Neuronal discharge of preoptic/ anterior hypothalamic thermosensitive neurons: relation to NREM sleep. *Am. J. Physiol.* **269**, R1240–9.

Alam, M. N., McGinty, D. & Szymusiak, R. (1997). Thermosensitive neurons of the diagonal band in rats: relation to wakefulness and non-rapid eye movement sleep. *Brain Res.* **752**, 81–9.

Alam, M. N., Szymusiak, R., Gong, H., King, J. & McGinty, D. (1999). Adenosinergic modulation of rat basal forebrain neurons during sleep and waking: Neuronal recording with microdialysis. *J. Physiol. Lond.* **521**, 679–90.

Amici, R., Sanford, L. D., Kearney, K. *et al.* (2004). A serotonergic (5-HT$_2$) receptor mechanism in the laterodorsal tegmental nucleus participates in regulating the pattern of rapid-eye-movement sleep occurrence in the rat. *Brain Res.* **996**, 9–18.

Araneda, R. & Andrade, R. (1991). 5-Hydroxytryptamine$_2$ and 5-hydroxytryptamine$_{1A}$ receptors mediate opposing responses on membrane excitability in rat association cortex. *Neuroscience* **40**, 399–412.

Armitage, R. (1996). Effects of antidepressant treatment on sleep EEG in depression. *J. Psychopharmacol.* **10** (Suppl. 1), 22–5.

Aston-Jones, G. & Bloom, F. E. (1981). Activity of norepinephrine-containing locus coeruleus neurons in behaving rats anticipates fluctuations in the sleep-waking cycle. *J. Neurosci.* **1**, 876–86.

Austin, M. C., Weikel, J. A., Arango, V. & Mann, J. J. (1994). Localization of serotonin 5-HT$_{1A}$ receptor mRNA in neurons of the human brainstem. *Synapse* **18**, 276–9.

Baez, M., Kursar, J. D., Helton, L. A., Wainscott, D. B. & Nelson, D. L. (1995). Molecular biology of serotonin receptors. *Obesity Res.* **3** (Suppl. 4), 441S–447S.

Baghdoyan, H. A. & Lydic, R. (2002). Neurotransmitters and neuromodulators regulating sleep. In *Sleep and Epilepsy: the Clinical Spectrum*, ed. C. W. Bazil, B. A. Marlow & M. R. Sammaritano, pp. 17–44. Amsterdam: Elsevier Science.

Baker, K. G., Halliday, G. M. & Tork, I. (1990). Cytoarchitecture of the human dorsal raphe nucleus. *J. Comp. Neurol* **301**, 147–61.

Behzadi, G., Kalen, P., Parvopassu, F. & Wiklund, L. (1990). Afferents to the median raphe nucleus of the rat: retrograde cholera toxin and wheat germ conjugated horseradish peroxidase tracing, and selective D-[^{3}H]aspartate labelling of possible excitatory amino acid inputs. *Neuroscience* **37**, 77–100.

Bidmon, H. J., Schleicher, A., Wicke, K., Gross, G. & Zilles, K. (2001). Localisation of mRNA for h5-HT$_{1B}$ and h5-HT$_{1D}$ receptors in human dorsal raphe. *Naunyn Schmiedebergs Arch. Pharmacol.* **363**, 364–8.

Bjorvatn, B. & Ursin, R. (1994). Effects of the selective 5-HT$_{1B}$ agonist, CGS 12066B, on sleep/waking stages and EEG power spectrum in rats. *J. Sleep Res.* **3**, 97–105.

Bjorvatn, B., Fornal, C. A., Martin, F. J., Metzler, C. W. & Jacobs, B. L. (1998). The 5-HT$_{1A}$ receptor antagonist p-MPPI blocks 5-HT$_{1A}$ autoreceptors and increases dorsal raphe unit activity in awake cats. *Eur. J. Pharmacol.* **356**, 167–78.

Borbély, A. A., Huston, J. P. & Waser, P. G. (1973). Physiological and behavioral effects of parachlorophenylalanine in the rat. *Psychopharmacologia* **31**, 131–42.

Bortolozzi, A., Díaz-Mataix, L., Scorza, M. C., Celada, P. & Artigas, F. (2005). The activation of 5-HT$_{2A}$ receptors in prefrontal cortex enhances dopaminergic activity. *J. Neurochem.* **95**, 1597–607.

Boutrel, B., Franc, B., Hen, R., Hamon, M. & Adrien, J. (1999) Key role of 5-HT$_{1B}$ receptors in the regulation of paradoxical sleep as evidenced in 5-HT$_{1B}$ knock-out mice. *J. Neurosci.* **19**, 3204–12.

Boutrel, B., Monaca, C., Hen, R., Hamon, M. & Adrien, J. (2002). Involvement of 5-HT$_{1A}$ receptors in homeostatic and stress-induced adaptive regulations of paradoxical sleep: studies in 5-HT$_{1A}$ knock-out mice. *J. Neurosci.* **22**, 4686–92.

Bruinvels, A. T., Landwehrmeyer, B., Gustafson, E. L. *et al.* (1994). Localization of the 5-HT$_{1B}$, 5-HT$_{1D\alpha}$, 5-HT$_{1E}$ and 5-HT$_{1F}$ receptor messenger RNA in rodent and primate brain. *Neuropharmacology* **33**, 367–86.

Bunin, M. A., Prioleau, C., Mailman, R. B. & Wightman, R. M. (1998). Release and uptake of 5-hydroxytryptamine in the dorsal raphe and substantia nigra reticulata of the rat brain. *J. Neurochem.* **70**, 1077–87.

Chan-Palay, V., Jonsson, G., Palay, S. L. (1978). Serotonin and substance P coexist in neurons of the rat's central nervous system. *Proc. Natl. Acad. Sci. USA* **75**, 1582–6.

Charara, A. & Parent, A. (1998). Chemoarchitecture of the primate dorsal raphe nucleus. *J. Chem. Neuroanat.* **15**, 111–27.

Clancy, J. J., Caldwell, D. F., Oberleas, D., Sangiah, S. & Villeneuve, M. J. (1978). Effect of chronic tryptophan dietary deficiency on the rat's sleep-wake cycle. *Brain Res. Bull.* **3**, 83–7.

Clements, J. R., Toth, D. D., Highfield, D. A. & Grant, S. J. (1991). Glutamate-like immunoreactivity is present within cholinergic neurons of the laterodorsal tegmental and pedunculopontine nuclei. *Adv. Exp. Med. Biolo.* **295**, 127–42.

Clemett, D. A., Punhani, T., Duxon, M. S., Blackburn, T. P. & Fone, K. C. F. (2000). Immunohistochemical localisation of the 5-HT$_{2C}$ receptor protein in the rat CNS. *Neuropharmacology* **39**, 123–32.

Coenen, A. M. L., Ates, N., Skarsfeldt, T. & Luijtelaar, E. L. J. M. (1995). Effects of sertindole on sleep-wake states, electroencephalogram, behavioral patterns, and epileptic activity in rats. *Pharmacol. Biochem. Behav.* **51**, 353–7.

Commons, K. G., Connolley, K. R. & Valentino R. J. (2003). A neurochemically distinct dorsal raphe-limbic circuit with a potential role in affective disorders. *Neuropsychopharmacology* **28**, 206–15.

Cooper, J. R., Bloom, F. E. and Roth, R. H. (1996). *The Biochemical Basis of Neuropharmacology*, 7th edn. Oxford: Oxford University Press.

Cornea-Hébert, V., Riad, M., Wu, C., Singh, S. K. & Descarries, L. (1999). Cellular and subcellular distribution of the serotonin 5-HT$_{2A}$ receptor in the central nervous system of adult rat. *J. Comp. Neurol.* **409**, 187–209.

Dement, W. C., Mitler, M. M. & Henriksen, S. J. (1972). Sleep changes during chronic administration of parachlorophenylalanine. *Can. J. Biol.* **31**, 239–46.

Detari, L., Rasmusson, D. D. & Semba, K. (1999). The role of basal forebrain neurons in tonic and phasic activation of the cerebral cortex. *Progr. Neurobiol.* **58**, 249–77.

Doucet, E., Pohl, M., Fattaccini, C. M. *et al.* (1995). In situ hybridization evidence for the synthesis of 5-HT$_{1B}$ receptor in serotoninergic neurons of anterior raphe nuclei in the rat brain. *Synapse* **19**, 18–28.

Driver, H. S., Flanigan, M. J., Bentley, A. J. *et al.* (1995). The influence of ipsapirone, a 5-HT$_{1A}$ agonist, on sleep patterns of healthy subjects. *Psychopharmacology* **117**, 186–92.

Dugovic, C. & Wauquier, A. (1987). 5-HT$_2$ receptors could be primarily involved in the regulation of slow wave sleep in the rat. *Eur. J. Pharmacol.* **137**, 145–6.

Dugovic, C., Wauquier, A., Leysen, J. E. & Janssen, P. A. J. (1989). Functional role of 5-HT$_2$ receptors in the regulation of sleep and wakefulness in the rat. *Psychopharmacology* **97**, 436–42.

Duxon, M. S., Flanigan, T. P., Reavley, A. C. *et al.* (1997). Evidence for the expression of the 5-hydroxytryptamine-2B receptor protein in the rat central nervous system. *Neuroscience* **76**, 323–9.

Fay, R. & Kubin, L. (2000). Pontomedullary distribution of 5-HT$_{2A}$ receptor-like protein in the rat. *J. Comp. Neurol.* **418**, 323–45.

Fletcher, A., Forster, E. A., Bill, D. J. *et al.* (1996). Electrophysiological, biochemical, neurohormonal and behavioral studies with WAY-100635, a potent, selective and silent 5-HT$_{1A}$ receptor antagonist. *Behav. Brain Res.* **73**, 337–53.

Forbes, I. T., Douglas, S., Gribble, A. D. *et al.* (2002). SB-656104-A: A novel 5-HT$_7$ receptor antagonist with improved *in vivo* properties. *Bioorgan. Med. Chem. Lett.* **12**, 334–44.

Ford, B., Holmes, C. J., Mainville, L. & Jones, B. E. (1995). GABAergic neurons in the rat pontomesencephalic tegmentum: codistribution with cholinergic and other tegmental neurons projecting to the posterior lateral hypothalamus. *J. Comp. Neurol.* **363**, 177–96.

Fornal, C. A., Metzler, C. W., Gallegos, R. A. *et al.* (1996). WAY-100635, a potent and selective 5-hydroxytryptamine$_{1A}$ antagonist increases serotonergic neuronal activity in behaving cats: Comparison with (S)-WAY-100635. *J. Pharmacol. Exp. Ther.* **278**, 752–62.

Forster, E. A., Cliffe, I. A., Bill, D. J. *et al.* (1995). A pharmacological profile of the selective silent 5-HT$_{1A}$ receptor antagonist WAY 100635. *Eur. J. Pharmacol.* **281**, 81–8.

Frank, M. G., Stryker, M. P. & Tecott, L. H. (2002). Sleep and sleep homeostasis in mice lacking the 5-HT$_{2C}$ receptor. *Neuropsychopharmacology* **27**, 869–73.

Gehlert, D. R., Gackenheimer, S. L., Wong, D. T. & Robertson, D. W. (1991). Localization of 5-HT$_3$ receptors in the rat brain using [^{3}H]LY278584. *Brain Res.* **553**, 149–54.

Gillin, J. C., Jernajczyk, W., Valladares-Neto, D. C. *et al.* (1994). Inhibition of REM sleep by ipsapirone, a 5-HT$_{1A}$ agonist, in normal volunteers. *Psychopharmacology* **116**, 433–6.

Glass, J. D., Grossman, G. H., Farnbauch L. & DiNardo, L. (2003). Midbrain raphe modulation of nonphotic circadian clock resetting and 5-HT release in the mammalian suprachiasmatic nucleus. *J. Neurosci.* **23**, 7451–60.

Gobert, A., Lejeune, F., Rivet, J. M. *et al.* (1995). Modulation of the activity of central serotoninergic neurons by novel serotonin$_{1A}$ receptor agonists and antagonists: a comparison to adrenergic and dopaminergic neurons in rats. *J. Pharmacol. Exp. Ther.* **273**, 1032–46.

Gonzalo-Ruiz, A., Lieberman, A. R. & Sanz-Anquela, J. M. (1995). Organization of serotoninergic projections from the raphe nuclei to the anterior thalamic nuclei in the rat: a combined retrograde tracing and 5-HT immuno-histochemical study. *J. Chem. Neuroanat.* **8**, 103–15.

Grace, A. A. (2002). Dopamine. In *Neuropsychopharmacology – The Fifth Generation of Progress*, ed. K. L. Davis, D. Charney, J. T. Coyle & C. Nemeroff, pp. 120–32. Philadelphia, PA: Lippincott Williams & Wilkins.

Gustafson, E. L., Durkin, M. M., Bard, J. A., Zgombick, J. & Branchek, T. A. (1996). A receptor autoradiographic and in situ hybridization analysis of the distribution of the 5-HT$_7$ receptor in rat brain. *Br. J. Pharmacol.* **117**, 657–66.

Hagan, J. J., Price, G. W., Jeffrey, P. *et al.* (2000). Characterization of SB-269970-A, a selective 5-HT$_7$ receptor antagonist. *Br. J. Pharmacol.* **130**, 539–48.

Hajós, M., Richards, C. D., Székely, A. D. & Sharp, T. (1998). An electrophysiological and neuroanatomical study of the medial prefrontal cortical projection to the midbrain raphe nuclei in the rat. *Neuroscience* **87**, 95–108.

Hamada, S., Senzaki, K., Hamaguchi-Hamada, K. *et al.* (1998). Localization of 5-HT$_{2A}$ receptor in rat cerebral cortex and olfactory system revealed by immuno-histochemistry using two antibodies raised in rabbit and chicken. *Molec. Brain Res.* **54**, 199–211.

Hedlund, P. B., Huitron-Resendiz, S., Henriksen, S. J. & Sutcliffe, J. G. (2005). 5-HT$_7$ receptor inhibition and inactivation induced antidepresssantlike behavior and sleep pattern. *Biol. Psychiatry* **58**, 831–7.

Hensler, J. G., Ferry, R. C., Labow, D. M., Kovachich, G. B. & Frazer, A. (1994). Quantitative autoradiography of the serotonin transporter to assess the distribution of serotonergic projections from the dorsal raphe nucleus. *Synapse* **17**, 1–15.

Hesen, W. & Joëls, M. (1996). Modulation of 5-HT$_{1A}$ responsiveness in CA$_1$ pyramidal neurons by in vivo activation of corticosteroid receptors. *J. Neuroendocrinol.* **8**, 433–8.

Hillegaart, V. (1990). Effects of local application of 5-HT and 8-OH-DPAT into the dorsal and median raphe nuclei on motor activity in the rat. *Physiol. Behav.* **48**, 143–8.

Horner, R. L., Sanford, L. D., Annis, D., Pack, A. I. & Morrison, A. R. (1997). Serotonin at the laterodorsal tegmental nucleus suppresses rapid-eye-movement sleep in freely behaving rats. *J. Neurosci.* **17**, 7541–52.

Hoyer, D. & Martin, G. R. (1996). Classification and nomenclature of 5-HT receptors: a comment on current issues. *Behav. Brain Res.* **73**, 263–8.

Hoyer, D., Clarke, D. E., Fozard, J. R. *et al.* (1994). International Union of Pharmacology classification of receptors for 5-hydroxytryptamine (serotonin). *Pharmacol. Rev.* **46**, 157–203.

Iwakiri, H., Matsuyama, K. & Mori, S. (1993). Extracellular levels of serotonin in the medial pontine reticular formation in relation to sleep-wake cycle in cats: a microdialysis study. *Neurosci. Res.* **18**, 157–70.

Jäkälä, P., Sirvio, J., Koivisto, E. *et al.* (1995). Modulation of rat neocortical high-voltage spindle activity by 5-HT$_1$/5-HT$_2$ receptor subtype specific drugs. *Eur. J. Pharmacol.* **282**, 39–55.

Janowski, M. P. & Sesack, S. R. (2004). Prefrontal cortical projections to the rat dorsal raphe nucleus: ultrastructural features and association with serotonin and gamma-aminobutyric acid neurons. *J. Comp. Neurol.* **468**, 518–29.

Jones, B. E. (2005). From waking to sleeping: neuronal and chemical substrates. *Trends Pharmacol. Sci.* **26**, 578–86.

Jones, F. J. (2003). Arousal systems. *Frontiers Biosci.* **8**, 438–51.

Jouvet, M. (1972). The role of monoamines and acetylcholine containing neurons in the regulation of the sleep–waking cycle. *Ergeb. Physiol.* **64**, 166–307.

Jouvet, M. (1984). Neuromediateurs et facteurs hypnogènes. *Rev. Neurol.* **140**, 389–400.

Kantor, S., Jakus, R., Bodizs, R., Halasz, P. & Bagdy, G. (2002). Acute and long-term effects of the 5-HT$_2$ receptor antagonist ritanserin on EEG power spectra, motor acivity, and sleep: changes at the light-dark phase shift. *Brain Res.* **943**, 105–11.

Kantor, S., Jakus, R., Balogh, B., Benko, A. & Bagdy, G. (2004). Increased wakefulness, motor activity and decreased theta activity after blockade of the 5-HT$_{2B}$ receptor by the subtype-selective antagonist SB-215505. *Br. J. Pharmacol.* **142**, 1332–42.

Kia, H. K., Brisorgueil, M. J., Hamon, M., Calas, A. & Vergé, D. (1996a). Ultrastructural localization of 5-hydroxytryptamine$_{1A}$ receptors in the rat brain. *J. Neurosci. Res.* **46**, 697–708.

Kia, H. K., Miquel, M. C., Brisorgueil, M. J. *et al.* (1996b). Immunocytochemical localization of 5-HT$_{1A}$ receptor in the rat central nervous system. *J. Comp. Neurol.* **365**, 289–205.

Kilpatrick, G. J. & Tyers, M. B. (1992). The pharmacological properties and functional roles of central 5-HT$_3$ receptors. In *Central and Peripheral 5-HT$_3$ Receptors*, ed. M. Hamon, pp. 33–57. London: Academic Press.

Kilpatrick, G. J., Jones, B. J. & Tyers, M. B. (1987). Identification and distribution of 5-HT$_3$ receptors in rat brain using radioligand binding. *Nature* **330**, 746–8.

Kilpatrick, G. J., Jones, B. J. & Tyers, M. B. (1988). The distribution and specific binding of the 5-HT$_3$ receptor ligand [^{3}H] GR65630 in rat brain using quantitative autoradiography. *Neurosci. Lett.* **94**, 156–60.

Kirov, R. & Moyanova, S. (1998a). Age-dependent effect of ketanserin on the sleep-waking phases in rats. *Int. J. Neurosci.* **93**, 257–64.

Kirov, R. & Moyanova, S. (1998b). Age-related effect of ritanserin on the sleep-waking phases in rats. *Int. J. Neurosci.* **93**, 265–78.

Kodama, T., Takahashi, Y. & Honda, Y. (1990). Enhancement of acetylcholine release during paradoxical sleep in the dorsal tegmental field of the cat brain stem. *Neurosci. Lett.* **114**, 277–82.

Laguzzi, R. F. & Adrien, J. (1980). Inversion de l'insomnie produite par la para-chlorophenylalanine chez le chat. *Arch. Ital. Biol.* **118**, 109–23.

Laporte, A. M., Koscielniak, T., Ponchant, M. *et al.* (1992). Quatitative autoradiographic mapping of 5-HT$_3$ receptors in the rat CNS using [^{125}I]iodo-zacopride and [^{3}H]zacopride as radioligands. *Synapse* **10**, 271–81.

Lebel, L. A. & Koe, B. K. (1992). Binding studies with the 5-HT$_{1B}$ receptor agonist [^{3}H]CP-96,501 in brain tissues. *Drug Devel. Res.* **27**, 253–64.

Lee, M. G., Hassani, O. K. & Jones, B. E. (2005). Discharge of identified orexin/ hypocretin neurons across the sleep-waking cycle. *J. Neurosci.* **25**, 6716–20.

Lerman, J. A., Kaitin, K. I., Dement, W. C. & Peroutka, S. J. (1986). The effects of buspirone on sleep in the rat. *Neurosci. Lett.* **72**, 64–8.

Li, Y. Q., Li, H., Kaneko, T. & Mizuno, N. (2001). Morphological features and electrophysiological properties of serotonergic and non-serotonergic projection neurons in the dorsal raphe nucleus. *Brain Res.* **900**, 110–18.

López-Giménez, J. F., Vilaró, M. T., Palacios, J. M. & Mengod, G. (2001). Mapping of 5-HT$_{2A}$ receptors and their mRNA in monkey brain: [^{3}H]MDL100,907 autoradiography and in situ hybridization studies. *J. Comp. Neurol.* **429**, 571–89.

Losier, B. J. & Semba, K. (1993). Dual projections of single cholinergic and aminergic brainstem neurons to the thalamus and basal forebrain in the rat. *Brain Res.* **604**, 41–52.

Lucas, E. A. & Sterman, M. B. (1975). Effect of a forebrain lesion on the polycyclic sleep-wake cycle and sleep-wake patterns in the cat. *Exp. Neurol.* **46**, 368–88.

Luebke, J. I., Greene, R. W., Semba, K. *et al.* (1992). Serotonin hyperpolarizes cholinergic low threshold burst neurons in the rat laterodorsal tegmental nuclei *in vitro*. *Proc. Natl. Acad. Sci. USA* **89**, 743–7.

Makarenko, I. G., Meguid, M. M. & Ugrumov, M. V. (2002). Distribution of serotonin 5-hydroxytryptamine$_{1B}$ (5-HT$_{1B}$) receptors in the normal rat hypothalamus. *Neurosci. Lett.* **328**, 156–9.

Mallick, B. N., Majumdar, S., Faisal, M. *et al.* (2002). Role of norepinephrine in the regulation of rapid eye movement sleep. *J. Biosci.* **27**, 539–51.

Manfredi, R. L., Kales, A., Vgontzas, A. N. *et al.* (1991). Buspirone: Sedative or stimulant effect? *Am. J. Psychiatry* **148**, 1213–17.

Marcinkiewicz, M., Morcos, R. & Chretien, M. (1989). CNS connections with the median raphe nucleus: retrograde tracing with WGA-apoHRP-gold complex in the rat. *J. Comp. Neurol.* **289**, 11–35.

Marrosu, F., Portas, C., Mascia, M. S. *et al.* (1995). Microdialysis measurement of cortical and hippocampal acetylcholine release during the sleep-wake cycle in freely moving cats. *Brain Res.* **671**, 329–32.

Martin, J. R., Bos, M., Jenck, F. *et al.* (1998). 5-HT$_{2C}$ receptor agonists: Pharmacological characteristics and therapeutic potential. *J. Pharmacol. Exp. Ther.* **286**, 913–24.

McCarley, R. W. & Hobson, J. A. (1975). Neuronal excitability modulation over the sleep cycle: a structural and mathematical model. *Science* **189**, 58–60.

McCarley, R. W., Nelson, J. P. & Hobson, J. A. (1978). PGO burst neurons: correlative evidence for neuronal generators of PGO waves. *Science* **201**, 209–62.

McGinty, D. & Szymusiak, R. (2001). Brain structures and mechanisms involved in the generation of NREM sleep: focus on the preoptic hypothalamus. *Sleep Med. Rev.* **5**, 323–42.

McQuade, R. & Sharp, T. (1997). Functional mapping of dorsal and median raphe 5-hydroxytryptamine pathways in forebrain of the rat using microdialysis. *J. Neurochem.* **69**, 791–6.

Mengod, G., Nguyen, H., Le, H. *et al.* (1990). The distribution and cellular localization of the serotonin 1C receptor mRNA in the rodent brain examined by in situ hybridization histochemistry. Comparison with receptor binding distribution. *Neuroscience* **35**, 577–91.

Mirkes, S. J. & Bethea, C. L. (2001). Oestrogen, progesterone and serotonin converge on GABAergic neurons in the monkey hypothalamus. *J. Neuroendocrinol.* **13**, 182–92.

Monaca, C., Boutrel, B., Hen, R., Hamon, M. & Adrien, J. (2003). 5-HT$_{1A/B}$ receptor-mediated effects of the selective serotonin reuptake inhibitor citalopram, on sleep: studies in 5-HT$_{1A}$ and 5-HT$_{1B}$ knockout mice. *Neuropharmacology* **28**, 850–6.

Monti, J. M. (2004). Primary and secondary insomnia: prevalence, causes and current therapeutics. *Curr. Med. Chem. Central Nerv. Syst. Agents*, **4**, 119–37.

Monti, J. M. & Jantos, H. (1992). Dose-dependent effects of the 5-HT$_{1A}$ receptor agonist 8-OHDPAT on sleep and wakefulness in the rat. *J. Sleep Res.* **1**, 169–75.

Monti, J. M. & Jantos, H. (2003). Differential effects of the 5-HT$_{1A}$ receptor agonist flesinoxan given locally or systemically on REM sleep in the rat. *Eur. J. Pharmacol.* **478**, 121–30.

Monti, J. M. & Jantos, H. (2004). Effects of the 5-HT$_{1A}$ receptor ligands flesinoxan and WAY 100635 given systemically or microinjected into the laterodorsal tegmental nucleus on REM sleep in the rat. *Behav. Brain Res.* **151**, 159–66.

Monti, J. M. & Jantos, H. (2006a). Effects of the 5-HT$_7$ receptor antagonist SB-269970 microinjected into the dorsal raphe nucleus on REM sleep in the rat. *Behav. Brain Res.* **167**, 245–50.

Monti, J. M. & Jantos, H. (2006b). Effects of the serotonin 5-HT$_{2A/2C}$ receptor agonist DOI and of the selective 5-HT$_{2A}$ or 5-HT$_{2C}$ receptor antagonists EMD 281014 and SB-243213, respectively, on sleep and waking in the rat. *Eur. J. Pharmacol.* **553**, 163–70.

Monti, J. M., Hawkins, M., Jantos, H., Labraga, P. & Fernández, J. (1988). Biphasic effects of dopamine D-2 receptor agonists on sleep and wakefulness in the rat. *Psychopharmacology* **95**, 395–400.

Monti, J. M., Orellana, C., Boussard, M. *et al.* (1990). 5-HT receptor agonists 1-(2,5-dimethoxy-4-iodophenyl)-2-aminopropane (DOI) and 8-OH-DPAT increase wakefulness in the rat. *Biogen. Amines* **7**, 145–51.

Monti, J. M., Jantos, H., Silveira, R. *et al.* (1994). Depletion of brain serotonin by 5,7-DHT: effects on the 8-OH-DPAT-induced changes of sleep and waking in the rat. *Psychopharmacology* **115**, 273–7.

Monti, J. M., Jantos, H., Silveira, R., Reyes-Parada, M. & Scorza, C. (1995a). Sleep and waking in 5,7-DHT-lesioned or (-)-pindolol-pretreated rats after administration of buspirone, ipsapirone, or gepirone. *Pharmacol. Biochem. Behav.* **52**, 305–12.

Monti, J. M., Monti, D., Jantos, H. & Ponzoni, A. (1995b). Effects of selective activation of the 5-HT$_{1B}$ receptor with CP-94,253 on sleep and wakefulness in the rat. *Neuropharmacology* **34**, 1647–51.

Monti, J. M., Ponzoni, A., Jantos, H. *et al.* (1999). Effects of accumbens m-chlorophenylbiguanide microinjection on sleep and waking in intact and 6-hydroxydopamine-treated rats. *Eur. J. Pharmacol.* **364**, 89–98.

Monti, J. M., Jantos, H. & Monti, D. (2000). Dorsal raphe nucleus administration of 5-HT$_{1A}$ receptor agonist and antagonists: effect on rapid eye movement sleep in the rat. *Sleep Res. Online* **3**, 29–34.

Monti, J. M., Jantos, H. & Monti, D. (2002). Increased REM sleep after intra-dorsal raphe nucleus injection of flesinoxan or 8-OHDPAT: prevention with WAY 100635. *Eur. Neuropsychopharmacol.* **12**, 47–55.

Morales, M., Battenberg, E. & Bloom, F. E. (1998). Distribution of neurons expressing immunoreactivity for the 5-HT$_3$ receptor subtype in the rat brain and spinal cord. *J. Comp. Neurol.* **402**, 385–401.

Morin, L. P. & Meyer-Bernstein, E. L. (1999). The ascending serotonergic system in the hamster: Comparison with projections of the dorsal and median raphe nuclei. *Neuroscience* **91**, 81–105.

Mouret, J., Bobillier, P. & Jouvet, M. (1968). Insomnia following parachloro-phenylalanine in the rat. *Eur. J. Pharmacol.* **5**, 17–22.

Mundey, M. K., Fletcher, A. & Marsden, C. A. (1996). Effects of 8-OHDPAT and 5-HT$_{1A}$ antagonists WAY 100135 and WAY 100635, on guinea-pig behavior and dorsal raphe 5-HT neurons firing. *Br. J. Pharmacol.* **117**, 750–8.

Nanopoulos, D., Belin, M. F., Maitre, M., Vincendon, G. & Pujol, J. F. (1982). Immunocytochemical evidence for the existence of GABAergic neurons in the nucleus raphe dorsalis. Possible existence of neurons containing serotonin and GABA. *Brain Res.* **232**, 375–89.

Neumaier, J. F., Sexton, T. J., Yracheta, J., Diaz, A. M. & Brownfield, M. (2001). Localization of 5-HT$_7$ receptors in rat brain by immunocytochemistry, in situ hybridization, and agonist stimulated cFos expression. *J. Chem. Neuroanat.* **21**, 63–73.

Newberry, N. R., Footitt, D. R., Papanastassiou, V. & Reynolds, D. J. (1999). Action of 5-HT on human neocortical neurones in vitro. *Brain Res.* **833**, 93–100.

Nichols, D. E. (2004). Hallucinogens. *Pharmacol. Ther.* **10**, 131–81.

Oberndorfer, S., Saletu-Zyhlarz, G. & Saletu, B. (2000). Effects of selective serotonin reuptake inhibitors on objective and subjective sleep quality. *Neuropsychobiology* **42**, 69–81.

Ochi, J. & Shimizu, K. (1978). Occurrence of dopamine-containing neurons in the midbrain raphe nuclei. *Neurosci. Lett.* **8**, 317–20.

Pace-Schott, E. F. & Hobson, J. A. (2002). Basic mechanisms of sleep: New evidence on the neuroanatomy and neuromodulation of the NREM-REM cycle. In *Neuropharmacology – The Fifth Generation of Progress*, ed. D. Charney and C. Nemeroff, pp. 1859–77. Philadelphia, PA: Lippincott Williams and Wilkins.

Parnavelas, J. G. (1990). Neurotransmitters in the cerebral cortex. In *Progress in Brain Research*, ed. H. B. M. Uylings, C. G. Van Eden, J. P. C. De Bruin, M. A. Corner & M. G. P. Feenstra, vol. 85, pp. 13–29. Amsterdam: Elsevier.

Pehec, E. A., McFarlane, H. G., Maguschak, K., Price, B. & Pluto, C. P. (2001). M100,907, a selective 5-HT$_{2A}$ antagonist, attenuates dopamine release in the rat medial prefrontal cortex. *Brain Res.* **888**, 51–9.

Peyron, C., Petit, J. M., Rampon, C., Jouvet, M. & Luppi, P. H. (1998). Forebrain afferents to the rat dorsal raphe nucleus demonstrated by retrograde and anterograde tracing methods. *Neuroscience* **82**, 443–68.

Pompeiano, M., Palacios, J. M. & Mengod, G. (1994). Distribution of the serotonin 5-HT$_2$ receptor family mRNAs: comparison between 5-HT$_{2A}$ and 5-HT$_{2C}$ receptors. *Molec. Brain Res.* **23**, 163–78.

Ponzoni, A., Monti, J. M. & Jantos, H. (1993). The effects of selective activation of the 5-HT$_3$ receptor with m-chlorophenylbiguanide on sleep and wakefulness in the rat. *Eur. J. Pharmacol.* **249**, 259–64.

Ponzoni, A., Monti, J. M., Jantos, H., Altier, H. & Monti, D. (1995). Increased waking after intra-accumbens injection of m-chlorophenylbiguanide: prevention with serotonin or dopamine receptor antagonists. *Eur. J. Pharmacol.* **278**, 111–15.

Portas, C. M., Thakkar, M., Rainnie, D. & McCarley, R. W. (1996). Microdialysis perfusion of 8-hydroxy-2-(di-n-propylamino)tetralin (8-OH-DPAT) in the dorsal raphe nucleus decreases serotonin release and increases rapid eye movement sleep in the freely moving cat. *J. Neurosci.* **16**, 2820–8.

Portas, C. M., Thakkar, M., Rainnie, D. G., Greene, R. W. & McCarley, R. W. (1997). Role of adenosine in behavioral state modulation: a microdialysis study in the freely moving cat. *Neuroscience* **79**, 225–35.

Pratt, G. D., Bowery, N. G., Kilpatrick, G. J. *et al.* (1990). Consensus meeting agrees distribution of 5-HT$_3$ receptors in mammalian hindbrain. *Trends Pharmacol. Sci.* **11**, 135–7.

Rechtschaffen, A., Lovell, R. A., Freedman, D. X., Whitehead, W. E. & Aldrich, M. (1973). The effects of parachlorophenylalanine in the rat: some implications for the serotonin-sleep hypothesis. In *Serotonin and Behavior*, ed. J. Barchas & E. Usdin, pp. 401–18. New York, NY: Academic Press.

Riad, M., García, S., Watkins, K. C. *et al.* (2000). Somatodendritic localization of 5-HT$_{1A}$ and preterminal axonal localization of 5-HT$_{1B}$ serotonin receptors in adult rat brain. *J. Comp. Neurol.* **417**, 181–94.

Roberts, C., Thomas, D. R., Bate, S. T. & Kew, J. N. C. (2004). GABAergic modulation of 5-HT$_7$ receptor-mediated effects on 5-HT efflux in the guinea-pig dorsal raphe nucleus. *Neuropharmacology* **46**, 935–41.

Ross, C. A., Trulson, M. E. & Jacobs, B. L. (1976). Depletion of brain 5-HT following intraventricular 5,7-dihydroxytryptamine fails to disrupt sleep in the rat. *Brain Res.* **114**, 517–23.

Rye, D. B. & Jankovic, J. (2002). Emerging views of dopamine in modulating sleep/ wake state from an unlikely source: PD. *Neurology* **58**, 341–6.

Sakai, K., El Mansari, M. & Jouvet, M. (1990). Inhibition by carbachol microinjections of presumptive cholinergic PGO-on neurons in freely moving cats. *Brain Res.* **527**, 213–23.

Sanford, L. D., Ross, R. J., Seggos, A. E. *et al.* (1994). Central administration of two 5-HT agonists: effect on REM sleep initiation and PGO waves. *Pharmacol. Biochem. Behav.* **49**, 93–100.

Saper, C. B., Sherin, J. E. & Elmquist, J. K. (1997). Role of the ventrolateral preoptic area in sleep induction. In *Sleep and Sleep Disorders: From Molecule to Behavior*, ed. O. Hayaishi & S. Inoué, pp. 281–94. Tokyo: Academic Press.

Sari, Y., Lefèvre, K., Bancila, M. *et al.* (1997). Light and electron microscopic immunocytochemical visualization of 5-HT$_{1B}$ receptors in the rat brain. *Brain Res.* **760**, 281–6.

Sari, Y., Miquel, M. C., Brisorgueil, M. J. *et al.* (1999). Cellular and subcellular localization of 5-hydroxytryptamine$_{1B}$ receptors in the rat central nervous system: immunocytochemical, autoradiographic and lesion studies. *Neuroscience* **88**, 899–915.

Seidel, W. F., Cohen, S. A., Bliwise, N. G. & Dement, W. C. (1985). Buspirone: An anxiolytic without sedative effect. *Psychopharmacology* **87**, 371–3.

Serrats, J., Mengod, G. & Cortés, R. (2005). Expression of serotonin 5-HT$_{2C}$ receptors in GABAergic cells of the anterior raphe nuclei. *J. Chem. Neuroanat.* **29**, 83–91.

Sheard, M. H. (1969). The effect of p-chlorophenylalanine on behavior in rats: relation to brain serotonin and 5-hydroxyindolacetic acid. *Brain Res.* **15**: 524–8.

Silhol, S., Glin, L. & Gottesmann, C. (1991). Study of the 5-HT$_2$ antagonist ritanserin on sleep-waking cycle in the rat. *Physiol. Behav.* **41**, 241–3.

Smith, M. I., Piper, D. C., Duxon, M. S. & Upton, N. (2002). Effect of SB-243213, a selective 5-HT$_{2C}$ receptor antagonist, on the rat sleep profile: A comparison to paroxetine. *Pharmacol. Biochem. Behav.* **71**, 599–605.

Sorensen, E., Gronli, J., Bjorvatn, B., Bjorkum, A. & Ursin, R. (2001). Sleep and waking following microdialysis perfusion of the selective 5-HT$_{1A}$ receptor antagonist p-MPPI into the dorsal raphe nucleus in the freely moving rat. *Brain Res.* **897**, 122–30.

Sprouse, J. S. & Aghajanian, G. K. (1987). Electrophysiological responses of serotoninergic dorsal raphe neurons to 5-HT$_{1A}$ and 5-HT$_{1B}$ agonists. *Synapse* **1**, 3–9.

Sprouse, J. S. & Aghajanian, G. K. (1988). Responses of hippocampal pyramidal cells to putative serotonin 5-HT$_{1A}$ and 5-HT$_{1B}$ agonists: a comparative study with dorsal raphe neurons. *Neuropsychopharmacology* **27**, 707–15.

Staner, L., Luthringer, R. & Macher, J. P. (1999). Effects of antidepressant drugs on sleep EEG in patients with major depression. *Central Nerv. Syst. Drugs* **11**, 49–60.

Stanford, S. C. (2001). 5-Hydroxytryptamine. In *Neurotransmitters, Drugs and Brain Function*, ed. R. A. Webster, pp. 187–209. Chichester: John Wiley & Sons.

Steinbusch, H. W. (1984). Serotonin-immunoreactive neurons and their projections in the CNS. In *Handbook of Chemical Neuroanatomy*, ed. A. Bjorklund & T. Hokfelt. New York, NY: Elsevier, vol. 3, pp. 68–125.

Steininger, T. L., Wainer, B. H., Blakely, R. D. & Rye, D. B. (1997). Serotonergic dorsal raphe nucleus projections to the cholinergic and noncholinergic neurons of the pedunculopontine tegmental region: a light and electron microscopic anterograde tracing and immunohistochemical study. *J. Comp. Neurol.* **382**, 302–22.

Steininger, T. L., Alam, M. N., Gong, H., Szymusiak, R. & McGinty, D. (1999). Sleep-waking discharge of neurons in the posterior lateral hypothalamus of the albino rat. *Brain Res.* **840**, 138–47.

Sterman, M. B. & Clemente, C. D. (1962). Forebrain inhibitory mechanisms: Sleep patterns induced by basal forebrain stimulation in the behaving cat. *Exp. Neurol.* **6**, 103–17.

Strecker, R. E., Moriarty, S., Thakkar, M. M. *et al.* (2000). Adenosinergic modulation of basal forebrain and preoptic/anterior hypothalamic neuronal activity in the control of behavioral state. *Behav. Brain Res.* **115**, 183–204.

Szymusiak, R., Steininger, T., Alam, N. & McGinty, D. (2001). Preoptic area sleep-regulating mechanisms. *Arch. Ital. Biol.* **139**, 77–92.

Tagliamonte, A., Tagliamonte, P., Gessa, G. & Brodie, B. (1969). Compulsive sexual activity induced by p-chlorophenylalanine in normal and pinealectomized male rats. *Science* **166**, 1433–5.

Takakusaki, K., Shiroyama, T. & Kitai, S. T. (1997). Two types of cholinergic neurons in the rat tegmental pedunculopontine nucleus: electrophysiological and morphological characterization. *Neuroscience* **79**, 1089–109.

Tenen, S. (1967). The effects of p-chlorophenylalanine, a serotonin depletor on avoidance adquisition, pain sensitivity and related behavior in the rat. *Psychopharmacologia* **10**, 204–19.

Thakkar, M. M., Strecker, R. E. & McCarley, R. W. (1998). Behavioral state control through differential serotonergic inhibition of the mesopontine cholinergic nuclei: a simultaneous unit recording and microdialysis study. *J. Neurosci.* **18**, 5490–7.

Tissier, M. H., Franc, B., Hamon, M. & Adrien, J. (1990). Effects of 5-HT$_{1A}$ and 5-HT$_3$-receptor ligands on sleep in the rat. In *Sleep '90*, ed. J. Horne, pp. 126–8. Bochum: Pontenagel Press.

Thomas, D. R. & Hagan, J. J. (2004). 5-HT$_7$ receptors. *Curr. Drug Targets, CNS Neurol. Dis.* **3**, 81–90.

Thomas, D. R., Melotto, S., Massagrande, M. *et al.* (2003). SB-656104-A, a novel selective 5-HT$_7$ receptor antagonist, modulates REM sleep in rats. *Br. J. Pharmacol.* **139**, 705–14.

To, Z. P., Bonhaus, D. W., Eglen, R. M. & Jakeman, L. B. (1995). Characterization and distribution of putative 5-ht7 receptors in guinea-pig brain. *Br. J. Pharmacol.* **115**, 107–16.

Tobler, I. & Borbély, A. A. (1982). Sleep regulation after reduction of brain serotonin: effect of p-chlorophenylalanine combined with sleep deprivation in the rat. *Sleep* **5**, 145–53.

Tohyama, M. & Takatsuji, K. (1998). *Atlas of Neuroactive Substances and Their Receptors in the Rat.* Oxford: Oxford University Press.

Tortella, F. C., Echevarria, E., Pastel, R. H., Cox, B. & Blackburn, T. P. (1989). Suppressant effects of selective 5-HT$_2$ antagonists on rapid eye movement sleep in rats. *Brain Res.* **485**, 294–300.

Trulson, M. E. & Jacobs, B. L. (1979). Raphe unit activity in freely moving cats: correlation with level of behavioral arousal. *Brain Res.* **163**, 135–50.

Vanhoenacker, P., Haegeman, G. & Leysen, J. E. (2000). 5-HT$_7$ receptors: current knowledge and future prospects. *Trends Pharmacol. Sci.* **21**, 70–7.

Van Bockstaele, E. J., Biswas, A. & Pickel, V. M. (1993). Topography of serotonin neurons in the dorsal raphe nucleus that send axon collaterals to the rat prefrontal cortex and nucleus accumbens. *Brain Res.* **624**, 188–98.

Varnäs, K., Hurd, Y. L. & Hall, H. (2005). Regional expression of 5-HT$_{1B}$ receptor mRNA in the human brain. *Synapse* **56**, 21–8.

Vergé, D. & Calas, A. (2000). Serotoninergic neurons and serotonin receptors: gains from cytochemical approaches. *J. Chem. Neuroanat.* **18**, 41–56.

Vertes, R. P. (1991). A PHA-L analysis of ascending projections of the dorsal raphe nucleus in the rat. *J. Comp. Neurol.* **313**, 643–68.

Vertes, R. P. & Kocsis, B. (1994). Projections of the dorsal raphe nucleus to the brainstem: PHA-L analysis of the rat. *J. Comp. Neurol.* **340**, 11–26.

Vertes, R. P., Fortin, W. J. & Crane, A. M. (1999). Projections of the median raphe nucleus in the rat. *J. Comp. Neurol.* **407**, 555–82.

Waeber, C., Dietl, M. M., Hoyer, D. & Palacios, J. M. (1989). 5-HT$_1$ receptors in the vertebrate brain. Regional distribution examined by autoradiography. *Naunyn Schmiedebergs Arch. Pharmacol.* **340**, 486–94.

Waeber, C., Pinkus, L. M. & Palacios, J. M. (1990). The (S)-isomer of [^{3}H]zacopride labels 5-HT$_3$ receptors with high affinity in rat brain. *Eur. J. Pharmacol.* **181**, 283–7.

Wang, R. Y. & Aghajanian, G. K. (1977). Antidromically identified serotoninergic neurons in the rat midbrain raphe: evidence for collateral inhibition. *Brain Res.* **132**, 186–93.

Wang, Q. P., Ochiai, H. & Nakai, Y. (1992). GABAergic innervation of serotonergic neurons in the dorsal raphe nucleus of the rat studied by electron microscopy double immunostaining. *Brain Res. Bull.* **29**, 943–8.

Wolf, W. A. & Schutz, L. J. (1997). The serotonin 5-HT$_{2C}$ receptor is a prominent serotonin receptor in basal ganglia: evidence from functional studies on serotonin-mediated phosphoinositide hydrolysis. *J. Neurochem.* **69**, 1449–58.

Wyatt, R. J., Engelman, K., Kupfer, D. J. *et al.* (1969). Effects of parachloro-phenylalanine on sleep in man. *Electroencephalogr. Clin. Neurophysiol.* **27**, 529–32.

Zeitzer, J. M., Buckmaster, C. I., Parker, K. J. *et al.* (2003). Circadian and homeostatic regulation of hypocretin in a primate model: implications for the consolidation of wakefulness. *J. Neurosci.* **23**, 3555–60.

Zoltoski, R. K., Cabeza, R. J. & Gillin, J. C. (1999). Biochemical pharmacology of sleep. In *Sleep Disorders Medicine: Basic Sciences, Technical Considerations and Clinical Aspects*, ed. S. Chokroverty and R. B. Daroff, 2nd edn, pp. 63–94. Boston, MA: Butterworth – Heinemann.

III CHANGING PERSPECTIVES

10

Melatonin and its receptors: biological function in circadian sleep–wake regulation

DANIEL P. CARDINALI, S. R. PANDI-PERUMAL, AND
LENNARD P. NILES

Biosynthesis and metabolism of melatonin

Melatonin was isolated in 1958 by Lerner and his associates, its chemical nature being identified as N-acetyl-5-methoxytryptamine (Lerner *et al.* 1958, 1959) (Fig. 10.1). In vertebrates, melatonin is primarily secreted by the pineal gland. Synthesis also occurs in other cells and organs including the retina (Cardinali and Rosner 1971; Tosini and Menaker 1998; Liu *et al.* 2004), human and murine bone marrow cells (Conti *et al.* 2000), platelets (Champier *et al.* 1997), gastrointestinal tract (Bubenik 2002), skin (Slominski *et al.* 2005a,b), or lymphocytes (Carrillo-Vico *et al.* 2004). However, circulating melatonin is derived only from the pineal gland, as shown by its disappearance after pineal removal. Since there is no storage of melatonin in the pineal gland, and since the circulating melatonin is degraded rapidly by the liver, plasma levels of melatonin reflect pineal biosynthetic activity.

Melatonin secretion is synchronized to the light/dark (LD) cycle, with a nocturnal maximum (in young humans, about 200 pg/ml plasma) and low diurnal baseline levels (about 10 pg/ml plasma). Studies have supported the value of the exogenous administration of melatonin in circadian rhythm sleep disorders, insomnia, cancer, neurodegenerative diseases, disorders of the immune function, and oxidative damage (Karasek *et al.* 2002; Pandi-Perumal *et al.* 2005, 2006; Srinivasan *et al.* 2005a,b, 2006; Hardeland *et al.* 2006).

Neurochemistry of Sleep and Wakefulness, ed. J. M. Monti *et al.* Published by Cambridge University Press.
© Cambridge University Press 2008.

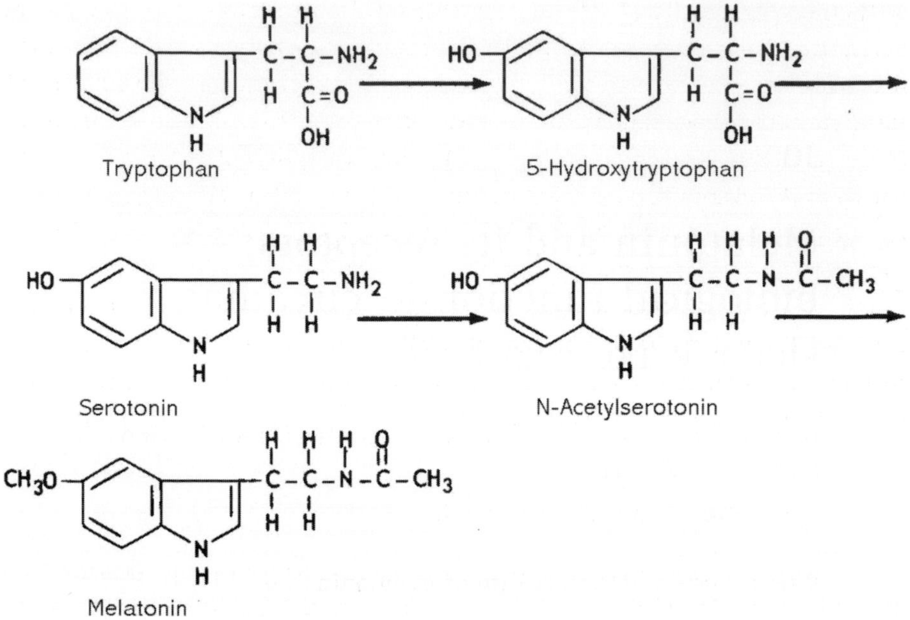

Figure 10.1 The biosynthesis of melatonin.

Soon after the identification of melatonin, Axelrod and co-workers demonstrated that the pinealocytes have the necessary enzymatic components for the biosynthesis of melatonin (Axelrod and Wurtman 1966; Axelrod 1974 p. 282). The sequence of events for the biosynthesis of melatonin is as follows (Fig. 10.1): (i) tryptophan is taken up from the circulation and is converted into serotonin; (ii) serotonin is converted into N-acetylserotonin by the SCN-regulated enzyme serotonin-N-acetyltransferase (NAT); (iii) N-acetylserotonin is converted to melatonin by the enzyme hydroxyindole-O-methyltransferase (HIOMT).

Once formed, melatonin is released into capillaries and can reach all tissues of the body within a very short period (Cardinali and Pevet 1998; Macchi and Bruce 2004). In the circulation, melatonin is bound to albumin (Cardinali *et al.* 1972). The secretion of melatonin occurs mainly during the night, with maximal plasma levels being found between 0200 and 0300 a.m. An episodic secretion of melatonin with peaks and troughs has also been noted (Claustrat *et al.* 1986, 2005). The half life of melatonin after intravenous infusion is about 30 min (Malloe *et al.* 1990) following a bi-exponential decay with first distribution half life of 2 min and a second metabolic half life of 20 min (Claustrat *et al.* 2005). A positron emission tomography study has shown that brain radioactivity is high within 6–8 min after injection of ^{11}C melatonin (Le Bars *et al.* 1991).

In the liver, melatonin is first hydroxylated and then conjugated with sulfate and glucuronide. In human urine, 6-sulphatoxymelatonin has been identified as the main metabolite. In the brain melatonin is metabolized into kynurenine derivatives (Hirata *et al.* 1974). It is of interest that the well-documented antioxidant properties of melatonin are shared by some of its metabolites, including cyclic 3-hydroxymelatonin, N^1-acetyl-N^2-formyl-5-methoxykynuramine (AFMK) (Tan *et al.* 2002, 2003; Allegra *et al.* 2003), and, with highest potency, N^1-acetyl-5-methoxykynuramine (AMK) (Ressmeyer *et al.* 2003; Silva *et al.* 2004). Contrary to initial claims in the literature that almost all melatonin is metabolized in the liver to 6-hydroxymelatonin followed by conjugation and excretion, recent estimates attribute about 30% of overall melatonin degradation to pyrrole ring cleavage (Ferry *et al.* 2005). The rate of AFMK formation may be even higher in certain tissues since extrahepatic P_{450} monooxygenase activities are frequently low and, consequently, smaller amounts of 6-hydroxymelatonin are produced.

Regulation of melatonin secretion

The circadian pattern of pineal NAT activity and consequently melatonin secretion is controlled by the suprachiasmatic nuclei (SCN) as it is abolished by lesions of the SCN, the major circadian oscillator (Klein and Moore 1979). Thus, the environmental L/D cycle acts as the pervasive and pre-eminent *Zeitgeber* that regulates melatonin synthesis (Scheer and Czeisler 2005).

The circadian activity of the SCN is synchronized to the LD cycle mainly by light through a monosynaptic retinohypothalamic tract originating from the ganglion cell layer in the retina and using glutamate as a neurotransmitter (Scheer and Czeisler 2005). Recently, it has been found that a subgroup of retinal ganglion cells containing melanopsin and that innervate the SCN are also involved in the photic transmission of light signals to the circadian clock (Berson *et al.* 2002). Light-induced suppression of pineal melatonin synthesis and secretion in humans has a peak sensitivity to short-wavelength light (446–477 nm) (Brainard *et al.* 2001). Melatonin secretion is suppressed by light intensities ranging from outdoor levels to, under certain circumstances, those seen indoors (Brainard *et al.* 2001; Lewy *et al.* 1980; McIntyre *et al.* 1989).

Animal studies have shown that the neural pathway connecting the SCN with the pineal gland starts with a γ-aminobutyric acid (GABA)-ergic projection from the SCN to the paraventricular nucleus (PVN) (Kalsbeek *et al.* 2000). Indeed, physiological and immunohistochemical studies have revealed that GABA is the principal transmitter in SCN cells (Cardinali and Golombek 1998). Efferent fibers from the PVN go through the medial forebrain bundle and reticular formation and make synaptic connections with the cells of the intermediolateral columns of the cervical spinal cord, from where preganglionic sympathetic fibers arise and project to the superior cervical ganglia (Moore 1996). NE release is inhibited by exposure to light (that stimulates the SCN) whereas its release is augmented during darkness, when the SCN is inhibited (Gerdin *et al.* 2004).

Norepinephrine (NE), by binding to β-adrenergic receptors on the pinealocytes, activates adenylate cyclase, via the α-subunit of G_s-protein. The increase in cAMP promotes the synthesis of proteins, among them the melatonin-synthesizing enzymes and in particular the rate-limiting NAT (Klein 2004). Melatonin synthesis in the pineal gland is also influenced by neuropeptides, such as vasoactive intestinal peptide, pituitary adenylate cyclase-activating peptide, and neuropeptide Y, which are partially co-released and seem to potentiate the NE response (Karolczak *et al.* 2005). Other receptors, e.g. for steroid hormones, are present in the pineal gland and may underlie the correlation that melatonin rhythm has with those of the reproductive hormones (Cardinali 1977; Vacas *et al.* 1979; Haldar and Gupta 1990; Luboshitzky *et al.* 1997; Sanchez *et al.* 2004).

Upregulation of melatonin formation is complex and also involves NAT activation by cAMP-dependent phosphorylation and NAT stabilization by a 14-3-3 protein (Hardeland *et al.* 2006). It is also subject to feedback mechanisms by cAMP-dependent inducible 3′,5′-cyclic adenosine monophosphate early repressor (ICER) expression and Ca^{2+}-dependent formation of DREAM (downstream regulatory element antagonist modulator) (Hardeland *et al.* 2006; Karolczak *et al.* 2005). Once formed, melatonin is not stored within the pineal gland but diffuses out into the capillary blood and cerebrospinal fluid (CSF) (Tricoire *et al.* 2003). Melatonin released to the CSF via the pineal recess attains concentrations in the third ventricle that are up to 20–30 times higher than those in blood. However, these concentrations rapidly diminish with increasing distance from the pineal gland (Tricoire *et al.* 2003), thus suggesting that melatonin is taken up by brain tissue.

The timing, duration, and amount of nocturnal melatonin production exhibit considerable interindividual differences (Macchi and Bruce 2004). There is greater than 10-fold variability in nocturnal melatonin concentrations among individuals (Zeitzer *et al.* 1999). A genetic cause of this variability is suggested by the lower variability found in siblings compared with the general population (Griefahn *et al.* 2003). Pineal melatonin production was shown to be independent of sleep deprivation (von Treuer *et al.* 1996). By applying deconvolution analysis to plasma melatonin concentration time series, Geoffriau and co-workers calculated a nocturnal melatonin production rate of 10–80 micrograms per night (Geoffriau *et al.* 1999).

Melatonin metabolism

Circulating melatonin is metabolized mainly in the liver, where it is first hydroxylated in the C6-position by cytochrome P_{450} monooxygenases (isoenzymes

CYP1A2, CYP1A1, and to a lesser extent CYP1B1) and thereafter conjugated with sulfate to be excreted as 6-sulphatoxymelatonin; glucuronide conjugation is extremely limited (Zeitzer *et al.* 1999). CYP2C19 and, at lower rates, CYP1A2 also demethylate melatonin to its precursor *N*-acetylserotonin, being otherwise its precursor (Ma *et al.* 2005). The metabolism in extrahepatic tissues exhibits substantial differences. Tissues of neural origin, including the pineal gland and retina, contain melatonin-deacetylating enzymes, which are either specific melatonin deacetylases (Hardeland *et al.* 1996) or less specific aryl acylamidases; since eserine-sensitive acetylcholinesterase has an aryl acylamidase side activity, melatonin can be deacetylated to 5-methoxytryptamine in any tissue carrying this enzyme (Hardeland *et al.* 1993, 1996).

Melatonin can be metabolized non-enzymatically in all cells, and extracellularly by free radicals and a few other oxidants. It is converted into cyclic 3-hydroxymelatonin when it directly scavenges two hydroxyl radicals (Tan *et al.* 1998). In the brain, a substantial fraction of melatonin is metabolized to kynuramine derivatives (Hirata *et al.* 1974). AFMK is produced by numerous non-enzymatic and enzymatic mechanisms (Hardeland *et al.* 2006); its formation by myeloperoxidase appears to be important in quantitative terms (Ferry *et al.* 2005).

Mechanism of action of melatonin

Inasmuch as melatonin diffuses easily through biological membranes, it can exert actions in almost every cell in the body. Some of its effects are receptor-mediated, whereas others are receptor-independent. Melatonin is involved in various physiological functions such as sleep propensity (Wurtman and Zhdanova 1995; Lavie 197; Zisapel 2001), control of sleep/wake rhythm (Doolen *et al.* 1998), blood pressure regulation (Doolen *et al.* 1998; Scheer *et al.* 2004), immune function (Guerrero and Reither 2002; Esquifino *et al.* 2004), circadian rhythm regulation (Armstrong 1989), retinal functions (Iuvone *et al.* 2005), detoxification of free radicals (Reiter *et al.* 2005), control of tumor growth (Blask *et al.* 2005), bone protection (Cardinali *et al.* 2003), and the regulation of bicarbonate secretion in the gastrointestinal tract (Bubenik 2002). Melatonin action involves interaction with specific receptors in the cell membrane (Dubocovich *et al.* 2000), with nuclear receptors (Carlberg and Wiesenberg 1995; Wiesenberg *et al.* 1998) and with intracellular proteins such as calmodulin (Anton-Tay *et al.* 1998; Benitez-King *et al.* 1996), dihydronicotinamide riboside:quinone reductase 2 (Mailliet *et al.* 2004), or tubulin-associated proteins (Cardinali *et al.* 1997). In addition, melatonin is a potent antioxidant, acting as a free radical scavenger as well as via induction of antioxidant enzymes, downregulation of pro-oxidant enzymes, or stabilization of mitochondrial membranes (Karasek *et al.* 2002; Pandi-Perumal *et al.* 2005, 2006; Srinivasan *et al.* 2005a,b, 2006; Hardeland *et al.* 2006).

Several major actions of melatonin are mediated by the membrane receptors MT_1 and MT_2 (Dubocovich *et al.* 2000; Reppert *et al.* 1994, 1995). They belong to the superfamily of G-protein-coupled receptors containing the typical seven transmembrane domains. These receptors are responsible for chronobiological effects in the SCN, the circadian pacemaker. MT_2 mainly acts by inducing phase shifts and MT_1 by suppressing neuronal firing activity. MT_1 and MT_2 are also expressed in peripheral organs and cells and contribute, for example, to several immunological actions or to vasomotor control (Dubocovich and Markowska 2005).

A third binding site, initially described as MT_3, has been subsequently characterized as the enzyme quinone reductase 2 (Nosjean *et al.* 2000). Quinone reductases participate in the protection against oxidative stress by preventing electron transfer reactions of quinones (Foster *et al.* 2000). Melatonin also binds to nuclear receptors of the retinoic acid receptor family, $ROR\alpha1$, $ROR\alpha2$, and $RZR\beta$ (Carlberg 2000). $ROR\alpha1$ and $ROR\alpha2$ seem to be involved in some aspects of immune modulation, whereas $RZR\beta$ is expressed in the central nervous system, including the pineal gland. Direct inhibition of the mitochondrial permeability transition pore by melatonin (Andrabi *et al.* 2004) may indicate that another, mitochondrial binding site is involved, although at the present time this has not been confirmed.

The melatonin MT_1 and MT_2 receptors mediate inhibition of the adenylate cyclase – cAMP pathway via pertussis-toxin-sensitive G_i proteins. In addition, the MT_1 receptor mediates the potentiating effect of melatonin on phospholipase C activation and arachidonate release following PGF_{2a} treatment (von Gall *et al.* 2002). This effect of melatonin is also sensitive to pertussis toxin, suggesting involvement of an inhibitory G protein. Similarly, the phase-shifting effect of melatonin on the firing rate rhythm in the SCN involves activation of protein kinase C (PKC), via a pertussis-toxin-sensitive pathway (Hunt *et al.* 2001). Melatonin has been reported to stimulate the mitogen-activated protein kinase – extracellular regulated kinase (ERK) pathway in MT_1-transfected Chinese hamster ovary (CHO) cells (Witt-Enderby *et al.* 2000) and in the mouse GT1-7 neuronal cell line, which expresses this receptor (Roy and Belsham 2002), indicating that the MT_1 receptor subtype is involved.

Recent studies in a model of ischemic stroke suggest that the acute neuroprotective effect of melatonin involves activation of the phosphatidylinositol-3-kinase/Akt pathway, whereas ERK-1/2 and c-Jun N-terminal kinase-1/2, in addition to Akt signaling, appear to be involved in its long-term effects (Kilic *et al.* 2005). These results indicate that melatonin can interact with multiple cellular pathways to produce its diverse physiological effects. Moreover, MT_1 and MT_2 receptors can interact with divergent signaling pathways, as shown by their ability to mediate stimulation or inhibition of GABAergic activity in the rat brain, respectively (Wan *et al.* 1999), or to couple to multiple G proteins (Brydon *et al.* 1999). In keeping with this view, the MT_2 but not the MT_1 receptor subtype is reportedly coupled to the cGMP pathway (Brydon *et al.* 2001).

Regulation of melatonin receptors

Several studies have demonstrated that exposure of receptors to their agonists results in desensitization so that there is a reduced response to subsequent stimulation. This attenuation of subsequent responses to a hormone or drug may be classified as either homologous (agonist-specific) or heterologous (agonist-non-specific) desensitization, and it may be due to various mechanisms including receptor phosphorylation, sequestration, and downregulation (Hausdorff *et al.* 1990). In accordance with the foregoing, a diurnal rhythm in the density of high-affinity receptors for melatonin, which is inversely related to its circulating levels, was observed in hamster and rat brain membranes (Vacas and Cardinali 1979) and in rat basal hypothalamic membranes containing the SCN (Tenn and Niles 1993). Thus, high-affinity binding was highest late in the light phase, following prolonged depletion of the endogenous agonist, and lowest during darkness when exposure to elevated melatonin concentrations presumably downregulated the high-affinity receptor (Vacas and Cardinali 1979; Tenn and Niles 1993). Similarly, a significant increase in high-affinity binding has been observed in the pars tuberalis/median eminence of rats sacrificed at the end of the light phase (when melatonin levels are low) compared with animals sacrificed in the morning (Vanecek *et al.* 1990). Suppression or depletion of circulating melatonin levels, by exposure to constant light or pinealectomy, caused a significant increase in the density of high-affinity sites in rat brain membranes (Cardinali and Vacas 1980) as well as in the pars tuberalis of the rat and hamster (Gauer *et al.* 1992). Conversely, a single injection of melatonin reversed the effect of constant light or pinealectomy on high-affinity binding in the rat pars tuberalis and SCN (Gauer *et al.* 1993). Moreover, preincubation of cultured ovine PT cells in the presence of melatonin (100 pM or 1 μM) for 24 h resulted in a significant decrease in melatonin binding in crude PT membranes (Hazlerigg *et al.* 1993).

The foregoing indicates that physiological concentrations of melatonin are involved in the homologous downregulation of its high-affinity G-protein-coupled receptors. However, other agents such as neurotransmitters, hormones, or clinically administered drugs may also be involved in the regulation of these receptors. For example, the potent steroid hormone 17β-estradiol causes a significant increase in the density of binding sites for the radiolabeled agonist

2-[^{125}I]iodomelatonin, in CHO cells transfected with the human MT$_2$ receptor and attenuates melatonin signalling via the human MT$_1$ subtype (Masana *et al.* 2005). Other recent studies show that valproic acid (VPA; 2-propylpentanoic acid), a short-chain branched fatty acid widely used as an anticonvulsant and mood stabilizer, can upregulate the MT$_1$ receptor in rat C6 glioma cells (Castro *et al.* 2005). VPA is known to increase the levels of GABA via stimulation of its biosynthesis while inhibiting enzymes involved in GABA degradation (Gould *et al.* 2002). There is evidence for an interaction between melatonin and GABAergic systems with implications for diverse aspects of brain function including sleep regulation (Rosenstein and Cardinali 1990; Golombek *et al.* 1996; Tenn and Niles 2002; Niles 2006). However, preliminary experiments with the GABAergic antagonist bicuculline do not support a GABAergic mechanism for induction of MT$_1$ receptors in C6 cells, which may lack functional GABA receptors (Castro *et al.* 2005). None the less, these novel findings raise interesting questions about the potential role of melatonin and its receptors in the diverse clinical effects of VPA. For example, it is possible that the anticonvulsant and mood-stabilizing effects of VPA may be enhanced by melatonin, as this hormone has been implicated in both of these areas (de Lima *et al.* 2005; Weil *et al.* 2006). Interestingly, add-on melatonin has been reported to improve sleep behavior in epileptic children treated with VPA (Gupta *et al.* 2005). As suggested by the authors, this approach may be useful in pediatric epilepsy, which is associated with sleep disorders.

Melatonin and human sleep

The finding that melatonin is secreted primarily during the night (Lynch *et al.* 1975), and the close relationship between the nocturnal increase of endogenous melatonin and the timing of human sleep, prompted many investigators to suggest that melatonin is involved in the regulation of sleep. The onset of night phase melatonin secretion occurs approximately 2 h before habitual bedtime and has been shown to correlate well with the onset of evening sleepiness (Tzischinksy *et al.* 1993; Zhdanova and Tucci 2003; Zhdanova *et al.* 1996). Suppression of melatonin production by procedures such as treatment with β-blockers has been shown to correlate with insomnia (Brismar *et al.* 1987, 1988; Van Den Heuvel *et al.* 1997). Conversely, increasing plasma melatonin concentrations by suppressing melatonin-metabolizing enzymes in the liver resulted in increased sleepiness (Hartter *et al.* 2001).

In a study conducted by Haimov & Lavie (Haimov and Lavie 1997) a temporal relation between the nocturnal increase of endogenous melatonin and "opening of the sleep gate" was found in all their subjects except one. After administration of melatonin in the afternoon, the sleep gate was advanced by 1–2 h, whereas exposure to 2 h of evening bright light between 08:00 and 10:00 p.m. delayed the subsequent rise in the nocturnal concentration of melatonin and the opening of the sleep gate (Haimov and Lavie 1997). The period of wakefulness immediately prior to the opening of the sleep gate is referred to as the wake-maintenance zone or "forbidden zone" for sleep (Strogatz *et al.* 1986; Lavie 1986]; during this time the sleep propensity is lowest, owing to the increased activity of SCN neurons (Buysse *et al.* 2004; Long *et al.* 2005). The transition phase from wakefulness and arousal to high sleep propensity coincides with the nocturnal rise in endogenous melatonin (Dijk and Cajochen 1997). It was therefore proposed that melatonin contributes to the opening of the gate of nocturnal sleepiness by inhibiting the circadian wakefulness-generating mechanism (Lavie 1997; Birkeland 1982; Sack *et al.* 1997). This effect is thought to be mediated by MT_1 receptors at the SCN level (Hunt *et al.* 2001; Liu *et al.* 1997). Melatonin is released in pulses during stages of light sleep and its function is to induce deep sleep and to prevent awakening by inhibiting the firing of SCN neurons.

Effects of exogenous melatonin administration on human sleep

Lerner (1960), in an attempt to treat patients suffering from vertigo, administered his newly discovered substance melatonin, and noticed that the patients became sleepy (Lerner and Case 1960). This was the first report of the sleep-promoting effects of melatonin in humans. By using polysomnography to study the change in sleep processes, Anton-Tay *et al.* (Anton-Tay *et al.* 1971) and Cramer *et al.* (Cramer *et al.* 1974), found that the administration of melatonin in pharmacological doses induced sleep with no significant changes in sleep architecture or side effects. An interesting fact that emerged from those studies, which employed very high doses of melatonin, was that they did not cause uncontrollable sedation or general anesthesia. The hypnotic effects of pharmacological doses (i.e. greater than 1 mg) of melatonin administered during the daytime has been confirmed by many investigators (Vollrath *et al.* 1981; Waldhauser *et al.* 1990; Dollins *et al.* 1993; Nave *et al.* 1995; Hughes and Badia 1997; Cajochen *et al.* 1998; Satomura *et al.* 2001). The ingestion of melatonin (0.1–0.3 mg) during the daytime, which increased the circulating melatonin levels to those usually observed during the night, also caused sleep induction (Dollins *et al.* 1994).

A reduced endogenous melatonin production seems to be a prerequisite for effective exogenous melatonin treatment of sleep disorders. A recent meta-analysis of the effects of melatonin in sleep disturbances, including all age groups, and presumably individuals with normal melatonin levels, failed to document significant and clinically meaningful effects of exogenous melatonin on sleep quality, efficiency, or latency (Buscemi *et al.* 2006). It must be noted that a statistically non-significant finding indicates that the alternative hypothesis (i.e. melatonin is effective in decreasing sleep onset latency) is not likely to be true, but that the null hypothesis might be false (which in this case is that melatonin has no effect on sleep onset latency) because of the possibility of a type II error. By combining several studies, meta-analyses provide better size effect estimates and reduce the probability of a type II error, making false negative results less likely. Nonetheless, this seems not to be the case in the study of Buscemi *et al.* (Buscemi *et al.* 2006). Firstly, sample size was fewer than 300 subjects. The papers reviewed showed significant variations in the route of administration of melatonin, the dose administered, and the way in which outcomes were measured. All of these drawbacks resulted in a significant heterogeneity index and in a low-quality size effect estimation, which was shown by the wide 95% confidence intervals reported (Buscemi *et al.* 2006).

In contrast, another meta-analysis undertaken by Brzezinski *et al.*, using 17 different studies involving 284 subjects, most of whom were older, concluded that melatonin is effective in increasing sleep efficiency and reducing sleep onset time (Brzezinski *et al.* 2005). Based on this meta-analysis the use of melatonin in the treatment of insomnia, particularly in aged individuals with nocturnal melatonin deficiency, was proposed.

The sedative or hypnotic effect of melatonin is dependent on the time of day when it is administered, according to the phase of the endogenous circadian oscillator. In a double-blind, placebo-controlled study on healthy human subjects, the effects of melatonin (0.1–10 mg) given at 11:30 p.m. on nocturnal sleep were compared with those of melatonin administered at 06:00 p.m. (Stone *et al.* 2000). EEG analysis, recording of core body temperature, and cognitive performance were all evaluated. Night phase administration of melatonin (1130 p.m.) had no significant effect on nocturnal sleep in healthy subjects whereas administration of melatonin at 06:00 p.m. had significant hypnotic activity. Assessment of the hypnotic action of melatonin during daytime administration and its comparison with triazolam indicated that a 6 mg dose of melatonin demonstrated hypnotic effects that were nearly equal to those of triazolam at 0.125 mg. Rectal temperature was significantly decreased by melatonin (Satomura *et al.* 2001). In another placebo-controlled and double-blind study with a cross-over design including temazepam (20 mg), the hypnotic activity of melatonin administered in the early evening (presumably in the absence of endogenous melatonin) was similar to that of 20 mg temazepam (Stone *et al.* 2000; Gilbert *et al.* 1999).

In another study (Tzischinsky and Lavie 1994), melatonin (5 mg) was administered four times during the day, at 12:00 a.m., 05:00 p.m., 07:00 p.m., and 09:00 p.m. Melatonin significantly increased sleep propensity at each time point as demonstrated by EEG measures, including increases in theta, delta, and spindle bursts. The subjective reports of sleepiness also increased following melatonin administration. However, the latency to maximal hypnotic effect varied linearly from 3 h 40 min at noon to 1 h after administration at 09:00 p.m. The time dependency of the hypnotic effects of melatonin has also been noted in other studies showing that melatonin administered at noon or in the early or late afternoon significantly promoted sleep onset in healthy subjects (Zhdanova et al. 1995, 1996; Terlo et al. 1997). Possibly, these variations indicate that the endogenous rise in melatonin at night obliterates the effects of the exogenously administered melatonin in healthy adults.

The circadian effects of melatonin in shifting the biological oscillator are manifested in its effects on the timing of sleep. Morning administration delays the onset of evening sleepiness; evening administration of melatonin advances sleep onset and other circadian rhythms (Lewy 1999). In a recent study (Rajaratnam et al. 2004) the phase shifting effect of prolonged-release melatonin (1.5 mg) given in the afternoon on polysomnographically recorded sleep was examined with special emphasis on the effects of melatonin on homeostatic sleep regulation. The results indicated that melatonin exerted both a direct (i.e. hypnotic) and circadian effect on sleep (Rajaratnam et al. 2004). The mean peak plasma melatonin concentration achieved was 626 pg/ml, approximately 10 times higher than the endogenous nocturnal peak level.

Phase-shifting by melatonin is attributed to its action at MT_2 receptors present in the SCN (Liu et al. 1997). The chronobiological effect of melatonin is due to its direct influence on the electrical and metabolic activity of the SCN, a finding that has been confirmed both in vivo and in vitro. The application of melatonin directly to the SCN significantly increases the amplitude of the melatonin peak, thereby suggesting that in addition to its phase-shifting effect melatonin directly acts on the amplitude of the oscillations (Pevet et al. 2002). However, this amplitude modulation seems to be unrelated to clock gene expression in the SCN (Poirel et al. 2003).

A number of studies have investigated the potential of melatonin to alleviate the symptoms of jet lag. Melatonin has been found to be effective in 11 placebo-controlled studies in reducing the subjective symptoms of jet lag such as sleepiness and impaired alertness (Arendt 2005). The most severe health effects of jet lag occur following eastbound flights, since this requires a phase advancement of the biological clock. In a recent study, phase advancement after melatonin administration (using 3 mg doses just before bedtime) occurred in all 11 subjects travelling from Tokyo to Los Angeles, as well as faster resynchronization, compared with controls. Melatonin increased the phase shift from about 1.1 to 1.4 h/day, causing complete entrainment of 7–8 h after 5 days of melatonin intake (Takahashi *et al.* 2000). Melatonin has been found useful in causing a 50% reduction in subjective assessment of jet lag symptoms in 474 subjects taking 5 mg fast-release tablets (Arendt 2005). Therefore, with few exceptions, compelling evidence indicates that melatonin is useful for ameliorating jet lag symptoms in air travellers [cf. meta-analysis at Cochrane Data Base (Herxheimer and Petrie 2002)].

One of us examined the timely use of three factors (melatonin treatment, exposure to light, physical exercise) to hasten the resynchronization of the sleep–wake cycle in a group of elite sports competitors after a transmeridian flight across 12 time zones (Cardinali *et al.* 2002). Outdoor light exposure and physical exercise were used to cover symmetrically the phase delay and the phase advance portions of the phase–response curve. Melatonin taken at local bedtime helped to resynchronize the circadian oscillator to the new time. Individual actograms taken from sleep log data showed that all subjects became synchronized in their sleep to the local time in 24–48 h, well in advance of what would be expected in the absence of any treatment (Cardinali *et al.* 2002). More recently, a retrospective analysis of the data obtained from 134 normal volunteers flying the Buenos Aires – Sydney transpolar route in the past 9 years was published; this further supports such a role for exogenous melatonin in resynchronization of sleep cycles (Cardinal! *et al.* 2006).

A number of clinical studies have now made use of the phase advancing property of melatonin for treating delayed sleep phase syndrome (DSPS). Melatonin, at a 5 mg dose, has been found beneficial in advancing the sleep onset time and wake time in DSPS subjects (Dahlitz *et al.* 1991; Nagtegaal *et al.* 1998; Kayumov *et al.* 2001). Melatonin was found to be effective when given five hours before its endogenous onset or seven hours before sleep onset.

Circadian rhythmicity is disrupted with age at several levels of biological organization (Pandi-Perumal *et al.* 2005). Age-related changes in the circadian system result in a decreased amplitude of the circadian rhythm of sleep and waking under a 12:12 LD cycle, as well as phase advance of several circadian rhythms. Melatonin administration at various doses (from 0.5 to 6.0 mg) has been found beneficial in improving subjective and objective sleep parameters (Olde Rikkert and Rigaud 2001). The beneficial effects of melatonin could be due to either its somnogenic or its phase shifting effects, or both. The efficacy of melatonin for entraining "free running" circadian rhythms in blind people has also been demonstrated.

Neuropharmacological mechanisms involved in sleep modulation by melatonin

Several studies have demonstrated that large doses of melatonin, which greatly exceed the endogenous levels of this hormone, produce sedative/hypnotic effects (Brzezinski *et al.* 2005) and can alleviate the symptoms of jet lag in humans (Herxheimer and Petrie 2002). At these pharmacological doses, melatonin could directly interact with benzodiazepine (BZD) receptors, which are allosterically linked to modulation of GABAergic activity via the BZ–GABA$_A$ receptor complex (Tenn and Niles 2002; Niles and Peace 1990). For example, melatonin competes for (^{3}H)diazepam binding sites in rat, human and bovine brain membranes with micromolar affinity (Niles 1991). Similarly, pharmacological doses of melatonin act on BZ-GABA$_A$ receptors to enhance both in vitro and in vivo binding of GABA, and to inhibit allosterically the binding of the caged convulsant t-butylbicyclophosphorothionate (TBPS) on GABA-gated chloride channels in rat brain (Niles and Peace 1990). In addition, pharmacological studies have shown that the anxiolytic, anticonvulsant, and other psychotropic actions of melatonin, which are similar to those exhibited by BZDs, involve the enhancement of GABAergic activity (Golombek *et al.* 1993, 1996; Golombek and Cardinali 1993; Tenn and Niles 1995). It is thought that GABA binds to specific sites at the interface of the α and β subunits on the BZ/GABA$_A$ receptor complex to induce opening of chloride channels, with consequent membrane hyperpolarization and neuronal inhibition (Sigel and Buhr 1997). Central-type BZDs, such as clonazepam, bind to other sites on the BZ/GABA$_A$ receptor complex, to enhance GABAergic activity allosterically. The binding site for melatonin on the BZ-GABA$_A$ receptor complex is not known, but its ability to competitively inhibit [^{3}H]diazepam binding suggests a direct interaction within the BZD binding pocket, which is located at the α/γ subunit interface of the BZ-GABA$_A$ receptor complex (Sigel and Buhr 1997; Baumann *et al.* 2003). In view of the importance of GABAergic mechanisms in sleep modulation, it is likely that the sedative effects of pharmacological doses of melatonin involve its allosteric interaction with BZ-GABA$_A$ receptors. This view is supported by evidence that BZ-GABA$_A$ antagonists block the sleep inducing effect of pharmacological doses of melatonin in experimental animals (Wang *et al.* 2003).

In addition to its interaction with central BZD receptors, pharmacological concentrations of melatonin can also bind to the peripheral-type BZ receptors (PBRs), which are involved in neurosteroidogenesis (Garcia-Ovejero *et al.* 2005). PBRs are primarily localized on the outer mitochondrial membrane; these sites are therefore also referred to as mitochondrial BZD receptors. Using the isoquinoline carboxamide, PK14105, for photoaffinity labelling, an 18 kDa isoquinoline binding protein (IBP) has been localized in diverse tissues that express PBRs. The melatonin binding site on the PBR complex is not known; however, it is reasonable to assume an interaction with the IBP subunit, where both isoquino-lines and BZDs are thought to bind (Joseph-Liauzun *et al.* 1997). Neurosteroids, which appear to be primarily produced by astrocytes (Zwain and Yen 1999), can exert potent modulatory effects on ion-gated neurotransmitter receptors, including the $GABA_A$ receptor complex (Mellon and Griffin 2002). Therefore, the pharmacological activation of PBRs by melatonin, with potential changes in neurosteroid production, provides another pathway for the pharmacological modulation of GABAergic activity by this hormone. Moreover, the ability of phar-macological concentrations of melatonin or BZDs to inhibit the AC-cAMP path-way via putative G protein-coupled BZ receptors (Tenn and Niles 1997) suggests yet another neuropharmacological mechanism for modulation of GABAergic activity.

In addition to the effects of pharmacological doses of melatonin, it is now known that relatively low doses of this hormone, equivalent to normal noc-turnal levels, can also promote sleep in humans (Dollins *et al.* 1994). In con-trast to the above data, the effects of these lower doses are not mediated by BZD receptors, as shown by the lack of antagonism by the central-type BZD antagonist, flumazenil (Nave *et al.* 1996). Although the physiological mechanisms underlying modulation of sleep by melatonin await clarification, an interaction with GABAergic systems appears to be implicated. There is *in vivo* electrophys-iological evidence that nanomolar concentrations of melatonin can potentiate GABAergic inhibition of neuronal activity in the mammalian cortex (Stankov *et al.* 1992). More recently, in vitro studies have indicated that the MT_1 receptor is coupled to stimulation of GABAergic activity in the hypothalamus, whereas the MT_2 receptor mediates an opposite effect in the hippocampus (Wan *et al.* 1999). Given the dominant inhibitory role of GABA in the central nervous sys-tem (CNS), the modulation of $GABA_A$ receptor function by melatonin appears to be the primary mechanism underlying its physiological effects on neuronal activity in the SCN and other brain areas. The primary effect of melatonin in the rat SCN appears to be inhibition of neuronal activity (Shibata *et al.* 1989; Stehle *et al.* 1989), which is consistent with the relatively high expression of the MT_1 subtype in the circadian clock and the fact that this receptor is linked to enhancement of GABAergic activity (Wan *et al.* 1999).

Immunohistochemical and electrophysiological studies of the hypothalamic preoptic area (POA), which plays a major role in sleep promotion, have identi-fied a subset of sleep-active ventrolateral POA (VLPO) neurons (Sherin *et al.* 1996; Szymusiak *et al.* 1998). A tightly clustered group of VLPO neurons appears to pro-mote non-REM sleep, by suppression of the histaminergic arousal system, which originates in the tuberomammillary nucleus of the posterior hypothalamus. Furthermore, a diffuse subgroup of VLPO neurons are thought to promote REM sleep through their inhibitory projection to monoaminergic dorsal raphe (serotonergic) and locus coeruleus (noradrenergic) nuclei in the brainstem (Lu *et al.* 2000). The inhibitory projections from the VLPO, to the histaminergic, serotonergic and noradrenergic components of the arousal system, utilize GABA and galanin which are present in nearly 80% of VLPO neurons (Sherin *et al.* 1998). In view of the ability of melatonin to modulate GABAergic activity, it is possible that VLPO neurons are activated by this hormone with consequent suppression of arousal systems and sleep induction. Such a scenario presumes that the G protein-coupled melatonin receptors that potentiate GABAergic activity are expressed on VLPO neurons. Studies with MT_1 receptor-deficient mice have demonstrated that this receptor subtype mediates acute physiological inhibition of spontaneous neuronal firing in the SCN (Liu *et al.* 1997). In addition, as noted above, the MT_1 receptor is coupled to stimulation of GABAergic activity in the SCN (Wan *et al.* 1999). Although these studies focused on the SCN, where MT_1 expression is relatively enriched, it is now known that this widely expressed receptor is present in hypothalamic areas outside the SCN and also in other mammalian or human CNS regions (Mazzucchelli *et al.* 1996; Al-Ghoul *et al.* 1998; Uz *et al.* 2005), which supports the possibility that melatonin acts directly on VLPO neurons to influence sleep. None the less, current evidence suggests that the SCN is the major hypothalamic target for melatonin, which acts at the predominantly expressed MT_1 receptor to acutely inhibit neuronal activity via enhancement of GABAergic activity (Wan *et al.* 1999). In addition, melatonin can activate an outward potassium current via G protein-coupled Kir3 channels in SCN neurons (Nelson *et al.* 1996; van den Pol *et al.* 2001), which would further inhibit neuronal activity, with associated sleep induction.

The effects of melatonin on SCN activity and sleep induction presumably involve the targets innervated by SCN efferents in various diencephalic regions, including the medial preoptic area (MPA), the dorsomedial hypothalamic nucleus (DMH) and the subparaventricular zone (Pace-Schott and Hobson 2002; Saper *et al.* 2005). These SCN targets, especially the MPA and DMH, which project to the VLPO, allow the SCN to regulate sleep promotion indirectly through the VLPO. In addition, the SCN is thought to have direct monosynaptic projections to the VLPO (Sun *et al.* 2000), although these are fewer than its efferents to the MPA and DMH (Saper *et al.* 2005). Since the predominant effect of melatonin in the SCN is suppression of neuronal GABAergic activity, this action presumably results in disinhibition of the MPA and DMH, which can then activate sleep-promoting neurons in the VLPO. This indirect activation of VLPO neurons

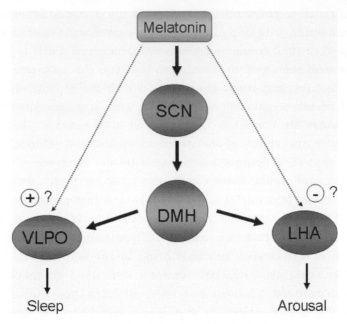

Figure 10.2 The suprachiasmatic nuclei (SCN) and other possible diencephalic targets for melatonin in sleep regulation. See text for details. VLPO, ventrolateral preoptic area; DMH, dorsomedial hypothalamus; LHA, lateral hypothalamic area.

may be augmented by further melatonin-induced disinhibition in the direct SCN–VLPO projection. The consequent activation of GABAergic projections from the VLPO would then induce sleep by inhibiting activity in the monoaminergic arousal system (Gervasoni *et al.* 1998). Other sites and/or mechanisms may also be involved in the sleep-promoting effects of melatonin. For example, this lipophilic hormone, which easily crosses cellular membranes, may inhibit the activity of intracellular targets such as Ca^{2+}/calmodulin-dependent kinase II (Benitez-King *et al.* 1996), with consequent changes in histaminergic, serotonergic, or noradrenergic neuronal activity in the arousal system, resulting in sleep. The hypocretin/ orexin system in the lateral hypothalamus, which is involved in arousal state control and sleep–wake regulation (Saper *et al.* 2005), may be influenced by melatonin acting via either membrane-bound G-protein-coupled receptors or intracellular targets, to modulate neuronal activity and promote sleep. The SCN and other possible diencephalic targets for melatonin in sleep regulation are illustrated in Fig. 10.2.

There is evidence that multiple kinases can phosphorylate several $GABA_A$ receptor subunits, to alter GABAergic activity in the brain (Browning *et al.* 1993; Poisbeau *et al.* 1999). Depending on the brain area and /or the receptor subunits involved, phosphorylation by kinases can result in either activation or inhibition of GABAergic function. For example, tyrosine phosphorylation, induced by intra-cellular application of protein tyrosine kinase (PTK), has been found to increase $GABA_A$-mediated currents in cultured CNS neurons (Wan et al. 1997). In contrast, protein kinase A (PKA)-induced phosphorylation of the $GABA_A$ receptor is usually associated with $GABA_A$ receptor desensitization in various CNS areas, and results in decreased GABAergic activity (Browning et al. 1993). Therefore, suppression of cAMP production by melatonin, which results in a decrease in PKA-induced phos-phorylation, may produce an opposite potentiating effect on GABAergic activ-ity with enhancement of sleep induction. Ca^{2+}/calmodulin-dependent kinase II, which is inhibited by physiological concentrations of melatonin (Benitez-King et al. 1996), can phosphorylate and modify $GABA_A$ receptor function (Churn et al. 2002). Various PKC isozymes have been reported to play critical roles in the regulation of $GABA_A$ receptor function and trafficking (Song and Messing 2005). Moreover, PKC-induced phosphorylation of $GABA_A$ subunits can alter the sensitivity of this receptor complex to allosteric modulators including neuros-teroids. Thus, the possible activation of the PKC pathway by melatonin via the MT_1 receptor (Brydon et al. 1999; MacKenzie et al. 2002) suggests an interplay between melatonin and neurosteroids in modulating GABAergic activity and sleep. Possible cellular pathways involved in the physiological modulation of GABAergic function by melatonin via its MT_1 receptor are shown in Fig. 10.3.

Melatonin receptor agonists in the treatment of sleep disorders

An ideal hypnotic agent should increase total sleep time and reduce sleep onset latency without significant side effects (Turek and Gillette 2004). Since melatonin has a short half life, an agonist with a longer half life, or a prolonged release melatonin formulation, may be more effective in activating brain melatonin receptors throughout the night, thus improving sleep efficiency and total sleep time (Turek and Gillette 2004). A number of melatonin agonists have been used successfully for the treatment of sleep disorders. Agomelatine, ramelteon, and LY 156735 are some of the melatonin agonists that have been found useful in the treatment of sleep problems primarily by shortening sleep onset latency (Fig. 10.4).

Agomelatine, an MT_1/MT_2 melatonin agonist and selective antagonist of $5\text{-}HT_{2C}$ receptors, has been demonstrated to be active in several animal models of depression. In a double-blind, randomized multicenter multinational placebo-controlled study, including 711 patients suffering from major depressive disor-der (MDD), agomelatine (25 mg) was significantly more effective (61.5%) than placebo (46.3%) in the treatment of MDD (Loo et al. 2002). Recently, this find-ing has been confirmed by two additional studies. The efficacy of agomelatine

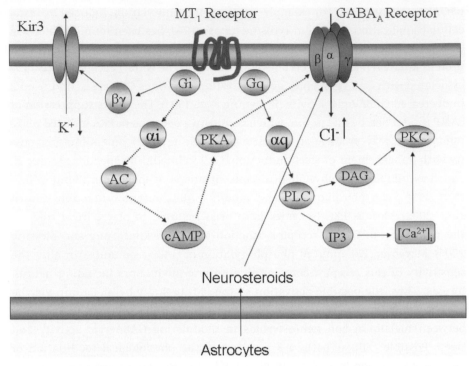

Figure 10.3 Possible cellular pathways involved in the physiological modulation of GABAergic function by melatonin via the MT_1 receptor. See text for explanation. (See also Plate 2.)

compared with placebo was noted after six weeks of treatment (at a dose of 25 mg/day) in MDD patients meeting DSM-IV criteria (Olie and Emsley 2005). In another clinical study, agomelatine (25 mg/day) was found to be significantly better than placebo in treating not only depressive symptomatology but also anxiety symptoms (Den Boer *et al.* 2006). From these studies, it is evident that agomelatine has emerged as a novel melatonergic antidepressant and may thus have value for the treatment of depression.

Ramelteon (Rozerem™), another non specific MT_1/MT_2 agonist, has a longer half life than melatonin, has high affinity for MT_1 and MT_2 receptors, and has been reported useful in promoting sleep in freely moving monkeys (Yukuhiro *et al.* 2004). Ramelteon is considered a new type of hypnotic without the adverse effects that are typically associated with BZDs (Hirai *et al.* 2005). In clinical trials, ramelteon has shown promising results in the treatment of transient and chronic insomnia (Cajochen 2005). In July 2005, the US Food and Drug Administration (FDA) approved Rozerem™ as 8 mg tablets for the treatment of insomnia characterized by sleep onset difficulty. Ramelteon is the first and only

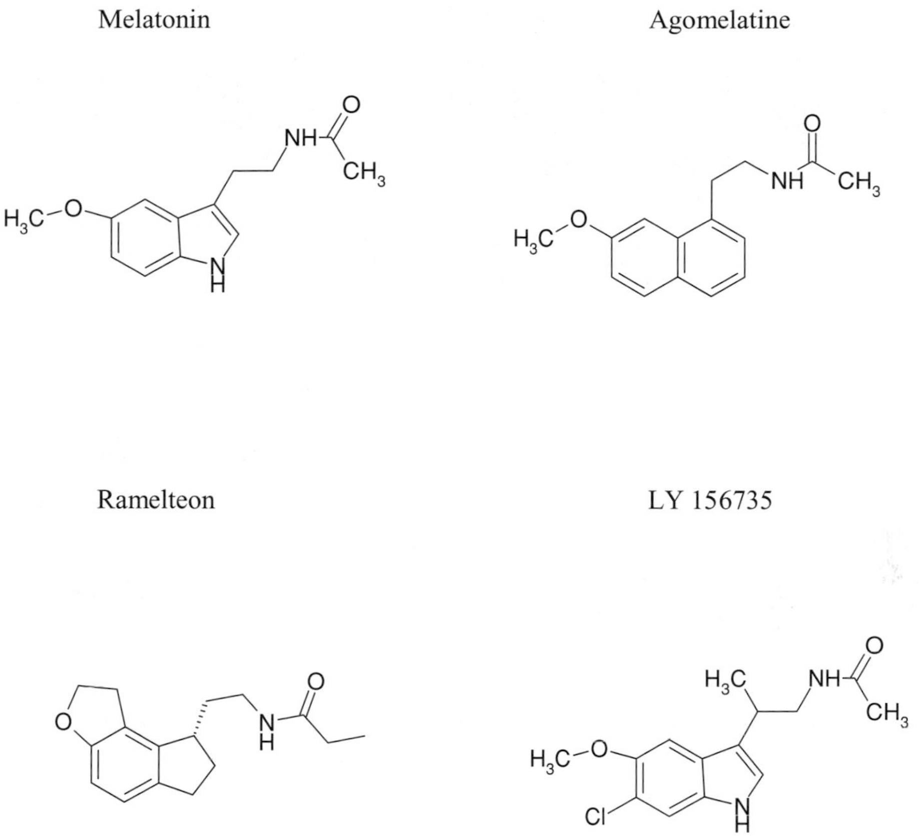

Melatonin   Agomelatine

Ramelteon   LY 156735

Figure 10.4 Chemical structures of the clinically relevant melatonin analogs, compared with melatonin (5-methoxy-N-acetyltryptamine). Agomelatine: N-(2-[7-methoxy-1-naphthalenyl]ethyl)acetamide. Ramelteon: (S)-N-[2-(1,6,7,8-tetrahydro-2H-indeno[5,4-b]furan-8-yl)-ethyl]propionamide. LY 156735: N-[2-(6-chloro-5-methoxy-1H-indol-3-yl)propyl]acetamide.

prescription sleep medication that has shown no evidence of abuse and dependence and, as a result, has not been designated as a controlled substance by the US Drug Enforcement Administration (DEA). The FDA approval allows physicians to prescribe Rozerem for long-term use in adults, based on the lack of abuse and dependence potential.

LY 156735 is a β-substituted analog of melatonin that has greater bioavailability than melatonin (Nickelsen *et al.* 2002). It is in an earlier stage of clinical trials; in initial trials, it reduced the sleep onset time in patients with moderate sleep-onset insomnia. Several other specific melatonin receptor agonists and antagonists are in development (Rivara *et al.* 2005; Zlotos 2005) and presumably will be clinically tested over the next few years.

References

Al-Ghoul, W. M., Herman, M. D. & Dubocovich, M. L. (1998). Melatonin receptor subtype expression in human cerebellum. *Neuroreport* **9**, 4063–8.

Allegra, M., Reiter, R. J., Tan, D. X. *et al.* (2003). The chemistry of melatonin's interaction with reactive species. *J. Pineal Res.* **34**, 1–10.

Andrabi, S. A., Sayeed, I., Siemen, D., Wolf, G. & Horn, T. F. (2004). Direct inhibition of the mitochondrial permeability transition pore: a possible mechanism responsible for anti-apoptotic effects of melatonin. *FASEB J.* **18**, 869–71.

Anton-Tay, F., Martinez, I., Tovar, R. & Benitez-King, G. (1998). Modulation of the subcellular distribution of calmodulin by melatonin in MDCK cells. *J. Pineal Res.* **24**, 35–42.

Anton-Tay, F., Diaz, J. L. & Fernandez-Guardiola, A. (1971). On the effect of melatonin upon human brain. Its possible therapeutic implications. *Life Sci.* [I] **10**, 841–50.

Arendt, J. (2005). Melatonin in humans: it's about time. *J. Neuroendocrinol.* **17**, 537–8.

Armstrong, S. M. (1989). Melatonin and circadian control in mammals. *Experientia* **45**, 932–8.

Axelrod, J. & Wurtman, R. J. (1966). The formation, metabolism and some actions of melatonin, a pineal gland substance. *Res. Publ. Assoc. Res. Nerv. Ment. Dis.* **43**, 200–11.

Axelrod, J. (1974). The pineal gland: a neurochemical transducer. *Science* **184**, 1341–8.

Baumann, S. W., Baur, R. & Sigel, E. (2003). Individual properties of the two functional agonist sites in GABA(A) receptors. *J. Neurosci.* **23**, 11158–66.

Benitez-King, G., Rios, A., Martinez, A. & Anton-Tay, F. (1996). In vitro inhibition of Ca^{2+}/calmodulin-dependent kinase II activity by melatonin. *Biochim. Biophys. Acta* **1290**, 191–6.

Berson, D. M., Dunn, F. A. & Takao, M. (2002). Phototransduction by retinal ganglion cells that set the circadian clock. *Science* **295**, 1070–3.

Birkeland, A. J. (1982). Plasma melatonin levels and nocturnal transitions between sleep and wakefulness. *Neuroendocrinology* **34**, 126–31.

Blask, D. E., Dauchy, R. T. & Sauer, L. A. (2005). Putting cancer to sleep at night: the neuroendocrine/circadian melatonin signal. *Endocrine* **27**, 179–88.

Brainard, G. C., Hanifin, J. P., Greeson, J. M. *et al.* (2001). Action spectrum for melatonin regulation in humans: evidence for a novel circadian photoreceptor. *J. Neurosci.* **21**, 6405–12.

Brismar, K., Hylander, B., Eliasson, K., Rossner, S. & Wetterberg, L. (1988). Melatonin secretion related to side-effects of beta-blockers from the central nervous system. *Acta Med. Scand.* **223**, 525–30.

Brismar, K., Mogensen, L. & Wetterberg, L. (1987). Depressed melatonin secretion in patients with nightmares due to beta-adrenoceptor blocking drugs. *Acta Med. Scand.* **221**, 155–8.

Browning, M. D., Endo, S., Smith, G. B., Dudek, E. M. & Olsen, R. W. (1993). Phosphorylation of the GABAA receptor by cAMP-dependent protein kinase and by protein kinase C: analysis of the substrate domain. *Neurochem. Res.* **18**, 95–100.

Brydon, L., Petit, L., P. deCoppet *et al.* (1999). Polymorphism and signalling of melatonin receptors. *Reprod. Nutr. Dev.* **39**, 315–24.

Brydon, L., Petit, L., Delagrange, P., Strosberg, A. D. & Jockers, R. (2001). Functional expression of mt2 (mel1b) melatonin receptors in human paz6 adipocytes. *Endocrinology* **142**, 4264–71.

Brydon, L., Roka, F., Petit, L. *et al.* (1999). Dual signaling of human Mel1a melatonin receptors via G(i2), G(i3), and G(q/11) proteins. *Mol. Endocrinol.* **13**, 2025–38.

Brzezinski, A., Vangel, M. G., Wurtman, R. J. *et al.* (2005). Effects of exogenous melatonin on sleep: a meta-analysis. *Sleep Med. Rev.* **9**, 41–50.

Bubenik, G. A. (2002). Gastrointestinal melatonin: localization, function, and clinical relevance. *Dig. Dis. Sci.* **47**, 2336–48.

Buscemi, N., Vandermeer, B., Hooton, N. *et al.* (2006). Efficacy and safety of exogenous melatonin for secondary sleep disorders and sleep disorders accompanying sleep restriction: meta-analysis. *Br. Med. J.* **332**, 385–93.

Buysse, D. J., Nofzinger, E. A., Germain, A. *et al.* (2004). Regional brain glucose metabolism during morning and evening wakefulness in humans: preliminary findings. *Sleep* **27**, 1245–54.

Cajochen, C. (2005). TAK-375 Takeda. *Curr. Opin. Investig. Drugs* **6**, 114–21.

Cajochen, C., Krauchi, K., Danilenko, K. V. & Wirz-Justice, A. (1998). Evening administration of melatonin and bright light: interactions on the EEG during sleep and wakefulness. *J. Sleep Res.* **7**, 145–57.

Cardinali, D. P. (1977). Nuclear receptor estrogen complex in the pineal gland. Modulation by sympathetic nerves. *Neuroendocrinology* **24**, 333–46.

Cardinali, D. P. & Golombek, D. A. (1998). The rhythmic gabaergic system. *Neurochem Res.* **23**, 607–14.

Cardinali, D. P. & Pevet, P. (1998). Basic aspects of melatonin action. *Sleep Med. Rev.* **2**, 175–90.

Cardinali, D. P. & Rosner, J. M. (1971). Metabolism of serotonin by the rat retina "in vitro". *J. Neurochem.* **18**, 1769–70.

Cardinali, D. P. & Vacas, M. I. (1980), Molecular endocrinology of melatonin: Receptor sites in brain and peripheral organs. *Adv. Biosci.* **29**, 237–46.

Cardinali, D. P., Bortman, G. P., Liotta, G. *et al.* (2002). A multifactorial approach employing melatonin to accelerate resynchronization of sleep-wake cycle after a 12 time-zone westerly transmeridian flight in elite soccer athletes. *J. Pineal Res.* **32**, 41–6.

Cardinali, D. P., Furio, A. M., Reyes, M. P. & Brusco, L. I. (2006). The use of chronobiotics in the resynchronization of the sleep/wake cycle. *Cancer Causes & Control* **17**,(4) 601–9.

Cardinali, D. P., Golombek, D. A., Rosenstein, R. E., Cutrera, R. A. & Esquifino, A. I. (1997). Melatonin site and mechanism of action: Single or multiple? *J. Pineal Res.* **23**, 32–9.

Cardinali, D. P., Lynch, H. J. & Wurtman, R. J. (1972). Binding of melatonin to human and rat plasma proteins. *Endocrinology* **91**, 1213–18.

Cardinali, D. P., Ladizesky, M. G., Boggio, V., Cutrera, R. A. & Mautalen, C. A. (2003). Melatonin effects on bone: Experimental facts and clinical perspectives. *J. Pineal Res.* **34**, 81–7.

Carlberg, C. (2000). Gene regulation by melatonin. *Ann. NY Acad. Sci.* **917**, 387–96.

Carlberg, C. & Wiesenberg, I. (1995). The orphan receptor family RZR/ROR, melatonin and 5-lipoxygenase: an unexpected relationship. *J. Pineal Res.* **18**, 171–8.

Carrillo-Vico, A., Calvo, J. R., Abreu, P. *et al.* (2004). Evidence of melatonin synthesis by human lymphocytes and its physiological significance: possible role as intracrine, autocrine, and/or paracrine substance. *FASEB J.* **18**, 537–9.

Castro, L. M., Gallant, M. & Niles, L. P. (2005). Novel targets for valproic acid: up-regulation of melatonin receptors and neurotrophic factors in C6 glioma cells. *J. Neurochem.* **95**, 1227–36.

Champier, J., Claustrat, B., Besancon, R. *et al.* (1997). Evidence for tryptophan hydroxylase and hydroxy-indol-O-methyl-transferase mRNAs in human blood platelets. *Life Sci.* **60**, 2191–7.

Churn, S. B., Rana, A., Lee, K. *et al.* (2002). Calcium/calmodulin-dependent kinase II phosphorylation of the $GABA_A$ receptor alpha1 subunit modulates benzodiazepine binding. *J. Neurochem.* **82**, 1065–76.

Claustrat, B., Brun, J. & Chazot, G. (2005). The basic physiology and pathophysiology of melatonin. *Sleep. Med. Rev.* **9**, 11–24.

Claustrat, B., Brun, J., Garry, P., Roussel, B. & Sassolas, G. (1986). A once-repeated study of nocturnal plasma melatonin patterns and sleep recordings in six normal young men. *J. Pineal Res.* **3**, 301–10.

Conti, A., Conconi, S., Hertens, E. *et al.* (2000). Evidence for melatonin synthesis in mouse and human bone marrow cells. *J. Pineal Res.* **28**, 193–202.

Cramer, H., Rudolph, J., Consbruch, U. & Kendel, K. (1974). On the effects of melatonin on sleep and behavior in man. *Adv. Biochem. Psychopharmacol.* **11**, 187–91.

Dahlitz, M., Alvarez, B., Vignau, J. *et al.* (1991). Delayed sleep phase syndrome response to melatonin. *Lancet* **337**, 1121–4.

Den Boer, J. A., Bosker, F. J. & Meesters, Y. (2006). Clinical efficacy of agomelatine in depression: the evidence. *Int. Clin. Psychopharmacol.* **21**, (Suppl. 1) S21–4.

Dijk, D. J. & Cajochen, C. (1997). Melatonin and the circadian regulation of sleep initiation, consolidation, structure, and the sleep EEG. *J. Biol. Rhythms* **12**, 627–35.

Dollins, A. B., Lynch, H. J., Wurtman, R. J. *et al.* (1993). Effect of pharmacological daytime doses of melatonin on human mood and performance. *Psychopharmacol. Berl.* **112**, 490–6.

Dollins, A. B., Zhdanova, I. V., Wurtman, R. J., Lynch, H. J. & Deng, M. H. (1994). Effect of inducing nocturnal serum melatonin concentrations in daytime on sleep, mood, body temperature, and performance. *Proc. Natl. Acad. Sci. USA* **91**, 1824–8.

Doolen, S., Krause, D. N., Dubocovich, M. L. & Duckles, S. P. (1998). Melatonin mediates two distinct responses in vascular smooth muscle. *Eur. J. Pharmacol.* **345**, 67–9.

Dubocovich, M. L. & Markowska, M. (2005). Functional MT_1 and MT_2 melatonin receptors in mammals. *Endocrine* **27**, 101–10.

Dubocovich, M. L., Cardinali, D. P., Delagrange, P. *et al.* (2000). Melatonin receptors; In ed. IUPHAR, *The IUPHAR Compendium of Receptor Characterization and Classification*, 2nd Edition. (London: IUPHAR Media) pp. 271–7.

Esquifino, A. I., Pandi-Perumal, S. R. & Cardinali, D. P. (2004). Circadian organization of the immune response: A role for melatonin. *Clin. Appl. Immunol. Rev.* **4**, 423–33.

Ferry, G., Ubeaud, C., Lambert, P. H. *et al.* (2005). Molecular evidence that melatonin is enzymatically oxidized in a different manner than tryptophan. Investigation on both indoleamine-2,3-dioxygenase and myeloperoxidase. *Biochem. J.* **388**, 205–15.

Foster, C. E., Bianchet, M. A., Talalay, P., Faig, M. & Amzel, L. M. (2000). Structures of mammalian cytosolic quinone reductases. *Free Radic. Biol. Med.* **29**, 241–5.

Gall, C. von, Stehle, J. H. & Weaver, D. R. (2002). Mammalian melatonin receptors: molecular biology and signal transduction. *Cell Tiss. Res.* **309**, 151–62.

Garcia-Ovejero, D., Azcoitia, I., Doncarlos, L. L., Melcangi, R. C. & Garcia-Segura, L. M. (2005). Glia-neuron crosstalk in the neuroprotective mechanisms of sex steroid hormones. *Brain Res. Brain. Res. Rev.* **48**, 273–86.

Gauer, F., Masson-Pevet, M. & Pevet, P. (1992). Pinealectomy and constant illumination increase the density of melatonin binding sites in the pars tuberalis of rodents. *Brain Res.* **575**, 32–8.

Gauer, F., Masson-Pevet, M. & Pevet, P. (1993). Melatonin receptor density is regulated in rat pars tuberalis and suprachiasmatic nuclei by melatonin itself. *Brain Res.* **602**, 153–6.

Geoffriau, M., Claustrat, B. & Veldhuis, J. (1999). Estimation of frequently sampled nocturnal melatonin production in humans by deconvolution analysis: evidence for episodic or ultradian secretion. *J. Pineal Res.* **27**, 139–44.

Gerdin, M. J., Masana, M. I., Rivera-Bermudez, M. A. *et al.* (2004). Melatonin desensitizes endogenous MT_2 melatonin receptors in the rat suprachiasmatic nucleus: relevance for defining the periods of sensitivity of the mammalian circadian clock to melatonin. *FASEB J.* **18**, 1646–56.

Gervasoni, D., Darracq, L., Fort, P. *et al.* (1998). Electrophysiological evidence that noradrenergic neurons of the rat locus coeruleus are tonically inhibited by GABA during sleep. *Eur. J. Neurosci.* **10**, 964–70.

Gilbert, S. S., VandenHeuvel, C. J. & Dawson, D. (1999). Daytime melatonin and temazepam in young adult humans: equivalent effects on sleep latency and body temperatures. *J. Physiol. Lond.* **514**, 905–14.

Golombek, D. A. & Cardinali, D. P. (1993). Melatonin accelerates re-entrainment after phase advance of the light-dark cycle in Syrian hamsters. Antagonism by flumazenil. *Chronobiol. Int.* **10**, 435–41.

Golombek, D. A., Martini, M. & Cardinali, D. P. (1993). Melatonin as an anxiolytic in rats: time-dependence and interaction with the central gabaergic system. *Eur. J. Pharmacol.* **237**, 231–6.

Golombek, D. A., Pevet, P. & Cardinali, D. P. (1996). Melatonin effects on behavior: possible mediation by the central GABAergic system. *Neurosci. Biobehav. Rev.* **20**, 403–12.

Gould, T. D., Chen, G. & Manji, H. K. (2002). Mood stabilizer psychopharmacology. *Clin. Neurosci. Res.* **2**, 193–212.

Griefahn, B., Brode, P., Remer, T. & Blaszkewicz, M. (2003). Excretion of 6-hydroxymelatonin sulfate (6-OHMS) in siblings during childhood and adolescence. *Neuroendocrinology* **78**, 241–3.

Guerrero, J. M. & Reiter, R. J. (2002). Melatonin-immune system relationships. *Curr. Top. Med. Chem.* **2**, 167–79.

Gupta, M., Aneja, S. & Kohli, K. (2005). Add-on melatonin improves sleep behavior in children with epilepsy: randomized, double-blind, placebo-controlled trial. *J. Child Neurol.* **20**, 112–15.

Haimov, I. & Lavie, P. (1997). Melatonin – a chronobiotic and soporific hormone. *Arch. Gerontol. Geriatr.* **24**, 167–73.

Haldar, C. & Gupta, D. (1990). Sex- and age-dependent nature of the cytoplasmic 5 alpha-dihydrotestosterone (DHT) binding site/receptor in bovine pineal gland. *J. Pineal Res.* **8**, 289–95.

Hardeland, R., Poeggeler, B., Behrmann, G. & Fuhrberg, B. (1996). Enzymatic and non-enzymatic metabolism of methoxyindoles. In ed. Hardeland, R. *Metabolism and Cellular Dynamics of Indoles.* (Goettingen: University of Goettingen) pp. 6–22.

Hardeland, R., Reiter, R. J., Poeggeler, B. & Tan, D. X. (1993). The significance of the metabolism of the neurohormone melatonin: antioxidative protection and formation of bioactive substances. *Neurosci. Biobehav. Rev.* **17**, 347–57.

Hardeland, R., Pandi-Perumal, S. R. & Cardinali, D. P. (2006). Melatonin. *Int. J. Biochem. Cell. Biol.* **38**, 313–16.

Hartter, S., Ursing, C., Morita, S., Tybring, G. *et al.* (2001). Orally given melatonin may serve as a probe drug for cytochrome P450 1A2 activity in vivo: a pilot study. *Clin. Pharmacol. Ther.* **70**, 10–16.

Hausdorff, W. P., Caron, M. G. & Lefkowitz, R. J. (1990). Turning off the signal: desensitization of beta-adrenergic receptor function. *FASEB J.* **4**, 2881–9.

Hazlerigg, D. G., Gonzalez-Brito, A., Lawson, W., Hastings, M. H. & Morgan, P. J. (1993). Prolonged exposure to melatonin leads to time-dependent sensitization of adenylate cyclase and down-regulates melatonin receptors in pars tuberalis cells from ovine pituitary. *Endocrinology* **132**, 285–92.

Herxheimer, A. & Petrie, K. J. (2002). Melatonin for the prevention and treatment of jet lag. *Cochrane Database Syst. Rev.* CD001520.

Hirai, K., Kita, M., Ohta, H. *et al.* (2005). Ramelteon (TAK-375) accelerates reentrainment of circadian rhythm after a phase advance of the light-dark cycle in rats. *J. Biol. Rhythms* **20**, 27–37.

Hirata, F., Hayaishi, O., Tokuyama, T. & Seno, S. (1974). In vitro and in vivo formation of two new metabolites of melatonin. *J. Biol. Chem.* **249**, 1311–13.

Hughes, R. J. & Badia, P. (1997). Sleep-promoting and hypothermic effects of daytime melatonin administration in humans. *Sleep* **20**, 124–31.

Hunt, A. E., Al Ghoul, W. M., Gillette, M. U. & Dubocovich, M. L. (2001). Activation of MT$_2$ melatonin receptors in rat suprachiasmatic nucleus phase advances the circadian clock. *Am. J. Physiol. Cell. Physiol.* **280**, C110–18.

Iuvone, P. M., Tosini, G., Pozdeyev, N. *et al.* (2005). Circadian clocks, clock networks, arylalkylamine N-acetyltransferase, and melatonin in the retina. *Prog. Retin. Eye Res.* **24**, 433–56.

Joseph-Liauzun, E., Farges, R., Delmas, P., Ferrara, P. & Loison, G. (1997). The Mr 18,000 subunit of the peripheral-type benzodiazepine receptor exhibits both benzodiazepine and isoquinoline carboxamide binding sites in the absence of the voltage-dependent anion channel or of the adenine nucleotide carrier. *J. Biol. Chem.* **272**, 28102–6.

Kalsbeek, A., Garidou, M. L., Palm, I. F. *et al.* (2000). Melatonin sees the light: blocking GABA-ergic transmission in the paraventricular nucleus induces daytime secretion of melatonin. *Eur. J. Neurosci.* **12**, 3146–54.

Karasek, M., Reiter, R. J., Cardinali, D. P. & Pawlikowski, M. (2002). Future of melatonin as a therapeutic agent. *Neuroendocrinol. Lett.* **23**, (Suppl. 1) 118–21.

Karolczak, M., Korf, H. W. & Stehle, J. H. (2005). The rhythm and blues of gene expression in the rodent pineal gland. *Endocrine* **27**, 89–100.

Kayumov, L., Brown, G., Jindal, R., Buttoo, K. & Shapiro, C. M. (2001). A randomized, double-blind, placebo-controlled crossover study of the effect of exogenous melatonin on delayed sleep phase syndrome. *Psychosom. Med.* **63**, 40–8.

Kilic, U., Kilic, E., Reiter, R. J., Bassetti, C. L. & Hermann, D. M. (2005). Signal transduction pathways involved in melatonin-induced neuroprotection after focal cerebral ischemia in mice. *J. Pineal Res.* **38**, 67–71.

Klein, D. C. & Moore, R. Y. (1979). Pineal N-acetyltransferase and hydroxyindole-O-methyltransferase: control by the retinohypothalamic tract and the suprachiasmatic nucleus. *Brain Res.* **174**, 245–62.

Klein, D. C. (2004). The 2004 Aschoff/Pittendrigh lecture: Theory of the origin of the pineal gland – a tale of conflict and resolution. *J. Biol. Rhythms* **19**, 264–79.

Lavie, P. (1986). Ultrashort sleep-waking schedule. III. 'Gates' and 'forbidden zones' for sleep. *Electroencephalogr. Clin. Neurophysiol.* **63**, 414–25.

Lavie, P. (1997). Melatonin: role in gating nocturnal rise in sleep propensity. *J. Biol. Rhythms* **12**, 657–65.

Le Bars, D., Thivolle, P., Vitte, P. A. *et al.* (1991). PET and plasma pharmacokinetic studies after bolus intravenous administration of [^{11}C]melatonin in humans. *Int. J. Rad. Appl. Instrum.* [B] **18**, 357–62.

Lerner, A. B. & Case, M. D. (1960). Melatonin. *Fed. Proc.* **19**, 590–2.

Lerner, A. B., Case, J. D. & Heinzelmann, R. V. (1959). Structure of melatonin. *J. Am. Chem. Soc.* **81**, 6085.

Lerner, A. B., Case, J. D., Takahashi, Y., Lee, T. H. & Mori, N. (1958). Isolation of melatonin, a pineal factor that lightens melanocytes. *J. Am. Chem. Soc.* **80**, 2587.

Lewy, A. J., Wehr, T. A., Goodwin, F. K., Newsome, D. A. & Markey, S. P. (1980). Light suppresses melatonin secretion in humans. *Science* **210**, 1267–9.

Lewy, A. J. (1999). Melatonin as a marker and phase-resetter of circadian rhythms in humans. *Adv. Exp. Med. Biol.* **460**, 425–34.

Lima, E. de, J. M. Soares, Jr., Carmen Sanabria, G. Y. *et al.* (2005). Effects of pinealectomy and the treatment with melatonin on the temporal lobe epilepsy in rats. *Brain Res.* **1043**, 24–31.

Liu, C., Fukuhara, C., Wessel, J. H. III, Iuvone, P. M. & Tosini, G. (2004). Localization of Aa-nat mRNA in the rat retina by fluorescence in situ hybridization and laser capture microdissection. *Cell Tiss. Res.* **315**, 197–201.

Liu, C., Weaver, D. R., Jin, X. *et al.* (1997). Molecular dissection of two distinct actions of melatonin on the suprachiasmatic circadian clock. *Neuron* **19**, 91–102.

Long, M. A., Jutras, M. J., Connors, B. W. & Burwell, R. D. (2005). Electrical synapses coordinate activity in the suprachiasmatic nucleus. *Nat. Neurosci.* **8**, 61–6.

Loo, H., Hale, A. & D'haenen, H. (2002). Determination of the dose of agomelatine, a melatoninergic agonist and selective 5-HT$_{2C}$ antagonist, in the treatment of major depressive disorder: a placebo-controlled dose range study. *Int. Clin. Psychopharmacol.* **17**, 239–47.

Lu, J., Greco, M. A., Shiromani, P. & Saper, C. B. (2000). Effect of lesions of the ventrolateral preoptic nucleus on NREM and REM sleep. *J. Neurosci.* **20**, 3830–42.

Luboshitzky, R., Dharan, M., Goldman, D. *et al.* (1997). Seasonal variation of gonadotropins and gonadal steroids receptors in the human pineal gland. *Brain Res. Bull.* **44**, 665–70.

Lynch, H. J., Wurtman, R. J., Moskowitz, M. A., Archer, M. C. & Ho, M. H. (1975). Daily rhythm in human urinary melatonin. *Science* **187**, 169–71.

Ma, X., Idle, J. R., Krausz, K. W. & Gonzalez, F. J. (2005). Metabolism of melatonin by human cytochromes p450. *Drug Metab. Dispos.* **33**, 489–94.

Macchi, M. M. & Bruce, J. N. (2004). Human pineal physiology and functional significance of melatonin. *Front. Neuroendocrinol.* **25**, 177–95.

MacKenzie, R. S., Melan, M. A., Passey, D. K. & Witt-Enderby, P. A. (2002). Dual coupling of MT$_1$ and MT$_2$ melatonin receptors to cyclic AMP and phosphoinositide signal transduction cascades and their regulation following melatonin exposure. *Biochem. Pharmacol.* **63**, 587–95.

Mailliet, F., Ferry, G., Vella, F. *et al.* (2004). Organs from mice deleted for NRH:quinone oxidoreductase 2 are deprived of the melatonin binding site MT$_3$. *FEBS Lett.* **578**, 116–20.

Mallo, C., Zaidan, R., Galy, G. *et al.* (1990). Pharmacokinetics of melatonin in man after intravenous infusion and bolus injection. *Eur. J. Clin. Pharmacol.* **38**, 297–301.

Masana, M. I., Soares, J. M. Jr & Dubocovich, M. L. (2005). 17beta-Estradiol modulates hMT(1) melatonin receptor function. *Neuroendocrinology* **81**, 87–95.

Mazzucchelli, C., Pannacci, M., Nonno, R. *et al.* (1996). The melatonin receptor in the human brain: cloning experiments and distribution studies. *Brain Res. Mol. Brain. Res.* **39**, 117–26.

McIntyre, I. M., Norman, T. R., Burrows, G. D. & Armstrong, S. M. (1989). Human melatonin suppression by light is intensity dependent. *J. Pineal Res.* **6**, 149–56.

Mellon, S. H. & Griffin, L. D. (2002). Neurosteroids: biochemistry and clinical significance. *Trends Endocrinol. Metab.* **13**, 35–43.

Moore, R. Y. (1996). Neural control of the pineal gland. *Behav. Brain Res.* **73**, 125–30.

Nagtegaal, J. E., Kerkhof, G. A., Smits, M. G., Swart, A. C. & van der Meer, Y. G. (1998). Delayed sleep phase syndrome: A placebo-controlled cross-over study on the effects of melatonin administered five hours before the individual dim light melatonin onset. *J. Sleep Res.* **7**, 135–43.

Nave, R., Herer, P., Haimov, I., Shlitner, A. & Lavie, P. (1996). Hypnotic and hypothermic effects of melatonin on daytime sleep in humans: lack of antagonism by flumazenil. *Neurosci. Lett.* **214**, 123–6.

Nave, R., Peled, R. & Lavie, P. (1995). Melatonin improves evening napping. *Eur. J. Pharmacol.* **275**, 213–16.

Nelson, C. S., Marino, J. L. & Allen, C. N. (1996). Melatonin receptors activate heteromeric G-protein coupled Kir3 channels. *Neuroreport* **7**, 717–20.

Nickelsen, T., Samel, A., Vejvoda, M. *et al.* (2002). Chronobiotic effects of the melatonin agonist LY 156735 following a simulated 9h time shift: results of a placebo-controlled trial. *Chronobiol. Int.* **19**, 915–36.

Niles, L. (1991). Melatonin interaction with the benzodiazepine-GABA receptor complex in the CNS. *Adv. Exp. Med. Biol.* **294**, 267–77.

Niles, L. P. (2006). Molecular mechanisms of melatonin action: Targets in sleep regulation. In ed. Cardinali, D. P. & Pandi-Perumal, S. R. *Neuroendocrine Correlates of Sleep/Wakefulness.* (New York, NY: Springer). pp. 119–35.

Niles, L. P. & Peace, C. H. (1990). Allosteric modulation of t-[35S]butylbicyclophosphorothionate binding in rat brain by melatonin. *Brain Res. Bull.* **24**, 635–8.

Nosjean, O., Ferro, M., Coge, F. *et al.* (2000). Identification of the melatonin binding site MT$_3$ as the quinone reductase 2. *J. Biol. Chem.* **275**, 31311–17.

Olde Rikkert, M. G. & Rigaud, A. S. (2001). Melatonin in elderly patients with insomnia. A systematic review. *Z. Gerontol. Geriatr.* **34**, 491–7.

Olie, P. & Emsley, R. (2005). Confirmed clinical efficacy of agomelatine (25–50 mg) in major depression; two randomized, double-blind controlled studies. *Eur. Neuropsychopharmacol.* **15**, (Suppl. 3) S416.

Pace-Schott, E. F. & Hobson, J. A. (2002). The neurobiology of sleep: genetics, cellular physiology and subcortical networks. *Nat. Neurosci. Rev.* **3**, 591–605.

Pandi-Perumal, S. R., Esquifino, A. I., Cardinali, D. P., Miller, S. C. & Maestroni, G. J. M. (2006). The role of melatonin in immunoenhancement: Potential application in cancer. *Int. J. Exp. Pathol.* **87**, 81–7.

Pandi-Perumal, S. R., Zisapel, N., Srinivasan, V. & Cardinali, D. P. (2005). Melatonin and sleep in aging population. *Exp. Gerontol.* **40**, 911–25.

Pandi-Perumal, S. R., Zisapel, N., Srinivasan, V. & Cardinali, D. P. (2005). Melatonin and sleep in aging population. *Exp. Gerontol.* **00**, 00–00.

Pevet, P., Bothorel, B., Slotten, H. & Saboureau, M. (2002). The chronobiotic properties of melatonin. *Cell. Tiss. Res.* **309**, 183–91.

Poirel, V. J., Boggio, V., Dardente, H. *et al.* (2003). Contrary to other non-photic cues, acute melatonin injection does not induce immediate changes of clock gene mrna expression in the rat suprachiasmatic nuclei. *Neuroscience* **120**, 745–55.

Poisbeau, P., Cheney, M. C., Browning, M. D. & Mody, I. (1999). Modulation of synaptic GABAA receptor function by PKA and PKC in adult hippocampal neurons. *J. Neurosci.* **19**, 674–83.

Rajaratnam, S. M., Middleton, B., Stone, B. M., Arendt, J. & Dijk, D. J. (2004). Melatonin advances the circadian timing of EEG sleep and directly facilitates sleep without altering its duration in extended sleep opportunities in humans. *J. Physiol.* **561**, 339–51.

Reiter, R. J., Tan, D. X. & Maldonado, M. D. (2005). Melatonin as an antioxidant: physiology versus pharmacology. *J. Pineal. Res.* **39**, 215–16.

Reppert, S. M., Godson, C., Mahle, C. D. *et al.* (1995). Molecular characterization of a second melatonin receptor expressed in human retina and brain: the Mel$_{1b}$ melatonin receptor. *Proc. Natl. Acad. Sci. USA* **92**, 8734–8.

Reppert, S. M., Weaver, D. R. & Ebisawa, T. (1994). Cloning and characterization of a mammalian melatonin receptor that mediates reproductive and circadian responses. *Neuron* **13**, 1177–85.

Ressmeyer, A. R., Mayo, J. C., Zelosko, V. *et al.* (2003). Antioxidant properties of the melatonin metabolite N^1-acetyl-5-methoxykynuramine (AMK): scavenging of free radicals and prevention of protein destruction. *Redox Rep.* **8**, 205–13.

Rivara, S., Lorenzi, S., Mor, M. *et al.* (2005). Analysis of structure-activity relationships for MT$_2$ selective antagonists by melatonin MT1 and MT$_2$ receptor models. *J. Med. Chem.* **48**, 4049–60.

Rosenstein, R. E. & Cardinali, D. P. (1990). Central gabaergic mechanisms as target for melatonin activity. *Neurochem. Int.* **17**, 373–9.

Roy, D. & Belsham, D. D. (2002). Melatonin receptor activation regulates GnRH gene expression and secretion in GT1–7 GnRH neurons. Signal transduction mechanisms. *J. Biol. Chem.* **277**, 251–8.

Sack, R. L., Hughes, R. J., Edgar, D. M. & Lewy, A. J. (1997). Sleep-promoting effects of melatonin: at what dose, in whom, under what conditions, and by what mechanisms? *Sleep* **20**, 908–15.

Sanchez, J. J., Abreu, P., Gonzalez-Hernandez, T. *et al.* (2004). Estrogen modulation of adrenoceptor responsiveness in the female rat pineal gland: differential expression of intracellular estrogen receptors. *J. Pineal Res.* **37**, 26–35.

Saper, C. B., Scammell, T. E. & Lu, J. (2005). Hypothalamic regulation of sleep and circadian rhythms. *Nature* **437**, 1257–63.

Satomura, T., Sakamoto, T., Shirakawa, S. *et al.* (2001). Hypnotic action of melatonin during daytime administration and its comparison with triazolam. *Psychiatry Clin. Neurosci.* **55**, 303–4.

Scheer, F. A. & Czeisler, C. A. (2005). Melatonin, sleep, and circadian rhythms. *Sleep. Med. Rev.* **9**, 5–9.

Scheer, F. A., Van Montfrans, G. A., Van Someren, E. J., Mairuhu, G. & Buijs, R. M. (2004). Daily nighttime melatonin reduces blood pressure in male patients with essential hypertension. *Hypertension* **43**, 192–7.

Sherin, J. E., Elmquist, J. K., Torrealba, F. & Saper, C. B. (1998). Innervation of histaminergic tuberomammillary neurons by GABAergic and galaninergic neurons in the ventrolateral preoptic nucleus of the rat. *J. Neurosci.* **18**, 4705–21.

Sherin, J. E., Shiromani, P. J., McCarley, R. W. & Saper, C. B. (1996). Activation of ventrolateral preoptic neurons during sleep. *Science* **271**, 216–19.

Shibata, S., Cassone, V. M. & Moore, R. Y. (1989). Effects of melatonin on neuronal activity in the rat suprachiasmatic nucleus in vitro. *Neurosci. Lett.* **97**, 140–4.

Sigel, E. & Buhr, A. (1997). The benzodiazepine binding site of GABAA receptors. *Trends Pharmacol. Sci.* **18**, 425–9.

Silva, S. O., Rodrigues, M. R., Carvalho, S. R. *et al.* (2004). Oxidation of melatonin and its catabolites, N^1-acetyl-N^2-formyl-5-methoxykynuramine and N^1-acetyl-5-methoxykynuramine, by activated leukocytes. *J. Pineal Res.* **37**, 171–5.

Slominski, A., Fischer, T. W., Zmijewski, M. A. *et al.* (2005a). On the role of melatonin in skin physiology and pathology. *Endocrine* **27**, 137–48.

Slominski, A., Wortsman, J. & Tobin, D. J. (2005b). The cutaneous serotoninergic/melatoninergic system: securing a place under the sun. *FASEB J.* **19**, 176–94.

Song, M. & Messing, R. O. (2005). Protein kinase C regulation of GABA$_A$ receptors. *Cell. Mol. Life Sci.* **62**, 119–27.

Srinivasan, V., Maestroni, G. J. M., Cardinali, D. P. *et al.* (2005a). Melatonin, immune function and aging. *Immun. Ageing* **2**, 17.

Srinivasan, V., Smits, M., Spence, W. *et al.* (2006). Melatonin in mood disorders. *World J. Biol. Psychiatry*. in press.

Srinivasan, V., Pandi-Perumal, S. R., Maestroni, G. J. M. *et al.* (2005b). Role of melatonin in neurodegenerative diseases. *Neurotox. Res.* **7**, 293–318.

Stankov, B., Biella, G., Panara, C. *et al.* (1992). Melatonin signal transduction and mechanism of action in the central nervous system: using the rabbit cortex as a model. *Endocrinology* **130**, 2152–9.

Stehle, J., Vanecek, J. & Vollrath, L. (1989). Effects of melatonin on spontaneous electrical activity of neurons in rat suprachiasmatic nuclei: an in vitro iontophoretic study. *J. Neural. Transm.* **78**, 173–7.

Stone, B. M., Turner, C., Mills, S. L. & Nicholson, A. N. (2000). Hypnotic activity of melatonin. *Sleep* **23**, 663–9.

Strogatz, S. H., Kronauer, R. E. & Czeisler, C. A. (1986). Circadian regulation dominates homeostatic control of sleep length and prior wake length in humans. *Sleep* **9**, 353–64.

Sun, X., Rusak, B. & Semba, K. (2000). Electrophysiology and pharmacology of projections from the suprachiasmatic nucleus to the ventromedial preoptic area in rat. *Neuroscience* **98**, 715–28.

Szymusiak, R., Alam, N., Steininger, T. L. & McGinty, D. (1998). Sleep-waking discharge patterns of ventrolateral preoptic/anterior hypothalamic neurons in rats. *Brain Res.* **803**, 178–88.

Takahashi, T., Sasaki, M., Itoh, H. *et al.* (2000). Effect of 3 mg melatonin on jet lag syndrome in an 8-h eastward flight. *Psychiatry Clin. Neurosci.* **54**, 377–8.

Tan, D. X., Hardeland, R., Manchester, L. C., *et al.* (2003). Mechanistic and comparative studies of melatonin and classic antioxidants in terms of their interactions with the ABTS cation radical. *J. Pineal Res.* **34**, 249–59.

Tan, D. X., Manchester, L. C., Reiter, R. J. *et al.* (1998). A novel melatonin metabolite, cyclic 3-hydroxymelatonin: a biomarker of in vivo hydroxyl radical generation. *Biochem. Biophys. Res. Comm.* **253**, 614–20.

Tan, D. X., Reiter, R. J., Manchester, L. C. *et al.* (2002). Chemical and physical properties and potential mechanisms: melatonin as a broad spectrum antioxidant and free radical scavenger. *Curr. Top. Med. Chem.* **2**, 181–97.

Tenn, C. & Niles, L. P. (1993). Physiological regulation of melatonin receptors in rat suprachiasmatic nuclei: diurnal rhythmicity and effects of stress. *Mol. Cell. Endocrinol.* **98**, 43–8.

Tenn, C. C. & Niles, L. P. (1995). Central-type benzodiazepine receptors mediate the antidopaminergic effect of clonazepam and melatonin in 6-hydroxydopamine lesioned rats: involvement of a GABAergic mechanism. *J. Pharmacol. Exp. Ther.* **274**, 84–9.

Tenn, C. C. & Niles, L. P. (1997). Mechanisms underlying the antidopaminergic effect of clonazepam and melatonin in striatum. *Neuropharmacology* **36**, 1659–63.

Tenn, C. C. & Niles, L. P. (2002). Modulation of dopaminergic activity in the striatum by benzodiazepines and melatonin. *Pharmacol. Rev. Commun.* **12**, 171.

Terlo, L., Laudon, M., Tarasch, R. *et al.* (1997). Effects of low doses of melatonin on late afternoon napping and mood. *Biol. Rhythm Res.* **28**, 2–15.

Tosini, G. & Menaker, M. (1998). The clock in the mouse retina: melatonin synthesis and photoreceptor degeneration. *Brain Res.* **789**, 221–8.

Treuer, K. von, Norman, T. R. & Armstrong, S. M. (1996). Overnight human plasma melatonin, cortisol, prolactin, TSH, under conditions of normal sleep, sleep deprivation, and sleep recovery. *J. Pineal Res.* **20**, 7–14.

Tricoire, H., Moller, M., Chemineau, P. & Malpaux, B. (2003). Origin of cerebrospinal fluid melatonin and possible function in the integration of photoperiod. *Reprod. Suppl.* **61**, 311–21.

Turek, F. W. & Gillette, M. U. (2004). Melatonin, sleep, and circadian rhythms: rationale for development of specific melatonin agonists. *Sleep Med.* **5**, 523–32.

Tzischinsky, O. & Lavie, P. (1994). Melatonin possesses time-dependent hypnotic effects. *Sleep* **17**, 638–45.

Tzischinsky, O., Shlitner, A. & Lavie, P. (1993). The association between the nocturnal sleep gate and nocturnal onset of urinary 6-sulfatoxymelatonin. *J. Biol. Rhythms* **8**, 199–209.

Uz, T., Arslan, A. D., Kurtuncu, M. *et al.* (2005). The regional and cellular expression profile of the melatonin receptor MT1 in the central dopaminergic system. *Brain Res. Mol. Brain Res.* **136**, 45–53.

Vacas, M. I. & Cardinali, D. P. (1979). Diurnal changes in melatonin binding sites of hamster and rat brains. Correlation with neuroendocrine responsiveness to melatonin. *Neurosci. Lett.* **15**, 259–63.

Vacas, M. I., Lowenstein, P. & Cardinali, D. P. (1979). Characterization of a cytosol progesterone receptor in bovine pineal gland. *Neuroendocrinology* **29**, 84–9.

Van Den Heuvel, C. J., Reid, K. J. & Dawson, D. (1997). Effect of atenolol on nocturnal sleep and temperature in young men: reversal by pharmacological doses of melatonin. *Physiol. Behav.* **61**, 795–802.

van den Pol, T. M., Buijs, R. M., Ruijter, J. M. *et al.* (2001). Melatonin generates an outward potassium current in rat suprachiasmatic nucleus neurones in vitro independent of their circadian rhythm. *Neuroscience* **107**, 99–108.

Vanecek, J., Kosar, E. & Vorlicek, J. (1990). Daily changes in melatonin binding sites and the effect of castration. *Mol. Cell. Endocrinol.* **73**, 165–70.

Vollrath, L., Semm, P. & Gammel, G. (1981). Sleep induction by intranasal administration of melatonin. *Adv. Biosci.* **29**, 327–9.

Waldhauser, F., Saletu, B. & Trinchard-Lugan, I. (1990). Sleep laboratory investigations on hypnotic properties of melatonin. *Psychopharmacol. Berl.* **100**, 222–6.

Wan, Q., Man, H. Y., Braunton, J. *et al.* (1997). Modulation of $GABA_A$ receptor function by tyrosine phosphorylation of beta subunits. *J. Neurosci.* **17**, 5062–9.

Wan, Q., Man, H. Y., Liu, F. *et al.* (1999). Differential modulation of GABAA receptor function by Mel_{1a} and Mel_{1b} receptors. *Nat. Neurosci.* **2**, 401–3.

Wang, F., Li, J., Wu, C. *et al.* (2003). The GABA(A) receptor mediates the hypnotic activity of melatonin in rats. *Pharmacol. Biochem. Behav.* **74**, 573–8.

Weil, Z. M., Hotchkiss, A. K., Gatien, M. L., Pieke-Dahl, S. & Nelson, R. J. (2006). Melatonin receptor (MT1) knockout mice display depression-like behaviors and deficits in sensorimotor gating. *Brain Res. Bull.* **68**, 425–9.

Wiesenberg, I., Missbach, M. & Carlberg, C. (1998). The potential role of the transcription factor RZR/ROR as a mediator of nuclear melatonin signaling. *Res. Neurol. Neurosci.* **12**, 143–50.

Witt-Enderby, P. A., MacKenzie, R. S., McKeon, R. M. *et al.* (2000). Melatonin induction of filamentous structures in non-neuronal cells that is dependent on expression of the human mt1 melatonin receptor. *Cell Motil. Cytoskeleton* **46**, 28–42.

Wurtman, R. J. & Zhdanova, I. (1995). Improvement of sleep quality by melatonin. *Lancet* **346**, 1491.

Yukuhiro, N., Kimura, H., Nishikawa, H. *et al.* (2004). Effects of ramelteon (TAK-375) on nocturnal sleep in freely moving monkeys. *Brain Res.* **1027**, 59–66.

Zeitzer, J. M., Daniels, J. E., Duffy, J. F. *et al.* (1999). Do plasma melatonin concentrations decline with age? *Am. J. Med.* **107**, 432–6.

Zhdanova, I. V. & Tucci, V. (2003). Melatonin, circadian rhythms, and sleep. *Curr. Treat. Options Neurol.* **5**, 225–9.

Zhdanova, I. V., Wurtman, R. J., Morabito, C., Piotrovska, V. R. & Lynch, H. J. (1996). Effects of low oral doses of melatonin, given 2–4 hours before habitual bedtime, on sleep in normal young humans. *Sleep* **19**, 423–31.

Zhdanova, I. V., Wurtman, R. J., Lynch, H. J. *et al.* (1995). Sleep-inducing effects of low doses of melatonin ingested in the evening. *Clin. Pharmacol. Ther.* **57**, 552–8.

Zisapel, N. (2001). Circadian rhythm sleep disorders: pathophysiology and potential approaches to management. *CNS Drugs* **15**, 311–28.

Zlotos, D. P. (2005). Recent advances in melatonin receptor ligands. *Arch. Pharm. Weinheim* **338**, 229–47.

Zwain, I. H. & Yen, S. S. (1999). Neurosteroidogenesis in astrocytes, oligodendrocytes, and neurons of cerebral cortex of rat brain. *Endocrinology* **140**, 3843–52.

11

Sleep regulatory factors

LEVENTE KAPÁS AND ÉVA SZENTIRMAI

Isolation of sleep factors from animals: historical perspectives

The concept of sleep factors stemmed from the commonplace observation that prolonged wakefulness makes people more sleepy. This led to the idea that, during wakefulness, an endogenously occurring sleep-inducing substance may accumulate in the body and this, in turn, would foster sleep. The first experiments addressing this hypothesis were performed independently in Japan by Ishimori (Ishimori 1909) and in France by Legendre and Piéron (Legendre and Piéron 1910, 1912) at the beginning of the twentieth century. In both series of experiments, cerebrospinal fluid (CSF) or serum of sleep-deprived dogs induced increased sleep in recipient animals. This suggested to the French scientists the accumulation of a "hypnotoxin" during wakefulness.

The quest for a key endogenous substance, the action of which is solely or mainly responsible for sleep, continued well into the 1980s. The heroic early era of endocrinology that yielded the discovery of key hormones that regulate various aspects of homeostasis, growth, and reproductive functions, also greatly influenced sleep research. Repeated attempts were made to try to identify and isolate the key hormone that may be responsible for sleep regulation. Schnedorf and Ivy successfully replicated the experiments of Legendre and Piéron 30 years later (Schnedorf and Ivy 1939). They concluded that ". . . the change or changes in 'fatigue' cerebrospinal fluid, if they are found, will only be a reflection of the underlying chemical changes in the brain conducive to fatigue or sleep". To investigate those chemical changes, they also tested for the presence of acetylcholine (ACh), an already known neurotransmitter at that time, in "fatigue CSF"

Neurochemistry of Sleep and Wakefulness, ed. J. M. Monti *et al.* Published by Cambridge University Press.
© Cambridge University Press 2008.

but could not detect any. This led to the conclusion that the endogenous substance that is responsible for the sleep-inducing effects of the samples is not ACh. They also noted that the body temperature of the dog rises after the intracisternal injection of "fatigue CSF". This observation is particularly interesting in the light of the finding of Pappenheimer and his co-workers, another 30 years or so later, that the active components of Factor S are muramyl peptides, immunoadjuvants with strong pyrogenic activities.

Pappenheimer reinvestigated the "Piéron phenomenon" by using sleep-deprived goats as CSF donors and cats and rats as recipients (Pappenheimer *et al.* 1967). The CSF of sleep-deprived goats produced profound depressant effects on motor activity for several hours and induced sleep-like behavior in the recipients. The finding that specimens from goats were active in two other species prompted Pappenheimer and colleagues to speculate that this putative sleep factor in the CSF is "of general and fundamental importance to the sleep mechanism". Subsequently, they named the sleep-promoting component Factor S and showed that its production increases progressively with the duration of sleep deprivation (Fencl *et al.* 1971) and that Factor S-induced sleep closely resembles the rebound sleep response after sleep deprivation (Pappenheimer *et al.* 1975). Eventually, the active component of Factor S was purified from human urine and identified as a muramyl peptide (Krueger *et al.* 1982). Since muramyl peptides induce the release of various cytokines, cytokines were tested as potential mediators of muramyl-peptide-induced sleep. The first cytokine that proved to have strong somnogenic properties was interleukin 1 (IL-1) (Krueger *et al.* 1984), followed by interferon alpha 2 (Krueger *et al.* 1987) and tumor necrosis factor α (TNFα) (Shoham *et al.* 1987). Mammalian brain is not known to be capable of producing muramyl peptides, and hence the physiological relevance of Factor S in sleep regulation is questionable. Nevertheless, the identification of muramyl peptides as sleep-inducing compounds had a lasting impact on sleep research. Muramyl peptides led to the discovery of the somnogenic action of cytokines and this opened a new chapter in sleep research and, more broadly, in our understanding of the interaction between the immune and nervous systems. Today, the most intensively studied sleep factors are the cytokines. One may regard TNFα as the best characterized sleep factor; it is the only known sleep factor the plasma level of which correlates with normal sleep–wake cycles and with certain sleep pathologies in humans (Krueger and Obal 2003).

At about the same time as Pappenheimer's studies, another approach emerged for finding the elusive hypnotoxin. Monnier, later joined by Schoenenberger, used somnogenic electrical stimulation of the thalamus in rabbit, instead of sleep deprivation (Monnier and Hösli 1964). Cross-stimulation experiments showed that the somnogenic actions of the thalamic stimulation could be humorally transmitted (Monnier and Hösli 1965; Monnier *et al.* 1972). From the blood dialysate of the stimulated rabbits, a somnogenic nonapeptide was isolated and named delta-sleep-inducing peptide (DSIP) (Schoenenberger *et al.* 1977). In the late 1970s and 1980s, DSIP was perhaps the most extensively studied sleep factor. The enthusiasm about DSIP, however, gradually faded because the somnogenic action of the peptide could not be confirmed consistently, and even sleep-inhibiting effects were reported by some groups [reviewed in (Borbély and Tobler 1989)].

The most recent attempt to purify sleep factor(s) from sleep-deprived animals started in the 1970s in Japan. A sleep-promoting substance (conveniently named "SPS") was purified from the brain stem of sleep-deprived rats (Nagasaki *et al.* 1974). The extract contained at least four somnogenic fractions. Subsequent analysis identified SPS-A as uridine (Iriki *et al.* 1983) and SPS-B as oxidized glutathione (Komoda *et al.* 1990).

Neurotransmitters and neuromodulators as sleep factors

The idea that a single, hormone-like substance has the central role in sleep regulation has substantially faded in the past 1–2 decades but remains alive in various forms. The inability to purify an endogenous substance that has a robust effect on sleep and may have a fundamental role in sleep regulation gradually made it more and more evident that it is unlikely that the regulation of sleep is the function of a single or only a few endogenous substances. The isolation of a yet unknown hypnotoxin gradually gave way to another approach: the role of the already well characterized, low-molecular-mass neurotransmitters in sleep regulation was investigated. This approach led to the characterization of such fundamental mechanisms as the serotonergic, noradrenergic, and cholinergic, and later the histaminergic, activating systems, the brainstem cholinergic rapid-eye-movement sleep (REMS) system, and to the expansion of the list of sleep factors by the monoamines and acetylcholine.

The characterization of a growing number of peptide neuromodulators in the brain further broadened the scope of the search for sleep factors. In addition to the already studied DSIP, various neuromodulators, neurohormones, and classic peptide hormones were shown to modulate sleep. It is beyond the scope of the present review to summarize the findings with these peptide sleep factors. Particularly well characterized are the members of the somatotropic axis, hypothalamic–pituitary–adrenal axis, and prolactin. Growth-hormone-releasing hormone is involved in the regulation of non-rapid-eye-movement sleep (NREMS) and somatostatin in REMS [reviewed in (Krueger and Obal 2003; Krueger *et al.* 2003)]. Corticotropin-releasing hormone (CRH) is involved in the function of arousal mechanisms [reviewed in (Chang and Opp 2001)] and prolactin has a strong REMS-promoting activity [reviewed in (Krueger *et al.* 2003)]. The identification of non-conventional signal molecules in the brain, such as nitric oxide (NO), adenosine, and prostaglandins produced another set of new molecules for sleep scientists to investigate as sleep factors. In the remainder of this review we summarize recent findings about a group of brain–gut peptides, the ghrelin–neuropeptide Y (NPY)–orexin system, and the gaseous signal molecule, NO. Other sleep factors are discussed in detail in various other chapters of this volume.

Orexin, NPY, and ghrelin as wake-promoting sleep factors

Orexin, ghrelin, and NPY are best known for their role in the hypothalamic food intake–regulatory circuit (Korbonits *et al.* 2004). Recent data suggest that the same network may also contribute to the maintenance of wakefulness and thus orexin, ghrelin and NPY may play a role as sleep factors. Among the three peptides, orexin was recognized first as a crucial factor in sleep–wake regulation when it was noticed that the disruption of the orexinergic system resulted in a narcoleptic state in mice (Chemelli *et al.* 1999). There is, however, further evidence for the role of orexin in the regulation of wakefulness: (a) orexin-containing neurons innervate forebrain and brainstem structures that are implicated in arousal, (b) central injections of orexins stimulate wakefulness, and (c) orexinergic neurons discharge during wakefulness and are silent in NREMS. For references and more details about the role of orexin in the regulation of vigilance, the reader is referred to the chapter by Sinton and Willie (this volume). Here, we focus on ghrelin and NPY, and their role in the regulation of sleep and wakefulness.

The major active form of ghrelin is a 28-amino-acid peptide with a fatty acid chain (octanoyl group) on the *N*-terminal third amino acid (Fig. 11.1); it is the first known peptide hormone with a fatty acid modification. Ghrelins are well conserved in mammals: rat and human ghrelins differ only in two amino acids [reviewed in (Korbonits *et al.* 2004)]. It is a classic gut–brain peptide with potent feeding-promoting and growth-hormone-releasing activities (Kojima *et al.* 1999). The main source of circulating ghrelin is the stomach (Kojima *et al.* 1999), but ghrelin is also produced by neurons of the arcuate nucleus (ARC) and by a distinct neuronal population in the internuclear space of the hypothalamus (Cowley *et al.* 2003). The actions of ghrelin are mediated through the growth hormone secretagogue receptor (GHS-R) (Kojima *et al.* 1999). GHS-R mRNA is widely distributed in hypothalamic nuclei that are implicated in the regulation of feeding and/or sleep–wake activity, such as the lateral hypothalamus

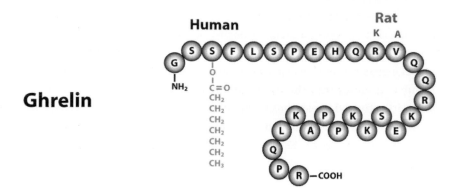

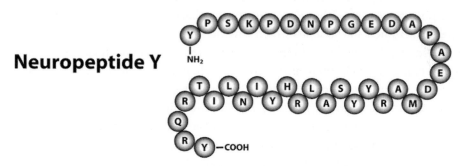

Figure 11.1 The amino acid sequence of ghrelin and neuropeptide Y.

(LH), paraventricular nucleus (PVN), ARC, dorsomedial hypothalamic nucleus (DMH), anteroventral preoptic nucleus, anterior hypothalamic area, suprachiasmatic nucleus (SCN), anterolateral hypothalamic nucleus, and the tuberomammillary nucleus (TMN) (Guan *et al.* 1997; Mitchell *et al.* 2001). In rats, hypothalamic ghrelin content displays diurnal rhythmicity and increases in response to sleep deprivation and feeding restriction (Bodosi *et al.* 2004).

There is a consensus among several studies that exogenous administration of ghrelin stimulates wakefulness in rats. Intracerebroventricular (i.c.v.) injection of ghrelin at light onset significantly increases the time spent awake and decreases NREMS and REMS duration in the first 2 h after injection (Szentirmai *et al.* 2006). Sleep almost completely disappears in response to 1 μg ghrelin in the first hour after ghrelin injection. NREMS-associated power of the electroencephalogram (EEG) is also affected by ghrelin: i.c.v. administration of ghrelin increases EEG slow-wave activity (SWA) for several hours after injection during the light period. EEG delta-wave activity during NREMS, commonly referred to as SWA, is regarded as a measure of NREMS intensity. Intravenous (i.v) injection of

10 μg/rat ghrelin decreases slow-wave sleep and increases wakefulness for 30 min after injection (Tolle *et al.* 2002). A positive correlation between plasma ghrelin levels and active wakefulness was found during the first 3 h of the dark period. The wake-promoting effect of ghrelin is also observed after microinjections of 0.2 and 1 μg doses into the hypothalamus. LH and medial preoptic area (MPA) ghrelin injections decrease both NREMS and REMS for 2 h; the PVN seems to be somewhat less sensitive than the MPA and LH to the wake-promoting action of ghrelin (Szentirmai *et al.* 2007). Ghrelin microinjections also affect EEG power. During NREMS, EEG power is attenuated, particularly the 1.5–4 Hz frequencies, but it is increased during wakefulness and REMS. The i.c.v. injection of ghrelin not only induces EEG-defined wakefulness, but also causes behavioral activation, such as increased locomotor activity in rats (Jásberényi *et al.* 2006).

The feeding-stimulating and sleep-suppressing effects of ghrelin are in the same dose-range after either i.c.v. or intrahypothalamic injections. Ghrelin promotes wakefulness in those rats which have no access to food, indicating that the increased wakefulness is not simply the consequence of increased eating activity (Szentirmai *et al.* 2006). There are several possible mechanisms that may mediate the wake-promoting effect of ghrelin. One is that ghrelin may activate orexinergic and NPY-ergic arousal mechanisms. Ghrelin-containing neurons innervate orexin-producing cells in the LH (Toshinai *et al.* 2003) and i.c.v. or local application of ghrelin into the LH of rats activates orexin neurons (Lawrence *et al.* 2002; Olszewski *et al.* 2003; Toshinai *et al.* 2003). The stimulatory effect of ghrelin on feeding is known to be mediated through NPY-ergic mechanisms in the ARC (Wren *et al.* 2002). In the PVN, the presynaptic terminals of NPY-producing neurons express GHS-R (Guan *et al.* 1997) and ghrelin-positive neuronal projections from the ARC stimulate NPY release (Cowley *et al.* 2003). Another possibility is that ghrelin acts through the activation of the hypothalamic–pituitary–adrenal axis; CRH release is stimulated by ghrelin in the PVN (Cowley *et al.* 2003) and CRH is known to inhibit sleep [reviewed in (Chang and Opp 2001)].

The effects of ghrelin and other GHS-R agonists on sleep is less clear in humans; increased and decreased sleep and no effect on sleep have been reported. In young healthy male subjects, i.v. bolus injections of ghrelin increase slow wave sleep during the first part and decrease REMS in the middle of the night. The increase in slow wave sleep is associated with an increase in the power of delta wave activity. No significant changes in the spectral power of other frequency bands were found (Weikel *et al.* 2003). MK-677, an orally active growth hormone secretagogue, increases the duration of stage 4 sleep by 50% and REMS by 20% in young male subjects and enhances REMS in elderly subjects after subchronic administration (Copinschi *et al.* 1997). A single intravenous bolus injection of growth-hormone-releasing peptide-2, given after the third REM period during the night, has no effect on sleep (Moreno-Reyes *et al.* 1998). Pulsatile administration of growth-hormone-releasing peptide-6 to young men induced a modest increase in stage 2 sleep, without any change in slow wave sleep and SWA (Frieboes *et al.* 1995). Hexarelin, the most potent agonist of the GHS-R in terms of growth hormone release, decreases stage 4 sleep and suppresses EEG delta power during NREMS, but does not affect REMS or sleep continuity (Frieboes *et al.* 1995).

The available data about the correlation between plasma ghrelin levels and sleep in humans are not consistent. In one study, no relation was found between plasma ghrelin levels and spontaneously occurring sleep stages (Schüssler *et al.* 2005). In another population-based longitudinal study, however, shorter sleep time correlated with elevated ghrelin levels (Taheri *et al.* 2004). Deprivation of sleep for one night did not affect plasma ghrelin levels during the subsequent, recovery night (Schüssler *et al.* 2006). Two days of sleep restriction, however, increased daytime plasma ghrelin levels in healthy men (Spiegel *et al.* 2004). Also, elevated nocturnal ghrelin levels were found in a patient with night-eating syndrome, a disorder that is characterized by repetitive awakenings (Rosenhagen *et al.* 2005). The differences in the effect of ghrelin on sleep between rats and humans may result from the different injection protocols or may reflect real species-specificity in the sleep-modulating effect of ghrelin.

Obestatin is a recently identified product of the ghrelin gene (Zhang *et al.* 2005). The effects of obestatin on feeding and body mass appear to be the opposite of those of ghrelin. A recent study suggests that, in rats, ghrelin and obestatin also have opposite effects on sleep (Szentirmai and Krueger 2006b). Central administration of obestatin induces an immediate increase in the amount of NREMS, which is followed by a decrease in NREMS and REMS. EEG SWA is suppressed after i.c.v. obestatin. Systemic injection of obestatin does not induce any changes in sleep in rats.

NPY is a 36-amino acid peptide that is highly conserved through evolution: the amino acid sequences of human and rat NPY are identical (Fig. 11.1). It is a widely distributed neuropeptide in the central nervous system. The main source of NPY in the brain is the hypothalamus. Its known physiological role is primarily related to feeding, but NPY is also implicated in the regulation of hormone secretion, thermoregulation and circadian rhythms [reviewed in (Kaga *et al.* 2001)]. NPY-ergic and orexinergic neurons in the LH and ARC are reciprocally innervated. An i.c.v. (2 and 10 μg) and LH (2 μg) injection of NPY at light onset induces wakefulness in rats (Szentirmai and Krueger 2006a). The sleep-suppressing effect of NPY is robust: both NREMS and REMS are significantly decreased in the first hour after injection, and REMS almost completely disappears. In another study, i.c.v. injection of *c.* 12 μg NPY decreased EEG power in all frequencies across all vigilance states in rats during a 40-min recording period. The latency to sleep onset and the amount of NREMS was not affected, but it should be noted that this experiment was not designed as a true test of sleep effects as the animals were not recorded in their home cages (Ehlers *et al.* 1997). In humans, repeated intravenous injections of NPY promote stage 2 sleep and reduce sleep latency in healthy subjects (Antonijevic *et al.* 2000). Using the same injection protocol, NPY induced only the shortening of NREMS and REMS latencies but did not affect the time spent in stage 2 sleep, slow wave sleep, REMS, or total sleep time in patients with depression and in age-matched controls (Held *et al.* 2006).

The mechanism by which NPY modulates sleep is unknown. Hypothalamic nuclei that are implicated in feeding and sleep–wake regulation, such as the ARC, PVN, SCN, DMH, and LH, all contain NPY-immunoreactive cell bodies. NPY receptors are also present in these hypothalamic nuclei (Wolak *et al.* 2003). NPY-positive fibers innervate orexinergic neurons in the LH. The activation of NPY Y4 receptors in the LH increases c-*fos* immunoreactivity locally in the orexinergic neurons (Campbell *et al.* 2003). It has been hypothesized that NPY-induced wakefulness is mediated through the activation of lateral hypothalamic orexinergic neurons (Szentirmai and Krueger 2006a). CRH is another potential mediator of the wakefulness-inducing activity of NPY. NPY stimulates CRH release and increases CRH gene expression in the PVN (Suda *et al.* 1993), and CRH is known to inhibit sleep (Chang and Opp 2001).

The sleep-suppressing and food-intake-promoting activities of central NPY, ghrelin, and orexin in rats are strikingly similar (see Fig. 11.2). The first hours of the active period in rats are characterized by increased time spent awake, increased duration of the individual wake episodes, and increased eating activity (i.e. the dark onset syndrome). Central administration of orexin, NPY, or ghrelin elicits all the symptoms of the dark onset syndrome. It is possible that the increased feeding activity and the stimulation of wakefulness are two parallel outputs of the activation of the same hypothalamic orexin-ghrelin-NPY circuit.

Nitric oxide as a sleep factor

NO is a gaseous neurotransmitter implicated in signaling in the central and peripheral nervous system as well as in the immune system and the vasculature. NO is formed from L-arginine by nitric oxide synthase (NOS). There are three isoforms of NOS. All isoforms require NADPH as a cofactor, use L-arginine as a substrate, and are inhibited by Nω-nitro-L-arginine methyl ester (L-NAME). The three isoforms are separate gene products. One isoform of NOS is a cytosolic, calcium/calmodulin-independent, inducible enzyme (iNOS). It is found in macrophages, neutrophils, vascular smooth muscle, and endothelia. The iNOS

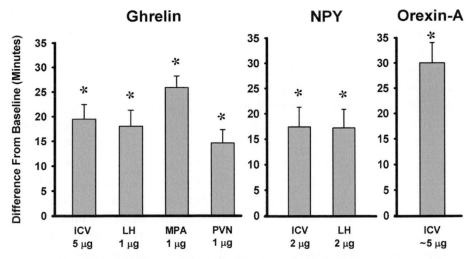

Figure 11.2   Increases in wakefulness after intracerebroventricular (ICV) or intrahypothalamic administration of ghrelin, neuropeptide Y (NPY), and orexin-A in the first hour of the light period in rats. LH, lateral hypothalamus; MPA, medial preoptic area; PVN, paraventricular nucleus; asterisks denote significant differences from baseline. Orexin data are extracted from Vogel *et al.*, *J. Neuroscience Methods*, 2002, **118**: 89–96.

is also expressed in the normal brain and its expression is greatly enhanced by endotoxin, gamma-interferon, IL-1 and TNFα [reviewed in (Alderton *et al.* 2001; Guix *et al.* 1999)]. The second isoform is expressed in neurons (nNOS). It is a constitutive, calcium-dependent, cytosolic enzyme. NO, released from neurons, serves a transmitter function and is implicated in a variety of basic neuronal functions; nNOS is selectively inhibited by 7-nitroindazole (7-NI). A third isoform is present in the endothelia (eNOS). It is constitutive and calcium-dependent, but unlike nNOS, it is membrane-bound. NO produced in the endothelia is a key factor in the homeostatic control of the vessels, and it elicits relaxation of the vascular smooth muscle.

Two sets of evidence suggested in the early 1990s that NO may serve as a sleep factor. First, it became evident that the enzyme NADPH diaphorase is the same as nNOS. NADPH diaphorase is regarded as a specific marker for pontine (Vincent *et al.* 1983) and basal forebrain cholinergic neurons (Ichikawa and Hirata 1986). Pontine cholinergic neurons are hypothesized to play a central role in wakefulness and REMS generation; corticopetal cholinergic projections from the basal forebrain are thought to contribute to the activation of the cortex. Second, it was shown that highly somnogenic cytokines, such as IL-1β and TNFα are strong stimulators of NO production. Five major approaches have since been used to address the role of NO as a sleep factor. The effects of (a) NOS inhibitors and (b) NO donors on sleep are studied, (c) the NO-producing activity of the brain is measured in vivo by voltammetry and microdialysis and ex vivo by essays for NOS enzyme activity, (d) the activity of NO-producing mechanisms is also assessed indirectly by measuring the protein or mRNA expression of various NOS isoforms, and (e) spontaneous sleep and sleep responses to various challenges are measured in NOS-deficient transgenic mice.

A growing body of evidence suggests that the role of NO in sleep regulation is more complex than that of most other sleep factors, since NO appears to be involved in the functioning of both sleep-promoting and arousal mechanisms. The first experiments tested the effects of systemic and i.c.v. injections of NOS inhibitors on sleep. L-NAME suppressed NREMS and REMS in rabbits after both i.c.v. and i.v. administration (Kapás *et al.* 1994b). In rats, the initial study reported a marked suppression of both NREMS and REMS after central and systemic administration of L-NAME; SWA was also strongly and dose-dependently suppressed (Kapás *et al.* 1994a). The majority of the subsequent studies reported similar sleep-suppressing effects after systemic administration of L-NAME (Monti *et al.* 1999, 2001; Ribeiro *et al.* 2000), or the injection of nNOS-specific inhibitors, 7-NI (Burlet *et al.* 1999; Dzoljic *et al.* 1996) or 3-bromo-7-NI (Cavas and Navarro 2006; Dzoljic *et al.* 1996). These results suggested that NO may be a sleep factor primarily involved in sleep-induction. Subsequently, however, it became evident that the picture was more complex. Sleep-promoting effects were also reported after the systemic injection of L-NAME (Burlet *et al.* 1999) or another NOS inhibitor, L-NMMA (Dzoljic and de Vries 1994). The fact that in the latter studies, NOS inhibitors were administered at dark onset or during the dark period, while in the other experiments NOS inhibitors were administered during the light phase, suggested that the effects of these inhibitors may depend on the circadian phase. A recent study specifically addressed this question (Ribeiro and Kapás 2005). Light onset intraperitoneal injection of 50 mg/kg L-NAME decreased NREMS and caused a delayed increases in REMS, whereas dark onset injections of 5–100 mg/kg L-NAME caused prompt increases in both REMS and NREMS. Interestingly, after both dark- and light-onset treatments, SWA was strongly suppressed. It seems that different NO-ergic mechanisms may be active during rest and activity periods and these mechanisms are likely to have opposite roles in sleep regulation (see below). The effects of the stimulation of NO-sensitive structures are usually tested by using NO donors, molecules that spontaneously decompose to release NO. The i.c.v. injection of 3-morpholino-sydnonimine (SIN-1) and S-nitroso-N-acetylpenicillamine, two commonly used NO donors, promotes NREMS and increases SWA in rats (Kapás and Krueger 1996). Similar to L-NAME, the effects of SIN-1 on sleep also depend on the circadian phase at the time of administration (Monti and Jantos 2004a).

The role of NO-ergic mechanisms in diencephalic and brainstem areas were further studied by microinjection experiments. The effects of NO donors and NOS inhibitors in the diencephalic area are complex, suggesting that various sites within this area express NOS and that the multiple target sites for NO may have different roles in sleep regulation. Nocturnal infusion of L-NAME into the subarachnoid ventral surface of the rostral basal forebrain (an area adjacent to the ventrolateral preoptic nucleus that is also sensitive to the sleep-promoting effects of prostaglandin D_2) markedly stimulates REMS (Matsumura *et al.* 1995). In addition, subarachnoidal dialysis of L-NAME into the "diencephalic region" stimulates, whereas infusion of a NO donor suppresses REMS (Matsumura *et al.* 1999). Injection of L-NAME into the horizontal limb of diagonal band of Broca, however, suppresses sleep (Monti and Jantos 2004b). In cats, lateral basal forebrain microinjection of Nω-nitro-L-arginine did not have any effect on sleep (Vazquez *et al.* 2002). Bilateral microinjections of NO donors into the SCN had robust wakefulness-promoting and REMS-suppressing effects (Ribeiro and Kapás 2003), whereas microinjections of L-NAME into the MPA and subparaventricular zone suppressed wakefulness and enhanced REMS (Ribeiro and Kapás 1999). Furthermore, injection of a NO donor into the MPA increased arousal and this effect was mimicked by the injection of 8-Br-cGMP (Ribeiro and Kapás 1999). Together, these results are consistent with the hypothesis that diencephalic NO-ergic mechanisms play a role in the regulation of vigilance, possibly by stimulating arousal mechanisms in the SCN, subparaventricular zone and MPA.

Cholinergic neurons of the brainstem pedunculopontine tegmental/ laterodorsal tegmental (PPT/LDT) region project to the medial pontine reticular formation (mPRF); these neurons also selectively stain for nNOS activity. Activation of the brainstem cholinergic system is thought to have a crucial role in REMS generation. In cats, microinjection of Nω-nitro-L-arginine into the cholinoceptive mPRF suppresses natural and neostigmine-induced REMS (Leonard and Lydic 1997), as well as ACh release from both the mPRF and PPT/LDT region (Leonard and Lydic 1995). Microinjection of L-NAME into the dorsal raphe nucleus suppresses NREMS (Monti *et al.* 1999, 2001) and REMS (Burlet *et al.* 1999; Monti *et al.* 2001) and administration of 7-NI reduces REMS (Burlet *et al.* 1999). Intra-PPT microinfusion of the NO donor *S*-nitroso-*N*-acetylpenicillamine in cats (Datta *et al.* 1997), or SIN-1 in rats (Hars 1999), stimulates both NREMS and REMS. It has been hypothesized that serotonin suppresses the activity of NOS-containing pontine neurons, and during REMS, when serotoninergic input is at its lowest level, NO production is disinhibited (Leonard *et al.* 2000). The brainstem mechanisms that mediate the actions of NO are currently under intense investigation. Cholinergic, adrenergic, prolactin, GABA, and adenosine mechanisms have been implicated in the brainstem actions of NO. NOS inhibitors decrease ACh release in the pontine reticular formation in cats (Leonard and Lydic 1997), and NO donors stimulate ACh release in mice by activating guanylyl cyclase (Lydic *et al.* 2006). NO also facilitates norepinephrine release from adrenergic terminals in the LDT (Kodama and Koyama 2006). The wake-promoting effects of dorsal raphe nucleus microinjections of L-NAME are prevented by $GABA_A$ and adenosine A_1 receptor antagonists (Monti *et al.* 2001). Prolactin mRNA levels are elevated in the brainstem of nNOS KO mice and increased in response to nNOS inhibitors in normal animals (Chen *et al.* 2004b), suggesting that NO may regulate brainstem prolactin production.

Sleep was also studied in mice with targeted disruption of nNOS or iNOS genes. Studying sleep in knockout (KO) animals often gives contradictory and unexpected results, which may even be misleading. The multiplicity of sleep factors and brain structures involved in the regulation of vigilance and the fact that the elimination of none of these mechanisms leads to permanent and complete loss of sleep suggest that there is a robust redundancy built into the sleep regulatory system. In KO animals, there is a possibility that compensatory mechanisms develop for the disrupted gene product. Therefore, negative findings need to be interpreted carefully, especially when they are related to spontaneous sleep. In nNOS KO mice, REMS is reduced, whereas iNOS KO animals show slightly decreased NREMS and increased REMS in the light period (Chen *et al.* 2003). This suggests that sleep may be differentially modulated by NO produced by various NOS isoforms. TNFα, a potent somnogen, failed to increase NREMS in nNOS KO mice (Chen *et al.* 2004c). This finding, together with prior results that the somnogenic effects of IL-1β (Kapás *et al.* 1994b) and acidic fibroblast growth factor (Galan *et al.* 1996) are attenuated by L-NAME and that viral challenge fails to induce sleep in nNOS and iNOS KO mice (Chen *et al.* 2004a), strongly suggests that cytokine-induced increased NREMS responses may be mediated, at least in part, by NO.

It has been suggested that basal forebrain NO-ergic mechanisms play a role in homeostatic sleep increases during the light phase in rats, but NO in the SCN may play a role in stimulating arousal mechanisms during the behaviorally active phase (Ribeiro and Kapás 2005). The most direct evidence that NO-ergic mechanisms are key players in the homeostatic regulation of sleep is that rebound increases in sleep after sleep deprivation are shorter in duration and lower in amplitude in NOS inhibitor-treated rats than sleep rebound in control animals (Ribeiro *et al.* 2000). Systemic injection of L-NAME suppresses NREMS only after light onset administration, when the homeostatic sleep pressure is highest in rats, but promotes sleep at night (Ribeiro and Kapás 2005). Also in line with this hypothesis, direct bilateral application of L-NAME into the nucleus of the horizontal limb of the diagonal band of Broca increases wakefulness and reduces slow wave sleep (Monti and Jantos 2004b). In a recent study, however, it was found that basal forebrain stimulation-induced cortical activation is attenuated by blocking NOS activity (Marino and Cudeiro 2003). This finding argues for the involvement of NO-ergic basal forebrain mechanisms in the maintenance of cortical activity.

It is expected that the production of a sleep factor that plays a role in inducing homeostatic increases in NREMS, is increased during both spontaneous and sleep deprivation-induced wakefulness and declines during sleep. The dynamics of NO release and NOS enzyme activity generally fit this pattern. NO is produced in an activity-dependent manner (Leonard et al. 2001), and both cortical (Burlet and Cespuglio 1997) and thalamic (107) release of NO are higher during wakefulness than in NREMS. NOS activity shows a marked diurnal rhythm in the hypothalamus, brainstem, hippocampus and cerebellum in rats, peaking at night, when the animals are behaviorally active. In fact, hypothalamic NOS activity increases by c. 100% from the middle of the day to the middle of the night (Ayers et al. 1996). Similarly, in rats, cortical release of NO increases throughout the night and declines during the day (Clément et al. 2004), and nNOS mRNA expression peaks during the night in rat pineal gland (Spessert and Rapp 2001). In mice, brain NOS activity and plasma nitrate/nitrite levels display circadian rhythm, with the highest levels during the dark phase (Tunctan et al. 2002). In the SCN, both NOS enzymatic activity (Ferreyra et al. 1998) and extracellular NO_2^-/NO_3^- concentrations (Mitome et al. 2001) show a marked diurnal rhythm, being elevated at night and reduced during the day. In rat visual cortex, NADPH-diaphorase activity, a measure of nNOS activity, is increased during the dark and decreased during the light period (Hilbig and Punkt 1997). Eight hours of sleep deprivation by gentle handling increases the expression of iNOS protein in the basal forebrain but not in the cerebellum, LDT, or SCN, suggesting a role for increased production of NO in the basal forebrain in rebound sleep responses to sleep deprivation (Ribeiro and Kapás 2005). REMS deprivation increases nNOS protein levels in the frontal cortex (Clément et al. 2004). Long-term sleep deprivation, however, suppresses nNOS expression in the hippocampus (Hsu et al. 2003).

NO is a crucial signaling molecule in the suprachiasmatic nucleus (SCN) [reviewed in (Golombek et al. 2004)]. Glutamate elevates NO levels in the SCN, which, in turn, activate soluble guanylyl cyclase, increasing cGMP levels. Intra-SCN microinjection, or in vitro application of glutamate (Ding et al. 1994; Meijer et al. 1988) or NO donors (Ding et al. 1994) to SCN slices, elicits phase shifts similar to those produced by in vivo light pulses. In contrast, cerebral injections of chemicals that block this signaling cascade prevent light-induced phase shifts [reviewed in (Ribeiro and Kapás 2005)]. Phase resetting by the light/glutamate/NO pathway is only active during the dark period (Gillette and Mitchell 2002), which is the phase when L-NAME strongly enhances NREMS and REMS. The actions of NO in the SCN suggest that NO-ergic mechanisms may also be part of the circadian process of sleep regulation. It has been hypothesized that, during the dark period when homeostatic sleep pressure is low, sleep responses to L-NAME are due to its effects on the light/glutamate/NO pathway in the SCN (Ribeiro and Kapás 2005). In fact, as discussed above, microinjection of NOS inhibitors into the medial preoptic region or anterior diencephalic area increases sleep, particularly REMS; and bilateral microinjections of an NO donor into the SCN suppress REMS.

During the light period, L-NAME may interfere with the sleep-promoting homeostatic effects of NO-ergic mechanisms. In vitro studies indicate that the SCN during this period is insensitive to NO (Gillette and Mitchell 2002). During the dark period, however, when homeostatic mechanisms are the least active but the SCN is sensitive to L-NAME, the target for L-NAME is most likely to be the SCN and increased sleep is due to the actions of L-NAME on the circadian process.

Conclusion

To provide a definition for sleep factors at the end of this review, rather than at the beginning, may seem somewhat misguided, but if one considers that there is not a single, universally accepted definition for sleep factors, and there does not necessarily have to be one, it is more understandable. It appears that the "hypnotoxin", a single, all-in-one sleep hormone, remains elusive and most of us researching in this field do not anticipate finding one. There are, however, numerous endogenous substances that are capable of modulating sleep: some may induce sleep, others may inhibit sleep, or have both effects, and the action may be specific to NREMS or REMS, or both. All of these endogenous substances that can affect sleep could be called "sleep factors".

To understand how sleep is modulated by endogenous substances, one needs to consider two related, fundamental observations regarding brain structures and sleep. One, the regulation and/or generation of sleep is not the function of a single brain structure; there are multiple brain sites, the manipulation of which affects sleep. Two, none of these multiple brain sites is absolutely necessary for the generation of sleep. Lesions of various structures may affect, or even completely eliminate sleep, but these changes are always temporary. If the animal survives the procedure, sleep will, inevitably, return in some form. It is clear that the function of those multiple brain regions that are already shown to be involved in sleep regulation, and the list is continuously growing, is driven and modulated by neurotransmitters, hormones, and other signal molecules. When these signals are experimentally manipulated, the functions – including generation, regulation or maintenance of sleep – of these neural networks will also be affected. It is becoming increasingly evident that, when manipulation of a certain messenger system affects sleep, it is not only the brain structure that is targeted, but also the timing, the right dose of agonist or antagonist, and the fortunate constellation of other experimental conditions that influence the outcome. Therefore, in the eyes of a significant number of researchers in the field, the agent in such a study would qualify for the title of "sleep factor".

There are two oft-cited criteria for sleep factors. One, a sleep factor is expected to cause a change in a sleep parameter, such as the amount or intensity of sleep; and two, the sleep factor should vary in association with sleeping or waking (Borbély and Tobler 1989). Recent advances in molecular and cellular neurobiology, however, have rendered this picture more complex. It is clear that a messenger per se does not necessarily have to change in concentration to exert varying effects: a variation in the sensitivity of the target structures may be sufficient. Also, a messenger may be an integral part of more than one key, sleep-regulatory network. If it plays a role in several networks with opposite function, if for example one is sleep-promoting and another arousal-facilitating, then routine screening of the putative sleep factor (e.g. by i.c.v. administration) might not yield a consistent change in sleep parameters. To test the effects of a receptor agonist or antagonist on sleep requires the local delivery of the messenger to the target site(s) by microinjection, microdialysis, or other similar technique. Considering the abundance of possible target sites, one soon comes to the realization that it is close to impossible to prove that a certain signal molecule is not a sleep factor.

References

Alderton, W. K., Cooper, C. E. & Knowles, R. G. (2001). Nitric oxide synthases: structure, function and inhibition. *Biochem. J.* **357**, 593–615.

Antonijevic, I. A., Murck, H., Bohlhalter, S. *et al.* (2000). Neuropeptide Y promotes sleep and inhibits ACTH and cortisol release in young men. *Neuropharmacology* **39**, 1474–81.

Ayers, N. A., Kapás, L. & Krueger, J. M. (1996). Circadian variation of nitric oxide synthase activity and cytosolic protein levels in rat brain. *Brain Res.* **707**, 127–30.

Bodosi, B., Gardi, J., Hajdu, I. *et al.* (2004). Rhythms of ghrelin, leptin, and sleep in rats: effects of the normal diurnal cycle, restricted feeding, and sleep deprivation. *Am. J. Physiol. Regul. Integr. Comp. Physiol.* **287**, R1071–9.

Borbély, A. A. & Tobler, I. (1989). Endogenous sleep-promoting substances and sleep regulation. *Physiol. Rev.* **69**, 605–70.

Burlet, S. & Cespuglio, R. (1997). Voltametric detection of nitric oxide (NO) in the rat brain: its variations throughout the sleep-wake cycle. *Neurosci. Lett.* **226**, 131–5.

Burlet, S., Leger, L. & Cespuglio, R. (1999). Nitric oxide and sleep in the rat: a puzzling relationship. *Neuroscience* **92**, 627–39.

Campbell, R. E., Smith, M. S., Allen, S. E. *et al.* (2003). Orexin neurons express a functional pancreatic polypeptide Y4 receptor. *J. Neurosci.* **23**, 1487–97.

Cavas, M. & Navarro, J. F. (2006). Effects of selective neuronal nitric oxide synthase inhibition on sleep and wakefulness in the rat. *Prog. Neuropsychopharmacol. Biol. Psychiatry* **30**, 56–67.

Chang, F. C. & Opp, M. R. (2001). Corticotropin-releasing hormone (CRH) as a regulator of waking. *Neurosci. Biobehav. Rev.* **25**, 445–53.

Chemelli, R. M., Willie, J. T., Sinton, C. M. *et al.* (1999). Narcolepsy in orexin knockout mice: molecular genetics of sleep regulation. *Cell* **98**, 437–51.

Chen, L., Duricka, D., Nelson, S. *et al.* (2004a). Influenza virus-induced sleep responses in mice with targeted disruptions in neuronal or inducible nitric oxide synthases. *J. Appl. Physiol.* **97**, 17–28.

Chen, L., Majde, J. A. & Krueger, J. M. (2003). Spontaneous sleep in mice with targeted disruptions of neuronal or inducible nitric oxide synthase genes. *Brain Res.* **973**, 214–22.

Chen, L., Taishi, P., Duricka, D. & Krueger, J. M. (2004b). Brainstem prolactin mRNA is enhanced in mice with suppressed neuronal nitric oxide synthase activity. *Brain Res. Mol. Brain Res.* **129**, 179–84.

Chen, L., Taishi, P., Majde, J. A. *et al.* (2004c). The role of nitric oxide synthases in the sleep responses to tumor necrosis factor-α. *Brain Behav. Immun.* **18**, 390–8.

Clément, P., Sarda, N., Cespuglio, R. & Gharib, A. (2004). Changes occurring in cortical NO release and brain NO-synthases during a paradoxical sleep deprivation and subsequent recovery in the rat. *J. Neurochem.* **90**, 848–56.

Copinschi, G., Leproult, R., Van, O. A. *et al.* (1997). Prolonged oral treatment with MK-677, a novel growth hormone secretagogue, improves sleep quality in man. *Neuroendocrinology* **66**, 278–86.

Cowley, M. A., Smith, R. G., Diano, S. *et al.* (2003). The distribution and mechanism of action of ghrelin in the CNS demonstrates a novel hypothalamic circuit regulating energy homeostasis. *Neuron* **37**, 649–61.

Datta, S., Patterson, E. H. & Siwek, D. F. (1997). Endogenous and exogenous nitric oxide in the pedunculopontine tegmentum induces sleep. *Synapse* **27**, 69–78.

Ding, J. M., Chen, D., Weber, E. T. *et al.* (1994). Resetting the biological clock: mediation of nocturnal circadian shifts by glutamate and NO. *Science* **266**, 1713–17.

Dzoljic, E., van Leeuwen, R., de Vries, R. & Dzoljic, M. R. (1997). Vigilance and EEG power in rats: effects of potent inhibitors of the neuronal nitric oxide synthase. *Naunyn Schmiedebergs Arch. Pharmacol.* **356**, 56–61.

Dzoljic, M. R. & de Vries, R. (1994). Nitric oxide synthase inhibition reduces wakefulness. *Neuropharmacology* **33**, 1505–9.

Dzoljic, M. R., de Vries, R. & van Leeuwen, R. (1996). Sleep and nitric oxide: effects of 7-nitro indazole, inhibitor of brain nitric oxide synthase. *Brain Res.* **718**, 145–50.

Ehlers, C. L., Somes, C., Lopez, A., Kirby, D. & Rivier, J. E. (1997). Electrophysiological actions of neuropeptide Y and its analogs: new measures for anxiolytic therapy? *Neuropsychopharmacology* **17**, 34–43.

Fencl, V., Koski, G. & Pappenheimer, J. R. (1971). Factors in cerebrospinal fluid from goats that affect sleep and activity in rats. *J. Physiol.* **216**, 565–89.

Ferreyra, G. A., Cammarota, M. P. & Golombek, D. A. (1998). Photic control of nitric oxide synthase activity in the hamster suprachiasmatic nuclei. *Brain Res.* **797**, 190–6.

Frieboes, R. M., Antonijevic, I. A., Held, K. *et al.* (2004). Hexarelin decreases slow-wave sleep and stimulates the secretion of GH, ACTH, cortisol and prolactin during sleep in healthy volunteers. *Psychoneuroendocrinology* **29**, 851–60.

Frieboes, R. M., Murck, H., Maier, P. *et al.* (1995). Growth hormone-releasing peptide-6 stimulates sleep, growth hormone, ACTH and cortisol release in normal man. *Neuroendocrinology* **61**, 584–9.

Galan, J. M., Cuevas, B., Dujovny, N., Gimenezgallego, G. & Cuevas, P. (1996). Sleep promoting effects of intravenously administered acidic fibroblast growth factor. *Neurol. Res.* **18**, 567–9.

Gillette, M. U. & Mitchell, J. W. (2002). Signaling in the suprachiasmatic nucleus: selectively responsive and integrative. *Cell Tiss. Res.* **309**, 99–107.

Gillette, M. U. & Tischkau, S. A. (1999). Suprachiasmatic nucleus: the brain's circadian clock. *Rec. Prog. Horm. Res.* **54**, 33–58.

Golombek, D. A., Agostino, P. V., Plano, S. A. & Ferreyra, G. A. (2004). Signaling in the mammalian circadian clock: the NO/cGMP pathway. *Neurochem. Int.* **45**, 929–36.

Guan, X. M., Yu, H., Palyha, O. C. *et al.* (1997). Distribution of mRNA encoding the growth hormone secretagogue receptor in brain and peripheral tissues. *Brain Res. Mol. Brain Res.* **48**, 23–9.

Guix, F. X., Uribesalgo, I., Coma, M. & Munoz, F. J. (2005). The physiology and pathophysiology of nitric oxide in the brain. *Prog. Neurobiol.* **76**, 126–52.

Hars, B. (1999). Endogenous nitric oxide in the rat pons promotes sleep. *Brain Res.* **816**, 209–19.

Held, K., Antonijevic, I., Murck, H., Kuenzel, H. & Steiger, A. (2006). Neuropeptide Y (NPY) shortens sleep latency but does not suppress ACTH and cortisol in depressed patients and normal controls. *Psychoneuroendocrinology* **31**, 100–7.

Hilbig, H. & Punkt, K. (1997). 24-hour rhythmicity of NADPH-diaphorase activity in the neuropil of rat visual cortex. *Brain Res. Bull.* **43**, 337–40.

Hsu, J. C., Lee, Y. S., Chang, C. N. *et al.* (2003). Sleep deprivation inhibits expression of NADPH-d and NOS while activating microglia and astroglia in the rat hippocampus. *Cell. Tiss. Org.* **173**, 242–54.

Ichikawa, T. & Hirata, Y. (1986). Organization of choline acetyltransferase-containing structures in the forebrain of the rat. *J. Neurosci.* **6**, 281–92.

Iriki, M., Honda, K., Inoue, S., Higashi, A. & Uchizono, K. (1983). Uridine, a sleep-promoting substance from brainstems of sleep-deprived rats. *Biomed. Res.* (Suppl.) **4**, 223–7.

Ishimori, K. (1909). True cause of sleep – a hypnogenic substance as evidenced in the brain of sleep-deprived animals. *Tokyo Igakkai Zasshi* **23**, 429–57.

Jászberényi, M., Bujdosó, E., Bagosi, Z. & Telegdy, G. (2006). Mediation of the behavioral, endocrine and thermoregulatory actions of ghrelin. *Horm. Behav.* **50**, 266–73.

Kaga, T., Fujimiya, M. & Inui, A. (2001). Emerging functions of neuropeptide Y Y(2) receptors in the brain. *Peptides* **22**, 501–6.

Kapás, L. & Krueger, J. M. (1996). Nitric oxide donors SIN-1 and SNAP promote nonrapid-eye-movement sleep in rats. *Brain Res. Bull.* **41**, 293–8.

Kapás, L., Fang, J. & Krueger, J. M. (1994a). Inhibition of nitric oxide synthesis inhibits rat sleep. *Brain Res.* **664**, 189–96.

Kapás, L., Shibata, M., Kimura, M. & Krueger, J. M. (1994b). Inhibition of nitric oxide synthesis suppresses sleep in rabbits. *Am. J. Physiol.* **266**, R151–7.

Kodama, T. & Koyama, Y. (2006). Nitric oxide from the laterodorsal tegmental neurons: its possible retrograde modulation on norepinephrine release from the axon terminal of the locus coeruleus neurons. *Neuroscience* **138**, 245–56.

Kojima, M., Hosoda, H., Date, Y. *et al.* (1999). Ghrelin is a growth-hormone-releasing acylated peptide from stomach. *Nature* **402**, 656–60.

Komoda, Y., Honda, K. & Inoue, S. (1990). SPS-B, a physiological sleep regulator, from the brainstems of sleep-deprived rats, identified as oxidized glutathione. *Chem. Pharm. Bull. (Tokyo)* **38**, 2057–9.

Korbonits, M., Goldstone, A. P., Gueorguiev, M. & Grossman, A. B. (2004). Ghrelin – a hormone with multiple functions. *Front. Neuroendocrinol.* **25**, 27–68.

Krueger, J. M. & Obal, F. Jr. (2003). Sleep function. *Front. Biosci.* **8**, d511–9.

Krueger, J. M., Dinarello, C. A., Shoham, S. *et al.* (1987). Interferon alpha-2 enhances slow-wave sleep in rabbits. *Int. J. Immunopharmacol.* **9**, 23–30.

Krueger, J. M., Majde, J. A. & Obál, F. (2003). Sleep in host defense. *Brain Behav. Immun.* **17** (Suppl. 1), S41–7.

Krueger, J. M., Pappenheimer, J. R. & Karnovsky, M. L. (1982). Sleep-promoting effects of muramyl peptides. *Proc. Natl. Acad. Sci. USA* **79**, 6102–6.

Krueger, J. M., Walter, J., Dinarello, C. A., Wolff, S. M. & Chedid, L. (1984). Sleep-promoting effects of endogenous pyrogen (interleukin-1). *Am. J. Physiol.* **246**, R994–9.

Lawrence, C. B., Snape, A. C., Baudoin, F. M. & Luckman, S. M. (2002). Acute central ghrelin and GH secretagogues induce feeding and activate brain appetite centers. *Endocrinology* **143**, 155–62.

Legendre, R. & Piéron, H. (1912). De la propriété hypnotoxique des humeurs dévéloppé au cours d'une veille prolongée. *C. R. Soc. Biol.* **72**, 210–2.

Legendre, R. & Piéron, H. (1910). Le probléme de facteurs de sommeil. Resultats d'injections vasculaires et intracérébrales des liquides insomniques. *C. R. Soc. Biol.* **68**, 1077–9.

Leonard, C. S., Michaelis, E. K. & Mitchell, K. M. (2001). Activity-dependent nitric oxide concentration dynamics in the laterodorsal tegmental nucleus in vitro. *J. Neurophysiol.* **86**, 2159–72.

Leonard, C. S., Rao, S. R. & Inoue, T. (2000). Serotonergic inhibition of action potential evoked calcium transients in NOS-containing mesopontine cholinergic neurons. *J. Neurophysiol.* **84**, 1558–72.

Leonard, T. O. & Lydic, R. (1995). Nitric oxide synthase inhibition decreases pontine acetylcholine release. *Neuroreport* **6**, 1525–9.

Leonard, T. O. & Lydic, R. (1997). Pontine nitric oxide modulates acetylcholine release, rapid eye movement sleep generation, and respiratory rate. *J. Neurosci.* **17**, 774–85.

Lydic, R., Garza-Grande, R., Struthers, R. & Baghdoyan, H. A. (2006). Nitric oxide in B6 mouse and nitric oxide-sensitive soluble guanylate cyclase in cat modulate acetylcholine release in pontine reticular formation. *J. Appl. Physiol.* **100**, 1666–73.

Marino, J. & Cudeiro, J. (2003). Nitric oxide-mediated cortical activation: a diffuse wake-up system. *J. Neurosci.* **23**, 4299–307.

Matsumura, H., Gerashchenko, D., Satoh, S. *et al.* (1995). Prostaglandin D2 and nitric oxide: key factors underlying the regulation of slow-wave sleep and paradoxical sleep in the rat brain. *Sleep Res.* **24A**, 134.

Matsumura, H., Maeda, T., Tokunaga, Y. *et al.* (1999). Evidence that nitric oxide acting in a diencephalic region is involved in the regulation of paradoxical sleep in rats. *Sleep Res. Online* **2** (Suppl. 1), 63.

Meijer, J. H., van der Zee, E. A. & Dietz, M. (1988). Glutamate phase shifts circadian activity rhythms in hamsters. *Neurosci. Lett.* **86**, 177–83.

Mitchell, V., Bouret, S., Beauvillain, J. C. *et al.* (2001). Comparative distribution of mRNA encoding the growth hormone secretagogue-receptor (GHS-R) in *Microcebus murinus* (Primate, lemurian) and rat forebrain and pituitary. *J. Comp. Neurol.* **429**, 469–89.

Mitome, M., Shirakawa, T., Oshima, S., Nakamura, W. & Oguchi, H. (2001). Circadian rhythm of nitric oxide production in the dorsal region of the suprachiasmatic nucleus in rats. *Neurosci. Lett.* **303**, 161–4.

Monnier, M. & Hösli, L. (1964). Dialysis of sleep and waking factors in blood of the rabbit. *Science* **146**, 796–8.

Monnier, M. & Hösli, L. (1965). Humoral regulation of sleep and wakefulness by hypnogenic and activating dialysable factors. *Prog. Brain Res.* **18**, 118–23.

Monnier, M., Hatt, A. M., Cueni, L. B. & Schoenenberger, G. A. (1972). Humoral transmission of sleep. VI. Purification and assessment of a hypnogenic fraction of "sleep Dialysate" (factor delta). *Pflugers Arch.* **331**, 257–65.

Monti, J. M. & Jantos, H. (2004a). Effects of L-arginine and SIN-1 on sleep and waking in the rat during both phases of the light-dark cycle. *Life Sci.* **75**, 2027–34.

Monti, J. M. & Jantos, H. (2004b). Microinjection of the nitric oxide synthase inhibitor L-NAME into the lateral basal forebrain alters the sleep/wake cycle of the rat. *Prog. Neuropsychopharmacol. Biol. Psychiatry.* **28**, 239–47.

Monti, J. M., Hantos, H., Ponzoni, A., Monti, D. & Banchero, P. (1999). Role of nitric oxide in sleep regulation: effects of L-NAME, an inhibitor of nitric oxide synthase, on sleep in rats. *Behav. Brain Res.* **100**, 197–205.

Monti, J. M., Jantos, H. & Monti, D. (2001). Increase of waking and reduction of NREM and REM sleep after nitric oxide synthase inhibition: prevention with $GABA_A$ or adenosine A_1 receptor agonists. *Behav. Brain Res.* **123**, 23–35.

Moreno-Reyes, R., Kerkhofs, M., L'Hermite-Baleriaux, M. *et al.* (1998). Evidence against a role for the growth hormone-releasing peptide axis in human slow-wave sleep regulation. *Am. J. Physiol.* **274**, E779–84.

Nagasaki, H., Iriki, M., Inoue, S. & Uchizono, K. (1974). The presence of a sleep-promoting material in the brain of sleep-deprived rats. *Proc. Japan Acad.* **50**, 241–6.

Olszewski, P. K., Li, D., Grace, M. K. *et al.* (2003). Neural basis of orexigenic effects of ghrelin acting within lateral hypothalamus. *Peptides* **24**, 597–602.

Pappenheimer, J. R., Koski, G., Fencl, V., Karnovsky, M. L. & Krueger, J. (1975). Extraction of sleep-promoting factor S from cerebrospinal fluid and from brains of sleep-deprived animals. *J. Neurophysiol.* **38**, 1299–311.

Pappenheimer, J. R., Miller, T. B. & Goodrich, C. A. (1967). Sleep-promoting effects of cerebrospinal fluid from sleep-deprived goats. *Proc. Natl. Acad. Sci. USA* **58**, 513–17.

Ribeiro, A. C. & Kapás, L. (2005). Day- and nighttime injection of a nitric oxide synthase inhibitor elicits opposite sleep responses in rats. *Am. J. Physiol. Regul. Integr. Comp. Physiol.* **289**, R521–31.

Ribeiro, A. C. & Kapás, L. (2003). Intra-suprachiasmatic nucleus (SCN) microinjection of a nitric oxide (NO) donor and NO synthase inhibitor affects sleep in rats. *Sleep* **26** (Abstr. Suppl.), 64.

Ribeiro, A. C. & Kapás, L. (1999). Nitric oxide in the preoptic region modulates sleep. *Sleep Res. Online* **2** (Suppl. 1), 75.

Ribeiro, A. C., Gilligan, J. G. & Kapás, L. (2000). Systemic injection of a nitric oxide synthase inhibitor suppresses sleep responses to sleep deprivation in rats. *Am. J. Physiol.* **278**, R1048–56.

Ribeiro, A. C. & Kapás, L. (2004). Sleep deprivation elicits changes in nitric oxide synthase activity and protein levels in rat brain. Abstract Viewer/Itinerary Planner. Washington, DC: Society for Neuroscience, Online, Program No. 546.17.

Rosenhagen, M. C., Uhr, M., Schüssler, P. & Steiger, A. (2005). Elevated plasma ghrelin levels in night-eating syndrome. *Am. J. Psychiatry* **162**, 813.

Schnedorf, J. G. & Ivy, A. C. (1939). An examination of the hypnotoxin theory of sleep. *Am. J. Physiol.* **125**, 491–505.

Schoenenberger, G. A., Maier, P. F., Tobler, J. H. & Monnier, M. (1977). A naturally occurring delta-EEG enhancing nonapeptide in rabbits. X. Final isolation, characterization and activity test. *Pflugers Arch.* **369**, 99–109.

Schüssler, P., Uhr, M., Ising, M. *et al.* (2005). Nocturnal ghrelin levels–relationship to sleep EEG, the levels of growth hormone, ACTH and cortisol – and gender differences. *J. Sleep Res.* **14**, 329–36.

Schüssler, P., Uhr, M., Ising, M. *et al.* (2006). Nocturnal ghrelin, ACTH, GH and cortisol secretion after sleep deprivation in humans. *Psychoneuroendocrinology* **31**, 915–23.

Shoham, S., Davenne, D., Cady, A. B., Dinarello, C. A. & Krueger, J. M. (1987). Recombinant tumor necrosis factor and interleukin 1 enhance slow-wave sleep. *Am. J. Physiol.* **253**, R142–9.

Spessert, R. & Rapp, M. (2001). Circadian rhythm in NO synthase I transcript expression and its photoperiodic regulation in the rat pineal gland. *Neuroreport* **12**, 781–5.

Spiegel, K., Tasali, E., Penev, P. & Van, C. E. (2004). Brief communication: Sleep curtailment in healthy young men is associated with decreased leptin levels, elevated ghrelin levels, and increased hunger and appetite. *Ann. Intern. Med.* **141**, 846–50.

Suda, T., Tozawa, F., Iwai, I. *et al.* (1993). Neuropeptide Y increases the corticotropin-releasing factor messenger ribonucleic acid level in the rat hypothalamus. *Brain Res. Mol. Brain Res.* **18**, 311–15.

Szentirmai, É., Kapás, L. & Krueger, J. M. (2007). Ghrelin microinjection into forebrain sites induces wakefulness and feeding in rats. *Am. J. Physiol. Regul. Integr. Comp. Physiol.* **292**, R575–85.

Szentirmai, E. & Krueger, J. M. (2006a). Central administration of neuropeptide Y induces wakefulness in rats. *Am. J. Physiol. Regul. Integr. Comp. Physiol.* **291**, R473–80.

Szentirmai, E. & Krueger, J. M. (2006b). Obestatin alters sleep in rats. *Neurosci. Lett.* **404**, 222–6.

Szentirmai, E., Hajdu, I., Obal, F., Jr. & Krueger, J. M. (2006). Ghrelin-induced sleep responses in ad libitum fed and food-restricted rats. *Brain Res.* **1088**, 131–40.

Taheri, S., Lin, L., Austin, D., Young, T. & Mignot, E. (2004). Short sleep duration is associated with reduced leptin, elevated ghrelin, and increased body mass index. *PLoS Med.* **1**, e62.

Tolle, V., Bassant, M. H., Zizzari, P. *et al.* (2002). Ultradian rhythmicity of ghrelin secretion in relation with GH, feeding behavior, and sleep-wake patterns in rats. *Endocrinology* **143**, 1353–61.

Toshinai, K., Date, Y., Murakami, N. *et al.* (2003). Ghrelin-induced food intake is mediated via the orexin pathway. *Endocrinology* **144**, 1506–12.

Tunctan, B., Weigl, Y., Dotan, A. *et al.* (2002). Circadian variation of nitric oxide synthase activity in mouse tissue. *Chronobiol. Int.* **19**, 393–404.

Vazquez, J., Lydic, R. & Baghdoyan, H. A. (2002). The nitric oxide synthase inhibitor N^G-Nitro-L-arginine increases basal forebrain acetylcholine release during sleep and wakefulness. *J. Neurosci.* **22**, 5597–605.

Vincent, S. R., Satoh, K., Armstrong, D. M. & Fibiger, H. C. (1983). NADPH-diaphorase: a selective histochemical marker for the cholinergic neurons of the pontine reticular formation. *Neurosci. Lett.* **43**, 31–6.

Weikel, J. C., Wichniak, A., Ising, M. *et al.* (2003). Ghrelin promotes slow-wave sleep in humans. *Am. J. Physiol. Endocrinol. Metab.* **284**, E407–15.

Williams, J. A., Vincent, S. R. & Reiner, P. B. (1997). Nitric oxide production in rat thalamus changes with behavioral state, local depolarization, and brainstem stimulation. *J. Neurosci.* **17**, 420–7.

Wolak, M. L., DeJoseph, M. R., Cator, A. D. *et al.* (2003). Comparative distribution of neuropeptide Y Y1 and Y5 receptors in the rat brain by using immunohistochemistry. *J. Comp. Neurol.* **464**, 285–311.

Wren, A. M., Small, C. J., Fribbens, C. V. *et al.* (2002). The hypothalamic mechanisms of the hypophysiotropic action of ghrelin. *Neuroendocrinology* **76**, 316–24.

Zhang, J. V., Ren, P. G., Avsian-Kretchmer, O. *et al.* (2005). Obestatin, a peptide encoded by the ghrelin gene, opposes ghrelin's effects on food intake. *Science* **310**, 996–9.

12

Adenosine and sleep–wake regulation

DAG STENBERG AND TARJA PORKKA-HEISKANEN

Introduction

The timing and amount of sleep is regulated by two main processes in order to optimize for the survival of the individual. A circadian process, driven by the internal clock in the brain, facilitates wakefulness at those times of the day when activity and foraging are possible, and facilitates sleep at those times when it is dangerous to leave the abode, or difficult to find nourishment. A homeostatic process ensures that the proper amount of sleep is acquired, according to the specific needs of the species and the individual. Insufficient sleep will cause "sleep pressure", which is expressed in increased propensity for sleep. If sleep is delayed, e.g. by activity, the accumulating sleep pressure will eventually result in "recovery sleep", characterized by increased duration and intensity, when sleep is again possible. To some extent the opposite is true: previous oversleeping may reduce sleep pressure to reduce sleep time. The interaction between these processes to regulate wake–sleep behavior has been formulated in Borbély's two-process theory (Borbély, 1982), the main tenet of which is still valid today. Adenosine has been shown to play a part in the homeostatic process, and this chapter will review that role.

As early as in 1909, it was recognized that some chemical factor in the brain was responsible for recovery sleep. Cerebrospinal fluid (Legendre & Piéron, 1911) or brain extract (Ishimori, 1909) from sleep-deprived dogs resulted in excess sleep when infused into the cerebral ventricles of recipient animals. The fact that the material was ineffective if heated or ultrafiltered pointed to a protein or peptide as sleep factor (Legendre & Piéron, 1911). Later studies have

Neurochemistry of Sleep and Wakefulness, ed. J. M. Monti *et al.* Published by Cambridge University Press.
© Cambridge University Press 2008.

suggested that there are several other putative "sleep factors" (cf. reviews in Borbély & Tobler, 1989; Obál & Krueger, 2003). A "sleep factor" meets the following criteria: (1) it can be shown to accumulate progressively in (part of) the brain during wakefulness, (2) it is removed or degraded during sleep, (3) it can induce or facilitate sleep. Jouvet divided putative sleep factors into two classes: sleep-inducing and sleep-promoting factors (Jouvet, 1982, 1984b). A sleep-inducing factor is directly involved in the executive mechanisms of sleep induction, whereas a sleep-promoting factor is only facilitatory, and sleep can be achieved even without it. On the basis of experimental findings, Jouvet also postulated separate homeostatic factors for non-REM (NREM) and rapid eye movement (REM) sleep (Jouvet, 1982, 1984a).

Another explanation for homeostatic sleep regulation would be "fatigue" of wake-maintaining mechanisms, such as the "ascending reticular activating system" (ARAS) of Moruzzi & Magoun (1949), for example, by depletion of cellular resources like transmitters or energy stores. This chapter will show how adenosine can be regarded as a homeostatic sleep factor that reflects both depletion of certain resources and the progressive accumulation of a sleep-inducing substance.

Adenosine physiology and receptors

Adenosine serves many functions in body and brain. It is the building block of ATP, the immediate energy store of cells. It relaxes smooth muscle in blood vessels and increases local circulation. In the central nervous system, adenosine is generally an inhibitory neuromodulator, being more potent as an inhibitor of excitatory transmission than of inhibitory transmission. In vitro experiments show that adenosine inhibits the firing of different neuron types, but especially that of cholinergic neurons from the basal forebrain or the mesopontine nuclei LDT and PPT, which are under tonic inhibitory control by adenosine acting through A1-type receptors (Rainnie et al., 1994; Arrigoni et al., 2001). As these cholinergic nuclei have been found to be wake-promoting and REM sleep-promoting, it is conceivable that locally increased adenosine concentrations could promote sleep by inhibiting the cholinergic neurons (Jones, 2004; Basheer et al., 2004). Disinhibition of sleep-active neurons, which have been found in the ventrolateral preoptic hypothalamic area, by inhibiting their presynaptic GABAergic inputs, is an additional possibility (Chamberlin et al., 2003; Morairty et al., 2004). These possible mechanisms are not mutually exclusive.

Adenosine exerts its cellular effects through G-protein-coupled cell membrane receptors, which are divided into classes A_1, A_{2A}, A_{2B}, and A_3 (for reviews, see Fredholm, 1995; Haas & Selbach, 2000; Dunwiddie & Masino, 2001). A_1 (A_1R)

and A_3 receptors (A_3R) are inhibitory to adenylyl cyclase and reduce cyclic AMP, whereas A_2 receptors (A_2R) have the opposite effect. A_1Rs are located both pre- and postsynaptically and are widely distributed in the nervous system. Post-synaptic A_1Rs are coupled to stimulation of K^+ channels, which results in hyper-polarization and inhibition of neural activity (Thompson *et al.*, 1992; Rainnie *et al.*, 1994; Strecker *et al.*, 2000). Another target of postsynaptic A_1Rs is phos-pholipase C (PLC), which can activate protein kinase C (PKC) via production of inositol triphosphate (IP_3) and mobilization of intracellular Ca^{2+} (Gerwins & Fredholm, 1992; Biber *et al.*, 1997). Presynaptic A_1Rs in the hippocampus reg-ulating acetylcholine release are not mediated by K^+ channels, but possibly by N-type Ca^{2+} channels (Fredholm, 1990a,b), whereas in the substantia gelati-nosa of rats the presynaptic A_1Rs seems to act through K^+ channels and not Ca^{2+} channels or PKC (Yang *et al.*, 2004). Adenosine can inhibit acetylcholine release (Fredholm, 1990b; Ribeiro *et al.*, 1996), and glutamate release (Oliet & Poulain, 1999) through presynaptic A_1Rs. Presynaptic A_1R-mediated inhibition of the release of the inhibitory transmitters GABA and glycine can disinhibit neurons (Oliet & Poulain, 1999; Yang *et al.*, 2004).

In contrast to A_1Rs, $A_{2A}Rs$ are located predominantly in the striatum, nucleus accumbens, and olfactory bulb and, at least in rodents, also in the leptomeninges. In the striatum, there is co-localization and interaction with dopamine D_2 receptors (Ferre *et al.*, 1991). $A_{2A}Rs$ are predominantly located post-synaptically in the striatum, but on presynaptic terminals in the hippocampus (Rebola *et al.*, 2005). $A_{2A}Rs$ mediate stimulation of acetylcholine release in rat striatum *in vivo* (Kurokawa *et al.*, 1996) and noradrenaline release in brainstem slices (Barraco *et al.*, 1995). Presynaptic $A_{2A}Rs$ on cholinergic nerve terminals enhance acetylcholine release in hippocampal synaptosomes (Cunha *et al.*, 1995). At least in the striatum, $A_{2A}Rs$ can also negatively modulate NMDA receptor con-ductance (Norenberg *et al.*, 1998). $A_{2B}Rs$ are found in both glial cells and neurons, and may have a widespread distribution in the brain (Sebastiao & Ribeiro, 1996). They increase a cAMP-dependent Ca^{2+} current in hippocampal pyramidal cells (Mogul *et al.*, 1993) and increase excitability in the CA3 region (Kessey & Mogul, 1998). Finally, it has been shown that A_3Rs can reduce A_1R-mediated inhibition of excitatory transmission in the hippocampus, although they seem to have no effect on their own (Dunwiddie *et al.*, 1997a).

Adenosine and vigilance

Pharmacological experiments have shown that adenosine and its recep-tor agonists promote, whereas its antagonists inhibit, sleep. Early experiments showed that injection into the cerebral ventricles of 2 μmol (0.5 mg) adenosine to cats caused a state resembling natural sleep of 30 min duration (Feldberg & Sherwood, 1954). Intracerebroventricular infusion of 0.2 µmol adenosine to dogs also caused sleep with a duration of an hour, alternating between slow wave and rapid wave sleep (Haulica et al., 1973). These authors suggested that adenosine might be the putative hypnotoxin (Legendre & Piéron, 1911) or a similar sleep factor. Systemic (i.p.) administration of the metabolically stable adenosine agonists N6-(L-phenylisopropyl)adenosine (L-PIA), N6-cyclohexyladenosine (CHA) and 5′-N-ethylcarboxamide (NECA) promoted NREM sleep in rats (Radulovacki et al., 1982, 1984; Radulovacki, 1985; Virus et al., 1990). The order of potency at A_1Rs of these drugs is L-PIA > CHA > NECA. All the drugs promoted deep slow wave sleep at moderate doses and inhibited REM sleep at high doses, but only L-PIA and CHA also increased waking at high doses. The A_1R agonist N6-cyclopentyladenosine (CPA) also dose-dependently (i.p. or i.c.v.) increased slow wave EEG activity, similarly to the effect of sleep deprivation (Benington et al., 1995). These findings suggested that the hypnogenic effect of adenosine was related to A_1Rs. However, the A_1R antagonist 8-cyclopentyltheophylline (CPT), when given i.p., promoted wakefulness and decreased sleep, but less than the optimum dose of the non-selective antagonist caffeine. When CPT was combined with the A_2R antagonist alloxazine, the increase in wakefulness and reduction of sleep was significantly enhanced (Radulovacki et al., 1985). The adenosine deaminase inhibitor deoxycoformycin also increased NREM and REM sleep in rats (Radulovacki et al., 1983). To increase adenosine concentrations and thus the hypnogenic effect, nucleoside transporter inhibitors were proposed as a treatment for insomnia. Of such molecules, orally administered mioflazine facilitated sleep in dogs for a duration of 8 h (Wauquier et al., 1987), and soluflazine increased sleep in rats when administered intracerebroventricularly (O'Connor et al., 1991) or microinjected into the ventrolateral hypothalamus (Sarda et al., 1989). The present knowledge of nucleoside transporter mechanisms may lead to more fruitful applications.

Caffeine, the stimulant drug apparently most widely used by humans, acts as a non-specific antagonist of adenosine receptors (Fredholm, 1995; Fredholm, et al., 1999; Dunwiddie & Masino, 2001). It also antagonizes cyclic nucleotide phosphodiesterase. The use of caffeine to reduce sleepiness and decrements in psychomotor performance has been documented in several human studies (De Valck & Cluydts, 2001; De Valck et al., 2003; McLellan et al., 2004; Wesensten et al., 2004, 2005; Beaumont et al., 2005; James et al., 2005; Kamimori et al., 2005; Rogers et al., 2005). In rats, caffeine dose-dependently increased wakefulness and increased all stages of sleep (Yanik et al., 1987) and was in addition able to counteract the increase in slow wave EEG activity caused by sleep deprivation (Schwierin et al., 1996). A plausible explanation is that this is due to the capability of caffeine to counteract the hypnogenic effect of adenosine by blocking A_1Rs,

$A_{2A}Rs$, or both in combination. Locomotor stimulation might also contribute to increased waking; and the combination of an A_1R and $A_{2A}R$ antagonist stimulates locomotion in mice, as does caffeine, and much more effectively than either antagonist alone (Kuzmin *et al.*, 2005).

Despite theoretical and experimental indications that adenosine has hypnogenic effects, it was necessary, in order to postulate adenosine as a homeostatic sleep factor, to show that its concentration in vivo depends on previous wakefulness and sleep, and to explain the mechanism of its hypnogenic effect.

In vivo measurements

Adenosine increased sleep in cats when infused by in vivo microdialysis into the basal forebrain (BF) area with the most cholinergic neurons (Portas *et al.*, 1997). By improving the sensitivity of the assay for adenosine by high-performance liquid chromatography coupled to ultraviolet light absorbance detection (HPLC–UV), it was shown that extracellular adenosine levels in various brain areas in the cat fluctuated with spontaneous vigilance cycles, being approximately 20% higher during wakefulness than during sleep (Porkka-Heiskanen *et al.*, 1997). However, when wakefulness was prolonged (by up to 6 h) by playing with the cats, adenosine levels increased further, even twofold compared to baseline in the BF, until deprivation ceased, whereupon the adenosine levels decreased during recovery sleep. The VA/VL nucleus of the thalamus was used for comparison: no progressive increase in extracellular adenosine was found there. Infusion of the nucleoside transporter (ENT1) blocker NBTI into the BF increased adenosine levels twofold over baseline and induced recovery sleep, whereas infusion into the thalamus only increased local adenosine levels twofold without inducing sleep. These findings provided powerful evidence for a homeostatic sleep-regulating role of adenosine with a special role for the BF, possibly its cholinergic, wake-promoting neurons (Porkka-Heiskanen *et al.*, 1997). A follow-up study (Fig. 12.1) showed that there was an early increase in adenosine during sleep deprivation in the cingulate cortex, but that levels started to decline even before the end of deprivation. In other regions tested (thalamus, preoptic area of hypothalamus, dorsal raphe, PPT) adenosine levels did not rise during sleep deprivation, but decreased further (Porkka-Heiskanen *et al.*, 2000). The microdialysis probe used, however, was rather large in relation to the size of small pontine nuclei such as LDT/PPT and the locus coeruleus, which precludes definitive statements regarding those structures. In vivo microdialysis in rats showed a similar, more than twofold increase in adenosine in the BF after 3 h of sleep deprivation and a decrease during recovery sleep, as well as a sleep-promoting effect of unilateral infusion of adenosine into the BF (Basheer *et al.*, 1999). This

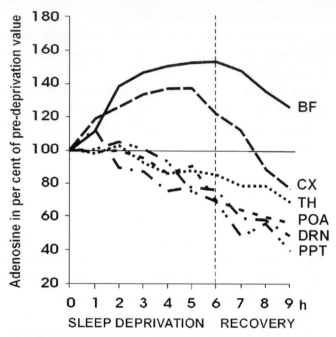

Figure 12.1 Extracellular adenosine concentrations in different brain areas, measured with in vivo microdialysis from cats during sleep deprivation (6 h gentle handling) and recovery sleep. Concentrations are given as a percentage of pre-deprivation values. BF, basal forebrain; CX, cingulate cortex; TH, VA/VL nucleus of thalamus; POA, preoptic hypothalamic area; DRN, dorsal raphe nucleus; PPT, pedunculopontine nucleus. In BF and CX; adenosine rises during sleep deprivation, but starts to decline during deprivation in CX, whereas the decline occurs during recovery in the BF. In other areas there is no accumulation during sleep deprivation. Modified from Porkka-Heiskanen *et al.* (2000).

was accompanied by increased expression of Fos and subsequent AP1 binding. In another study, an average increase in extracellular adenosine of 297% over baseline values was seen after 3 h sleep deprivation in the cholinergic BF area (diagonal band and substantia innominata), but no increase was seen outside that area (Kalinchuk *et al.*, 2003b). In vivo measurements thus supported the notion of adenosine as a homeostatic sleep factor acting in the BF.

Metabolism and transport of adenosine

The main source of brain energy metabolism is the continuous availability of glucose from the blood. To some extent, energy can be derived from glycogen, stored in astrocytes. Neurons also use lactate as an energy source, even under normoxic conditions. During neuronal activation, lactate may even be the

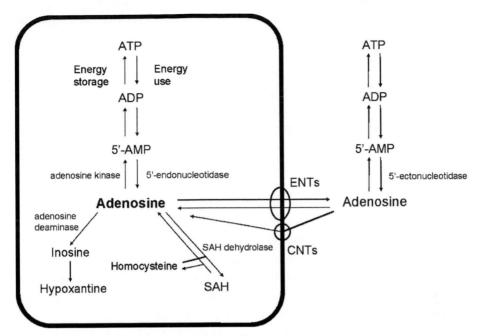

Figure 12.2 Adenosine metabolism. Intracellular adenosine concentrations depend on the balance between energy storage and breakdown. The most important enzymes catalyzing the reactions are indicated. SAH, S-adenosyl-homocysteine; ENTs, equilibrative nucleoside transporters; CNTs, concentrating nucleoside transporters.

preferred substrate. Astrocytes convert glucose to lactate, which is transported to neurons and there converted to pyruvate, which is further oxidized to yield ATP (for a review on neuroenergetics, see Pellerin & Magistretti, 2004). When the stored energy is used during neuronal activity, intracellular ATPase, ADPase and endo-5′-nucleotidases catalyze the breakdown of ATP to adenosine. Intracellular adenosine formation is thus largely a result of the rate of energy utilization and the availability of metabolizable substrate. Hydrolysis of S-adenosylhomocysteine (SAH) by SAH hydrolase could also produce adenosine intracellularly, but is thought to have little role in the brain (Pak *et al.*, 1994; Brundege & Dunwiddie, 1997).

Adenosine metabolism (Fig. 12.2) is reviewed in Dunwiddie & Masino (2001) and Ribeiro *et al.* (2002). The phosphorylation of intracellular adenosine to AMP is catalyzed by adenosine kinase. Intracellularly, adenosine can also be deaminated to inosine by adenosine deaminase. Free intracellular adenosine is normally low. Excess adenosine, which cannot be regenerated to ATP, is extruded to the extracellular space by equilibrative nucleoside transporters (ENTs) in the cell membrane. During electrical stimulation or energy depletion, adenosine is thus released into the extracellular space (Lloyd *et al.*, 1993). Ischemia, hypoxia, and acidosis can increase extracellular levels a hundredfold by inhibiting adenosine kinase. Under conditions that provide adequate oxygen and glucose, adenosine kinase is the most effective regulator of intracellular adenosine levels, and prevents extracellular concentrations from rising (Pak *et al.*, 1994), but when adenosine formation is increased by energy depletion, adenosine deaminase becomes important in regulating extracellular adenosine concentrations (Ballarin *et al.*, 1991; Lloyd & Fredholm, 1995). This is because the affinity for adenosine of adenosine kinase is in the physiological, nanomolar range (K_m optimum 0.2 μM, inhibited by concentrations over 0.5 μM) (Yamada *et al.*, 1980), but that of adenosine deaminase in the micromolar range (K_m optimum 17–45 μM), (Phillips & Newsholme, 1979). The selective inhibitor of adenosine deaminase, deoxycoformycin, has been shown to increase extracellular adenosine levels in vivo both under basal conditions and under hypoxia (Phillis *et al.*, 1988; Ballarin *et al.*, 1991). However, during basal conditions the increase was larger with the adenosine kinase inhibitor iodotubericine than with the deaminase inhibitor erythro-2-(2-hydroxy-3-nonyl)adenine (EHNA) (Sciotti & Van Wylen, 1993).

Adenosine can also be formed extracellularly from ATP, which is released from nerve endings and degraded via AMP to adenosine by ecto-5′-nucleotidase (Zimmermann & Braun, 1999), where the ectonucleotidase-catalyzed last step is rate-limiting (Dunwiddie *et al.*, 1997b). Agents that block extracellular AMP hydrolysis do not significantly affect the rate of adenosine release (Lloyd *et al.*, 1993), so extracellular adenosine formation is probably less important quantitatively. Extracellular accumulation of cAMP could also result in conversion to adenosine (Rosenberg & Dichter, 1989), but it has been speculated that extracellular accumulation occurs only with longer exposure to stimulation (Brundege *et al.*, 1997).

Extracellular adenosine concentrations in the brain under basal conditions have been found to be from 40 to 270 nM from in vivo microdialysis measurements (Pazzagli *et al.*, 1994; Ballarin *et al.*, 1991; Porkka-Heiskanen *et al.*, 2000). Under normal conditions, the main route of disposal of adenosine is transport into cells, either by the ENTs or by active transport through high-affinity concentrative transporters (CNTs) (Thorn & Jarvis, 1996). The CNTs that are expressed in the rat brain are CNT1 and CNT2 (Anderson *et al.*, 1996). ENTs were originally divided according to their sensitivity to the drug nitrobenzylthioinosine (NBTI, aka NBMPR): NBTI-sensitive (es) transporters are inhibited by nanomolar concentrations, and NBTI-insensitive (ei) transporters only by micromolar concentrations. When these were cloned from humans and rats, they were renamed ENT1 (es) and ENT2 (ei) (Yao *et al.*, 1997). In vivo, NBTI causes increased extracellular adenosine concentrations (Porkka-Heiskanen *et al.*, 1997), which indicates that under normal conditions there is a net uptake of adenosine into the cells due to an inward concentration gradient. The lack of specific pharmacological tools has hindered research on ENT2 and the CNTs.

Sleep deprivation and adenosine: source of the increased adenosine

As shown by in vivo microdialysis, extracellular adenosine levels are higher during wakefulness than sleep in all brain areas studied, but only in the BF does adenosine progressively increase during prolonged wakefulness (Porkka-Heiskanen et al., 1997). This indicates that in this area there may be specific local mechanisms causing adenosine accumulation, which become activated only during prolonged wakefulness. Possible sources of this extracellular adenosine include: increased intracellular breakdown of ATP, inhibition of adenosine kinase, inhibition of SAH hydrolase or adenosine deaminase, decreased transporter activity, or increased extracellular formation of adenosine.

Experimental data show that changes in enzyme activity might affect sleep–wake patterns, but such changes might not occur during prolonged wakefulness. Quantitative trait loci analyses in mice showed that the rate of accumulation of slow EEG waves during wakefulness, indicating increased sleep pressure, was related to a genomic region containing the genes of adenosine deaminase and S-adenosyl-homocysteine hydrolase (Franken et al., 2001). Of several variants of adenosine deaminase in the human genome, some are related to severe immunodeficiency, but the most frequent asymptomatic variant, a G-to-A transition at nucleotide 22, is related to increased slow wave sleep and less nocturnal awakenings than in persons with the major isoform of the enzyme (Rétey et al., 2005). Such findings point to a possible source for interindividual variations in sleep length and sleep patterns. Furthermore, a novel selective adenosine kinase inhibitor, ABT-702, which produces increases in extracellular adenosine, increased slow wave sleep and decreased REM sleep when given intraperitoneally to rats (Radek et al., 2004). ABT-702 dose-dependently increased slow EEG waves. This increase could be antagonized by the centrally active, non-selective adenosine antagonist theophylline, but not by the peripherally active antagonist 8-(p-sulfophenyl)-theophylline (8-PST), which indicates a central action.

During experimental sleep deprivation, however, it was found that there are no changes in the activity of adenosine kinase, ecto- and endonucleotidases (Alanko et al., 2003a,b), or adenosine deaminase (Mackiewicz et al., 2003), despite diurnal variations in activity. It can be concluded that changes in adenosine with sleep deprivation are not a consequence of alterations in adenosine enzyme activity. In the rat, 6 h of sleep deprivation led to a decrease in NBTI binding (to ENT1) in BF but not cortex, which could mean decreased ENT1 activity, although there was no change in ENT1 mRNA (Alanko *et al.*, 2003a,b). With the aid of poly-clonal antibodies, raised in rabbits, it was shown that ENT1 is located mainly in neuronal and glial cell membranes, whereas ENT2 also stains the soma of cells (Alanko, 2005). ENT1 would thus be the more important equilibrative trans-porter in the regulation of extracellular adenosine levels. Decreased ENT1 activ-ity should increase extracellular adenosine levels as does local administration of NBTI (Porkka-Heiskanen, 1999).

Increased extracellular ATP breakdown has been seen in vitro during elec-trical field stimulation and during hypoxia (Lloyd *et al.*, 1993). Although this source of extracellular adenosine accumulation remains a possibility, it has been found that inhibition of extracellular AMP hydrolysis does not significantly affect adenosine levels (Rosenberg *et al.*, 2000). The main source of adenosine is thus probably intracellular, and possibly related to increased energy consumption.

Energy depletion and nitric oxide as a cause of the rise in adenosine

Experimental energy depletion in vivo supports the notion that sleep deprivation causes energy imbalance. Microdialysis of dinitrophenol (DNP) into the BF dose-dependently increased adenosine, pyruvate, and lactate levels, and caused a subsequent increase in sleep, quite similar to the effect of sleep depri-vation applied according to the same time schedule (Kalinchuk *et al.*, 2003b). A control experiment showed that energy depletion by local potassium cyanate had the same consequences. If the infusion site was outside the BF area with a high proportion of cholinergic neurons, the increase in adenosine and metabo-lites was seen, but there was no subsequent increase in sleep. This constitutes part of the evidence that sleep deprivation causes recovery sleep by local energy depletion in the BF, which increases extracellular adenosine in that area.

Nitric oxide (NO) is an intercellular signaling molecule that can inhibit neu-ronal energy production (Brorson *et al.*, 1999; Maletic *et al.*, 2004). It has been found that NO donors cause large increases in extracellular adenosine in cul-tures of forebrain neurons (Rosenberg *et al.*, 2000). These were shown to be caused by NO release, and the accumulation of adenosine was not blocked by probenecid (ENT blocker) or GMP (a blocker of AMP hydrolysis), suggesting that adenosine was likely of intracellular origin. Indeed, it was found that NO donors caused a decrease in intracellular ATP and the inhibition of adenosine kinase activity, possibly due to the rise in adenosine.

Nitric oxide has been implicated in sleep regulation. NO concentrations undergo state-dependent modulation during the sleep–wake cycle in the cortex (Burlet & Cespuglio, 1997) and thalamus (Williams *et al.*, 1997). Intraperitoneal, subcutaneous or intracerebroventricular administrations of inhibitors of NO synthase (NOS) decrease spontaneous sleep (Kapás et al., 1994a,b; Dzoljic et al., 1996; Monti et al., 1999; Ribeiro & Kapás, 2005) as well as NREM recovery sleep after sleep deprivation (Ribeiro et al., 2000), whereas NO donors increase sleep (Kapás & Krueger, 1996). Local injections of NOS inhibitors into the PPT reduced NREM and REM sleep, whereas an NO precursor and NO donors had the opposite effect (Datta et al., 1997; Hars, 1999). Injection into the pontine reticular formation of the NOS inhibitor NLA decreased local acetylcholine release and REM sleep (Leonard & Lydic, 1997). The NOS inhibitor L-NAME given subcutaneously or into the dorsal raphe nucleus (DRN) reduced sleep and increased waking, and the effects were partly antagonized by subcutaneous administration of either the GABA$_A$ agonist muscimol or the A$_1$R antagonist L-PIA, indicating that part of the effect of reduction in NO might be through decreased GABAergic transmission and/or decreased adenosine (Monti et al., 2001). Direct bilateral application of L-NAME into the lateral BF reduced NREM sleep and increased wakefulness, and this could be prevented by pretreatment with the precursor, L-arginine or the NO donor molsamine (Monti & Jantos, 2004). However, in another study, microdialysis delivery of the NOS inhibitor NLA into cat BF had no effect on sleep, although it increased acetylcholine release in lateral BF regions, contrary to the effect on acetylcholine in the pons (Vazquez et al., 2002). In vivo microdialysis experiments in rat showed that infusion into the BF of the NO donor DETA-NONOate both increased extracellular adenosine and caused a subsequent sleep increase, supporting the notion that sleep deprivation causes recovery sleep through local BF energy depletion, NO formation, and adenosine release from cells (Kalinchuk et al., 2003a).

Neural mechanisms of the hypnogenic effect of adenosine: the case for an A$_1$-receptor-mediated action in the BF

Different lines of evidence point to involvement of both A$_1$ and A$_{2A}$ receptors in the hypnogenic action of adenosine. In vivo experiments involving microdialysis of specific agonists into the BF point to A$_1$R involvement. Thus infusion into BF of the A$_1$R antagonist cyclopentyltheophylline (CPT) decreased sleep (Strecker et al., 2000; Steriade & McCarley, 2006). Drugs acting on A$_{2A}$ receptors were, on the contrary, quite inefficient in the BF area. Microdialysis of the A$_1$R antagonist 8-cyclopentyl-1,3-dimethylxanthine (CPDX) into the BF increased the discharge rate of BF neurons (Alam et al., 1999). Microdialysis of the A$_1$R agonist N^6-cyclohexyladenosine (CHA) decreased the firing rate of wake-active neurons, and the A$_1$R antagonist CPT increased it dose-dependently (Thakkar et al., 2003a). Microdialysis perfusion into the BF of antisense oligonucleotides to A$_1$R mRNA significantly reduced spontaneous NREM sleep in the rat, and also reduced by half the recovery sleep after sleep deprivation (Thakkar *et al.*, 2003b).

The involvement of A_1Rs is also suggested by the fact that prolonged sleep deprivation upregulates A_1Rs by increasing the transcription of A_1R mRNA, whereas A_{2A}R mRNA was undetectable (Basheer *et al.*, 2001a). A_1R-dependent G-protein activity is transiently upregulated by sleep deprivation in rat cortex, but not in the BF (Alanko *et al.*, 2004). Adenosine can activate phospholipase C (PLC) in the cell membrane through A_1Rs, causing intracellular release of IP_3 and the consequent increase in intracellular Ca^{2+} (Gerwins & Fredholm, 1992). Adenosine-mediated mobilization of intracellular Ca^{2+} apparently occurs almost exclusively in cholinergic neurons (Steriade & McCarley, 2006). This mechanism can induce translocation of the nuclear factor NF-κB, which stimulates the expression of several sleep-regulatory substances, including nitric oxide synthase (Xie *et al.*, 1994) and A_1Rs (Nie *et al.*, 1998). Sleep deprivation has been shown to increase NF-κB DNA-binding activity in cortex (Chen *et al.*, 1999) and in the BF of rats after sleep deprivation (Basheer *et al.*, 2001b). In vitro studies show that the adenosine-mediated increase in NF-κB activation can be blocked by the A_1R antagonist CPT. Thus although adenosine may activate NF-κB by acting through A_1Rs, NF-κB can induce A_1R gene expression, increasing cellular sensitivity to adenosine (upregulation), which would maintain A_1R-mediated signaling efficiency during prolonged sleep deprivation (Porkka-Heiskanen *et al.*, 2002). The upregulation of A_1R mRNA after sleep deprivation can be blocked by injection of a cell-permeable protein inhibitor, which prevents NF-κB activation and translocation, and this occurred almost exclusively in cholinergic BF neurons (R. Basheer, unpublished, cited in Steriade & McCarley, 2006). Using both in situ hybridization for adenosine receptor mRNA and an autoradiographical assay of receptor protein, it was found that A_1Rs but not A_{2A}Rs were upregulated by sleep deprivation in the BF of rats. On the other hand, A_{2A}R mRNA was reduced by sleep deprivation in the olfactory tubercle area on the ventral surface of the forebrain, supporting the possibility of regulation through those structures by A_{2A}Rs (Basheer *et al.*, 2001b). Likewise, in mice with constitutive knockout of A_1Rs, spontaneous sleep–wake patterns and the homeostatic response to sleep deprivation were equal to those of wild-type controls, also supporting the involvement of adenosine receptors, other than A_1Rs, in sleep–wake regulation (Stenberg *et al.*, 2003).

The site-specificity of the adenosine A_1R-mediated hypnogenic effect in the BF (Fig. 12.3) implies an inhibiting effect on state-regulating neurons in this area. In the magnocellular BF, several types of neuron project to the cortex. Of these, about one third are cholinergic, one third GABAergic, and one third unidentified (Gritti *et al.*, 1997). The cholinergic neurons are thought to be essential

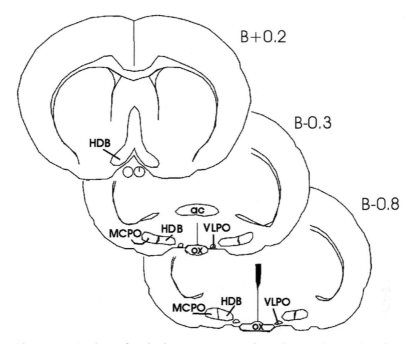

Figure 12.3 Sections of rat brain at 0.2 mm anterior to bregma (B + 0.2), and 0.3 and 0.8 mm posterior (B − 0.3, B − 0.8), showing areas relevant to adenosine influences on sleep induction. HDB, horizontal diagonal band; MCPO, magnocellular preoptic nucleus; VLPO, ventrolateral preoptic nucleus; ac, anterior commissure; ox, optic chiasm.

for the induction of cortical EEG arousal (Steriade, 1992; Steriade & McCarley, 2006). Neuronal activity recording in vitro and in vivo with identification of the neurotransmitter shows that cholinergic neurons discharge at higher rates during cortical activation than during slow wave activity, whereas GABAergic neurons have an opposite pattern of activity (Jones, 2004). The activity of the cholinergic neurons was stimulated by noradrenaline, and noradrenaline infused into the BF induces cortical arousal and decreases NREM sleep (Jones, 2004). Cholinergic neurons are effectively inhibited by adenosine in vitro (Rainnie *et al.*, 1994). It would seem that inhibition of the arousal-promoting cholinergic BF neurons is the most obvious explanation for the hypnogenic effect of adenosine in the BF. Selective and discrete lesions of BF cholinergic neurons can be achieved by injection of the immunotoxin IgG192-saporin (Wiley *et al.*, 1991; Waite, 1994). Application of this technique to the study of behavior and attention shows that different tasks are differentially influenced (Wenk, 1997). EEG gamma activity is reduced, indicating decreased activation of the cortex (Berntson *et al.*, 2002).

Neural mechanisms of the hypnogenic effect of adenosine: the case for an $A_{2A}R$-mediated action in the VLPO

A_{2A} receptors are abundant in the striatum, and play an important role there in motor functions. Other important areas include, in rodents, the nucleus accumbens, the olfactory tubercle, and the leptomeninges (Haas & Selbach, 2000; Dunwiddie & Masino, 2001). Infusion of CGS 21680 into the subarachnoid space close to the BF dose-dependently promoted NREM and REM sleep, and the effect could be blocked by the $A_{2A}R$ antagonist (E)-1,3-dipropyl-7-methyl-8-(3,4-dimethoxystyryl)xanthine (KF17837) (Satoh et al., 1996). The same effect was found with the specific $A_{2A}R$ agonist 2-(4-(2-(2-aminoethylaminocarbonyl)ethyl)phenylethylamino)-5′-N-ethylcarboxamidoadenosine (APEC), and with the $A_1R/A_{2A}R$ agonist 5′-N-ethylcarboxamidoadenosine (NECA) (Satoh et al., 1998). In contrast, the A_1R agonists CHA and CPA infused into this space did not increase sleep, but instead inhibited it (Satoh et al., 1996, 1998). In addition to promoting sleep, subarachnoidally infused CGS 21680, but not CPA, induced robust Fos expression in the leptomeninges neighbouring the BF, as well as in the ventrolateroposterior area (VLPO). The VLPO (Fig. 12.3) contains a population of sleep-active neurons (Sherin et al., 1996; Szymusiak et al., 1998) which co-localize galanin and GABA, indicating inhibitory action in projection sites, which include the tuberomamillary histaminergic neurons (Sherin et al., 1998) and other arousal systems (see McGinty & Szymusiak, 2001). The $A_{2A}R$ agonist CGS 21680, when infused into the subarachnoid space adjacent to BF, induced Fos expression in VLPO neurons and increased sleep (Scammell et al., 2001). Similar infusion increased GABA release in the tuberomamillary nucleus but not in the frontal cortex, while inhibiting histamine release in the frontal cortex, suggesting that $A_{2A}R$ activation increased GABAergic inhibition of the histaminergic wakefulness system (Hong et al., 2005).

In vivo microdialysis infusion of CGS 21680 into the sleep-promoting lateral preoptic area (LPOA) of rats reduced waking and increased NREM sleep, whereas infusion of CPA induced waking and decreased NREM sleep (Methippara et al., 2005). In the same experiments, the $A_{2A}R$ antagonist 8-(3-chlorostyryl)caffeine (CSC) increased wakefulness and suppressed NREM sleep, whereas the A_1R antagonist CPDX had no effect on sleep, alone or in combination with CSC. This would indicate that in the LPOA, adenosine can induce sleep by exciting sleep-active neurons through $A_{2A}Rs$ or inhibit sleep by inhibiting them through A_1Rs. When the ENT1 inhibitor NBTI, which has been shown to increase extracellular adenosine concentrations and increase sleep when infused into the BF (Porkka-Heiskanen et al., 1997), was infused into the LPOA at 20 μM, waking was induced, whereas infusion into the BF confirmed the previous finding of sleep induction in that location (Methippara *et al.*, 2005). The higher dose of 50 μM NBTI was ineffective; this result could be explained by preferential action through A_1Rs at the lower dose, and opposing effects of A_1Rs and A_{2A}Rs at the higher dose.

In VLPO slices, adenosine blocked spontaneous IPSPs determined to be GABAergic in most neurons recorded, without changing their resting potential. This indicates an effect of adenosine on afferent inhibitory GABAergic input rather than a postsynaptic action. The effect on afferent excitatory inputs was less predictable. These data are consistent with the possibility that adenosine could promote sleep also by disinhibiting sleep-active VLPO neurons, provided that the disinhibited neurons were actually sleep-active (Morairty *et al.*, 2004). Examination of the actions of A_1R and A_{2A}R agonists and antagonists on neurons in slices from rat VLPO revealed, however, that putative sleep-active neurons (identified as such through inhibition by noradrenaline) that were excited by serotonin (i.e. Type-2 neurons) were also excited by the A_{2A}R agonist CGS21680 acting postsynaptically, whereas the sleep-active neurons that were inhibited by serotonin (i.e. Type-1) were insensitive to the A_{2A}R agonist. Both types of neuron were inhibited by adenosine and the A_1R agonist CPA, but in the presence of the A_1R antagonist CPDX, adenosine was without effect on Type-1 neurons and excited Type-2 neurons, unmasking the A_{2A}R excitation of the latter (Gallopin *et al.*, 2005).

A role for A_{2A}Rs in sleep–wake regulation was also supported by studies in mice with constitutional knockout of A_{2A}Rs (Urade *et al.*, 2003). Infusion into the lateral ventricle of CGS 21680 increased NREM and REM sleep in wild-type mice, but not in the knockouts. In contrast, the A_1R agonist CPA did not affect sleep in either genotype, which indicated that A_1Rs could not compensate for the absence of A_{2A}Rs under these conditions.

The same leptomeningeal area surrounding the BF is also the target for the hypnogenic action of prostaglandin D_2 (PGD_2) (Urade & Hayaishi, 1999; Hayaishi, 2002; Mizoguchi *et al.*, 2001). When PGD_2 was infused into the subarachnoid space below the rostral BF, NREM sleep was increased and there was a striking expression of Fos in the VLPO in addition to Fos expression in the leptomeninges (Scammell *et al.*, 1998). This hypnogenic effect of PGD_2 is apparently mediated by adenosine. Local infusion of PGD_2 into the subarachnoid space has been found to increase local adenosine concentration (Mizoguchi *et al.*, 2001). The hypnogenic effect of subarachnoidally infused PGD_2 could be attenuated by the A_{2A}R antagonist KF17837 (Satoh *et al.*, 1996). In A_{2A}R knockout mice, the hypnogenic response to PGD_2 infusion into the lateral ventricle was attenuated to 40% of that in the wild-type mice, and the recovery sleep after sleep deprivation was inhibited (Urade *et al.*, 2003).

There is thus evidence that leptomeningeal PGD$_2$ promotes sleep through adenosine acting at A$_{2A}$Rs, possibly activating sleep-active neurons in the VLPO, which in turn inhibit waking systems through a GABAergic action. In vitro studies showed that neither type of sleep-active neuron in the VLPO was sensitive to PGD$_2$ when directly applied (Gallopin *et al.*, 2005). PGD$_2$ production in the leptomeninges has been found in inflammatory conditions (Roberts *et al.*, 1980) including African sleeping sickness (Pentreath *et al.*, 1990). It is thus possible that the A$_{2A}$R system is specialized for the mediation of sleepiness that occurs with leptomeningeal inflammation in contrast to the more homeostatically regulated A$_1$R system (Steriade & McCarley, 2006).

Possible applications

Sleep disorders, especially those of diminished or unsatisfying sleep, are exceedingly common in the human population. Daytime sleepiness, either due to sleep disorder or to voluntary sleep restriction, is also common. Restoration of sleep and counteracting sleepiness are targets of possible applications of the knowledge about adenosine in sleep–wake regulation. Given the ubiquitous nature of the actions of adenosine, it is, however, difficult to devise a drug that would affect only sleep mechanisms without carrying side effects relating to the heart and circulation, respiration, gastrointestinal function, etc.

The use of caffeine as a stimulant is widespread; several studies have documented that caffeine temporarily improves performance during prolonged wakefulness (McLellan *et al.*, 2004; Wesensten *et al.*, 2004, 2005; James *et al.*, 2005; Kamimori *et al.*, 2005; Rogers *et al.*, 2005). For practical purposes, a long-acting caffeine preparation seems more useful than the common beverages (De Valck & Cluydts, 2001; De Valck *et al.*, 2003; Beaumont *et al.*, 2005). Caffeine is also the only agent shown to decrease significantly sleep inertia (the adverse effect on performance of a nap) (Van Dongen *et al.*, 2001), and should preferably be taken just before the nap (Hayashi *et al.*, 2003).

As mentioned above, inhibition of adenosine kinase increases extracellular adenosine concentrations. Interest in enhancement of the neuroprotective, antinociceptive, and anti-inflammatory actions of adenosine has encouraged development of systemically applicable adenosine kinase inhibitor drugs. For example, it was found recently that the specific adenosine kinase inhibitor ABT-702, when given intraperitoneally, increases sleep and slow wave EEG activity of rats (Radek *et al.*, 2004), a finding that encourages further research into the hypnogenic effect of this type of drug.

Increasing extracellular adenosine levels by blocking the nucleoside transporter system has been suggested to improve sleep. The nucleoside transport blocker mioflazine, given orally, increased sleep in dogs (Wauquier *et al.*, 1987), and a 60 mg oral dose improved sleep quality but did not extend sleep in humans (Hoppenbrouwers & Van den Busche, 1987). A similar substance, soluflazine, has been proposed as an antiepileptic (Ashton *et al.*, 1988). Given the new knowledge on nucleoside transporters in sleep (Alanko, 2005), this approach might yet lead to useful applications.

Acknowledgements

The work was funded by Academy of Finland, EU grants MCRTN_CT_2004_512362 and LSHM_CT_2005_518189, NIH grant P50 HL060292, and Finska Läkaresällskapet.

References

Alam, M. N., Szymusiak, R., Gong, H., King, J. & McGinty, D. (1999). Adenosinergic modulation of rat basal forebrain neurons during sleep and waking: neuronal recording with microdialysis. *J. Physiol.* **521** (3), 679–90.

Alanko, L. (2005). Adenosine during prolonged wakefulness in the rat brain. Ph.D. Thesis, University of Helsinki.

Alanko, L., Heiskanen, S., Stenberg, D. & Porkka-Heiskanen, T. (2003a). Adenosine kinase and 5′-nucleotidase activity after prolonged wakefulness in the cortex and the basal forebrain of rat. *Neurochem. Int.* **42** (6), 449–54.

Alanko, L., Stenberg, D. & Porkka-Heiskanen, T. (2003b). Nitrobenzylthioinosine (NBMPR) binding and nucleoside transporter ENT1 mRNA expression after prolonged wakefulness and recovery sleep in the cortex and basal forebrain of rat. *J. Sleep Res.* **12** (4), 299–304.

Alanko, L., Laitinen, J. T., Stenberg, D. & Porkka-Heiskanen, T. (2004). Adenosine A1 receptor-dependent G-protein activity in the rat brain during prolonged wakefulness. *Neuroreport* **15** (13), 2133–7.

Anderson, C. M., Xiong, W., Young, J. D., Cass, C. E. & Parkinson, F. E. (1996). Demonstration of the existence of mRNAs encoding N1/cif and N2/cit sodium/nucleoside cotransporters in rat brain. *Brain Res. Mol.Brain Res.* **42** (2), 358–61.

Arrigoni, E., Rainnie, D. G., McCarley, R. W. & Greene, R. W. (2001). Adenosine-mediated presynaptic modulation of glutamatergic transmission in the laterodorsal tegmentum. *J. Neurosci.* **21** (3), 1076–85.

Ashton, D., De Prins, E., Willems, R., Van Belle, H. & Wauquier, A. (1988). Anticonvulsant action of the nucleoside transport inhibitor, soluflazine, on synaptic and non-synaptic epileptogenesis in the guinea-pig hippocampus. *Epilepsy Res.* **2** (2), 65–71.

Ballarin, M., Fredholm, B. B., Ambrosio, S. & Mahy, N. (1991). Extracellular levels of adenosine and its metabolites in the striatum of awake rats: inhibition of uptake and metabolism. *Acta Physiol. Scand.* **142** (1), 97–103.

Barraco, R. A., Clough-Helfman, C., Goodwin, B. P. & Anderson, G. F. (1995). Evidence for presynaptic adenosine A2a receptors associated with norepinephrine release and their desensitization in the rat nucleus tractus solitarius. *J. Neurochem.* **65** (4), 1604–11.

Basheer, R., Porkka-Heiskanen, T., Stenberg, D. & McCarley, R. W. (1999). Adenosine and behavioral state control: adenosine increases c-Fos protein and AP1 binding in basal forebrain of rats. *Brain Res. Mol. Brain Res.* **73** (1–2), 1–10.

Basheer, R., Halldner, L., Alanko, L. *et al.* (2001a). Opposite changes in adenosine A1 and A2A receptor mRNA in the rat following sleep deprivation. *Neuroreport* **12** (8), 1577–80.

Basheer, R., Rainnie, D. G., Porkka-Heiskanen, T., Ramesh, V. & McCarley, R. W. (2001b). Adenosine, prolonged wakefulness, and A1-activated NF-kappaB DNA binding in the basal forebrain of the rat. *Neuroscience* **104** (3), 731–9.

Basheer, R., Strecker, R. E., Thakkar, M. M. & McCarley, R. W. (2004). Adenosine and sleep-wake regulation. *Prog. Neurobiol.* **73** (6), 379–96.

Beaumont, M., Batejat, D., Coste, O. *et al.* (2005). Recovery after prolonged sleep deprivation: residual effects of slow-release caffeine on recovery sleep, sleepiness and cognitive functions. *Neuropsychobiology* **51** (1), 16–27.

Benington, J. H., Kodali, S. K. & Heller, H. C. (1995). Stimulation of A1 adenosine receptors mimics the electroencephalographic effects of sleep deprivation. *Brain Res.* **692** (1–2), 79–85.

Berntson, G. G., Shafi, R. & Sarter, M. (2002). Specific contributions of the basal forebrain corticopetal cholinergic system to electroencephalographic activity and sleep/waking behaviour. *Eur. J. Neurosci.* **16** (12), 2453–61.

Biber, K., Klotz, K.-N., Berger, M., Gebicke-Härter, P. J. & van Calker, X. (1997). Adenosine A1 receptor-mediated activation of phospholipase C in cultured astrocytes depends on the level of receptor expression. *J. Neurosci.* **17**, 4956–64.

Borbély, A. A. (1982). A two process model of sleep regulation. *Hum. Neurobiol.* **1**, 195–204.

Borbély, A. A. & Tobler, I. (1989). Endogenous sleep-promoting substances and sleep regulation. *Physiol. Rev.* **69**, 605–70.

Brorson, J. R., Schumacker, P. T. & Zhang, H. (1999). Nitric oxide acutely inhibits neuronal energy production. The Committees on Neurobiology and Cell Physiology. *J. Neurosci.* **19** (1), 147–58.

Brundege, J. M. & Dunwiddie, T. V. (1997). Role of adenosine as a modulator of synaptic activity in the central nervous system. *Adv. Pharmacol.* **39** 353–91.

Brundege, J. M., Diao, L., Proctor, W. R. & Dunwiddie, T. V. (1997). The role of cyclic AMP as a precursor of extracellular adenosine in the rat hippocampus. *Neuropharmacology* **36** (9), 1201–10.

Burlet, S. & Cespuglio, R. (1997). Voltammetric detection of nitric oxide (NO) in the rat brain: its variations throughout the sleep-wake cycle. *Neurosci. Lett.* **226** (2), 131–5.

Chamberlin, N. L., Arrigoni, E., Chou, T. C. *et al.* (2003). Effects of adenosine on gabaergic synaptic inputs to identified ventrolateral preoptic neurons. *Neuroscience* **119** (4), 913–18.

Chen, Z., Gardi, J., Kushikata, T., Fang, J. & Krueger, J. M. (1999). Nuclear factor kB -like activity increases in murine cerebral cortex after sleep deprivation. *Am. J. Physiol.* **276**, R1812–18.

Cunha, R. A., Johansson, B., Fredholm, B. B., Ribeiro, J. A. & Sebastiao, A. M. (1995). Adenosine A2A receptors stimulate acetylcholine release from nerve terminals of the rat hippocampus. *Neurosci. Lett.* **196** (1–2), 41–4.

Datta, S., Patterson, E. H. & Siwek, D. F. (1997). Endogenous and exogenous nitric oxide in the pedunculopontine tegmentum induces sleep. *Synapse* **27** (1), 69–78.

De Valck, E. & Cluydts, R. (2001). Slow-release caffeine as a countermeasure to driver sleepiness induced by partial sleep deprivation. *J. Sleep Res.* **10** (3), 203–9.

De Valck, E., De Groot, E. & Cluydts, R. (2003). Effects of slow-release caffeine and a nap on driving simulator performance after partial sleep deprivation. *Percept. Mot. Skills* **96** (1), 67–78.

Dunwiddie, T. V. & Masino, S. A. (2001). The role and regulation of adenosine in the central nervous system. *An. Rev. Neurosci.* **24**, 31–55.

Dunwiddie, T. V., Diao, L., Kim, H. O., Jiang, J. L. & Jacobson, K. A. (1997a). Activation of hippocampal adenosine A3 receptors produces a desensitization of A1 receptor-mediated responses in rat hippocampus. *J. Neurosci.* **17** (2), 607–14.

Dunwiddie, T. V., Diao, L. & Proctor, W. R. (1997b). Adenine nucleotides undergo rapid, quantitative conversion to adenosine in the extracellular space in rat hippocampus. *J. Neurosci.* **17** (20), 7673–82.

Dzoljic, M. R., de Vries, R. & van Leeuwen, R. (1996). Sleep and nitric oxide: effects of 7-nitro indazole, inhibitor of brain nitric oxide synthase. *Brain Res.* **718** (1–2), 145–50.

Feldberg, W. & Sherwood, S. L. (1954). Injections of drugs into the lateral ventricle of the cat. *J. Physiol.* **123** (1), 148–67.

Ferre, S., von Euler, G., Johansson, B., Fredholm, B. B. & Fuxe, K. (1991). Stimulation of high-affinity adenosine A2 receptors decreases the affinity of dopamine D2 receptors in rat striatal membranes. *Proc. Natl. Acad. Sci. USA* **88** (16), 7238–41.

Franken, P., Chollet, D. & Tafti, M. (2001). The homeostatic regulation of sleep need is under genetic control. *J. Neurosci.* **21** (8), 2610–21.

Fredholm, B. B. (1990a). Adenosine A1-receptor-mediated inhibition of evoked acetylcholine release in the rat hippocampus does not depend on protein kinase C. *Acta Physiol. Scand.* **140** (2), 245–55.

Fredholm, B. B. (1990b). Differential sensitivity to blockade by 4-aminopyridine of presynaptic receptors regulating [3H]acetylcholine release from rat hippocampus. *J. Neurochem.* **54** (4), 1386–90.

Fredholm, B. B. (1995). Adenosine receptors in the central nervous system. *News Physiol. Sci.* **10**, 122–8.

Fredholm, B. B., Battig, K., Holmen, J., Nehlig, A. & Zvartau, E. E. (1999). Actions of caffeine in the brain with special reference to factors that contribute to its widespread use. *Pharmacol. Rev.* **51** (1), 83–133.

Gallopin, T., Luppi, P. H., Cauli, B. *et al.* (2005). The endogenous somnogen adenosine excites a subset of sleep-promoting neurons via A2A receptors in the ventrolateral preoptic nucleus. *Neuroscience* **134** (4), 1377–90.

Gerwins, P. & Fredholm, B. B. (1992). ATP and its metabolite adenosine act synergistically to mobilize intracellular calcium via the formation of inositol 1,4,5-triphosphate and intracellular free calcium in DDT 1 MF-2 smooth muscle cells. *Proc. Natl. Acad. Sci. USA* **89**, 7330–4.

Gritti, I., Mainville, L., Mancia, M. & Jones, B. E. (1997). GABAergic and other noncholinergic basal forebrain neurons, together with cholinergic neurons, project to the mesocortex and isocortex in the rat. *J. Comp. Neurol.* **383** (2), 163–77.

Haas, H. L. & Selbach, O. (2000). Functions of neuronal adenosine receptors. *Naunyn Schmiedebergs Arch. Pharmacol.* **362** (4–5), 375–81.

Hars, B. (1999). Endogenous nitric oxide in the rat pons promotes sleep. *Brain Res.* **816** (1), 209–19.

Haulica, I., Ababei, L., Branisteanu, D. & Topoliceanu, F. (1973). Letter: Preliminary data on the possible hypnogenic role of adenosine. *J. Neurochem.* **21** (4), 1019–20.

Hayaishi, O. (2002). Molecular genetic studies on sleep-wake regulation, with special emphasis on the prostaglandin D(2) system. *J. Appl. Physiol.* **92** (2), 863–8.

Hayashi, M., Masuda, A. & Hori, T. (2003). The alerting effects of caffeine, bright light and face washing after a short daytime nap. *Clin. Neurophysiol.* **114** (12), 2268–78.

Hong, Z. Y., Huang, Z. L., Qu, W. M. *et al.* (2005). An adenosine A receptor agonist induces sleep by increasing GABA release in the tuberomammillary nucleus to inhibit histaminergic systems in rats. *J. Neurochem.* **92** (6), 1542–9.

Hoppenbrouwers, M. L. & Van den Busche, G. (1987). Mioflazine, a nucleoside transport inhibitor effective as sleep promotor in humans?. Abstract, International Symposium *Current Trends in Slow Wave Sleep Research*, Beerse, Belgium, p. 38.

Ishimori, K. (1909). True cause of sleep: a hypnogenic substance as evidenced in the brain of sleep-deprived animals. *Tokyo Igakkai Zasshi* **23**, 429–57.

James, J. E., Gregg, M. E., Kane, M. & Harte, F. (2005). Dietary caffeine, performance and mood: enhancing and restorative effects after controlling for withdrawal reversal. *Neuropsychobiology* **52** (1), 1–10.

Jones, B. E. (2004). Activity, modulation and role of basal forebrain cholinergic neurons innervating the cerebral cortex. *Prog. Brain Res.* **145**, 157–69.

Jouvet, M. (1982). Hypnogenic indolamine-dependent factors and paradoxical sleep rebound. In *Sleep*, ed. W. P. Koella, pp. 2–18. Basel: Karger.

Jouvet, M. (1984a). Indolamines and sleep-inducing factors. In *Sleep Mechanisms*, ed. A. Borbély & J.-L. Valatx, pp. 81–94. Berlin: Springer-Verlag.

Jouvet, M. (1984b). Neuromediateurs et facteurs hypnogenes. *Rev. Neurol. Paris* **140** (6–7), 389–400.

Kalinchuk, A. V., Hokkanen, M., Stenberg, D., Rosenberg, P. A. & Porkka-Heiskanen, T. (2003a). The role of nitric oxide in regulation of sleep need. *J. Neurophysiol.* **26**, (suppl), A32–3.

Kalinchuk, A. V., Urrila, A. S., Alanko, L. *et al.* (2003b). Local energy depletion in the basal forebrain increases sleep. *Eur. J. Neurosci.* **17** (4), 863–9.

Kamimori, G. H., Johnson, D., Thorne, D. & Belenky, G. (2005). Multiple caffeine doses maintain vigilance during early morning operations. *Aviat. Space Environ. Med.* **76** (11), 1046–50.

Kapás, L. & Krueger, J. M. (1996). Nitric oxide donors SIN-1 and SNAP promote nonrapid-eye-movement sleep in rats. *Brain Res. Bull.* **41** (5), 293–8.

Kapás, L., Fang, J. & Krueger, J. M. (1994a). Inhibition of nitric oxide synthesis inhibits rat sleep. *Brain Res.* **664** (1–2), 189–96.

Kapás, L., Shibata, M., Kimura, M. & Krueger, J. M. (1994b). Inhibition of nitric oxide synthesis suppresses sleep in rabbits. *Am. J. Physiol.* **266** (1), R151–7.

Kessey, K. & Mogul, D. J. (1998). Adenosine A2 receptors modulate hippocampal synaptic transmission via a cyclic-AMP-dependent pathway. *Neuroscience* **84** (1), 59–69.

Kurokawa, M., Koga, K., Kase, H., Nakamura, J. & Kuwana, Y. (1996). Adenosine A2a receptor-mediated modulation of striatal acetylcholine release in vivo. *J. Neurochem.* **66** (5), 1882–8.

Kuzmin, A., Johansson, B., Gimenez, L., Ogren, S. O. & Fredholm, B. B. (2005). Combination of adenosine A(1) and A(2A) receptor blocking agents induces caffeine-like locomotor stimulation in mice. *Eur. Neuropsychopharmacol.* **00**, 000–000.

Legendre, R. & Piéron, H. (1911). Du développement, au cours de l'insomnie expérimentale, de propriétés hypnotoxiques des humeurs en relation avec le besoin croissant de sommeil. *C. R. Soc. Biol.* **70**, 190–2.

Leonard, T. O. & Lydic, R. (1997). Pontine nitric oxide modulates acetylcholine release, rapid eye movement sleep generation, and respiratory rate. *J. Neurosci.* **17** (2), 774–85.

Lloyd, H. G. & Fredholm, B. B. (1995). Involvement of adenosine deaminase and adenosine kinase in regulating extracellular adenosine concentration in rat hippocampal slices. *Neurochem. Int.* **26** (4), 387–95.

Lloyd, H. G., Lindstrom, K. & Fredholm, B. B. (1993). Intracellular formation and release of adenosine from rat hippocampal slices evoked by electrical stimulation or energy depletion. *Neurochem. Int.* **23** (2), 173–85.

Mackiewicz, M., Nikonova, E. V., Zimmerman, J. E. *et al.* (2003). Enzymes of adenosine metabolism in the brain: diurnal rhythm and the effect of sleep deprivation. *J. Neurochem.* **85** (2), 348–57.

Maletic, S. D., Dragicevic-Djokovic, L. M., Ognjanovic, B. L. *et al.* (2004). Effects of exogenous donor of nitric oxide-sodium nitroprusside on energy production of rat reticulocytes. *Physiol. Res.* **53** (4), 439–47.

McGinty, D. & Szymusiak, R. (2001). Brain structures and mechanisms involved in the generation of NREM sleep: focus on the preoptic hypothalamus. *Sleep Med. Rev.* **5** (4), 323–42.

McLellan, T. M., Bell, D. G., & Kamimori, G. H. (2004). Caffeine improves physical performance during 24 h of active wakefulness. *Aviat. Space Environ. Med.* **75** (8), 666–72.

Methippara, M. M., Kumar, S., Alam, M. N., Szymusiak, R. & McGinty, D. (2005). Effects on sleep of microdialysis of adenosine A1 and A2a receptor analogs into the lateral preoptic area of rats. *Am. J. Physiol Regul. Integr. Comp. Physiol.* **289** (6), R1715–23.

Mizoguchi, A., Eguchi, N., Kimura, K. *et al.* (2001). Dominant localization of prostaglandin D receptors on arachnoid trabecular cells in mouse basal forebrain and their involvement in the regulation of non-rapid eye movement sleep. *Proc. Natl. Acad. Sci. USA* **98** (20), 11674–9.

Mogul, D. J., Adams, M. E. & Fox, A. P. (1993). Differential activation of adenosine receptors decreases N-type but potentiates P-type Ca2+ current in hippocampal CA3 neurons. *Neuron* **10** (2), 327–34.

Monti, J. M. & Jantos, H. (2004). Microinjection of the nitric oxide synthase inhibitor L-NAME into the lateral basal forebrain alters the sleep/wake cycle of the rat. *Prog. Neuropsychopharmacol. Biol. Psychiatry* **28** (2), 239–47.

Monti, J. M., Jantos, H., Ponzoni, A., Monti, D. & Banchero, P. (1999). Role of nitric oxide in sleep regulation: effects of L-NAME, an inhibitor of nitric oxide synthase, on sleep in rats. *Behav. Brain Res.* **100** (1–2), 197–205.

Monti, J. M., Jantos, H. & Monti, D. (2001). Increase of waking and reduction of NREM and REM sleep after nitric oxide synthase inhibition: prevention with GABA(A) or adenosine A(1) receptor agonists. *Behav. Brain Res.* **123** (1), 23–35.

Morairty, S., Rainnie, D., McCarley, R. & Greene, R. (2004). Disinhibition of ventrolateral preoptic area sleep-active neurons by adenosine: a new mechanism for sleep promotion. *Neuroscience* **123** (2), 451–7.

Moruzzi, G. & Magoun, H. (1949). Brain stem reticular formation and activation of the EEG. *Electroenceph. Clin. Neurophysiol.* **1**, 455–73.

Nie, Z., Mei, Y., Ford, M. *et al.* (1998). Oxidative stress increases A1 adenosine receptor expression by activationg nuclear factor kappa B. *Mol. Pharmacol.* **53** (4), 663–9.

Norenberg, W., Wirkner, K., Assmann, H., Richter, M. & Illes, P. (1998). Adenosine A2A receptors inhibit the conductance of NMDA receptor channels in rat neostriatal neurons. *Amino. Acids* **14** (1–3), 33–9.

O'Connor, S. D., Stojanovic, M. & Radulovacki, M. (1991). The effect of soluflazine on sleep in rats. *Neuropharmacology* **30** (6), 671–4.

Obál, F. Jr. & Krueger, J. M. (2003). Biochemical regulation of non-rapid-eye-movement sleep. *Front. Biosci.* **8**, d520–50.

Oliet, S. H. & Poulain, D. A. (1999). Adenosine-induced presynaptic inhibition of IPSCs and EPSCs in rat hypothalamic supraoptic nucleus neurones. *J. Physiol.* **520** (3), 815–25.

Pak, M. A., Haas, H. L., Decking, U. K. & Schrader, J. (1994). Inhibition of adenosine kinase increases endogenous adenosine and depresses neuronal activity in hippocampal slices. *Neuropharmacology* **33** (9), 1049–53.

Pazzagli, M., Corsi, C., Latini, S., Pedata, F. & Pepeu, G. (1994). In vivo regulation of extracellular adenosine levels in the cerebral cortex by NMDA and muscarinic receptors. *Eur. J. Pharmacol.* **254** (3), 277–82.

Pellerin, L. & Magistretti, P. J. (2004). Neuroenergetics: calling upon astrocytes to satisfy hungry neurons. *Neuroscientist.* **10** (1), 53–62.

Pentreath, V. W., Rees, K., Owolabi, O. A., Philip, K. A. & Doua, F. (1990). The somnogenic T lymphocyte suppressor prostaglandin D2 is selectively elevated in cerebrospinal fluid of advanced sleeping sickness patients. *Trans. R. Soc. Trop. Med. Hyg.* **84** (6), 795–9.

Phillips, E. & Newsholme, E. A. (1979). Maximum activities, properties and distribution of 5' nucleotidase, adenosine kinase and adenosine deaminase in rat and human brain. *J. Neurochem.* **33** (2), 553–8.

Phillis, J. W., O'Regan, M. H. & Walter, G. A. (1988). Effects of deoxycoformycin on adenosine, inosine, hypoxanthine, xanthine, and uric acid release from the hypoxemic rat cerebral cortex. *J. Cereb. Blood Flow Metab.* **8** (5), 733–41.

Porkka-Heiskanen, T. (1999). Adenosine in sleep and wakefulness. *Ann. Med.* **31** (2), 125–9.

Porkka-Heiskanen, T., Strecker, R. E., Thakkar, M. *et al.* (1997). Adenosine: a mediator of the sleep-inducing effects of prolonged wakefulness. *Science* **276** (5316), 1265–8.

Porkka-Heiskanen, T., Strecker, R. E. & McCarley, R. W. (2000). Brain site-specificity of extracellular adenosine concentration changes during sleep deprivation and spontaneous sleep: an in vivo microdialysis study. *Neuroscience* **99** (3), 507–17.

Porkka-Heiskanen, T., Alanko, L., Kalinchuk, A. & Stenberg, D. (2002). Adenosine and sleep. *Sleep Med. Rev.* **6** (4), 321–32.

Portas, C. M., Thakkar, M., Rainnie, D. G., Greene, R. W. & McCarley, R. W. (1997). Role of adenosine in behavioral state modulation: a microdialysis study in the freely moving cat. *Neuroscience* **79** (1), 225–35.

Radek, R. J., Decker, M. W. & Jarvis, M. F. (2004). The adenosine kinase inhibitor ABT-702 augments EEG slow waves in rats. *Brain Res.* **1026** (1), 74–83.

Radulovacki, M. (1985). Role of adenosine in sleep in rats. *Rev. Clin. Basic Pharm.* **5** (3–4), 327–39.

Radulovacki, M., Miletich, R. S. & Green, R. D. (1982). N6 (L-phenylisopropyl) adenosine (L-PHA) increases slow-wave sleep (S2) and decreases wakefulness in rats. *Brain Res.* **246** (1), 178–80.

Radulovacki, M., Virus, R. M., Djuricic-Nedelson, M. & Green, R. D. (1983). Hypnotic effects of deoxycorformycin in rats. *Brain Res.* **271** (2), 392–5.

Radulovacki, M., Virus, R. M., Djuricic-Nedelson, M. & Green, R. D. (1984). Adenosine analogs and sleep in rats. *J. Pharmacol. Exp. Ther.* **228** (2), 268–74.

Radulovacki, M., Virus, R. M., Rapoza, D. & Crane, R. A. (1985). A comparison of the dose response effects of pyrimidine ribonucleosides and adenosine on sleep in rats. *Psychopharmacology* **87** (2), 136–40.

Rainnie, D. G., Grunze, H. C., McCarley, R. W. & Greene, R. W. (1994). Adenosine inhibition of mesopontine cholinergic neurons: implications for EEG arousal. *Science* **263** (5147), 689–92.

Rebola, N., Rodrigues, R. J., Lopes, L. V. *et al.* (2005). Adenosine A1 and A2A receptors are co-expressed in pyramidal neurons and co-localized in glutamatergic nerve terminals of the rat hippocampus. *Neuroscience* **133** (1), 79–83.

Rétey, J. V., Adam, M., Honegger, E. *et al.* (2005). A functional genetic variation of adenosine deaminase affects the duration and intensity of deep sleep in humans. *Proc. Natl. Acad. Sci. USA* **102** (43), 15676–81.

Ribeiro, A. C. & Kapás, L. (2005). Day- and nighttime injection of a nitric oxide synthase inhibitor elicits opposite sleep responses in rats. *Am. J. Physiol. Regul. Integr. Comp. Physiol.* **289** (2), R521–31.

Ribeiro, J. A., Cunha, R. A., Correia-de-Sa, P. & Sebastiao, A. M. (1996). Purinergic regulation of acetylcholine release. *Prog. Brain Res.* **109**, 231–41.

Ribeiro, A. C., Gilligan, J. G. & Kapás, L. (2000). Systemic injection of a nitric oxide synthase inhibitor suppresses sleep responses to sleep deprivation in rats. *Am. J. Physiol. Regul. Integr. Comp. Physiol.* **278** (4), R1048–56.

Ribeiro, J. A., Sebastiao, A. M. & de Mendonca, A. (2002). Adenosine receptors in the nervous system: pathophysiological implications. *Prog. Neurobiol.* **68** (6), 377–92.

Roberts, L. J., Sweetman, B. J., Lewis, R. A. *et al.* (1980). Markedly increased synthesis of prostaglandin D2 in systemic mastocytosis. *Trans. Assoc. Am. Physicians* **93**, 141–7.

Rogers, P. J., Heatherley, S. V., Hayward, R. C. *et al.* (2005). Effects of caffeine and caffeine withdrawal on mood and cognitive performance degraded by sleep restriction. *Psychopharmacology* **179** (4), 742–52.

Rosenberg, P. A. & Dichter, M. A. (1989). Extracellular cAMP accumulation and degradation in rat cerebral cortex in dissociated cell culture. *J. Neurosci.* **9**, 2654–63.

Rosenberg, P. A., Li, Y., Le, M. & Zhang, Y. (2000). Nitric oxide-stimulated increase in extracellular adenosine accumulation in rat forebrain neurons in culture is associated with ATP hydrolysis and inhibition of adenosine kinase activity. *J. Neurosci.* **20** (16), 6294–301.

Sarda, N., Cespuglio, R., Gharib, A. & Reynaud, D. (1989). Rôles des systemes adénosinergiques hypothalamiques dans la régulation des états de vigilance chez le chat. *C. R. Acad. Sci.[III]* **308**, 473–8.

Satoh, S., Matsumura, H., Suzuki, F. & Hayaishi, O. (1996). Promotion of sleep mediated by the A2a-adenosine receptor and possible involvement of this receptor in the sleep induced by prostaglandin D2 in rats. *Proc. Natl. Acad. Sci. USA* **93** (12), 5980–4.

Satoh, S., Matsumura, H. & Hayaishi, O. (1998). Involvement of adenosine A2A receptor in sleep promotion. *Eur. J. Pharmacol.* **351** (2), 155–62.

Scammell, T., Gerashchenko, D., Urade, Y. *et al.* (1998). Activation of ventrolateral preoptic neurons by the somnogen prostaglandin D2. *Proc. Natl. Acad. Sci. USA* **95** (13), 7754–9.

Scammell, T. E., Gerashchenko, D. Y., Mochizuki, T. *et al.* (2001). An adenosine A2a agonist increases sleep and induces Fos in ventrolateral preoptic neurons. *Neuroscience* **107** (4), 653–63.

Schwierin, B., Borbély, A. A. & Tobler, I. (1996). Effects of N6-cyclopentyladenosine and caffeine on sleep regulation in the rat. *Eur. J. Pharmacol.* **300** (3), 163–71.

Sciotti, V. M. & Van Wylen, D. G. (1993). Increases in interstitial adenosine and cerebral blood flow with inhibition of adenosine kinase and adenosine deaminase. *J. Cereb. Blood Flow Metab.* **13** (2), 201–7.

Sebastiao, A. M. & Ribeiro, J. A. (1996). Adenosine A2 receptor-mediated excitatory actions on the nervous system. *Prog. Neurobiol.* **48** (3), 167–89.

Sherin, J. E., Shiromani, P. J., McCarley, R. W. & Saper, C. B. (1996). Activation of ventrolateral preoptic neurons during sleep. *Science* **271** (5246), 216–19.

Sherin, J. E., Elmquist, J. K., Torrealba, F. & Saper, C. B. (1998). Innervation of histaminergic tuberomammillary neurons by GABAergic and galaninergic neurons in the ventrolateral preoptic nucleus of the rat. *J. Neurosci.* **18** (12), 4705–21.

Stenberg, D., Litonius, E., Halldner, L. *et al.* (2003). Sleep and its homeostatic regulation in mice lacking the adenosine A1 receptor. *J. Sleep Res.* **12** (4), 283–90.

Steriade, M. (1992). Basic mechanisms of sleep generation. *Neurology* **42** (7, suppl. 6), 9–17.

Steriade, M. & McCarley, R. W. (2006). The role of active forebrain and humoral systems in sleep control. In *Brain Control of Wakefulness and Sleep*, pp. 561–610. Berlin: Springer.

Strecker, R. E., Morairty, S., Thakkar, M. M. *et al.* (2000). Adenosinergic modulation of basal forebrain and preoptic/anterior hypothalamic neuronal activity in the control of behavioral state. *Behav. Brain Res.* **115** (2), 183–204.

Szymusiak, R., Alam, N., Steininger, T. L. & McGinty, D. (1998). Sleep-waking discharge patterns of ventrolateral preoptic/anterior hypothalamic neurons in rats. *Brain Res.* **803** (1–2), 178–88.

Thakkar, M. M., Delgiacco, R. A., Strecker, R. E. & McCarley, R. W. (2003a). Adenosinergic inhibition of basal forebrain wakefulness-active neurons: a simultaneous unit recording and microdialysis study in freely behaving cats. *Neuroscience* **122** (4), 1107–13.

Thakkar, M. M., Winston, S. & McCarley, R. W. (2003b). A1 receptor and adenosinergic homeostatic regulation of sleep-wakefulness: effects of antisense to the A1 receptor in the cholinergic basal forebrain. *J. Neurosci.* **23** (10), 4278–87.

Thompson, S. M., Haas, H. L. & Gahwiler, B. H. (1992). Comparison of the actions of adenosine at pre- and postsynaptic receptors in the rat hippocampus in vitro. *J. Physiol.* **451**, 347–63.

Thorn, J. A. & Jarvis, S. M. (1996). Adenosine transporters. *Gen. Pharmacol.* **27** (4), 613–20.

Urade, Y. & Hayaishi, O. (1999). Prostaglandin D2 and sleep regulation. *Biochim. Biophys. Acta* **1436** (3), 606–15.

Urade, Y., Eguchi, N., Qu, W. M. *et al.* (2003). Sleep regulation in adenosine A2A receptor-deficient mice. *Neurology* **61** (11, suppl. 6), S94–6.

Van Dongen, H. P., Price, N. J., Mullington, J. M. *et al.* (2001). Caffeine eliminates psychomotor vigilance deficits from sleep inertia. *J. Neurophysiol.* **24** (7), 813–19.

Vazquez, J., Lydic, R. & Baghdoyan, H. A. (2002). The nitric oxide synthase inhibitor NG-Nitro-L-arginine increases basal forebrain acetylcholine release during sleep and wakefulness. *J. Neurosci.* **22** (13), 5597–605.

Virus, R. M., Ticho, S., Pilditch, M. & Radulovacki, M. (1990). A comparison of the effects of caffeine, 8-cyclopentyltheophylline, and alloxazine on sleep in rats. Possible roles of central nervous system adenosine receptors. *Neuropsychopharmacology* **3** (4), 243–9.

Waite, J. J., Wardlow, M. L., Chen, A. C. *et al.* (1994). Time course of cholinergic and monoaminergic changes in rat brain after immunolesioning with 192 IgG-saporin. *Neurosci. Lett.* **169** (1–2), 154–8.

Wauquier, A., Van Belle, H., Van den Broeck, W. A. & Janssen, P. A. (1987). Sleep improvement in dogs after oral administration of mioflazine, a nucleoside transport inhibitor. *Psychopharmacology* **91** (4), 434–9.

Wenk, G. L. (1997). The nucleus basalis magnocellularis cholinergic system: one hundred years of progress. *Neurobiol. Learn. Mem.* **67** (2), 85–95.

Wesensten, N. J., Belenky, G., Thorne, D. R., Kautz, M. A. & Balkin, T. J. (2004). Modafinil vs. caffeine: effects on fatigue during sleep deprivation. *Aviat. Space Environ. Med.* **75** (6), 520–5.

Wesensten, N. J., Killgore, W. D. & Balkin, T. J. (2005). Performance and alertness effects of caffeine, dextroamphetamine, and modafinil during sleep deprivation. *J. Sleep Res.* **14** (3), 255–66.

Wiley, R. G., Oeltmann, T. N. & Lappi, D. A. (1991). Immunolesioning: selective destruction of neurons using immunotoxin to rat NGF receptor. *Brain Res.* **562** (1), 149–53.

Williams, J. A., Vincent, S. R. & Reiner, P. B. (1997). Nitric oxide production in rat thalamus changes with behavioral state, local depolarization, and brainstem stimulation. *J. Neurosci.* **17** (1), 420–7.

Xie, Q., Kashiwabara, Y. & Nathan, C. (1994). Role of transcription factor NF.kB/Rel in induction of nitric oxide synthase. *J. Biol. Chem.* **269**, 4705–8.

Yamada, Y., Goto, H. & Ogasawara, N. (1980). Purification and properties of adenosine kinase from rat brain. *Biochim. Biophys. Acta* **616** (2), 199–207.

Yang, K., Fujita, T. & Kumamoto, E. (2004). Adenosine inhibits GABAergic and glycinergic transmission in adult rat substantia gelatinosa neurons. *J. Neurophysiol.* **92** (5), 2867–77.

Yanik, G., Glaum, S. & Radulovacki, M. (1987). The dose-response effects of caffeine on sleep in rats. *Brain Res.* **403** (1), 177–80.

Yao, S. Y., Ng, A. M., Muzyka, W. R. *et al.* (1997). Molecular cloning and functional characterization of nitrobenzylthioinosine (NBMPR)-sensitive (es) and NBMPR-insensitive (ei) equilibrative nucleoside transporter proteins (rENT1 and rENT2) from rat tissues. *J. Biol. Chem.* **272** (45), 28423–30.

Zimmermann, H. & Braun, N. (1999). Ecto-nucleotidases – molecular structures, catalytic properties, and functional roles in the nervous system. *Prog. Brain Res.* **120**, 371–85.

13

Prostaglandins and the regulation of sleep and wakefulness

OSAMU HAYAISHI AND YOSHIHIRO URADE

Introduction

Sleep substances

The humoral theory of sleep regulation, the concept that sleep and wakefulness are induced and regulated by a hormone-like chemical substance rather than by a neural network, was initially proposed by Kuniomi Ishimori of Nagoya, Japan, and independently and concurrently by the French neuroscientist Henri Piéron of Paris, in the first decade of the twentieth century. They took samples of cerebrospinal fluid (CSF) from sleep-deprived dogs and infused them into the brains of normal dogs. The recipient dogs soon fell asleep. Thus these researchers became the first to demonstrate the existence of endogenous sleep-promoting substances. However, the chemical nature of these sleep substance(s) was not identified. During the following 90 years, more than 30 so-called endogenous sleep and wake substances were reported by numerous investigators to exist in the brain, CSF, urine, and other organs and tissues of animals. For example, delta-sleep-inducing peptide, muramyl peptides, uridine, oxidized glutathione, and vitamin B12 have been proposed as endogenous somnogenic substances. The detailed account of these substances is described in an excellent treatise by Inoué (1989). During the early 1980s, Professor Jouvet and his colleagues in Lyon also found a sleep-inducing factor produced by the periventricular structures including the choroid plexus in the central nervous system (CNS) of cats (Bobillier et al., 1982; Jouvet et al., 1983). However, the physiological relevance of these substances has remained uncertain in most instances.

Neurochemistry of Sleep and Wakefulness, ed. J. M. Monti *et al.* Published by Cambridge University Press.
© Cambridge University Press 2008.

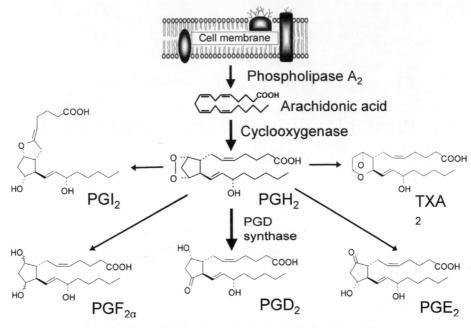

Figure 13.1 The arachidonate cascade system (TX, thromboxane).

Prostanoids

Prostanoids are a group of 20-carbon polyunsaturated fatty acids containing a unique 5-carbon ring structure. Prostanoids are produced from arachidonate ($C_{20:4}$ fatty acid) and other polyunsaturated fatty acids by the action of a unique dioxygenase, cyclooxygenase (COX; prostaglandin [PG] endoperoxide synthase, EC 1.14.99.1), which incorporates 2 mol of molecular oxygen into the substrate, followed by a hydroperoxidase-catalyzed step and subsequent specific synthetase-catalyzed steps, as shown in Fig. 13.1.

Although PGs were initially discovered in human semen, they are now known to be widely distributed in virtually all types of cell in almost all tissues and organs and to act as local hormones, exhibiting numerous and diverse biological effects on a large variety of physiological and pathological activities such as contraction and relaxation of smooth muscles, inflammation, platelet aggregation, etc. However, relatively little was known about PGs in the CNS of mammals until the late 1970s.

PGD$_2$ and sleep

Sleep-inducing activity of PGD$_2$

We found PGD$_2$ to be the most abundant prostanoid in the brains of rats (Narumiya *et al.*, 1982; Hiroshima *et al.*, 1986) and other mammals, including

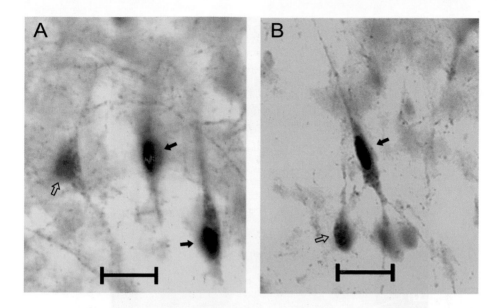

Plate 1 Examples of immunostaining for c-Fos IR (dark nuclear staining) and GAD (light cytoplasmic staining) in the MnPN. A higher percentage of GAD-positive cells (arrows) also expressed c-Fos IR (black arrows) following high (A) compared with low spontaneous sleep (B). From Gong *et al.* (2004b).

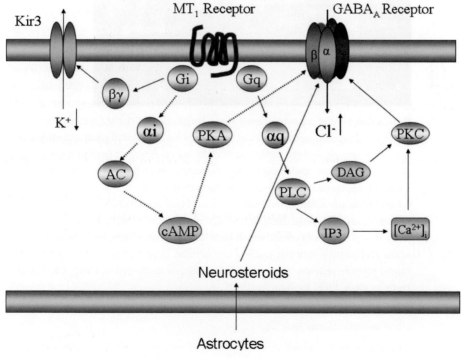

Plate 2 Possible cellular pathways involved in the physiological modulation of GABAergic function by melatonin via the MT$_1$ receptor. See text for explanation.

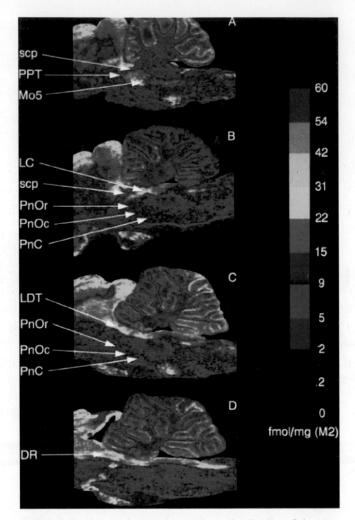

Plate 3 Color-coded autoradiograms show distribution of the M2 muscarinic receptor subtype in sagittal views of rat brain stem. M2 binding was quantified as fmol/mg tissue equivalent. Color bar at right indicates higher (red) to lower (purple) M2 binding. Images labeled (A)–(D) show a section every 0.5 mm and progress from lateral (A, approximately 1.9 mm from the midline) to medial (D, approximately 0.4 mm from the midline), according to a rat brain atlas (Paxinos & Watson, 1998). Abbreviations: PPT, pedunculopontine tegmental nucleus; Mo5, motor trigeminal nucleus; scp, superior cerebellar peduncle; LC, locus coeruleus; PnOr, rostral portion of the oral pontine reticular nucleus (PnO); PnOc, caudal portion of the PnO; PnC, caudal pontine reticular nucleus; LDT, laterodorsal tegmental nucleus; DR, dorsal raphe nucleus. From Baghdoyan (1997).

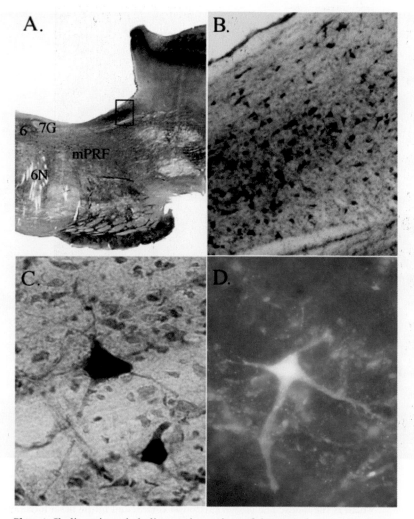

Plate 4 Cholinergic and cholinoceptive regions of the pons that contribute to the regulation of sleep and wakefulness. (A) A sagittal view of cat pons with caudal to the left. Abbreviations: 6, abducens nucleus; 7G, the genu of the facial nerve; 6N, the sixth cranial nerve; mPRF, medial pontine reticular formation. The boxed area in (A) includes laterodorsal and pedunculopontine tegmental (LDT/PPT) neurons that synthesize acetylcholine (Jones & Beaudet, 1987). The region of the black box is enlarged in (B) to show cells stained positively for NADPH-diaphorase (black dots). In the LDT/PPT, 100% of the cholinergic neurons stain positively for NADPH-diaphorase (Vincent *et al.*, 1983; Steriade and McCarley, 2005). These LDT/PPT cells project to cholinoceptive cells in the medial pontine reticular formation that contain muscarinic cholinergic receptors. Muscarinic receptors are present in medial regions of the pontine reticular formation of cat (Baghdoyan *et al.*, 1994), rat (Baghdoyan, 1997; Capece *et al.*, 1998), and C57BL/6J mouse (DeMarco *et al.*, 2003). (C) and (D) highlight a cholinergic LDT/PPT neuron (C) that was identified via retrograde fluorescent tracer (D) as projecting to the medial pontine reticular formation. (Modified from Lydic & Baghdoyan, 2005).

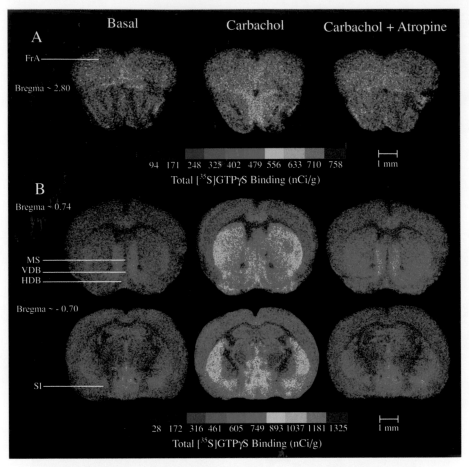

Plate 5 Cholinergic activation of G proteins in the forebrain of C57BL/6J mouse. Color-coded G protein activation is shown (A) for the frontal association cortex (FrA), which is the mouse homolog of prefrontal cortex, and for (B) basal forebrain. Color-coded autoradiograms of coronal sections show total [^{35}S]GTPγS binding (representing activation of G proteins) for three conditions (columns). Note the difference in the color scale between the FrA (A) and the basal forebrain (B), indicating higher total binding in the basal forebrain. In sections treated with carbachol plus atropine, [^{35}S]GTPγS binding was similar to basal levels. Additional data showed that carbachol caused a concentration-dependent increase in G protein activation. Together, these data demonstrate that G protein activation was mediated by muscarinic receptors. Abbreviations: FrA, frontal association cortex; MS, medial septum; VDB, vertical and HDB, horizontal limbs of the diagonal band of Broca; SI, substantia innominata. From DeMarco *et al.* (2004).

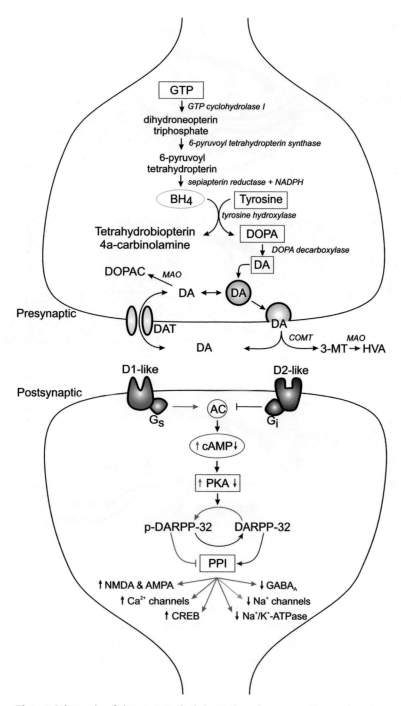

Plate 6 Schematic of the prototypical dopaminergic synapse. Pre- and postsynaptic components of a dopaminergic synapse summarizing molecular pathways for dopamine synthesis, metabolism, and second messenger effects following D1-like or D2-like receptor activation.

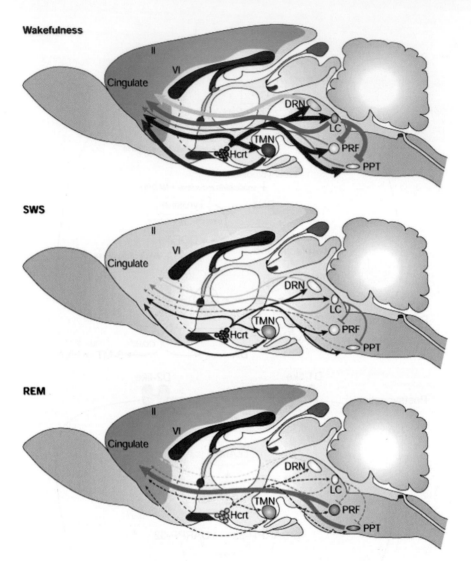

Plate 7 Hypocretinergic activity dependent on the states of vigilance. During wakefulness, metabolic, circadian, and behavioral inputs converge on hypocretin neurons, which activate noradrenergic neurons in the locus coeruleus and promote arousal. During non-REM sleep, the activity of hypocretin neurons decreases, but the inhibitory influence of REM−off neurons on REM-on cells is still effective. During REM sleep, hypocretin and REM-off cells are silent, disinhibiting REM-on cells. Reprinted with permission from Sutcliffe & de Lecea (2002).

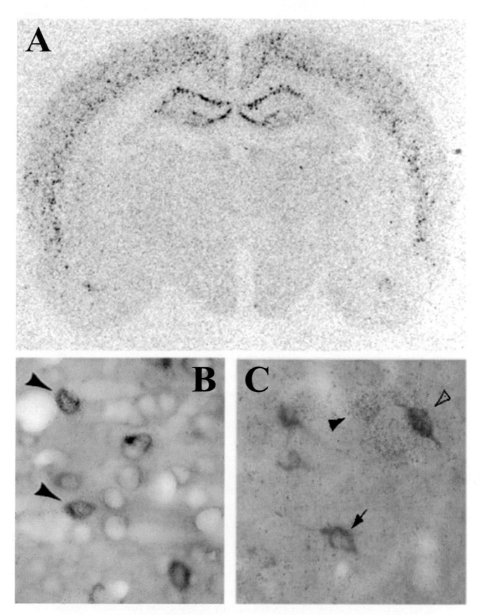

Plate 8 Cortistatin is expressed in cortical interneurons and may provide an intrinsic mechanism of cortical synchronization by increasing Ih. A. In situ hybridization showing preprocortistatin mRNA signals in sparse non-principal neurons throughout the cerebral cortex, hippocampus and amygdala. B. Double in situ hybridization of preprocortistatin and GAD65 demonstrating that all cortistatin-positive cells in the neocortex are GABAergic. C. Combined in situ hybridization to preprocortistatin and immunocytochemistry to somatostatin, showing that preprocortistatin labels a partially overlapping although distinct population of GABAergic neurons.

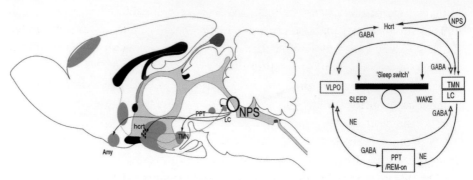

Plate 9 NPS and the sleep-switch model. NPS projects to the main circuits involved in arousal, including the TMN, PPT, hcrt, and basal forebrain. Areas with high density of NPS terminals and NPS receptors are shown in blue. Reciprocal connections between NPS, hcrt, and the TMN are the substrate of the "flip–flop" sleep-switch model (Saper *et al.*, 2001), which consists of a bistable system that prevents intermediate states. Aminergic regions such as the TMN, LC, and cholinergic neurons in the basal forebrain promote wakefulness by direct excitatory effects on the cortex and by inhibition of sleep–promoting neurons of the VLPO. As sleep demand increases, adenosine concentrations increase and inhibit arousal centers. During sleep, the VLPO inhibits amine-mediated arousal regions through GABAergic projections (shown in red). This inhibition of the amine-mediated arousal system disinhibits VLPO neurons, further stabilizing the production of sleep. The PPT also contains REM-promoting cholinergic neurons. The extended VLPO might promote REM sleep by disinhibiting the PPT region; its axons innervate interneurons within the PPT area, as well as aminergic neurons that normally inhibit REM-promoting cells in the PPT nucleus. Hypocretin neurons stabilize behavioral state by increasing the activity of aminergic neurons, thus maintaining consistent inhibition of sleep-promoting neurons in the VLPO and REM-promoting neurons in the PPT. Neuropeptide S may further stabilize this bistable circuitry by transiently increasing the activity of both hcrt and aminergic neurons. The transient wake promoting of NPS may be advantageous in situations of high alertness.

humans (Ogorochi *et al.*, 1984). PGD_2 had long been considered as a minor and biologically relatively inactive prostanoid, and therefore our findings suggested that PGD_2 may be a unique constituent of the brain of mammals and that it may play some important and rather specific function in the CNS.

In an attempt to determine the neural function of PGD_2, we microinjected nanomolar quantities of PGD_2 into the preoptic area (POA) of rats and discovered that the amount of slow wave sleep (SWS) was increased dose-dependently up to approximately six-fold with a concomitant drop in the colonic temperature, exactly as occurs during normal, physiological sleep (Ueno *et al.*, 1982). Encouraged by this unexpected finding, we proceeded to examine the somnogenic activity of PGD_2 in collaboration with Professor Inoué and collaborators by using their circadian sleep bioassay system involving continuous intracerebroventricular (i.c.v.) infusion. The somnogenic activity of PGD_2 was found to be dose- and time-dependent, and as little as 60 fmol/min of PGD_2 was sufficient to induce both SWS and rapid eye movement (REM) sleep. This effect was specific to PGD_2; other PGs were inactive except for PGD_1 and PGD_3, which were weakly active. Most importantly, however, sleep induced by PGD_2 was indistinguishable from physiological sleep as judged by several electrophysiological and behavioral criteria such as body and brain temperature, heart rate, locomotor activity, and the general behavior of the rat (Ueno *et al.*, 1983). During the infusion of PGD_2, rats were easily aroused by a brief sound stimulation and their sleep was episodic, indicating that PGD_2 does not interfere with the minimum waking time for survival. Essentially similar results were subsequently obtained when the rhesus monkey, *Macaca mulatta*, was the subject (Onoe *et al.*, 1988). However, the sleep induced by sleeping pills such as benzodiazepine derivatives under the same conditions was clearly different from the natural sleep, as judged by power spectral analysis of the electroencephalogram (EEG) (Onoe *et al.*, 1988).

Furthermore, the PGD_2 concentration in rat CSF showed a circadian fluctuation that paralleled the sleep–wake cycle (Pandey *et al.*, 1995), as well as an elevation with an increase in sleep propensity during sleep deprivation (Ram *et al.*, 1997). Infusion of an antagonist of the PGD_2 receptor (ONO-4127) into rat brain (Hayaishi, 2005; Qu *et al.*, 2006) and the i.c.v. or intraperitoneal administration of a selective inhibitor of PGD synthase (PGDS), $SeCl_4$, to rats (Matsumura *et al.*, 1991; Takahata *et al.*, 1993) (Qu *et al.*, 2006) inhibited their sleep in a dose-dependent manner. These results clearly showed that PGD_2 is an endogenous sleep-promoting substance, i.e. a sleep hormone, in rodents. Furthermore, the presence of lipocalin-type PGD synthase (L-PGDS/β-trace) protein in the CSF of fetal sheep in late gestation and the $SeCl_4$ effect of increasing the incidence of arousal-like behavior indicated that PGD_2 also plays a role in the induction or maintenance of prenatal sleep in sheep (Lee *et al.*, 2002).

PGD$_2$ was reported to be involved in the pathogenesis of mastocytosis, a disorder characterized by episodic and endogenous production of PGD$_2$ accompanied by deep sleep episodes (Roberts *et al.*, 1980). Members of the genus *Trypanosoma* cause African sleeping sickness, which is lethal in humans and animals, especially cows. Pentreath and co-workers (Pentreath *et al.*, 1990) determined the levels of interleukin-1, PGD$_2$, and PGE$_2$ by radioimmunoassay in samples of CSF from 24 severe cases of sleeping sickness caused by *Trypanosoma* and from 12 patients without neurological symptoms. PGD$_2$ concentrations were selectively and time-dependently elevated in the advanced-stage patients with parasites in their CSF. This correlation indicates that sleep in the late stage of sleeping sickness is caused at least in part by increased endogenous production of PGD$_2$. Whether this excessive production of PGD$_2$ was due to enzymatic formation in the host cells, in the parasites, or both, has not been clearly understood, because recent evidence from several laboratories indicated that PGs are not only present and widely distributed in higher animals but also in parasites, such as cestodes, trematodes, nematodes, and protozoa (Kubata *et al.*, 2000, 2007; Hervé *et al.*, 2003). These findings show that PGD$_2$ induces sleep not only in rodents and monkeys but also in humans as well.

PGD synthase

Structure and Function

In 1985, we isolated L-PGDS from rat brain as a monomeric protein with a relative molecular mass of 26 000 (Urade *et al.*, 1985), although the enzyme (PGH$_2$ D-isomerase, EC 5.3.99.2) had previously been misidentified as a protein with a relative molecular mass of 80 000–85 000 (Shimizu *et al.*, 1979). L-PGDS catalyzes the isomerization of the 9,11-endoperoxide of PGH$_2$ to produce PGD$_2$ with 9-hydroxy and 11-keto groups at the low turnover number of 170 min^{-1} in the presence of various sulfhydryl compounds, such as glutathione (GSH), dithiothreitol, or β-mercaptoethanol (Fig. 13.1). L-PGDS is the only molecule associated with enzyme activity among members of the lipocalin gene family, which is composed of various secretary proteins that bind and transport small hydrophobic substances (Urade & Hayaishi, 2000a; Urade *et al.*, 2006a). L-PGDS was previously designated as brain-type PGDS or GSH-independent PGDS to distinguish it from GSH-requiring PGDS purified from rat spleen (Christ-Hazelhof & Nugteren, 1979; Urade *et al.*, 1987b), which is now termed hematopoietic PGDS (H-PGDS) (Kanaoka & Urade, 2003; Urade *et al.*, 2006b). L-PGDS and H-PGDS are quite different from each other in terms of their amino acid sequence, tertiary structure, evolutionary origin, cellular distribution, etc., although both enzymes catalyze essentially the same reaction (Urade & Hayaishi, 2000b; Urade *et al.*, 2002). During a 20-year period after the first report of the purification of L-PGDS (Urade *et al.*, 1985), we extensively studied the chemical and functional properties of L-PGDS and reported the cloning of its cDNA and the chromosomal gene of the human and mouse enzymes, its X-ray crystallographic structure, and its immunohisto-chemical localization. We also reported the functional abnormalities of L-PGDS gene knockout (KO) mice and human enzyme-overexpressing transgenic (TG) mice for L-PGDS. Some of these findings have previously been reviewed elsewhere (Urade & Hayaishi, 2000a; Urade *et al.*, 2006a).

The cDNA for L-PGDS was first isolated from a rat brain cDNA library (Urade *et al.*, 1989) and subsequently from many other mammalian species, including human (Nagata *et al.*, 1991) and mouse (Eguchi *et al.*, 1999), and also from several amphibians (Achen *et al.*, 1992; Lepperdinger *et al.*, 1996; Irikura *et al.*, 2006). L-PGDS cDNA encodes a protein composed of 189 and 190 amino acid residues in the mouse and human enzyme, respectively. L-PGDS is post-translationally modified by the cleavage of an N-terminal hydrophobic signal peptide comprising 24 and 22 amino acid residues in the mouse and human enzyme, respectively. Two N-glycosylation sites, at positions of Asn51 and Asn78, of the mouse and human enzymes (Urade *et al.*, 1989) are conserved in all mammalian enzymes thus far identified but are not found in the amphibian homologs. Mammalian L-PGDS is highly glycosylated, with two N-glycosylated sugar chains, each with a relative molecular mass of 3,000. The carbohydrate structures of L-PGDS were determined in samples purified from human CSF (Hoffmann *et al.*, 1994), serum (Hoffmann *et al.*, 1997), urine (Hoffmann *et al.*, 1997; Manya *et al.*, 2000), and amniotic fluid (Manya *et al.*, 2000). However, the functional significance of these sugar chains remains to be determined.

Chemical and structural properties of the L-PGDS protein have been analyzed by using the recombinant protein heterologously expressed in *E. coli* or yeast. L-PGDS is a very stable enzyme and is highly resistant to heat treatment (Urade *et al.*, 1985) and protease digestion (Urade *et al.*, 1990). Circular dichroism spectroscopy of the recombinant rat L-PGDS revealed that the enzyme is composed of mainly β-strands (Inui *et al.*, 2003), similar to other proteins in the lipocalin family. We crystallized the recombinant mouse L-PGDS (Urade & Hayaishi, 2000a). Recently, by modifying the crystallization conditions and using the selenomethionyl Cys[65]Ala mutant (Irikura *et al.*, 2003), we successfully determined the X-ray crystallographic structure of L-PGDS with two different conformers of L-PGDS, i.e. one with an open and the other with a closed calyx at 2.1Å resolution (T. Kumasaka, D. Irikura, H. Ago *et al.*, unpublished results). We also determined the solution structure of mouse L-PGDS by NMR (Shimamoto *et al.*, 2007). X-ray crystallographic analysis and NMR analysis revealed that L-PGDS possesses a typical lipocalin-fold, β-barrel structure. However, L-PGDS contains two pockets in the large central cavity: one is the hydrophobic pocket corresponding to the ligand-binding pocket of other lipocalins; and the other, the hydrophlic pocket containing the catalytic Cys65, located on the upper part of the central cavity of the L-PGDS molecule.

Localization

L-PGDS is localized in the CNS and male genital organs of various mammals (Ujihara et al., 1988), as well as in the human heart (Eguchi et al., 1997). The cellular localization of L-PGDS has been extensively studied in these tissues from several mammals. The results of the in situ hybridization studies revealed that the mRNA was expressed intensely in the membrane system surrounding the brain rather than in the brain parenchyma, namely, in the leptomeninges, i.e. in the arachnoid membrane of the brain and spinal cord, and also in the choroid plexus in the ventricles (Urade et al., 1993). The mRNA was only faintly and diffusely expressed in the brain parenchyma, mainly in the white matter rather than in the gray matter, especially in the corpus callosum. Immunohistochemical detection of the L-PGDS protein also revealed essentially the same results (Urade et al., 1993; Yamashima et al., 1997; Beuckmann et al., 2000). The oligodendrocytes were positive for both mRNA and protein staining, but little, if any, of either was observed in other types of cell, including neurons, in adult rats (Urade et al., 1987a). Further studies in the mouse brain were in essential agreement with the results obtained with rats and clearly showed that mRNA and the immunoreactive protein for L-PGDS were mainly localized in the trabecular cells of the entire leptomeninges and also in the epithelial cells of the choroid plexus (Eguchi et al., 1999). These results gave us new insights into the mechanism of the somnogenic activity of PGD_2 dominantly produced in the leptomeninges, choroid plexus, and oligodendrocytes and secreted into the CSF.

In the testis and epididymis of humans (Tokugawa et al., 1998) and other mammals (Gerena et al., 1998, 2000a,b; Rodriguez et al., 2000; Samy et al., 2000; Fouchecourt et al., 2002a,b; Zhu et al., 2004; Malki et al., 2005), L-PGDS is localized in Leydig cells, Sertoli cells, and ductal epithelial cells and is secreted from them into the seminal plasma. Among other human tissues, the heart expresses L-PGDS mRNA most intensely (Eguchi et al., 1997).

L-PGDS is the same protein as β-trace (Hoffmann et al., 1993; Watanabe et al., 1994), which was originally discovered in 1961 as a major protein of human CSF (Clausen, 1961) and later identified in the seminal plasma, serum, and urine. Therefore, the L-PGDS/β-trace concentration in body fluids may be a useful clinical marker for various diseases (Urade & Hayaishi, 2000a; Urade et al., 2002, 2006). The L-PGDS/β-trace concentrations in seminal plasma, serum, and urine have been extensively evaluated in recent years as a biomarker for the diagnosis of several neurological disorders (Melegos *et al.*, 1997; Hiraoka *et al.*, 1998, 2001; Tumani *et al.*, 1998; Mase *et al.*, 1999, 2003; Brettschneider *et al.*, 2004), dysfunctional sperm formation (Tokugawa *et al.*, 1998), cardiovascular (Eguchi *et al.*, 1997; Taba *et al.*, 2000; Hirawa *et al.*, 2002; Ragolia *et al.*, 2003; Cipollone *et al.*, 2004) and renal (Melegos *et al.*, 1999; Priem *et al.*, 1999; Giessing, 1999; Hirawa *et al.*, 2001; Oda *et al.*, 2002; Hamano *et al.*, 2002) diseases, and pregnancy (Shiki *et al.*, 2004).

The serum L-PGDS/β-trace concentration shows a circadian variation with a nocturnal increase, which is suppressed during total sleep deprivation but not affected by deprivation of REM sleep (Jordan *et al.*, 2004). Whether or not L-PGDS is a dual-function protein in vivo and is involved in the production of PGD_2 as well as in the transport of PGD_2 or some other compound(s) remains to be elucidated.

Genetic studies

The gene for L-PGDS was cloned from rat (Igarashi *et al.*, 1992), human (White *et al.*, 1992), and mouse (Eguchi *et al.*, 1999) sources and shown to span about 3 kb and to contain seven exons split by six introns. The gene organization is remarkably analogous to that of other members of the lipocalin family in terms of number and size of exons and phase of splicing of introns (Igarashi *et al.*, 1992; White *et al.*, 1992). The human and mouse genes were mapped to chromosome 9q34.2–34.3 (White *et al.*, 1992) and 2B-C1 (Chan *et al.*, 1994), respectively, both regions being within the lipocalin gene cluster.

The transcriptional regulation of the L-PGDS gene has been studied after stimulation with various hormones. For example, the thyroid hormone activates L-PGDS expression through a thyroid hormone response element in human brain-derived TE671 cells (White *et al.*, 1997). In addition, dexamethasone, a synthetic glucocorticoid, induces L-PGDS expression via glucocorticoid receptors in mouse neuronal GT1-7 cells (Garcia-Fernandez *et al.*, 2000). 17β-Estradiol regulates L-PGDS gene expression in a tissue- and region-specific manner. It activates the expression via estrogen β receptors in the mouse heart (Otsuki *et al.*, 2003) and increases the L-PGDS expression in the arcuate and ventromedial nuclei of the rat hypothalamus, but decreases it in the ventrolateral preoptic area (VLPO) of the hypothalamus, an area that contains sleep-active neurons (Mong *et al.*, 2003a,b). Expression of L-PGDS is downregulated by Notch-HES signaling in primary cultures of rat leptomeningeal cells (Fujimori *et al.*, 2003) and in human TE671 cells (Fujimori *et al.*, 2005). In contrast, L-PGDS expression is activated by protein kinase C signaling through de-repression of the Notch-HES signaling and enhancement of AP-2β function in the TE671 cells (Fujimori *et al.*, 2005). The latter occurs by the binding of c-Fos and c-Jun to the AP-1 binding site of the promoter after addition of shear stress to human vascular endothelial cells (Miyagi *et al.*, 2005), and by the binding of microphthalmia-associated transcription factor to E-box motifs of the promoter in mouse melanocytes (Takeda *et al.*, 2006).

We generated L-PGDS KO mice with the null mutation by homologous recombination (Eguchi *et al.*, 1999) and demonstrated that the KO mice grow normally but exhibit several functional abnormalities in their regulation of nociception (Eguchi *et al.*, 1999), sleep (Eguchi *et al.*, 2002; Hayaishi *et al.*, 2004), and energy metabolism (Ragolia *et al.*, 2005). These KO mice do not exhibit allodynia (touch-evoked pain), which is a typical phenomenon of neuropathic pain, after an intrathecal administration of PGE_2 or bicuculline, a γ-aminobutyric acid ($GABA_A$) receptor antagonist (Eguchi *et al.*, 1999). The KO mice do not accumulate PGD_2 in their brain during sleep deprivation nor do they show the non-REM (NREM) sleep rebound after sleep deprivation, whereas the wild-type (WT) mice show an increase in the PGD_2 content in their brain during sleep deprivation, which induces the NREM sleep rebound (Eguchi *et al.*, 2002; Hayaishi *et al.*, 2004). L-PGDS KO mice become glucose-intolerant and insulin-resistant at an accelerated rate compared with their WT counterparts (Ragolia *et al.*, 2005). The KO mice possess adipocytes of larger size than the WT mice, and develop nephropathy and an aortic thickening when fed a high-fat diet (Ragolia *et al.*, 2005).

We also generated TG mice (Pinzar *et al.*, 2000) that overexpressed the human L-PGDS under the control of the β-actin promoter. Serendipitously, we discovered that these TG mice showed a transient increase in NREM sleep after their tails had been clipped for DNA sampling used for genetic analysis (Pinzar *et al.*, 2000; Eguchi *et al.*, 2002). We showed that the noxious stimulation of tail clipping induced a remarkable increase in the PGD_2 content in the brain of the TG mice but not in that of the WT mice, although we do not yet understand in detail the mechanism responsible for this increase. Similarly, in an ovalbumin-induced asthma model, the TG-mice showed notably increased PGD_2 production in the lung after the antigen challenge and developed pronounced eosinophilic lung inflammation and Th2 cytokine release compared with their WT littermates (Fujitani *et al.*, 2002). These TG mice also exhibited accelerated adipogenesis (Y. Fujitani, K. Aritake, and Y. U., unpublished results). Therefore, L-PGDS TG mice are useful as a unique animal model to study the functional abnormalities caused by the overproduction of PGD_2.

PGD receptors (D-type PG receptors, DPR)

Earlier autoradiographic studies using computerized densitometry and color coding of the binding ^{3}H-labeled PGD_2 showed PGD_2 binding in the POA of rat brain (Yamashita *et al.*, 1983). In agreement with this result, when a picomolar amount of PGD_2 was infused through a microdialysis probe into more than 200 different areas in the rat brain, PGD_2 failed to induce sleep in all parts of the brain parenchyma except in the POA, where a weak somnogenic activity was consistently observed. The most pronounced sleep-inducing activity was observed, however, when PGD_2 was applied to the subarachnoid space in the medial ventral region of the rostral basal forebrain (Matsumura et al., 1994).

Two distinct subtypes of receptor for PGD_2 have been identified: one is the DP (DP_1) receptor (DPR) originally identified as a homolog of other prostanoid receptors (Hirata et al., 1994), and the other is the CRTH2 (DP_2) receptor more recently identified as a chemoattractant receptor for PGD_2 (Hirai et al., 2001). DPR mRNA expression was shown to be significantly abundant in the leptomeninges of rat brain (Gerashchenko et al., 1998). Finally, the location of DPR in the mouse brain was visualized by using an antibody highly specific for DPR (Mizoguchi et al., 2001). The DPR-immunoreactivity was localized almost exclusively in the leptomeninges on the ventral surface of the basal forebrain, with weak immunoreactivity in the pia/arachnoid membrane in the choroid plexus of the lateral and third ventricles. In contrast, L-PGDS-immunoreactivity was localized in the leptomeninges surrounding the entire brain and in the choroid plexus, in good agreement with our previous studies in rat brain (Urade et al., 1993; Beuckmann et al., 2000). Little, if any, DPR-immunoreactivity was found in the dura mater, pia mater, or brain parenchyma. Electron microscopic studies in mouse brain clearly showed that DPR-expressing cells were arachnoid trabecular cells and that the immunogold particles were mainly located on the plasma membranes and, less frequently, on the intracellular membrane structures such as the vesicles and endoplasmic reticulum (Mizoguchi et al., 2001). Most DPR-expressing cells were also positive for L-PGDS, indicating that PGD_2 acts as an autocrine as well as a paracrine agent, although PGD_2 produced in other parts of the brain, such as the CSF, may also contribute to promoting sleep.

More than 700 serial coronal sections were used to find the exact location of DPR-expressing cells in the mouse brain (Mizoguchi et al., 2001). The DPR-positive cells were highly concentrated in the ventral surface of the rostral basal forebrain, whereas other areas were almost completely negative. The region with concentrated DPRs was clearly defined as bilateral wings in the rostral basal forebrain lateral to the optic chiasm in the proximity of the ventrolateral preoptic (VLPO) area, an important sleep center, and the tuberomammillary nucleus (TMN), a center of wakefulness-inducing cells. The rostral and main portions of this region were associated with the visual pathway composed of the optic nerves, optic chiasm, and optic tracts.

PGD_2 infusion into the lateral ventricle of mice increased NREM sleep preferentially over REM sleep (Mizoguchi et al., 2001), in good agreement with our previous observation that NREM sleep was selectively induced by PGD$_2$ infusion into the DPR-rich area in the basal forebrain of rats (Matsumura *et al.*, 1994). In the DPR KO mice, the amount of NREM sleep did not increase after PGD$_2$ infusion into the brain (Mizoguchi *et al.*, 2001). These results taken together clearly show that PGD$_2$ produced in the leptomeninges and choroid plexus, and possibly in the CSF, circulates in the ventricular and subarachnoid space, and binds to DPR in the basal forebrain to initiate NREM sleep.

Adenosine and receptors

To find out how the sleep signal initiated by the binding of PGD$_2$ to the DPR in the surface of the basal forebrain is transduced into the brain parenchyma, we applied numerous neurotransmitters, peptides, hormones, and other bioactive substances to the DPR-rich sleep-promoting zone to see whether any of these compounds could replace or mimic the somnogenic activity of PGD$_2$. Among several hundred test compounds, only adenosine and adenosine A$_{2A}$ receptor (A$_{2A}$R) agonists such as 2-(4(2-carboxyethyl) phenylethylamino) adenosine-5′-N-ethylcarboxamideadenosine (CGS21680) and 2-(4-(2-(2-aminoethylamino-carbonyl)ethyl) phenylethylamino)-5′-N-ethylcarboxamidoadenosine (APEC) were effective and induced NREM, but not REM, sleep when infused into rats during the dark phase (Satoh *et al.*, 1998). In contrast, A$_1$-receptor (A$_1$R) agonists, such as N^6-cyclohexyladenosine and N^6-cyclopentyladenosine, were ineffective. In rats pretreated by intraperitoneal infusion of a selective A$_{2A}$R antagonist, KF17837, the sleep-inducing effects of both A$_{2A}$R agonists and PGD$_2$ were attenuated, indicating that the somnogenic effect of PGD$_2$ may be mediated by adenosine via the A$_{2A}$R. Furthermore, the extracellular level of adenosine in the subarachnoid space of the basal forebrain was increased dose-dependently by the infusion of PGD$_2$ or the DPR agonist BW245C in rats, and this effect was attenuated by the simultaneous treatment of animals with a DPR antagonist, BWA868C. The PGD$_2$-induced increase in extracellular adenosine was also found in WT mice, but was not observed in the DPR KO mice (Mizoguchi *et al.*, 2001).

The biosynthesis of adenosine is theoretically controlled by several processes; namely (1) the biosynthesis of adenosine from AMP by 5′-nucleotidase [EC 3.1.3.5], (2) from S-adenosyl homocysteine by S-adenosyl homocystine hydrolase [EC 3.3.1.1], (3) the metabolism of adenosine to AMP by adenosine kinase [EC 2.7.1.20], and (4) to inosine by adenosine deaminase (ADA) [EC 3.5.4.2]. Interestingly, both 5′-nucleotidase and ADA activities were found to be highest in the leptomeninges of rat brain; in contrast, the adenosine kinase activity was widely distributed throughout the brain parenchyma, which has negligible ADA activity

(Okada *et al.*, 2003). More recent experiments in humans (Rétey *et al.*, 2005) confirmed and extended our observation and showed that genetic variation of ADA specifically increases deep sleep and SWS and that the $A_{2A}R$ is involved in this process.

The leptomeninges is a membrane system that encloses the brain to form the subarachnoid space. It is generally recognized only as a cushion to protect the brain from physical impact. However, the co-localization of 5'-nucleotidase, ADA, L-PGDS, and DPR in the leptomeninges indicates that this membrane system plays a crucial role in the regulation of sleep by producing and sensing two endogenous somnogenic substances, adenosine and PGD_2, both of which circulate in the subarachnoid space and act as humoral sleep regulators. This suggestion is also supported by the fact that PGD_2 and $A_{2A}R$ agonists exhibit potent somnogenic effects when administered in the subarachnoid space below the rostral basal forebrain, but no such effect is observed when they are administered in any other brain region.

Adenosine has been known to be an endogenous sleep substance based on the experimental evidence of a variety of pharmacological and behavioral studies. A number of stable adenosine analogs are known to induce sleep when administered to rats and other experimental animals (Satoh *et al.*, 1998; Strecker *et al.*, 2000). Caffeine is considered to inhibit sleep by acting as an adenosine antagonist in man (Landolt *et al.*, 2004). We previously showed that PGD_2 induced NREM sleep by producing excess amounts of adenosine, which in turn binds to the $A_{2A}R$, rather than to the A_1R, and promotes sleep (Satoh *et al.*, 1998). However, previous investigators have shown that the A_1R is involved in this process (Rainnie *et al.*, 1994; Mignot *et al.*, 2002), and thus this question has long been considered controversial (Basheer *et al.*, 2004).

In order to provide a definitive answer to this long-standing question, we compared the sleep–wake patterns of WT mice and $A_{2A}R$ KO mice of the inbred C57BL/6 strain generated by Chen and collaborators (Urade *et al.*, 2003). When CGS21680, an $A_{2A}R$ agonist, was infused into the lateral ventricle of WT mice, NREM sleep was induced dose-dependently, whereas the A_1R-selective agonist N^6-cyclopentyladenosine was totally inactive, indicating that the $A_{2A}R$, but not the A_1R, is involved in NREM sleep regulation. $A_{2A}R$ KO mice showed clear circadian variations of sleep-stage distribution during basal conditions, similar to WT mice, but were completely insensitive to CGS21680. Interestingly, the amount of sleep increase induced by the infusion of PGD_2 in the $A_{2A}R$ KO mice was about 60% of that observed in the WT mice, suggesting a possibility that the somnogenic effect of PGD_2 was partially independent of the $A_{2A}R$.

Caffeine binds, as an antagonist, to both A_1R and $A_{2A}R$ with almost the same affinity and induces wakefulness (Fredholm *et al.*, 1999, 2001). The receptor subtype involved in caffeine-induced wakefulness had remained unidentified until recently. In 2005, we compared the effect of caffeine on the sleep–wake cycle of WT, A_1R KO, and $A_{2A}R$ KO mice and showed that caffeine induced wakefulness in WT mice and A_1R KO mice but not in $A_{2A}R$ KO mice (Huang et al., 2005). These results clearly indicate that caffeine-induced wakefulness also depends on $A_{2A}Rs$.

Sleep (VLPO) and wake (TMN) centers in the hypothalamus

The immediate early gene product c-Fos (cellular feline osteosarcoma) has widely been used as a useful marker of neuronal activation. Fos, the protein encoded by the *c-fos* gene, is a transcription factor that triggers transcription in a cascade of cellular responses. To determine which neuron groups are involved in the response to PGD_2 and/or adenosine, especially $A_{2A}R$ agonists, we examined Fos-immunoreactivity under these conditions (Scammell et al., 1998, 2001; Satoh et al., 1999).

When PGD_2 or the $A_{2A}R$ agonist CGS21680 was infused for 2 h into the PGD_2-sensitive zone of the subarachnoid space, a marked increase in the number of Fos-positive cells was observed in the leptomeningeal membrane on the ventral surface of the basal forebrain as well as in the VLPO area concomitant with the induction of NREM sleep. In contrast, the number of Fos-positive neurons decreased markedly in the TMN of the posterior hypothalamus. Using Fos-immunoreactivity, Sherin et al. (1996) showed a discrete cluster of neurons in the VLPO to play a critical role in the generation of sleep. The VLPO is known to send specific inhibitory GABAergic and galaninergic efferents to the TMN, the histaminergic neurons of which contribute to the ascending arousal system (Fig. 13.2).

PGD_2 does not induce sleep when infused into the TMN (Matsumura et al., 1994), and therefore it is unlikely that putative wake neurons in the TMN are directly inhibited by PGD_2. On the other hand, PGD_2 induces sleep most effectively when infused into the subarachnoid space in the PGD_2-sensitive zone (Matsumura et al., 1994). PGD_2 increased the firing rates of sleep-active neurons in the preoptic area (POA) (Koyama & Hayaishi, 1994), where these neurons are most abundant in the VLPO. The VLPO may induce sleep by inhibiting wake-promoting neurons in the TMN, for both GABA and galanin were shown to inhibit the firing rate of wake-active TMN neurons (Sherin et al., 1996).

PGD_2 also induced the expression of Fos-immunoreactivity in the leptomeninges (Scammell et al., 1998), suggesting that PGD_2 activates the VLPO via leptomeningeal DPR. Taken together, these results indicate that PGD_2 binds to DPR in the PGD_2-sensitive zone, where meningeal cells release paracrine

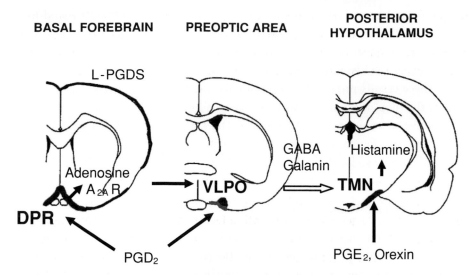

Figure 13.2 Schematic representation of the molecular mechanisms of sleep–wake regulation by PGD_2, PGE_2, adenosine, histamine, and orexin.

signaling molecules such as adenosine, which subsequently excite neighboring sleep-active VLPO neurons. These VLPO neurons may directly induce NREM sleep or send inhibitory signals to the TMN to downregulate the wake-active neurons. Thus the sleep–wake cycle is regulated by a "flip–flop" mechanism involving the interaction between these two centers (Saper *et al.*, 2001, 2005; Hayaishi & Huang, 2004).

Disinhibition of VLPO sleep-active neurons through presynaptic reduction of GABA release by adenosine was suggested by the intracellular recording of VLPO neurons in vitro (Morairty *et al.*, 2004). More recent studies, using intracellular recording of VLPO neurons in rat brain slices, demonstrated the existence of two distinct types of VLPO neuron in terms of their responses to serotonin and adenosine. VLPO neurons are inhibited uniformly by the two arousal neurotransmitters, noradrenaline and acetylcholine, and mostly by an adenosine A_1R agonist. However, serotonin inhibits the Type-1 neurons but excites the Type-2 neurons. An $A_{2A}R$ agonist postsynaptically excited the Type-2, but not the Type-1 neurons. These results suggest that the Type-2 neurons are involved in the initiation of sleep and that the Type-1 neurons contribute to sleep consolidation, since they are activated only when released from inhibition by the arousal systems (Gallopin *et al.*, 2005).

We recently demonstrated that CGS21680, an adenosine $A_{2A}R$ agonist, inhibited histamine release in both the frontal cortex and medial POA in a dose-dependent manner, and increased GABA release specifically in the TMN but not in the frontal cortex (Hong *et al.*, 2005). Furthermore, the CGS21680-induced inhibition of histamine release was antagonized by perfusion of the TMN with a $GABA_A$ antagonist, picrotoxin, suggesting that the $A_{2A}R$ agonist induced sleep by inhibiting the histaminergic system through increasing GABA release in the TMN. These results provide further evidence to support the original hypothesis of the "flip–flop" mechanism, whereby sleep is promoted by upregulation of the sleep-active neurons in the VLPO and at the same time by downregulation of the wake-active neurons in the TMN (Saper *et al.*, 2001, 2005), a hypothesis that was extended by subsequent work in our laboratory (Hayaishi & Huang, 2004).

PGE_2 and wakefulness

PGE_2 and PGD_2 are positional isomers (Fig. 13.1) and are known to exhibit occasionally opposite biological effects. For example, PGD_2 lowers body temperature, suppresses secretion of luteinizing hormone-releasing hormone, and decreases the transmucosal potential difference in rat colon mucosa, whereas PGE_2 has the opposite effects: it causes an increase in body temperature, stimulates the hormone secretion, and increases the transmucosal potential difference. Concerning the effect of the E-series of PGs on sleep, reports by previous investigators have been inconsistent, probably due to differences in animal species, site of application, and other conditions.

Matsumura *et al.* (1988) demonstrated that microinjection of PGE_2 into the POA reduced the amount of diurnal sleep of rats, indicating that PGE_2 may induce wakefulness. The awakening effect of this PG was further examined by using the long-term sleep bioassay system of i.c.v. infusion (Matsumura *et al.*, 1989). Under more physiological conditions, both NREM and REM sleep were dose-dependently reduced during PGE_2 infusion. A rebound of both NREM and REM sleep was subsequently observed during the dark phase after the PGE_2 infusion. The reduction in NREM sleep was due to a shortened episode duration, whereas that in REM sleep resulted from both a shortened duration and a decreased number of episodes. Under these experimental conditions, PGE_2 also induced hyperthermia. However, there seems to be no evidence to support a cause–effect relationship between the changes in sleep–wakefulness and body temperature changes.

To explore the neural mechanisms involved in PGE_2-induced wakefulness in rats, the effect of PGE_2 on the activity of the histaminergic system and the involvement of PGE_2 receptor subtypes in the response were examined (Huang *et al.*, 2003). The TMN of the posterior hypothalamus is the sole source of histaminergic innervation of the mammalian CNS, and this histaminergic system is considered to play a central role in mediating wakefulness, as described above.

PGE_2 perfusion of the TMN significantly increased both the synthesis and release of histamine. Among the agonists of the four distinct subtypes of PGE_2 receptors (EP_{1-4}) tested, only the EP_4 receptor-agonist (ONO-AE1-329) mimicked the excitatory effect of PGE_2. In situ hybridization revealed that EP_4 receptor mRNA was expressed in the TMN region. Furthermore, perfusion of the TMN with the EP_4 agonist induced wakefulness. These findings thus indicate that PGE_2 induced wakefulness through activation of the histaminergic system via EP_4 receptors.

Other activators of the histaminergic system may also be involved in wakefulness. The orexin (i.e. hypocretin) A and B neuropeptides were isolated from rat hypothalamic extracts. A mutation in the orexin-2 receptor gene was found to be associated with canine narcolepsy, and mice lacking the orexin peptide display increases in REM and NREM sleep and a decrease in wakefulness time during the active period of normal rodents. However, the exact role of orexin in physiological sleep and the mechanisms involved have not yet been elucidated.

Orexin neurons are exclusively localized in the lateral hypothalamic area and their fibers project to the entire CNS including the TMN, which is enriched in orexin-2 receptors. Perfusion of orexin A (5–25 pmol/min) for 1 h into the TMN of rats through a microdialysis probe promptly increased wakefulness, concomitant with a reduction in REM and NREM sleep (Huang et al., 2001). Furthermore, microdialysis studies showed that orexin A increased histamine release from both the medial POA and the frontal cortex approximately two-fold over the baseline in a dose-dependent manner. Infusion of orexin A (1.5 pmol/min) for 6 h into the lateral ventricle of mice produced a significant increase in wakefulness during the first 8 h after the start of infusion to the same level seen during the active period in WT mice. However, in H1R KO mice, no effect of orexin infusion was observed under these conditions. These results indicate that orexin is a potent waking substance acting upon orexin-2 receptors in the TMN and that the arousing effect of orexin A depends on histaminergic neurotransmission mediated by H_1Rs.

Conclusions

The concept of humoral, rather than neural, regulation of sleep dates back almost 100 years when Kuniomi Ishimori and Henri Piéron demonstrated the presence of endogenous sleep-promoting substance(s) that had accumulated in the CSF of sleep-deprived dogs. PGD_2 is the most plausible candidate of their endogenous sleep-promoting substance, based on the data obtained in our own and other laboratories over the past 20 years, as summarized in this chapter.

We have drawn the following tentative conclusions as a working hypothesis for future studies. (i) PGD_2 and PGE_2 are endogenous sleep and wake substances, respectively, involved in the regulation of sleep and wakefulness under physiological conditions not only in rodents but also in monkeys and possibly in humans as well. (ii) PGD_2 is produced by L-PGDS mainly present in the arachnoid membrane surrounding the brain, secreted into the CSF, and circulates within the CSF as a sleep hormone. (iii) Binding of PGD_2 to DPR on the arachnoid membrane of the rostral basal forebrain increases the extracellular concentration of adenosine, which transduces the somnogenic information from the CSF to the brain parenchyma including the VLPO and TMN, putative sleep and wake centers, respectively, through the adenosine A_{2A} receptor. (iv) The L-PGDS/PGD_2/DPR system plays a crucial role in the homeostatic regulation of NREM sleep, as indicated by recent studies, including those in L-PGDS-KO and DPR-KO mice (Hayaishi *et al.*, 2004; Qu *et al.*, 2006).

We have thus witnessed significant progress in sleep research as to the humoral mechanisms of sleep regulation, and have opened up a new research frontier by elucidating the interplay between humoral regulation and the neural network. Although many important questions remain to be answered, we hope that our studies described here will provide a basis for further work on solving the remaining difficult problems. In this way, we believe, we may eventually uncover some of the mysteries of sleep.

Acknowledgements

The authors are indebted to Drs. Z.-L. Huang and L. Frye for their help during the preparation of this manuscript and illustrations and to N. Ueda, M. Yamada and M. Yamaguchi for secretarial assistance. We also express deep gratitude to all collaborators, past and present, on this project during the past 20 years. The work from this laboratory was supported mainly by grants-in-aid from the Ministry of Health, Labour, and Welfare of Japan, the Ministry of Education, Culture, Sports, Science, and Technology of Japan, the Bio-oriented Technology Research Advancement Institution, Takeda Pharmaceutical Co., Ltd., Ono Pharmaceutical Co., Ltd., and the Osaka Bioscience Institute.

References

Achen, M. G., *et al.* (1992). Protein synthesis at the blood-brain barrier. The major protein secreted by amphibian choroid plexus is a lipocalin. *J. Biol. Chem.* **267**, 23170–4.

Basheer, R., *et al.* (2004). Adenosine and sleep-wake regulation. *Prog. Neurobiol.* **73**, 79–96.

Beuckmann, C. T., *et al.* (2000). Cellular localization of lipocalin-type prostaglandin D synthase (beta-trace) in the central nervous system of the adult rat. *J. Comp. Neurol.* **428**, 62–78.

Bobillier, P., et al. (1982). Glucose utilization increases in choroid plexus during slow wave sleep. A [^{14}C] deoxyglucose study in the cat. Brain Res. 240, 359–63.

Brettschneider, J., et al. (2004). Meningeal derived cerebrospinal fluid proteins in different forms of dementia: is a meningopathy involved in normal pressure hydrocephalus? J. Neurol. Neurosurg. Psychiatry 75, 1614–16.

Chan, P., et al. (1994). Comparative mapping of lipocalin genes in human and mouse: the four genes for complement C8 gamma chain, prostaglandin-D-synthase, oncogene-24p3, and progestagen-associated endometrial protein map to HSA9 and MMU2. Genomics 23, 145–50.

Christ-Hazelhof, E. & Nugteren, D. H. (1979). Purification and characterisation of prostaglandin endoperoxide D-isomerase, a cytoplasmic, glutathione-requiring enzyme. Biochim. Biophys. Acta 572, 43–51.

Cipollone, F., et al. (2004). Balance between PGD synthase and PGE synthase is a major determinant of atherosclerotic plaque instability in humans. Arteriosclerosis Thrombosis Vasc. Biol. 24, 1259–65.

Clausen, J. (1961). Proteins in normal cerebrospinal fluid not found in serum. Proc. Soc. Exp. Biol. Med. 107, 170–2.

Eguchi, Y., et al. (1997). Expression of lipocalin-type prostaglandin D synthase (beta-trace) in human heart and its accumulation in the coronary circulation of angina patients. Proc. Natl. Acad. Sci. USA 94, 14689–94.

Eguchi, N., et al. (1999). Lack of tactile pain (allodynia) in lipocalin-type prostaglandin D synthase-deficient mice. Proc. Natl. Acad. Sci. USA, 96, 726–30.

Eguchi, N., et al. (2002). Sleep in transgenic and gene-knockout mice for lipocalin-type prostaglandin D synthase. In Oxygen and Life: Oxygenases, Oxidases, and Lipid Mediators, ed. Y. Ishimura, M. Nozak, S. Yamamoto et al., International Congress Series 1233. Amsterdam: Elsevier Science, pp. 429–33.

Fouchecourt, S., et al. (2002a). Mammalian lipocalin-type prostaglandin D$_2$ synthase in the fluids of the male genital tract: putative biochemical and physiological functions. Biol. Reprod. 66, 458–67.

Fouchecourt, S., et al. (2002b). Epididymal lipocalin-type prostaglandin D$_2$ synthase: identification using mass spectrometry, messenger RNA localization, and immunodetection in mouse, rat, hamster, and monkey. Biol. Reprod. 66, 524–33.

Fredholm, B. B., et al. (1999). Actions of caffeine in the brain with special reference to factors that contribute to its widespread use. Pharmacol. Rev. 51, 83–133.

Fredholm, B. B., et al. (2001). International Union of Pharmacology. XXV. Nomenclature and classification of adenosine receptors. Pharmacol. Rev. 53, 527–52.

Fujimori, K., et al. (2003). Regulation of lipocalin-type prostaglandin D synthase gene expression by Hes-1 through E-box and interleukin-1 beta via two NF-kappa B elements in rat leptomeningeal cells. J. Biol. Chem. 278, 6018–26.

Fujimori, K., et al. (2005). Protein kinase C activates human lipocalin-type prostaglandin D synthase gene expression through de-repression of notch-HES signaling and enhancement of AP-2 beta function in brain-derived TE671 cells. J. Biol. Chem. 280, 18452–61.

Fujitani, Y., *et al.* (2002). Pronounced eosinophilic lung inflammation and Th2 cytokine release in human lipocalin-type prostaglandin D synthase transgenic mice. *J. Immunol.* **168**, 443–9.

Gallopin, T., *et al.* (2005). The endogenous somnogen adenosine excites a subset of sleep-promoting neurons via A_{2A} receptors in the ventrolateral preoptic nucleus. *Neuroscience* **134**, 1377–90.

Garcia-Fernandez, L. F., *et al.* (2000). Dexamethasone induces lipocalin-type prostaglandin D synthase gene expression in mouse neuronal cells. *J. Neurochem.* **75**, 460–70.

Gerena, R. L., *et al.* (1998). Identification of a fertility-associated protein in bull seminal plasma as lipocalin-type prostaglandin D synthase. *Biol. Reprod.* **58**, 826–33.

Gerena, R. L., *et al.* (2000a). Stage and region-specific localization of lipocalin-type prostaglandin D synthase in the adult murine testis and epididymis. *J. Androl.* **21**, 848–54.

Gerena, R. L., *et al.* (2000b). Immunocytochemical localization of lipocalin-type prostaglandin D synthase in the bull testis and epididymis and on ejaculated sperm. *Biol. Reprod.* **62**, 547–56.

Gerashchenko, D., *et al.* (1998). Dominant expression of rat prostanoid DP receptor mRNA in leptomeninges, inner segments of photoreceptor cells, iris epithelium, and ciliary processes. *J. Neurochem.* **71**, 937–45.

Giessing, M. (1999). Beta-trace protein as indicator of glomerular filtration rate. *Urology* **54**, 940–1.

Hamano, K., *et al.* (2002). Blood sugar control reverses the increase in urinary excretion of prostaglandin D synthase in diabetic patients. *Nephron* **92**, 77–85.

Hayaishi, O. (2005). Molecular mechanisms of sleep-wake regulation. In *Sleep: Circuits and Functions*, ed. P.-H. Luppi, Boca Raton, FL: CRC Press, pp. 65–82.

Hayaishi, O. & Huang, Z. L. (2004). Role of orexin and prostaglandin E_2 in activating histaminergic neurotransmission. *Drug News Perspec.* **17**, 105–9.

Hayaishi, O., *et al.* (2004). Genes for prostaglandin D synthase and receptor as well as adenosine A_{2A} receptor are involved in the homeostatic regulation of nrem sleep. *Arch. Ital. Biol.* **142**, 533–9.

Hervé, M., *et al.* (2003). Pivotal roles of the parasite PGD_2 synthase and of the host D prostanoid receptor 1 in schistosome immune evasion. *Eur. J. Immunol.* **33**, 2764–72.

Hirai, H., *et al.* (2001). Prostaglandin D_2 selectively induces chemotaxis in T helper type 2 cells, eosinophils, and basophils via seven-transmembrane receptor CRTH2. *J. Exp. Med.* **193**, 255–61.

Hiraoka, A., *et al.* (1998). Sodium dodecyl sulfate-capillary gel electrophoretic analysis of molecular mass microheterogeneity of beta-trace protein in cerebrospinal fluid from patients with central nervous system diseases. *J. Chromatogr. A* **802**, 143–8.

Hiraoka, A., *et al.* (2001). Charge microheterogeneity of the beta-trace proteins (lipocalin-type prostaglandin D synthase) in the cerebrospinal fluid of patients with neurological disorders analyzed by capillary isoelectrofocusing. *Electrophoresis* **22**, 3433–7.

Hirata, M., *et al.* (1994). Molecular characterization of a mouse prostaglandin D receptor and functional expression of the cloned gene. *Proc. Natl. Acad. Sci. USA* **91**, 11192–6.

Hirawa, N., *et al.* (2001). Urinary prostaglandin D synthase (beta-trace) excretion increases in the early stage of diabetes mellitus. *Nephron* **87**, 321–7.

Hirawa, N., *et al.* (2002). Lipocalin-type prostaglandin D synthase in essential hypertension. *Hypertension* **39**, 449–54.

Hiroshima, O., *et al.* (1986). Basal level of prostaglandin D_2 in rat brain by a solid-phase enzyme immunoassay. *Prostaglandins* **32**, 63–80.

Hoffmann, A., *et al.* (1993). Purification and chemical characterization of beta-trace protein from human cerebrospinal fluid: its identification as prostaglandin D synthase. *J. Neurochem.* **61**, 451–6.

Hoffmann, A., *et al.* (1994). Carbohydrate structures of beta-trace protein from human cerebrospinal fluid: evidence for "brain-type" N-glycosylation. *J. Neurochem.* **63**, 2185–96.

Hoffmann, A., *et al.* (1997). Molecular characterization of beta-trace protein in human serum and urine: a potential diagnostic marker for renal diseases. *Glycobiology* **7**, 499–506.

Hong, Z. Y., *et al.* (2005). An adenosine A receptor agonist induces sleep by increasing GABA release in the tuberomammillary nucleus to inhibit histaminergic systems in rats. *J. Neurochem.* **92**, 1542–9.

Huang, Z. L., *et al.* (2001). Arousal effect of orexin A depends on activation of the histaminergic system. *Proc. Natl. Acad. Sci. USA* **98**, 9965–70.

Huang, Z. L., *et al.* (2003). Prostaglandin E2 activates the histaminergic system via EP_4 receptor to induce wakefulness in rats. *J. Neurosci.* **23**, 5975–83.

Huang, Z. L., *et al.* (2005). Adenosine A_{2A}, but not A1, receptors mediate the arousal effect of caffeine. *Nat. Neurosci.* **8**, 858–9.

Igarashi, M., *et al.* (1992). Structural organization of the gene for prostaglandin D synthase in the rat brain. *Proc. Natl. Acad. Sci. USA* **89**, 5376–80.

Inoué, S. (1989). *Biology of Sleep Substances.* Boca Raton, FL: CRC Press.

Inui, T., *et al.* (2003). Characterization of the unfolding process of lipocalin-type prostaglandin D synthase. *J. Biol. Chem.* **278**, 2845–52.

Irikura, D., *et al.* (2003). Cloning, expression, crystallization, and preliminary X-ray analysis of recombinant mouse lipocalin-type prostaglandin D synthase, a somnogen-producing enzyme. *J. Biochem.* **133**, 29–32.

Irikura, D., *et at.* (2007). Characterization of a major secretory protein in the cane toad (*Bufo marinus*) choroid plexus as an amphibian lipocalin-type prostaglandin D synthase. *J. Biochem.* **141**, 173–80.

Jordan, W., *et al.* (2004). Prostaglandin D synthase (beta-trace) in healthy human sleep. *Sleep* **27**, 867–74.

Jouvet, M., *et al.* (1983). Serotonergic and nonserotonergic mechanisms in sleep. In *Sleep Disorders; Basic and Clinical Research*, ed. Gibson, C. J. and Chase, M. H., New York, NY: Spectrum, pp. 557–71.

Kanaoka, Y. & Urade, Y. (2003). Hematopoietic prostaglandin D synthase. *Prostagland. Leukotrienes Essent. Fatty Acids* **69**, 163-7.

Koyama, Y. & Hayaishi, O. (1994). Modulation by prostaglandins of activity of sleep-related neurons in the preoptic/anterior hypothalamic areas in rats. *Brain Res. Bull.* **33**, 367-72.

Kubata, B. K., *et al.* (2000). Identification of a novel prostaglandin $F_{2\alpha}$ synthase in *Trypanosoma brucei. J. Exp. Med.* **192**, 1327-38.

Kubata, B. K., *et al.* (2007). Molecular basis for prostaglandin production in hosts and parasites. *Trends Parasitol.* **23**, 325-31.

Landolt, H. P., *et al.* (2004). Caffeine attenuates waking and sleep electroencephalographic markers of sleep homeostasis in humans. *Neuropsychopharmacology* **29**, 1933-9.

Lee, B., *et al.* (2002). Prostaglandin D synthase in the prenatal ovine brain and effects of its inhibition with selenium chloride on fetal sleep/wake activity in utero. *J. Neurosci.* **22**, 5679-86.

Lepperdinger, G., *et al.* (1996). The lipocalin X1cpll expressed in the neural plate of Xenopus laevis embryos is a secreted retinaldehyde binding protein. *Protein Sci.* **5**, 1250-60.

Malki, S., *et al.* (2005). Prostaglandin D2 induces nuclear import of the sex-determining factor SOX9 via its cAMP-PKA phosphorylation. *EMBO J.* **24**, 1798-809.

Manya, H., *et al.* (2000). Comparative study of the asparagine-linked sugar chains of human lipocalin-type prostaglandin D synthase purified from urine and amniotic fluid, and recombinantly expressed in Chinese hamster ovary cells. *J. Biochem.* **127**, 1001-11.

Mase, M., *et al.* (1999). Acute and transient increase of lipocalin-type prostaglandin D synthase (beta-trace) level in cerebrospinal fluid of patients with aneurysmal subarachnoid hemorrhage. *Neurosci. Lett.* **270**, 188-90.

Mase, M., *et al.* (2003). Lipocalin-type prostaglandin D synthase (beta-trace) in cerebrospinal fluid: a useful marker for the diagnosis of normal pressure hydrocephalus. *Neurosci. Res.* **47**, 455-9.

Matsumura, H., *et al.* (1988). Awaking effect of PGE_2 microinjected into the preoptic area of rats. *Brain Res.* **444**, 265-72.

Matsumura, H., *et al.* (1989). Awaking effect of prostaglandin E_2 in freely moving rats. *Brain Res.* **481**, 242-9.

Matsumura, H., *et al.* (1991). Inhibition of sleep in rats by inorganic selenium compounds, inhibitors of prostaglandin D synthase. *Proc. Natl. Acad. Sci. USA* **88**, 9046-50.

Matsumura, H., *et al.* (1994). Prostaglandin D_2-sensitive, sleep-promoting zone defined in the ventral surface of the rostral basal forebrain. *Proc. Natl. Acad. Sci. USA* **91**, 11998-2002.

Melegos, D. N., *et al.* (1997). Prostaglandin D synthase concentration in cerebrospinal fluid and serum of patients with neurological disorders. *Prostaglandins* **54**, 463-74.

Melegos, D. N., *et al.* (1999). Highly elevated levels of prostaglandin D synthase in the serum of patients with renal failure. *Urology* **53**, 32–7.

Mignot, E., *et al.* (2002). Sleeping with the hypothalamus: emerging therapeutic targets for sleep disorders. *Nat. Neurosci.* **5** (Suppl.), 1071–5.

Miyagi, M., *et al.* (2005). Activator protein-1 mediates shear stress-induced prostaglandin d synthase gene expression in vascular endothelial cells. *Arterioscler. Thromb. Vasc. Biol.* **25**, 970–5.

Mizoguchi, A., *et al.* (2001). Dominant localization of prostaglandin D receptors on arachnoid trabecular cells in mouse basal forebrain and their involvement in the regulation of non-rapid eye movement sleep. *Proc. Natl. Acad. Sci. USA* **98**, 11674–9.

Mong, J. A., *et al.* (2003a). Estradiol differentially regulates lipocalin-type prostaglandin D synthase transcript levels in the rodent brain: evidence from high-density oligonucleotide arrays and in situ hybridization. *Proc. Natl. Acad. Sci. USA* **100**, 318–23.

Mong, J. A., *et al.* (2003b). Reduction of lipocalin-type prostaglandin D synthase in the preoptic area of female mice mimics estradiol effects on arousal and sex behavior. *Proc. Natl. Acad. Sci. USA* **100**, 15206–11.

Morairty, S., *et al.* (2004). Disinhibition of ventrolateral preoptic area sleep-active neurons by adenosine: a new mechanism for sleep promotion. *Neuroscience* **123**, 451–7.

Nagata, A., *et al.* (1991). Human brain prostaglandin D synthase has been evolutionarily differentiated from lipophilic-ligand carrier proteins. *Proc. Natl. Acad. Sci. USA* **88**, 4020–4.

Narumiya, S., *et al.* (1982). Prostaglandin D2 in rat brain, spinal cord and pituitary: basal level and regional distribution. *Life Sci.* **31**, 2093–103.

Oda, H., *et al.* (2002). Development and evaluation of a practical ELISA for human urinary lipocalin-type prostaglandin D synthase. *Clin. Chem.* **48**, 1445–53.

Ogorochi, T., *et al.* (1984). Regional distribution of prostaglandins D_2, E_2, and E_2 and related enzymes in postmortem human brain. *J. Neurochem.* **43**, 71–82.

Okada, T., *et al.* (2003). Dominant localization of adenosine deaminase in leptomeninges and involvement of the enzyme in sleep. *Biochem. Biophys. Res. Commun.* **312**, 29–34.

Onoe, H., *et al.* (1988). Prostaglandin D2, a cerebral sleep-inducing substance in monkeys. *Proc. Natl. Acad. Sci. USA* **85**, 4082–6.

Otsuki, M., *et al.* (2003). Specific regulation of lipocalin-type prostaglandin D synthase in mouse heart by estrogen receptor beta. *Molec. Endocrinol.* **17**, 1844–55.

Pandey, H. P., *et al.* (1995). Concentration of prostaglandin D2 in cerebrospinal fluid exhibits a circadian alteration in conscious rats. *Biochem. Molec. Biol. Int.* **37**, 431–7.

Pentreath, V. W., *et al.* (1990). The somnogenic T lymphocyte suppressor prostaglandin D_2 is selectively elevated in cerebrospinal fluid of advanced sleeping sickness patients. *Trans. R. Soc. Trop. Med. Hyg.* **84**, 795–9.

Pinzar, E., *et al.* (2000). Prostaglandin D synthase gene is involved in the regulation of non-rapid eye movement sleep. *Proc. Natl. Acad. Sci. USA* **97**, 4903–7.

Priem, F., *et al.* (1999). Beta-trace protein in serum: a new marker of glomerular filtration rate in the creatinine-blind range. *Clin. Chem.* **45**, 567–8.

Qu, W. M., *et al.* (2006). Lipocalin-type prostaglandin D synthase prozduces prostaglandin D_2 involved in regulation of physiological sleep. *Proc. Natl. Acad. Sci. USA* **103**, 17949–54.

Ragolia, L., *et al.* (2003). Prostaglandin D_2 synthase inhibits the exaggerated growth phenotype of spontaneously hypertensive rat vascular smooth muscle cells. *J. Biol. Chem.* **278**, 22175–81.

Ragolia, L., *et al.* (2005). Accelerated glucose intolerance, nephropathy, and atherosclerosis in prostaglandin D_2 synthase knock-out mice. *J. Biol. Chem.* **280**, 29946–55.

Rainnie, D. G., *et al.* (1994). Adenosine inhibition of mesopontine cholinergic neurons: implications for EEG arousal. *Science* **263**, 689–92.

Ram, A., *et al.* (1997). CSF levels of prostaglandins, especially the level of prostaglandin D_2, are correlated with increasing propensity towards sleep in rats. *Brain Res.* **751**, 81–9.

Rétey, J. V., *et al.* (2005). A functional genetic variation of adenosine deaminase affects the duration and intensity of deep sleep in humans. *Proc. Natl. Acad. Sci. USA* **102**, 15676–81.

Roberts, J. L. II, *et al.* (1980). Increased production of prostaglandin D_2 in patients with systemic mastocytosis. *New Engl. J. Med.* **303**, 1400–4.

Rodriguez, C. M., *et al.* (2000). Expression of the lipocalin-type prostaglandin D synthase gene in the reproductive tracts of Holstein bulls. *J. Reprod. Fert.* **120**, 303–9.

Samy, E. T., *et al.* (2000). Sertoli cell prostaglandin D2 synthetase is a multifunctional molecule: its expression and regulation. *Endocrinology* **141**, 710–21.

Saper, C. B., *et al.* (2001). The sleep switch: hypothalamic control of sleep and wakefulness. *Trends Neurosci.* **24**, 726–31.

Saper, C. B., *et al.* (2005). Hypothalamic regulation of sleep and circadian rhythms. *Nature* **437**, 1257–63.

Satoh, S., *et al.* (1996). Promotion of sleep mediated by the A2a-adenosine receptor and possible involvement of this receptor in the sleep induced by prostaglandin D2 in rats. *Proc. Natl. Acad. Sci. USA* **93**, 5980–4.

Satoh, S., *et al.* (1998). Involvement of adenosine A_{2A} receptor in sleep promotion. *Eur. J. Pharmacol.* **351**, 155–62.

Satoh, S., *et al.* (1999). Region-dependent difference in the sleep-promoting potency of an adenosine A_{2A} receptor agonist. *Eur. J. Neurosci.* **11**, 1587–97.

Scammell, T., *et al.* (1998). Activation of ventrolateral preoptic neurons by the somnogen prostaglandin D_2. *Proc. Natl. Acad. Sci. USA* **95**, 7754–9.

Scammell, T. E., *et al.* (2001). An adenosine A_{2a} agonist increases sleep and induces Fos in ventrolateral preoptic neurons. *Neuroscience* **107**, 653–63.

Sherin, J. E., *et al.* (1996). Activation of ventrolateral preoptic neurons during sleep. *Science* **271**, 216–19.

Shiki, Y., *et al.* (2004). Changes of lipocalin-type prostaglandin D synthase level during pregnancy. *J. Obstet. Gynaecol. Res.* **30**, 65–70.

Shimamoto, S., *et al.* (2007). NMR solution structure of lipocalin-type prostaglandin D synthase: Evidence for partial overlapping of catalytic pocket and retinoic acid-binding pocket within the central cavity. *J. Biol. Chem.* (in press)

Shimizu, T., *et al.* (1979). Purification and properties of prostaglandin D synthetase from rat brain. *J. Biol. Chem.* **254**, 5222–8.

Strecker, R. E., *et al.* (2000). Adenosinergic modulation of basal forebrain and preoptic/anterior hypothalamic neuronal activity in the control of behavioral state. *Behav. Brain Res.* **115**, 183–204.

Taba, Y., *et al.* (2000). Fluid shear stress induces lipocalin-type prostaglandin D_2 synthase expression in vascular endothelial cells. *Circul. Res.* **86**, 967–73.

Takahata, Y., *et al.* (1993). Intravenous administration of inorganic selenium compounds, inhibitors of prostaglandin D synthase, inhibits sleep in freely moving rats. *Brain Res.* **623**, 65–71.

Takeda, K., *et al.* (2006). Lipocalin-type prostaglandin D synthase as a melanocyte marker regulated by MITF. *Biochem. Biophys. Res. Commun.* **339**, 1098–106.

Tokugawa, Y., *et al.* (1998). Lipocalin-type prostaglandin D synthase in human male reproductive organs and seminal plasma. *Biol. Reprod.* **58**, 600–7.

Tumani, H., *et al.* (1998). Beta-trace protein in cerebrospinal fluid: a blood-CSF barrier-related evaluation in neurological diseases. *Ann. Neurol.* **44**, 882–9.

Ueno, R., *et al.* (1982). Prostaglandin D_2 induces sleep when microinjected into the preoptic area of conscious rats. *Biochem. Biophys. Res. Commun.* **109**, 576–82.

Ueno, R., *et al.* (1983). Prostaglandin D2, a cerebral sleep-inducing substance in rats. *Proc. Natl. Acad. Sci. USA* **80**, 1735–7.

Ujihara, M., *et al.* (1988). Prostaglandin D2 formation and characterization of its synthetases in various tissues of adult rats. *Arch. Biochem. Biophys.* **260**, 521–31.

Urade, Y. & Hayaishi, O. (2000a). Biochemical, structural, genetic, physiological, and pathophysiological features of lipocalin-type prostaglandin D synthase. *Biochim. Biophys. Acta* **1482**, 259–71.

Urade, Y. & Hayaishi, O. (2000b). Prostaglandin D synthase: structure and function. *Vitam. Horm.* **58**, 89–120.

Urade, Y., *et al.* (1985). Purification and characterization of rat brain prostaglandin D synthetase. *J. Biol. Chem.* **260**, 12410–15.

Urade, Y., *et al.* (1987a). Postnatal changes in the localization of prostaglandin D synthetase from neurons to oligodendrocytes in the rat brain. *J. Biol. Chem.* **262**, 15132–6.

Urade, Y., *et al.* (1987b). Biochemical and immunological characterization of rat spleen prostaglandin D synthetase. *J. Biol. Chem.* **262**, 3820–5.

Urade, Y., *et al.* (1989). Primary structure of rat brain prostaglandin D synthetase deduced from cDNA sequence. *J. Biol. Chem.* **264**, 1041–5.

Urade, Y., *et al.* (1990). Mast cells contain spleen-type prostaglandin D synthetase. *J. Biol. Chem.* **265**, 371–5.

Urade, Y., *et al.* (1993). Dominant expression of mRNA for prostaglandin D synthase in leptomeninges, choroid plexus, and oligodendrocytes of the adult rat brain. *Proc. Natl. Acad. Sci. USA* **90**, 9070–4.

Urade, Y., *et al.* (2002). Lipocalin-type and hematopoietic prostaglandin D synthases as a novel example of functional convergence. *Prostaglandins Other Lipid Mediators* **68–9**, 375–82.

Urade, Y., *et al.* (2003). Sleep regulation in adenosine A2A receptor-deficient mice. *Neurology* **61**, S94–6.

Urade, Y., *et al.* (2006a). Lipocalin-type prostaglandin D synthase as an enzymic lipocalin. In *Lipocalins*, ed. B. Åkersröm, N. Borregaard, D. R. Flower & J-P, Salier. Georgetown, TX: Eurekah, pp. 99–109.

Urade, Y., *et al.* (2006b). Biochemical and structural characteristics of hematopoietic prostaglandin D synthase: from evolutionary analysis to drug designing. *Functional and Structural Biology on the Lipo-network*, *2006*, Transworld Research Network, Kerala, India, pp. 135–64.

Watanabe, K., *et al.* (1994). Identification of beta-trace as prostaglandin D synthase. *Biochem. Biophys. Res. Commun.* **203**, 1110–16.

White, D. M., *et al.* (1992). Structure and chromosomal localization of the human gene for a brain form of prostaglandin D_2 synthase. *J. Biol. Chem.* **267**, 23202–8.

White, D. M., *et al.* (1997). Beta-trace gene expression is regulated by a core promoter and a distal thyroid hormone response element. *J. Biol. Chem.* **272**, 14387–93.

Yamashima, T., *et al.* (1997). Prostaglandin D synthase (beta-trace) in human arachnoid and meningioma cells: roles as a cell marker or in cerebrospinal fluid absorption, tumorigenesis, and calcification process. *J. Neurosci.* **17**, 2376–82.

Yamashita, A., *et al.* (1983). Autoradiographic localization of a binding protein(s) specific for prostaglandin D_2 in rat brain. *Proc. Natl. Acad. Sci. USA* **80**, 6114–18.

Zhu, H., *et al.* (2004). Expression and regulation of lipocalin-type prostaglandin D synthase in rat testis and epididymis. *Biol. Reprod.* **70**, 1088–95.

14

Neuropeptides and sleep–wake regulation

LUIS DE LECEA

Introduction

The importance of peptide transmitters in the modulation of sleep and wakefulness has become apparent in recent years. Previous work had focused on the role of monoamines in the circuitry that regulates the transitions between states of vigilance. Histaminergic neurons in the tuberomammillary nucleus are known to be key players in the activation of subcortical afferents during wakefulness (Wada *et al.*, 1991). Activity of noradrenergic neurons in the locus coeruleus correlates with the state of vigilance (Jones, 1991). The role of serotonergic neurons in rapid eye movement (REM) sleep has also been established (Lydic *et al.*, 1987; Monti & Jantos, 1992; Fabre *et al.*, 2000).

In spite of major advances in our understanding of the neuronal circuits that govern the sleep–wakefulness cycle (Pace-Schott & Hobson, 2002), the cell groups involved in the coordination of the different stages of sleep and in the control of the boundaries between sleep states are poorly understood. The development of molecular markers that define neuronal cell groups with distinct physiological properties is expected to enhance our understanding of the regulation of the states of vigilance.

With this in mind, the search for molecular markers that define populations of neurons in areas important for arousal is clearly warranted. In this chapter we describe the identification of four peptidergic systems that modulate different aspects of the sleep–wakefulness cycle. The success of this strategy demonstrates the need for new markers of neuronal cell types, which may define populations of neurons critical for our understanding of cortical activity and sleep.

Neurochemistry of Sleep and Wakefulness, ed. J. M. Monti *et al.* Published by Cambridge University Press.
© Cambridge University Press 2008.

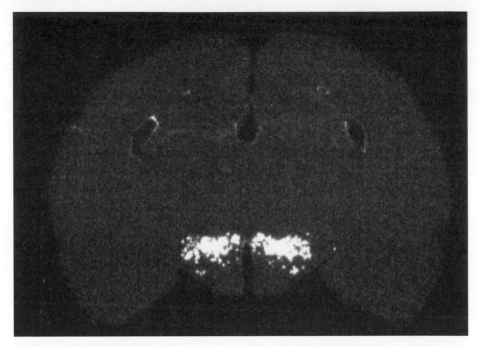

Figure 14.1 The hypocretins are produced in about 4,000 neurons in the rodent posterior hypothalamus.

The hypocretins (orexins): two hypothalamus-specific peptides

The hypothalamus can be considered a federation of nuclei with distinct functions that include energy homeostasis, circadian rhythms, sexual behavior and arousal. It is thus expected that mRNAs specifically expressed in restricted areas of the hypothalamus will affect selective functions. Analysis of a collection of the most prevalent cDNAs expressed in the hypothalamus revealed that as many as 40% of these sequences encode secreted proteins (Gautvik *et al.*, 1996). Further characterization of a cDNA encoding a novel putative secreted protein revealed that it was restricted to the perifornical area of the lateral hypothalamus (Fig. 14.1). The deduced protein sequence contained a putative signal secretory sequence and several pairs of dibasic residues that were possible substrates of prohormone convertases. Cleavage at these sites would generate two putative products of proteolysis of 28 and 33 residues in length, which had 13 amino acid identities across 19 residues. This region of one of the peptides contained a 7/7 match with secretin, suggesting that the prepropeptide gave rise to two peptide products that were structurally related both to each other and to secretin. These putative peptides were named hypocretin (hcrt) 1 and 2 to reflect their hypothalamic origin and the similarity to the incretin neuropeptide family (de

Lecea *et al.*, 1998). The peptides showed neuroexcitatory activity in mature cultured hypothalamic neurons and were localized in large dense core vesicles by immuno-electron microscopy. Shortly after the peptides were discovered, Sakurai *et al.* (1998) reported the isolation of the orexins, which are identical to the hypocretins, as the endogenous ligands of two orphan G-protein coupled receptors. These authors named the peptides orexins because they induced feeding activity when injected into the brain ventricles. A great deal of interest was sparked by three reports linking the hypocretinergic system with narcolepsy. In sum, the discovery that canine narcolepsy is caused by mutations in hypocretin receptor 2, together with the narcolepsy-like phenotype of hypocretin-deficient mice, and the absence of hypocretin neurons in the hypothalamus of narcoleptic patients, has demonstrated that this system is involved in state boundary control. Comprehensive reviews of the hypocretinergic system are available elsewhere in the literature (Hungs & Mignot, 2001; Willie *et al.*, 2001; Sutcliffe & de Lecea, 2002).

The hypocretins in the normal sleep–wake cycle

The actions of hcrt on sleep may be integrated into the reciprocal interaction model of REM sleep generation by McCarley & Hobson (1975). This model considers two populations of neurons: REM-off cells, which are silent during REM sleep, and REM-on neurons, which generate REM sleep bouts. REM-off cells, which include noradrenergic neurons of the LC, serotoninergic neurons of the raphe nucleus, and the histaminergic neurons of the tuberomammilary nucleus (TMN), are active during wakefulness and silent during REM sleep. During wakefulness, REM-off neurons inhibit REM-on cells, which include cholinergic neurons of the laterodorsal tegmentum and pedunculopontine nucleus (LDT/PPT). During REM sleep, REM-on cells show higher activity after the inhibitory action of REM-off cells is removed. Considering the wake-promoting properties of hcrt1, it has been suggested that hcrt increases arousal and inhibits REM sleep by activating REM-off cells, in particular noradrenergic cells in the LC, which receive the densest hcrt innervation (Peyron *et al.*, 1998; Date *et al.*, 1999) (Fig. 14.2). This hypothesis is in line with in vitro and in vivo experiments, which have shown that hcrt1 excites this cell population (Hagan *et al.*, 1999; Horvath *et al.*, 1999; Bourgin *et al.*, 2000). Further, local administration of hcrt1 promotes wakefulness and suppresses REM sleep (Bourgin *et al.*, 2000). Several studies have revealed the ability of hcrt to excite other REM-off neurons (Bayer *et al.*, 2001; Brown *et al.*, 2001; Eriksson *et al.*, 2001; Huang *et al.*, 2001), as well as REM-on cells in the LDT/PPT (Xi *et al.*, 2001) and cholinergic neurons in the basal forebrain (Espana *et al.*, 2001; Thakkar *et al.*, 2001). Some of the wake-promoting effects of hcrt seem

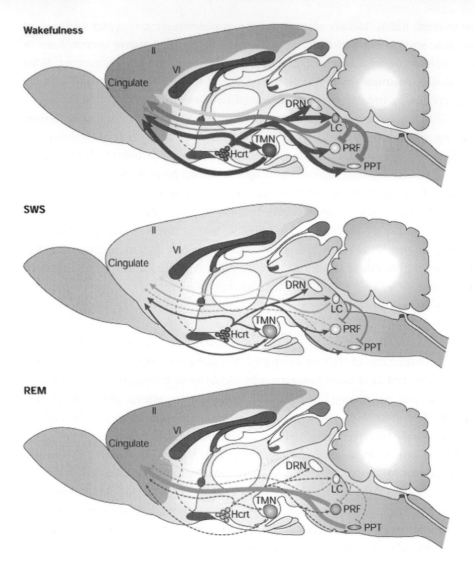

Figure 14.2 Hypocretinergic activity dependent on the states of vigilance. During wakefulness, metabolic, circadian, and behavioral inputs converge on hypocretin neurons, which activate noradrenergic neurons in the locus coeruleus and promote arousal. During non-REM sleep, the activity of hypocretin neurons decreases, but the inhibitory influence of REM–off neurons on REM-on cells is still effective. During REM sleep, hypocretin and REM-off cells are silent, disinhibiting REM-on cells. Reprinted with permission from Sutcliffe & de Lecea (2002). (See also Plate 7.)

to be mediated by histaminergic neurons in the tuberomammilary nucleus, as histamine H1 receptor knockout mice are unaffected by hcrt administration (Huang *et al.*, 2001). Clearly, similar analyses in mutant animals with alterations in specific neurotransmitter systems will lead to a better understanding of the interaction of the hcrts with sleep–wake circuitry.

Investigating the activity of hcrt neurons during states of vigilance is essential for understanding the physiological role of hcrt in the regulation of sleep–wakefulness. Several studies have correlated hcrt release with the sleep–wakefulness cycle. Prolonged waking produced by pharmacological or instrumental sleep deprivation produces an increase in extracellular hcrt levels or c-fos/hcrt mRNA-positive cells (Scammell *et al.*, 2000; Estabrooke *et al.*, 2001; Yoshida *et al.*, 2001). This initially suggested that hcrt may be a factor that accumulates during wakefulness. However, there is no correlation between hcrt levels and wakefulness or sleep amounts (Yoshida *et al.*, 2001), strongly suggesting that hcrt may be primarily related to the regulation of the transitions between states of vigilance, rather than a particular sleep–wake stage. Recent electrophysiological studies have investigated the activity of neurons in the lateral hypothalamus in parallel with sleep recording in restrained (Lee *et al.*, 2005) and freely moving rats (Mileykovskiy *et al.*, 2005). Both studies show that hcrt cells are relatively inactive in quiet waking but are transiently activated during sensory stimulation. Hcrt cells are silent in slow-wave sleep and tonic periods of REM sleep, with occasional burst discharge during phasic REM sleep. Hcrt cells discharge in active waking and have moderate and approximately equal levels of activity during grooming and eating and maximal activity during exploratory behavior. This pattern of activity is consistent with the idea that discharge of hcrt generates an "alarm" signal and engages multiple networks that result in cortical activation and locomotor activity. Hcrt neurons integrate multiple signals (including metabolic, circadian, and limbic afferents) that result in a coherent output that activates arousal networks. Hcrt neurons have also been proposed as modulators of the states of vigilance in the "sleep-switch" model (Saper *et al.*, 2001). The hypocretin system provides overall stability to the flip–flop switch by activating wake-promoting circuits (e.g. TMN, cholinergic basal forebrain), REM-on neurons (in the PPT) and REM-off cells (in the LC and raphe). Hypocretin neurons appear to act as a "finger" on the switch, reinforcing the awake component, and thus consolidating both wakefulness and sleep. Recent data have shown that the responsiveness of hypocretin neurons to norepinephrine is dependent on sleep demand, from excitatory under awake conditions to inhibitory after sleep deprivation, suggesting that a signaling switch is turned on or off for hcrt as a function of sleep homeostasis (Grivel *et al.*, 2005).

Cortistatin: a cortical neuropeptide with sleep-modulating activity

Cortistatin was discovered as a result of the effort to characterize cortex-specific gene expression modulated by synaptic activity. It was named after its cortical expression and sequence homology to somatostatin (de Lecea *et al.*, 1996). The characterization of this peptide is yet another example of the use of reverse genetics to study the molecular components of the sleep machinery.

Cortistatin is synthesized as a precursor of 116 amino acids that gives rise to a C-terminal mature peptide, cortistatin-14 (CST-14), that shares 11 of its 14 residues with the neuropeptide somatostatin. However, the similarities between cortistatin and somatostatin are restricted to the mature peptides, which are the products of different genes. CST-14 binds to all five somatostatin receptors in vitro, although several authors suggest that CST-14 exerts its actions in vivo by binding to its own specific receptor (Spier & de Lecea, 2000).

Cortistatin expression is restricted to scattered cells in the cerebral cortex and hippocampus. These neurons express GABA as their neurotransmitter, and are different from the population of cortical neurons that express somatostatin (de Lecea *et al.*, 1997) (Fig. 14.3). Networks of GABAergic inhibitory neurons are known to be critical for synchronization of cortical activity, and have been proposed as having a major role in the maintenance of slow wave sleep (Whittington *et al.*, 1995; Jefferys & Whittington, 1996; Traub *et al.*, 1996, 1997). Experiments and models have shown how the network frequency depends on excitation of the interneurons, and on the conductance and time course parameters of $GABA_A$-mediated IPSCs between the interneurons (Amzica & Steriade, 1998). The discharge properties of interneurons are substantially different from those of pyramidal cells, and are thought to be based on the expression of particular ionic conductances (e.g. HCN2, KCNQ2-4, Kv3.1, etc). Further proof that cortical GABAergic neurons and these conductances are important for cortical activity and slow wave sleep was provided by a study showing significant differences in delta power in mice deficient in Kv3.1 channels (Joho *et al.*, 1999).

Intracerebroventricular infusion of CST-14 dramatically increases the amount of slow wave activity in rats, at the expense of wakefulness. The mechanism by which CST-14 enhances cortical synchronization has been established through the interaction of CST-14 with acetylcholine, a neurotransmitter known to be involved in the maintenance of cortical desynchronization. Application of acetylcholine (ACh) in the anesthetized animal increases fast activity, and this effect is blocked with the simultaneous addition of CST-14. These data suggest that CST-14 increases slow wave sleep by antagonizing the effects of ACh on cortical excitability. In addition to this mechanism, cortistatin may enhance cortical

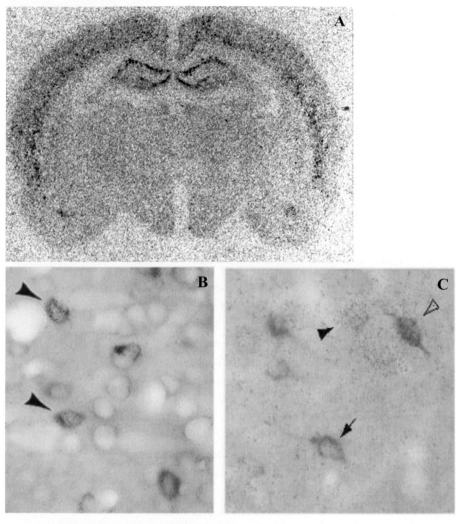

Figure 14.3 Cortistatin is expressed in cortical interneurons and may provide an intrinsic mechanism of cortical synchronization by increasing Ih. A. In situ hybridization showing preprocortistatin mRNA signals in sparse non-principal neurons throughout the cerebral cortex, hippocampus and amygdala. B. Double in situ hybridization of preprocortistatin and GAD65 demonstrating that all cortistatin-positive cells in the neocortex are GABAergic. C. Combined in situ hybridization to preprocortistatin and immunocytochemistry to somatostatin, showing that preprocortistatin labels a partially overlapping although distinct population of GABAergic neurons. (See also Plate 8.)

synchronization by enhancing Ih, a cation conductance shown to be important in thalamocortical synchronization (Spier & de Lecea, 2000).

Several studies suggest that cortistatin expression correlates with the sleep homeostat. The concentration of cortistatin mRNA oscillates with the light–dark cycle in rats, with maximal levels at the end of the dark (i.e. active) period. Further, the steady-state concentration of cortistatin mRNA increases four-fold after sleep deprivation, and returns to normal levels after sleep rebound, indicating that the expression of the peptide is associated with sleep demand (Spier & de Lecea, 2000). Preliminary studies in cortical slices suggest that cortistatin-14 increases cortical synchronization by enhancing the H-current. Thus, cortistatin and somatostatin may be part of the intrinsic mechanisms of the cerebral cortex that are involved in the maintenance of excitability.

Urotensin II: a modulator of REM sleep

Urotensin II (UII) is a cyclic neuropeptide with some structural similarity to somatostatin and cortistatin. It exhibits marked vasoconstrictive activity in the peripheral vasculature (Gibson et al., 1986). The urotensin II receptor mRNA is also expressed in the central nervous system, in particular on cholinergic neurons located in the mesopontine tegmental area, including the pedunculo-pontine tegmental (PPT) and lateral dorsal tegmental (LDT) nuclei (Clark et al., 2001). This distribution suggests that the UII system is involved in functions regulated by ACh, such as the sleep–wake cycle. Recent data provide evidence that UII in fact acts as a modulator of REM sleep (Huitron-Resendiz et al., 2005). Local administration of UII into the PPT leads to a significant increase in the number of REM sleep episodes; this increase can be blocked by intracerebroven-tricular (i.c.v.) coadministration of a UII antagonist. Wakefulness and slow-wave sleep do not seem to be affected by local application of UII. This profile appears to be unique to UII. Similar effects of UII on REM sleep episodes were observed following i.c.v. administration (Huitron-Resendiz et al., 2005).

An important consideration when monitoring the activity of UII is the well known effect of the peptide in the peripheral vasculature (Bohm & Pernow, 2002). Huitron-Resendiz and colleagues tested whether UII administered locally or i.c.v. could affect regional cerebrovascular blood flow by using a Doppler flowme-ter (Huitron-Resendiz et al., 2005). Intracerebroventricular infusion of UII signifi-cantly increased blood flow in the cerebral cortex, suggesting direct activation of cerebral vasculature or the activation of brain areas that are involved in cardio-vascular regulation. The noradrenergic A1 area, located in the lower medulla, has been identified as a possible neural substrate of the central cardiovascu-lar action of UII because microinjections of UII into A1 cause strong systemic cardiovascular responses in anesthetized rats (Clark *et al.*, 2005; Nothacker & Clark, 2005).

Huitron-Resendiz *et al.* (2005) reported that when UII was applied i.c.v., a significant increase in wakefulness was observed during the first hour post-injection. The amount of wakefulness returned to control levels after two hours, whereas the increase in the number of REM sleep episodes could be observed for up to five hours. Local UII application into the PPT did not produce any effect on wakefulness, nor was there an increase in cerebral blood flow, suggesting that the effect on wakefulness was not due to the action of UII in the PPT. Therefore, the acute effects that have been measured and interpreted as anxiogenic, or stress-related, may be due to UII-induced changes in cerebral blood flow or other cardiovascular changes that follow a more rapid time course. The most direct evidence for UII neuromodulatory properties in the PPT comes from electrophysiological studies (Huitron-Resendiz *et al.*, 2005). Whole-cell recordings from rat-brain slices showed that UII selectively excites cholinergic PPT neurons via an inward current and membrane depolarization accompanied by a decrease in membrane conductance. This effect does not depend on action potential generation or fast synaptic transmission because it persisted in the presence of TTX and antagonists of ionotropic glutamate, GABA, and glycine receptors. Together, these results are consistent with the hypothesis that, in addition to its cerebrovascular properties, UII plays a significant role in the modulation of REM sleep by directly depolarizing cholinergic neurons. However, it is still unclear whether the endogenous ligand for GPR14 in the PPT nucleus is UII or urotensin II related-peptide (URP) (Nothacker & Clark, 2005).

Neuropeptide S: another component of the sleep-switch?

Neuropeptide S (NPS) is a recently discovered bioactive peptide that has emerged as a new signaling molecule in the complex circuitry that modulates sleep–wakefulness and anxiety-like behavior. The peptide precursor is expressed most prominently in a novel nucleus located in the perilocus coeruleus, a brain structure with well-defined functions in arousal, stress, and anxiety. NPS was also found to induce anxiolytic-like behavior in a battery of four different tests of innate responses to stress. Infusion of NPS potently increases wakefulness and suppresses non-REM (NREM) and REM sleep (Xu *et al.*, 2004). NPS binds to a G-protein-coupled receptor, the NPS receptor, with nanomolar affinity; activation of the receptor mobilizes intracellular calcium. The NPS receptor is expressed throughout the brain, particularly in regions relevant to the modulation of sleep and waking, in the tuberomammillary region, lateral hypothalamus, and medial thalamic nuclei.

Infusion of NPS may increase wakefulness by inhibiting NREM sleep and activating wake-promoting circuits. NPS may inhibit sleep-promoting circuits by activating GABAergic neurons in the area surrounding the ventrolateral preoptic area and median preoptic area, which are known to be active during NREM sleep (Sherin *et al.*, 1996). After the initial phase of NPS activity, neurotransmitters that correlate with sleep demand (e.g. adenosine (Mackiewicz *et al.*, 2000; Thakkar *et al.*, 2003)) may accumulate in the basal forebrain; when their concentrations reach a certain threshold, excitation of sleep-promoting circuits may occur at the transitions from wakefulness to NREM sleep. NPS may thus serve as a transient enhancer of the wake component of the sleep-switch (Saper *et al.*, 2001), therefore preventing intermediate states (cf. Fig. 14.4).

Since the effect of NPS on waking is strong, but short lasting, NPS may provide additional stability through a strong excitatory drive over a short period of time on hcrt neurons themselves and on many of the common targets of hcrt, including awake-, sleep-, and REM sleep-promoting areas. According to the "flip–flop" model of sleep regulation, if either side of the switch is weakened, there are more transitions in both directions, but if either side is strengthened, transitions become less frequent (Saper *et al.*, 2001). This appears to be the case in the first hour after i.c.v. injection of NPS, a fast and robust increase in wakefulness that dramatically reduces the number of transitions between states of vigilance. The resulting transient increase in wakefulness may be advantageous in situations that demand high levels of alertness. It is also noteworthy that another prominent aspect of NPS is its anxiolytic properties (Xu *et al.*, 2004). This activity would counterbalance the anxiogenic properties of transmitters released as a result of activation of the HPA axis and the stress response.

Neuropeptides and the control of sleep

Here we have described a few examples of novel neuropeptides that have different activities and regulate different aspects of the sleep–wakefulness cycle. The use of reverse genetics has uncovered basic properties of the peptides (e.g. structure, distribution, electrophysiological activity, and connectivity). The development of mouse models has allowed a better understanding of their function and their role in sleep regulation. It is not surprising that neuropeptides have a major role in the modulation of sleep circuits. First, most peptidergic systems are localized in small populations of neurons that modulate the activity of multiple brain regions. This provides a physical means of integration of activity, hence controlling a single coherent output on many brain networks. Second, the time frame and kinetics of peptidergic action (seconds to minutes) is consistent with the reversible modification of synaptic transmission that would be required

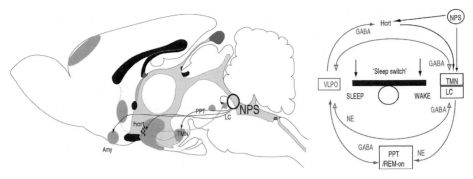

Figure 14.4 NPS and the sleep-switch model. NPS projects to the main circuits involved in arousal, including the TMN, PPT, hcrt, and basal forebrain. Areas with high density of NPS terminals and NPS receptors are shown in blue. Reciprocal connections between NPS, hcrt, and the TMN are the substrate of the "flip–flop" sleep-switch model (Saper *et al.*, 2001), which consists of a bistable system that prevents intermediate states. Aminergic regions such as the TMN, LC, and cholinergic neurons in the basal forebrain promote wakefulness by direct excitatory effects on the cortex and by inhibition of sleep–promoting neurons of the VLPO. As sleep demand increases, adenosine concentrations increase and inhibit arousal centers. During sleep, the VLPO inhibits amine-mediated arousal regions through GABAergic projections (shown in red). This inhibition of the amine-mediated arousal system disinhibits VLPO neurons, further stabilizing the production of sleep. The PPT also contains REM-promoting cholinergic neurons. The extended VLPO might promote REM sleep by disinhibiting the PPT region; its axons innervate interneurons within the PPT area, as well as aminergic neurons that normally inhibit REM-promoting cells in the PPT nucleus. Hypocretin neurons stabilize behavioral state by increasing the activity of aminergic neurons, thus maintaining consistent inhibition of sleep-promoting neurons in the VLPO and REM-promoting neurons in the PPT. Neuropeptide S may further stabilize this bistable circuitry by transiently increasing the activity of both hcrt and aminergic neurons. The transient wake promoting of NPS may be advantageous in situations of high alertness. (See also Plate 9.)

during sleep. Third, peptide release is associated with high-frequency firing of presynaptic neurons, which provides another code for the stability of neuronal systems. Fourth, recent data seem to indicate that cortical neuropeptides signif-icantly affect local blood flow by directly acting on the neurovasculature (Cauli *et al.*, 2004). Reduction in cortical blood flow is a well known attribute of REM sleep and could be modulated by a balance between neuroexcitatory and inhibitory peptides. Additional peptidergic systems with restricted localizations in areas critical for sleep–wakefulness regulation are likely to be discovered and may yield more clues about the mechanisms underlying sleep and waking.

Acknowledgements

This work was supported by grants from NIH.

References

Amzica, F. & Steriade, M. (1998). Electrophysiological correlates of sleep delta waves. *Electroencephalogr. Clin. Neurophysiol.* **107**, 69–83.

Bayer, L., Eggermann, E., Serafin, M. *et al.* (2001). Orexins (hypocretins) directly excite tuberomammillary neurons. *Eur. J. Neurosci.* **14**, 1571–5.

Bohm, F. & Pernow, J. (2002). Urotensin II evokes potent vasoconstriction in humans in vivo. *Br. J. Pharmacol.* **135**, 25–7.

Bourgin, P., Huitrón-Reséndiz, S., Spier, A. *et al.* (2000). Hypocretin-1 modulates REM sleep through activation of locus coeruleus neurons. *J. Neurosci.* **20**, 7760–5.

Brown, R. E., Sergeeva, O. A., Eriksson, K. S. & Haas, S. L. (2001). Orexin A excites serotonergic neurons in the dorsal raphe nucleus of the rat. *Neuropharmacology* **00**, 000–00.

Cauli, B., Tong, X. K., Rancillac, A. *et al.* (2004). Cortical GABA interneurons in neurovascular coupling: relays for subcortical vasoactive pathways. *J. Neurosci.* **24**, 8940–9.

Clark, S. D., Nothacker, H. P., Wang, Z. *et al.* (2001). The urotensin II receptor is expressed in the cholinergic mesopontine tegmentum of the rat. *Brain Res.* **923**, 120–7.

Clark, S. D., Nothacker, H. P., Blaha, C. D. *et al.* (2005). Urotensin II acts as a modulator of mesopontine cholinergic neurons. *Brain Res.* **1059**, 139–48.

Date, Y., Ueta, Y., Yamashita, H. *et al.* (1999). Orexins, orexigenic hypothalamic peptides, interact with autonomic, neuroendocrine and neuroregulatory systems. *Proc. Natl. Acad. Sci. USA* **96**, 748–53.

de Lecea, L., Criado, J. R., Prospero-Garcia, O. *et al.* (1996). A cortical neuropeptide with neuronal depressant and sleep-modulating properties. *Nature* **381**, 242–5.

de Lecea, L., del Rio, J. A., Criado, J. R. *et al.* (1997). Cortistatin is expressed in a distinct subset of cortical interneurons. *J. Neurosci.* **17**, 5868–80.

de Lecea, L., Kilduff, T. S., Peyron, C. *et al.* (1998). The hypocretins: hypothalamus-specific peptides with neuroexcitatory activity. *Proc. Natl. Acad. Sci. USA* **95**, 322–7.

Eriksson, K. S., Sergeeva, O., Brown, R. E. & Haas, H. L. (2001). Orexin/hypocretin excites the histaminergic neurons of the tuberomammillary nucleus. *J. Neurosci.* **21**, 9273–9.

Espana, R. A., Baldo, B. A., Kelley, A. E. & Berridge, C. W. (2001). Wake-promoting and sleep-suppressing actions of hypocretin (orexin): basal forebrain sites of action. *Neuroscience* **106**, 699–715.

Estabrooke, I. V., McCarthy, M. T., Ko, E. *et al.* (2001). Fos expression in orexin neurons varies with behavioral state. *J. Neurosci.* **21**, 1656–62.

Fabre, V., Boutrel, B., Hanoun, N. *et al.* (2000). Homeostatic regulation of serotonergic function by the serotonin transporter as revealed by nonviral gene transfer. *J. Neurosci.* **20**, 5065–75.

Gautvik, K. M., de Lecea, L., Gautvik, V. T. *et al.* (1996). Overview of the most prevalent hypothalamus-specific mRNAs, as identified by directional tag PCR subtraction. *Proc. Natl. Acad. Sci. USA* **93**, 8733–8.

Gibson, A., Wallace, P. & Bern, H. A. (1986). Cardiovascular effects of urotensin II in anesthetized and pithed rats. *Gen. Comp. Endocrinol.* **64**, 435–9.

Grivel, J., Cvetkovic, V., Bayer, L. *et al.* (2005). The wake-promoting hypocretin/orexin neurons change their response to noradrenaline after sleep deprivation. *J. Neurosci.* **25**, 4127–30.

Hagan, J. J., Leslie, R. A., Patel, S. *et al.* (1999). Orexin A activates locus coeruleus cell firing and increases arousal in the rat. *Proc. Natl. Acad. Sci. USA* **96**, 10911–16.

Horvath, T. L., Peyron, C., Diano, S. *et al.* (1999). Hypocretin (orexin) activation and synaptic innervation of the locus coeruleus noradrenergic system. *J. Comp. Neurol.* **415**, 145–59.

Huang, Z. L., Qu, W. M., Li, W. D. *et al.* (2001). Arousal effect of orexin A depends on activation of the histaminergic system. *Proc. Natl. Acad. Sci. USA* **98**, 9965–70.

Huitron-Resendiz, S., Kristensen, M. P., Sanchez-Alavez, M. *et al.* (2005). Urotensin II modulates rapid eye movement sleep through activation of brainstem cholinergic neurons. *J. Neurosci.* **25**, 5465–74.

Hungs, M. & Mignot, E. (2001). Hypocretin/orexin, sleep and narcolepsy. *Bioessays* **23**, 397–408.

Jefferys, J. G. & Whittington, M. A. (1996). Review of the role of inhibitory neurons in chronic epileptic foci induced by intracerebral tetanus toxin. *Epilepsy Res.* **26**, 59–66.

Joho, R. H., Ho, C. S. & Marks, G. A. (1999). Increased gamma – and decreased delta – oscillations in a mouse deficient for a potassium channel expressed in fast-spiking interneurons. *J. Neurophysiol.* **82**, 1855–64.

Jones, B. E. (1991). The role of noradrenergic locus coeruleus neurons and neighboring cholinergic neurons of the pontomesencephalic tegmentum in sleep-wake states. *Prog. Brain Res.* **88**, 533–43.

Lee, M. G., Hassani, O. K. & Jones, B. E. (2005). Discharge of identified orexin/hypocretin neurons across the sleep-waking cycle. *J. Neurosci.* **25**, 6716–20.

Lydic, R., McCarley, R. W. & Hobson, J. A. (1987). Serotonin neurons and sleep. I. Long term recordings of dorsal raphe discharge frequency and PGO waves. *Arch. Ital. Biol.* **125**, 317–43.

Mackiewicz, M., Nikonova, E. V., Bell, C. C. *et al.* (2000). Activity of adenosine deaminase in the sleep regulatory areas of the rat CNS. *Brain Res. Mol. Brain Res.* **80**, 252–5.

McCarley, R. W. & Hobson, J. A. (1975). Neuronal excitability modulation over the sleep cycle: a structural and mathematical model. *Science* **189**, 58–60.

Mileykovskiy, B. Y., Kiyashchenko, L. I. & Siegel, J. M. (2005). Behavioral correlates of activity in identified hypocretin/orexin neurons. *Neuron* **46**, 787–98.

Monti, J. M. & Jantos, H. (1992). Dose-dependent effects of the 5-HT1A receptor agonist 8-OH-DPAT on sleep and wakefulness in the rat. *J. Sleep Res.* **1**, 169–75.

Nothacker, H. P. & Clark, S. (2005). From heart to mind. The urotensin II system and its evolving neurophysiological role. *FEBS J.* **272**, 5694–702.

Pace-Schott, E. F. & Hobson, J. A. (2002). The neurobiology of sleep: genetics, cellular physiology and subcortical networks. *Nat. Rev. Neurosci.* **3**, 591–605.

Peyron, C., Tighe, D. K., van den Pol, A. N. *et al.* (1998). Neurons containing hypocretin (orexin) project to multiple neuronal systems. *J. Neurosci.* **18**, 9,996–10,015.

Sakurai, T., Amemiya, A., Ishii, M. *et al.* (1998). Orexins and orexin receptors: a family of hypothalamic neuropeptides and G protein-coupled receptors that regulate feeding behavior. *Cell* **92**, 573–85.

Saper, C. B., Chou, T. C. & Scammell, T. E. (2001). The sleep switch: hypothalamic control of sleep and wakefulness. *Trends Neurosci.* **24**, 726–31.

Scammell, T. E., Estabrooke, I. V., McCarthy, M. T. *et al.* (2000). Hypothalamic arousal regions are activated during modafinil-induced wakefulness. *J. Neurosci.* **20**, 8620–8.

Sherin, J. E., Shiromani, P. J., McCarley, R. W. & Saper, C. B. (1996). Activation of ventrolateral preoptic neurons during sleep. *Science* **271**, 216–19.

Spier, A. D. & de Lecea, L. (2000). Cortistatin: a member of the somatostatin neuropeptide family with distinct physiological functions. *Brain Res. Brain Res. Rev.* **33**, 228–41.

Sutcliffe, J. G. & de Lecea, L. (2002). The hypocretins: setting the arousal threshold. *Nat. Rev. Neurosci.* **3**, 339–49.

Thakkar, M. M., Ramesh, V., Strecker, R. E. & McCarley, R. W. (2001). Microdialysis perfusion of orexin-A in the basal forebrain increases wakefulness in freely behaving rats. *Arch. Ital. Biol.* **139**, 313–28.

Thakkar, M. M., Winston, S. & McCarley, R. W. (2003). A1 receptor and adenosinergic homeostatic regulation of sleep-wakefulness: effects of antisense to the A1 receptor in the cholinergic basal forebrain. *J. Neurosci.* **23**, 4278–87.

Traub, R. D., Whittington, M. A., Stanford, I. M. & Jefferys, J. G. (1996). A mechanism for generation of long-range synchronous fast oscillations in the cortex. *Nature* **383**, 621–4.

Traub, R. D., Jefferys, J. G. & Whittington, M. A. (1997). Simulation of gamma rhythms in networks of interneurons and pyramidal cells. *J. Comput. Neurosci.* **4**, 141–50.

Wada, H., Inagaki, N., Itowi, N. & Yamatodani, A. (1991). Histaminergic neuron system in the brain: distribution and possible functions. *Brain Res. Bull.* **27**, 367–70.

Whittington, M. A., Traub, R. D. & Jefferys, J. G. (1995). Synchronized oscillations in interneuron networks driven by metabotropic glutamate receptor activation. *Nature* **373**, 612–15.

Willie, J. T., Chemelli, R. M., Sinton, C. M. & Yanagisawa, M. (2001). To eat or to sleep? Orexin in the regulation of feeding and wakefulness. *A. Rev. Neurosci.* **24**, 429–58.

Xi, M., Morales, F. R. & Chase, M. H. (2001). Effects on sleep and wakefulness of the injection of hypocretin-1 (orexin-A) into the laterodorsal tegmental nucleus of the cat. *Brain Res.* **901**, 259–64.

Xu, Y. L., Reinscheid, R. K., Huitron-Resendiz, S. *et al.* (2004). Neuropeptide S: a neuropeptide promoting arousal and anxiolytic-like effects. *Neuron* **43**, 487–97.

Yoshida, Y., Fujiki, N., Nakajima, T. *et al.* (2001). Fluctuation of extracellular hypocretin-1 (orexin A) levels in the rat in relation to the light-dark cycle and sleep-wake activities. *Eur. J. Neurosci.* **14**, 1075–81.

15

Orexins in sleep and wakefulness: rodent models of narcolepsy–cataplexy

CHRISTOPHER M. SINTON AND JON T. WILLIE

Introduction

Although the past decade has witnessed many advances in the basic science and clinical practice of sleep medicine, perhaps none has been more significant than the discovery of the orexin (also called hypocretin) neuropeptides that are produced in the lateral hypothalamus (LH). Failure of orexin signaling causes narcolepsy–cataplexy in humans and animals. In this chapter, we briefly review current knowledge about orexins and the symptoms of narcolepsy–cataplexy in humans. We discuss the molecular genetic analysis of the narcolepsy–cataplexy syndrome through phenotypic characterization of rodents genetically modified to be deficient in orexins or orexin receptors. These studies point to the mechanisms by which orexins promote arousal and gate sleep in normal animals; they thus have important therapeutic implications for disorders of sleep and wakefulness. We conclude with recent data implicating melanin-concentrating hormone (MCH), a related hypothalamic neuropeptide system, in the modulation of arousal. Orexin and MCH may act in concert to stabilize vigilance states, suggesting a more significant role for the LH in sleep–wakefulness regulation than previously appreciated.

The orexin neuropeptide system

Orexins are two hypothalamically expressed neuropeptide sequences, the gene for which was described concurrently and independently by two groups using different biochemical and genetic approaches (de Lecea, This volume, de

Neurochemistry of Sleep and Wakefulness, ed. J. M. Monti *et al.* Published by Cambridge University Press.
© Cambridge University Press 2008.

Lecea *et al.*, 1998; Sakurai *et al.*, 1998). One of these reports (Sakurai *et al.*, 1998) showed that orexins were endogenous ligands at two orphan G-protein coupled receptors of previously unknown significance. Termed orexin-A and orexin-B (i.e. hypocretin-1 and hypocretin-2), the neuropeptides comprise 33 and 28 amino acids, respectively, with 46% homology. They are both products of the *prepro-orexin* (*prepro-hypocretin*) gene that is uniquely expressed in a discrete popula-tion of neurons, concentrated in the lateral and perifornical hypothalamic areas (Fig. 15.1). Significantly, orexin neurons project throughout the neuraxis with particularly dense innervation of the brainstem monoaminergic and cholin-ergic nuclei that have been implicated in a variety of behaviors, including sleep–wakefulness (Peyron *et al.*, 1998). The original orphan receptor used in a functional biochemical assay to purify orexins was named the orexin type 1 receptor (i.e. OX_1R). It exhibits moderately higher affinity for orexin-A (20 nM versus 420 nM for orexin-B, IC_{50} values against $[^{125}I\text{-}Tyr^{17}]$orexin-A) (Sakurai *et al.*, 1998). The orexin type 2 receptor (OX_2R), which shows equal affinity for orexin-A and orexin-B (30–40 nM), was then cloned on the basis of sequence homology with OX_1R. The two receptors are differentially distributed throughout the cen-tral nervous system (Marcus *et al.*, 2001; Marcus & Elmquist, 2006), suggesting distinct roles for each in the functions of orexin. Several studies have shown that the orexins are primarily excitatory in their actions and couple typically to intracellular Gq signaling proteins, although coupling through Gs and Gi has also been reported in some cells (Hoang *et al.*, 2003; Karteris *et al.*, 2005).

Narcolepsy in humans and the loss of orexin signaling

A patient with attacks of sleep associated with motor incapacity was first described by Westphal (1877). Three years later, the French neurologist Gélineau (1880) recognized that the disorder was a clinical entity rather than symp-tomatic of another condition. He proposed the term narcolepsy in describing a patient who fell asleep suddenly and also had cataplectic episodes whenever he became emotional. The narcolepsy–cataplexy syndrome is now recognized as having these two principal symptoms, excessive daytime sleepiness and cat-aplexy. In addition, the disorder has secondary signs and symptoms, including hypnagogic or hypnopompic hallucinations, sleep paralysis, automatic behav-iors, and fragmented nocturnal sleep (Choo & Guilleminault, 1998). Increased body mass index has also been suggested as being a feature of the disorder (Dahmen *et al.*, 2001).

Excessive daytime sleepiness, the irresistible need for sleep during the day, is associated with a chronically low level of alertness. The term "sleep attack" describes these unavoidable brief naps. Cataplexy, an abrupt decrease or loss in

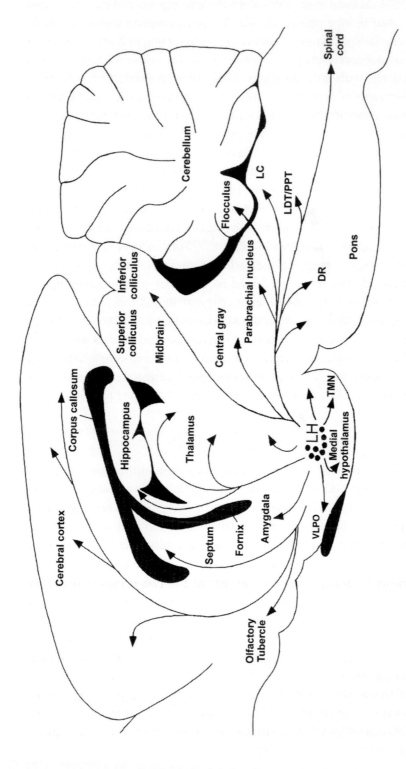

Figure 15.1 A schematic of a sagittal section of the rodent brain, displaying the location of the orexin-containing cell bodies in the lateral hypothalamus (LH) and the principal projections of the orexin system throughout the neuraxis, particularly to regions known to be critically involved in the control and expression of sleep and wakefulness: DR, dorsal raphe; LC, locus coeruleus; LDT/PPT, laterodorsal tegmentum/pedunculopontine tegmentum; TMN, tuberomamillary nucleus; VLPO, ventrolateral preoptic nucleus. Adapted from Nambu *et al.* (1999).

muscle tone, is most often triggered by strong emotions, occurs without alteration in the level of consciousness, lasts from seconds to minutes, generally
reverses with sudden resumption of normal muscle tone, and responds specifically to treatment with tricyclic antidepressants (Guilleminault & Gelb, 1995).
Excessive daytime sleepiness is an important diagnostic criterion for narcolepsy,
but its presence alone is not specific. In contrast, cataplexy, though not expressed
in all narcoleptic patients, is highly specific to narcolepsy when clearly documented (cf. Table 15.1). Hishikawa & Shimizu (1995) hypothesized that cataplexy
could be a transition between, or mixed state of, rapid eye movement (REM) sleep
and wakefulness. About a quarter of narcoleptic patients report hallucinations
that are hypnagogic or hypnopompic (i.e. occurring at the onset or offset of
sleep, respectively), and these are primarily auditory or visual. Complete loss of
muscle tone during the onset of nocturnal sleep or a daytime nap or abnormal
prolongation of atonia upon awakening are experienced as sleep paralysis. Lasting from seconds to minutes, sleep paralysis can be associated with hypnagogic
or hypnopompic hallucinations. Automatic behaviors are semipurposeful; they
occur without full awareness and often with total amnesia for the period in
which they occurred. Nocturnal sleep fragmentation and complaints of insomnia are seemingly paradoxical symptoms of narcolepsy. Although the narcoleptic
patient readily initiates sleep episodes, nocturnal sleep, including REM sleep,
is often fragmented by awakenings. Both excessive daytime sleepiness and disrupted nocturnal sleep reflect the poor regulation of sleep–wakefulness in narcolepsy (Aldrich, 1992). An exemplar nocturnal hypnogram of a narcoleptic
patient, showing these multiple awakenings and fragmented sleep, and compared with that of a normal control subject, is displayed in Fig. 15.2.

At a mechanistic level, the symptoms of narcolepsy result from a primary disruption of sleep–wakefulness regulation. They can be summarized as an expression of the features of REM sleep intruding into wakefulness or at sleep onset,
combined with difficulty maintaining prolonged wakefulness or sleep episodes.
Varying sensitivities and specificities of the principal and secondary symptoms
of the disorder complicate the diagnosis of narcolepsy in the individual patient.
Clinical diagnosis is ideally based on a history of the two principal symptoms
(Honda, 1988). Alternatively, excessive daytime sleepiness can be diagnostic if
it is associated with one of the secondary symptoms, as well as a polysomnographic indication such as that provided by the multiple sleep latency test (MSLT)
(International Classification of Sleep Disorders, 1990). Typically, this would be
the occurrence of two or more episodes of REM sleep within 15 min of sleep
onset during polysomnographic recordings of daytime naps. Such an occurrence
is defined as a sleep-onset REM sleep (SOREM) period. In fact, further evaluation
with the MSLT is usually indicated in cases of clinical diagnostic uncertainty.

Table 15.1 *Diagnostic certainty in the evaluation of narcolepsy*

Symptom	Sensitivity[a] (%)	Specificity[b] (%)	Differential diagnosis	Comment
Cataplexy and cataplexy-like symptoms	Moderate (60)	High (80)	Infrequent association with Niemann–Pick disease, Norrie disease, or brain tumors	Variable severity; diagnosed clinically or electrophysiologically
Excessive daytime sleepiness and "sleep attacks"	Very high (95)	Very low (5)	Wide differential diagnosis for this complaint	Diagnosed clinically; very disabling symptom
Hypnagogic[1]/hypnopompic[2] hallucinations	Moderate (60[1], 40[2])	High (90)	If frequent (i.e., several times/week) unlikely to be associated with other disorders	Diagnosed clinically; occur with both nocturnal sleep and daytime naps
Sleep paralysis	Moderate (50)	High (80)	Induced easily in normal controls with sleep deprivation	Diagnosed clinically or electrophysiologically
Fragmented nocturnal sleep	High (70)	Moderate (60)	Wide differential diagnosis for this complaint	Diagnosed electrophysiologically
Automatic behaviors	Moderate (50)	High (80)	Severe sleepiness including idiopathic hypersomnia	Comparable with sleepwalking

Approximate percentages are derived from Sturzenegger & Bassetti (2004).

[a] Percentage of patients with narcolepsy who demonstrate the sign or complain of the symptom.

[b] Presenting with the complaint of hypersomnolence, the percentage of patients who do not have narcolepsy and who do not have the sign or symptom.

Interestingly, diagnostic confirmation may be aided by profiling major histocompatibility complex (MHC) proteins. This analysis was based initially on serological studies, which showed a genetic linkage between narcolepsy and two major histocompatibility human leukocyte antigen (HLA) class II alleles, DR2 and DQw1. Despite subsequent extension and refinement of the nomenclature for HLA typing, and inclusion of diverse patient populations in the analysis, this basic finding remains valid. In fact, recent studies have confirmed that HLA haplotypes influence predisposition to the disorder, and have also reported that susceptibility is significantly affected by interactions between specific HLA-DR and HLA-DQ alleles, most importantly DQB1*0602, but also DRB1*1501 and DQA1*0102 (Honda et al., 1997; Mignot, 1998; Mignot et al., 2001). Although exceptions to these associations are relatively rare, the presence of DQB1*0602, the major HLA susceptibility allele across different population groups, increases the relative risk of contracting the disorder only about twofold (for narcolepsy) or fourfold (for narcolepsy–cataplexy) (Chabas et al., 2003; Mignot, 1998). Factors other than HLA alleles must therefore be involved in the etiology of the disorder. Although the mechanisms by which HLA alleles influence susceptibility to narcolepsy remain to be determined, HLA typing currently remains an important clinical tool for confirming a diagnosis of narcolepsy in patients with excessive daytime sleepiness but without cataplexy. If these histocompatibility antigens are not found in these patients, narcolepsy can usually be eliminated as a diagnosis.

Studies of orexin knockout mice and orexin receptor mutant canines in which narcoleptic traits are transmitted in an autosomally recessive manner first implicated dysfunction of the orexin system in the etiology of narcolepsy–cataplexy (Chemelli et al., 1999; Lin et al., 1999). A landmark study confirmed the near or total absence of orexin-A in the CSF of several narcoleptic patients compared with normal controls (Nishino et al., 2000b). Subsequent work demonstrated that the human disorder does not typically involve highly penetrant orexin-gene mutations (Peyron et al., 2000). Nevertheless, nearly all human cases of narcolepsy–cataplexy are now known to result from a selective loss of the orexin signal, probably reflecting a loss of the population of hypothalamic neurons that contain orexin (Peyron et al., 2000; Thannickal et al., 2000). However, narcolepsy without cataplexy is less closely associated with orexin deficiency (cf. review by Baumann & Bassetti, 2005), a result that may either reflect diagnostic uncertainty within this group or indicate a pathophysiologically unique subset of narcolepsy.

The cause of the orexin-containing cell loss in typical narcolepsy–cataplexy remains unknown, but the HLA association is intriguing because it suggests that autoimmunity could mediate a central disease process. This is not

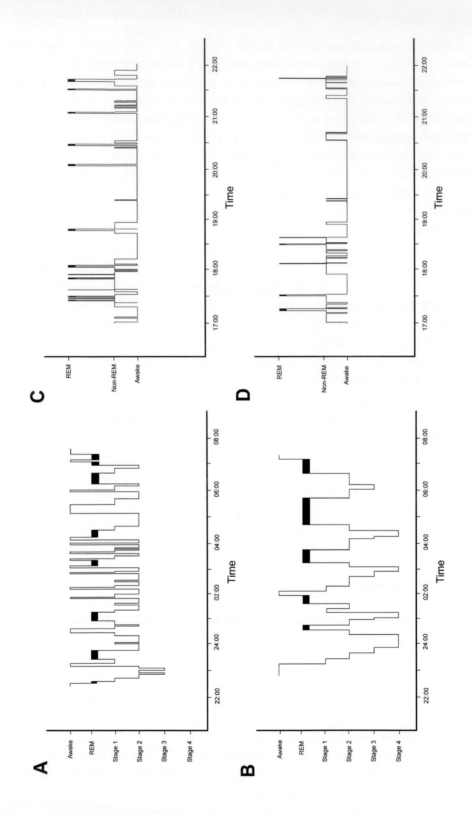

unprecedented: pediatric autoimmune neuropsychiatric disorders associated with streptococcal infections (PANDAS), including a form of obsessive–compulsive disorder, are increasingly recognized in children (Snider & Swedo, 2004; Swedo *et al.*, 1998). Although no antiserum reactive against orexins, orexin receptors, or orexin neuron-containing tissues has successfully been purified from patients to date, these studies may have been limited by serum collection after peak autoimmunity had subsided, when the destruction of orexin neurons was essentially complete (Taheri *et al.*, 2006). The identification of molecular markers other than orexin peptides that are unique to this cell population may be the key to identifying a putative molecular target for autoimmunity in the future. Possible support for the autoimmune hypothesis is provided by a recent report indicating that treatment with intravenous immunoglobulin may halt symptom progression in patients showing early signs of narcolepsy (Dauvilliers *et al.*, 2004). However, this initial study must be viewed skeptically in light of diagnostic uncertainties and the uncontrolled nature of the study.

Vigilance state characterization of orexin- and orexin receptor-deficient rodents

The phenotypic characterization of genetically modified rodents has advanced the understanding of both the basis of narcolepsy–cataplexy and the functions of the orexin system in the normal animal. Here we review the

---

Figure 15.2 Example hypnograms comparing nocturnal sleep in a narcoleptic patient with that in a healthy normal control, and vigilance state transitions in an *orexin*$^{-/-}$ mouse with a wild-type littermate. (A) A typical hypnogram displaying the progression of sleep stages in a narcoleptic patient. Note the fragmented sleep, the multiple awakenings, and the direct transitions from wakefulness to REM sleep. The fragmented sleep results in less slow wave sleep in these patients than normal: in this example, no stage 4 is evident and there is little stage 3. Note also the appearance of a REM sleep episode at sleep onset, and also at the end of the sleep phase, both of which might be accompanied by hallucinations. (B) For comparison, an example hypnogram from a healthy young adult showing the normal progression of sleep during the night. Note the presence of both stages 3 and 4, principally at the beginning of the night, and the concentration of REM sleep at the end of the night. (C) Vigilance state transitions in an *orexin*$^{-/-}$ mouse across the dark phase boundary, which occurs at 19:00. Note the direct transitions from wakefulness to REM sleep and the increased vigilance state fragmentation when compared with the corresponding hypnogram from a wild-type mouse (D). For clarity, the time scales are different in the display of the mouse and human data and non-REM is condensed to a single stage in the mouse.

principal effects of orexin- and orexin receptor-deficiency in rodents; these differences are summarized in Table 15.2.

Orexin$^{-/-}$ mice

Chemelli *et al.* (1999) first noted that *orexin*$^{-/-}$ mice exhibited a phenotype that was remarkably similar to human narcolepsy. Abrupt behavioral arrests with postural collapse were observed from video records obtained during the dark, normally active, period in these mice. Seizure activity was considered as a possible cause of these arrests, but subsequent electroencephalogram/electromyogram (EEG/EMG) recording revealed that these changes in behavior corresponded to direct transitions from wakefulness to REM sleep (Figs. 15.2C, 15.3A), a pathognomonic characteristic of narcolepsy. Less frequently, these behavioral arrests corresponded to episodic bursts of rhythmic spindles, 14–16 Hz waves, which are normally observed just prior to REM sleep in the rodent (Chemelli *et al.*, 1999). As detailed below, evidence was accumulated later to show that abrupt arrests fulfill criteria that are comparable to those used clinically to define cataplexy, including muscle atonia, preserved consciousness, an association with emotional arousal, and amelioration by clomipramine (Willie *et al.*, 2003; Willie & Yanagisawa, 2006). Vigilance state characterization of the *orexin*$^{-/-}$ mice from the EEG/EMG recordings also showed sleep and wakefulness fragmentation, together with a reduced mean latency to REM sleep, and increased REM sleep time during the dark phase. Figure 15.2 (C, D) displays exemplar hypnograms across the dark phase photoperiod boundary in *orexin*$^{-/-}$ and wild-type mice to highlight these vigilance state differences and to contrast them with the human hypnograms from a narcoleptic patient and a normal control subject.

Additional observational studies of *orexin*$^{-/-}$ mice revealed a second type of behavioral arrest with a gradual loss of head and neck posture not unlike the "nodding off" in sleepy humans and narcoleptic dogs (Willie *et al.*, 2003). This type of arrest appeared distinct from cataplexy, not only because of the gradual onset (Fig. 15.3B), but also because it began from quiet wakefulness rather than active or emotional states, it was correlated with the onset of non-REM sleep and preservation of basal muscle tone, and it was specifically suppressed by caffeine but not by clomipramine. These arrests were also clearly distinguished from normal sleep, as they were not preceded by stereotypical rest-associated behaviors such as nesting or sleep posturing. They were also frequently associated with an abnormally rapid progression to atonia and REM sleep, analogous to human SOREM periods. Importantly, wild-type mice did not exhibit these attacks under the same experimental conditions. It was therefore concluded that these gradual

Table 15.2 *Genetic modifications of orexin in rodents and studies of narcolepsy-cataplexy*[*].

Genetic modification	Pathophysiology	Relevant findings	Interpretations
Prepro-orexin gene knockout (*orexin*$^{-/-}$)	Loss of orexin-A and -B function throughout development	Inability to maintain wakefulness bouts *Severe decrease in REM sleep latency* *Frequent cataplexy and direct transitions to REM sleep*	Severe narcolepsy-cataplexy comparable to the human disorder.
Orexin receptor type 1 gene knockout (*OX$_1$R*$^{-/-}$)	Loss of OX$_1$R function throughout development	Mild decrease in REM sleep latency Absence of cataplexy or direct transitions to REM sleep	OX$_1$R signaling contributes to REM sleep gating
Orexin receptor type 2 gene knockout (*OX$_2$R*$^{-/-}$)	Loss of OX$_2$R function throughout development	Inability to maintain wakefulness bouts Mild decrease in REM sleep latency Occasional cataplexy and direct transitions to REM sleep	Milder narcolepsy-cataplexy comparable to canine narcolepsy. OX$_2$R signaling stabilizes wakefulness and also contributes to REM sleep gating
Double receptor gene knockout (*OX$_1$R*$^{-/-}$;*OX$_2$R*$^{-/-}$)	Loss of OX$_1$R and OX$_2$R function throughout development	Inability to maintain wakefulness bouts *Severe decrease in REM sleep latency* *Frequent cataplexy and direct transitions to REM sleep*	Severe narcolepsy-cataplexy indistinguishable from *orexin*$^{-/-}$ mice
Orexin/ataxin-3 transgenic mouse	Selective postnatal degeneration of orexin neurons, complete by early adulthood	Inability to maintain wakefulness bouts *Severe decrease in REM sleep latency* *Frequent cataplexy and direct transitions to REM sleep*	Severe narcolepsy-cataplexy indistinguishable from *orexin*$^{-/-}$ mice
Orexin/ataxin-3 transgenic rat	Selective postnatal degeneration of orexin neurons, complete by early adulthood	Inability to maintain wakefulness bouts *Severe decrease in REM latency* *Frequent cataplexy and separable direct transitions to REM sleep*	Severe narcolepsy-cataplexy comparable to the human disorder. Cataplectic episodes can be separated from wakefulness–REM sleep transitions

[*] Adapted from Willie & Yanagisawa (2006)

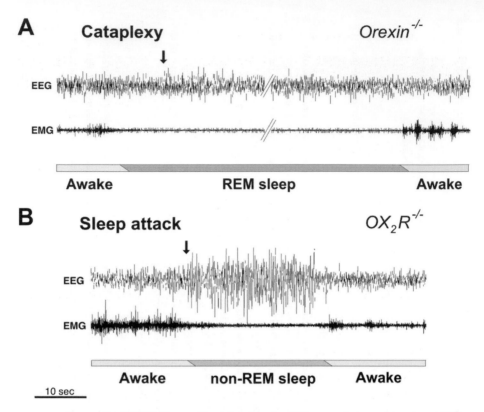

Figure 15.3 EEG/EMG recordings showing the differences between cataplexy (A) in an *orexin*$^{-/-}$ mouse, and a sleep attack (B) in an *OX$_2$R*$^{-/-}$ mouse. Note how cataplexy (i.e. an abrupt arrest) is associated with a transition to REM sleep, but the sleep attack (i.e. a gradual arrest) shows the characteristics of non-REM sleep after the transition. In fact, based only on these EEG/EMG records, the sleep attack would not appear unusual, and it is the associated behavior, as revealed on the concurrent video recordings (i.e. the collapse into sleep without the typical preparatory behaviors), that reveals how this type of attack is similar to the overwhelming sleepiness experienced by the narcoleptic patient. Vertical arrows denote the times at which an arrest is behaviorally evident. Scale bar is 10 sec. Adapted from Willie *et al.* (2003).

arrests corresponded most closely to the sleep attacks observed in narcoleptic patients.

Although human narcolepsy is not typically associated with orexin gene mutations, the *orexin*$^{-/-}$ model is most similar to the case of a narcoleptic-cataplectic child, severely symptomatic from infancy, who has a genetic defect in orexin production and release (Peyron *et al.*, 2000). Thus, constitutive orexin deficiency alone in the presence of otherwise histologically normal orexin neurons

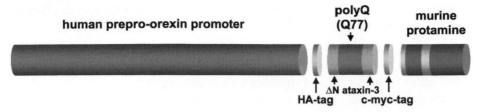

Figure 15.4 Schematic representation of the transgene used for generating *orexin/ataxin-3* rodents. The DNA fragment of the human prepro-orexin gene was ligated to a cDNA fragment encoding the N-terminally truncated human elongated ataxin-3 gene, expressing the toxic Q77 polyglutamine stretch. The 5′ terminus of this fragment has the HA-epitope, and the 3′ terminus has the myc-epitope for histological immunofluorescence. The 3′ end of the ataxin-3 cDNA was followed by a murine protamine-1 fragment to provide an intron and polyadenylation signal. Adapted from Hara *et al.* (2001).

seems to be sufficient to reproduce the primary symptoms of narcolepsy–cataplexy.

Orexin/ataxin-3 *transgenic mice and rats*

A human *ataxin-3* gene fragment, cloned from a patient with Muchado–Joseph disorder (i.e. cerebellar ataxia type 3) and containing an expanded polyglutamine repeat, is neurotoxic. Hence expression of the fragment by neuron-selective promoters can be used for targeted neurodegeneration. Driven by the orexin gene promoter, this fragment, as schematically represented in Fig. 15.4, caused specific postnatal degeneration of orexin neurons in *orexin/ataxin-3* transgenic mice (Hara *et al.*, 2001) and rats (Beuckmann *et al.*, 2004). These models are important because they mimic more closely the timing and specificity of the putative neuronal loss as it is believed to occur in most cases of human narcolepsy–cataplexy. Thus *orexin/ataxin-3* transgenic mice were found to express essentially the same sleep phenotype as *orexin*$^{-/-}$ mice although it developed later, at about 6 weeks of age (Hara *et al.*, 2001). Similarly, by 17 weeks of age, *orexin/ataxin-3* rats (Beuckmann *et al.*, 2004) exhibited postnatal loss of orexin neurons, and orexin-containing projections were essentially undetectable at this age. This loss of orexin in the rat resulted in a sleep phenotype during the dark phase that paralleled that seen in the mouse, including abrupt arrests, some of which corresponded to direct transitions from wakefulness to REM sleep (see below), a decreased latency to REM sleep, and increased REM sleep time. Although typical posture and behavior in *orexin/ataxin-3* rats made visual differentiation of gradual arrests more difficult than in the mouse, concurrent video and EEG/EMG monitoring revealed episodes in which the onset of non-REM sleep occurred during ongoing motivated behaviors in association with SOREM episodes (Beuck-mann *et al.*, 2004). These episodes have the characteristics, therefore, of gradual arrests as described in the *orexin$^{-/-}$* mice (Willie *et al.*, 2003), and are likely to be the analogs in the rat of sleep attacks. O*rexin/ataxin-3* rats also showed decreased dark-phase wakefulness and vigilance state fragmentation.

Significantly, *orexin/ataxin-3* mice respond to intracerebroventricular injection of orexin-A with increased wakefulness and suppression of REM sleep and cat-aplexy. This pharmacological reversal indicated that orexin receptors remain functional in the absence of orexin neurons, and that these narcoleptic mice can respond to orexin agonists, a finding with significant therapeutic implica-tions (Mieda *et al.*, 2004b).

The orexin receptor null mice: $OX_1R^{-/-}$, $OX_2R^{-/-}$ *and* $OX_1R^{-/-};OX_2R^{-/-}$

Characterization of the receptor knockout mice ($OX_1R^{-/-}$ and $OX_2R^{-/-}$) provided important information about the differential roles of the two recep-tors in both vigilance state control and the symptoms of narcolepsy (Kisanuki *et al.*, 2000; Willie *et al.*, 2003). In contrast to the direct transitions to REM sleep and abrupt behavioral arrests that characterized *orexin$^{-/-}$* mice, $OX_1R^{-/-}$ mice exhibited no direct transitions to REM sleep and only a modest decrease in REM sleep latency (Kisanuki *et al.*, 2000). $OX_1R^{-/-}$ mice also showed slight fragmenta-tion of vigilance states when compared with the normal animals (Kisanuki *et al.*, 2000).

Two lines of narcoleptic canines had been found to express mutations of the OX_2R gene, and the absence of OX_2R-mediated signaling was therefore proposed as a critical pathophysiological mediator of the narcolepsy-cataplexy phenotype (Lin *et al.*, 1999). However, although $OX_2R^{-/-}$ mice showed signs of narcolepsy–cataplexy, the phenotype was considerably milder than that expressed by the orexin-deficient animals. In addition to less severe REM sleep abnormalities, a carefully controlled comparison of videotaped behavioral arrests in $OX_2R^{-/-}$ and *orexin$^{-/-}$* mice, combined with concurrent EEG/EMG recording and EEG spectral analysis, showed that the previously characterized cataplexy-like arrests, though displaying similar features, were approximately 30 times less frequent in $OX_2R^{-/-}$ mice than in the orexin null animals (Willie *et al.*, 2003).

Like *orexin$^{-/-}$* mice, the $OX_2R^{-/-}$ mice also exhibited gradual arrests analo-gous to sleep attacks. In both mutants, gradual arrests occurred with similar frequency, and caffeine was similarly effective in suppressing them. In con-trast, $OX_1R^{-/-}$ mice were found to exhibit possible sleep attacks so infrequently that detailed characterization has not been possible. Notably, the sleep attacks of $OX_2R^{-/-}$ mice did not exhibit the abnormally rapid progressions to REM sleep observed during these attacks in *orexin$^{-/-}$* mice. However, the equivalent frequency of sleep attacks and comparable levels of vigilance state fragmentation recorded in $orexin^{-/-}$ and $OX_2R^{-/-}$ mice indicated that these mice expressed similar levels of sleepiness. But the high incidence of SOREM-like phenomena unique to $orexin^{-/-}$ mice suggested that abnormal REM sleep intrusion may not be the cause of sleepiness per se (Willie & Yanagisawa, 2006). This is generally consistent with the clinical management of narcolepsy–cataplexy by utilizing different classes of drugs (i.e. stimulants and antidepressants) to treat sleepiness and REM sleep-associated symptoms, respectively (Aldrich, 1998).

In finalizing this series of studies, the double receptor knockout mouse $(OX_1R^{-/-};OX_2R^{-/-})$ was shown to be phenotypically indistinguishable from $orexin^{-/-}$ mice (Kisanuki et al., 2001), a result that makes the existence of additional orexin receptors unlikely.

Summary of the findings in orexin- and receptor-deficient rodents

In the absence of OX_2R, considerable functional control for REM sleep is provided by OX_1R, and thus normal gating of REM sleep must depend on both OX_1R and OX_2R signaling. Hence an important conclusion from these studies is that the absence of orexin signaling through both receptor pathways is required to produce severe narcolepsy–cataplexy and profound dysregulation of REM sleep (Kisanuki et al., 2000, 2001; Willie et al., 2003). In contrast, OX_2R signaling appears to be critical for regulating the transition from wakefulness to non-REM sleep. Hence the hypersomnolence, as well as the sleep attacks in the human disorder, are more closely linked with the lack of an orexin signal at the OX_2R receptor. These conclusions were supported by complementary experiments in which the non-selective agonist orexin-A was administered intracerebroventricularly to the knockout murine models (Mieda & Yanagisawa, 2006). Administration of orexin-A to wild-type mice increased wakefulness and suppressed both non-REM and REM sleep in a dose-dependent manner, and OX_1R deficiency did not significantly decrease these effects over the dose range tested. In contrast, OX_2R deficiency resulted in a significant attenuation of the wakefulness-promoting action of orexin-A, but notably, the effect of orexin-A was still observable. Thus, although OX_2R mediates most of the arousing effects of orexin-A, the orexin signal at OX_1R is still effective in the absence of OX_2R. With respect to the changes in REM sleep induced by orexin-A administration, however, no significant differences between wild-type, $OX_1R^{-/-}$, and $OX_2R^{-/-}$ mice were noted. These results are consistent with the hypothesis that both receptors function in a complementary manner to gate REM sleep, at least under these conditions. Importantly, administration of high doses of orexin-A to the double receptor knockout mice $(OX_1R^{-/-};OX_2R^{-/-})$ was without observable effect. In summary, these data not only confirm that deficient signaling through both pathways reproduces the complete narcolepsy–cataplexy syndrome, but also that *only* these two receptor pathways mediate both the wakefulness-promoting and REM sleep gating effects of the orexins.

Animal models and the nature of cataplexy

Clinical observations originally led to the hypotheses that cataplexy could reflect a fragmentary manifestation of REM sleep muscle atonia, or alternatively, a transitional state between wakefulness and REM sleep (Hishikawa & Shimizu, 1995). Thus during prolonged episodes of cataplexy in humans, the awake EEG can transition through an EEG more closely resembling that of REM sleep but with continued awareness, and even to unambiguous REM sleep (Hishikawa & Shimizu, 1995). However, the underlying neuronal substrates for the onset and progression of human cataplexy have been inferred primarily from recent studies in OX_2R-deficient canines (John et al., 2004; Nishino et al., 2000a; Wu et al., 2004), a model in which cataplexy is only infrequently associated with an EEG resembling that of REM sleep. These canine studies have shown that the brain sites and mechanisms for triggering cataplexy may be distinct from those that trigger REM sleep. The results have thus been interpreted as supporting an alternative hypothesis that cataplexy is a unique state not directly related to REM sleep, despite spinally mediated muscle tone inhibition being the final common pathway in both states. Hence this conceptualization of cataplexy requires that muscle atonia per se can exist as a physiological state independent of its occurrence as one of the cardinal, separable signs of REM sleep.

A detailed analysis of the similarities between murine abrupt arrests and cataplexy in humans has shown that abrupt behavioral arrests in the mouse fulfill most, if not all, of the accepted clinical criteria for the definition of cataplexy (Willie & Yanagisawa, 2006). These include the time course, emotional triggering, muscle atonia, and, as noted above, the response to clomipramine. Interestingly, evidence of briefly preserved consciousness in mice has also been documented (Willie et al., 2003), although this state was invariably followed by REM sleep. This important finding led to the recognition that abrupt arrests in the mouse are initiated as a bout of muscle atonia during wakefulness (i.e. cataplexy) which then transitions rapidly to REM sleep. Hence the EEG recorded during murine cataplexy is almost always indistinguishable from REM sleep within seconds of the onset of cataplexy, even in those episodes with concurrent behavioral evidence of preserved consciousness.

In contrast, the *orexin/ataxin*-3 rat exhibited more diversity in episodes of behavioral arrest than had been observed in the mice (Beuckmann et al., 2004). Video recording and observation of these rats revealed that during ongoing motivated behaviors, such as ambulation and drinking, an abrupt change occurred

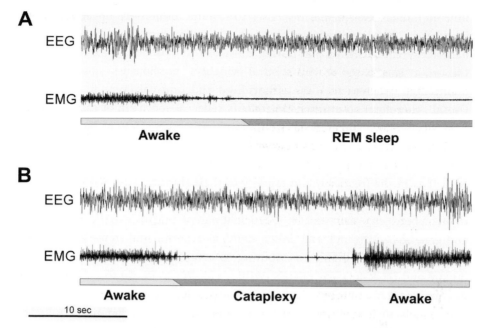

Figure 15.5 Exemplar EEG/EMG recordings, from an *orexin/ataxin-3* rat, to show the differences between two episodes of behavioral arrest (i.e. cataplexy): (A) associated with complete muscle atonia and accompanied by an EEG with the characteristics of REM sleep, and (B) also associated with complete muscle atonia, but with minimal change to the EEG. Both of these episodes are therefore cataplectic, as characterized in the mouse and human, but only in (B) is wakefulness, and therefore consciousness, likely to be maintained. The existence of both types of episode in the rat adds support to the conceptualization of cataplexy in the human as a transitional state between wakefulness and REM sleep, or a fragmentary occurrence of REM sleep (Hishikawa & Shimizu, 1995). The visual differences evident between the EEG signals recorded in these two examples were subsequently confirmed by spectral analysis. Adapted from Beuckmann *et al.* (2004).

that was characterized by a sudden loss of muscle tone and posture. Correlated with EEG/EMG recordings, muscle atonia was evident during all these episodes, but the spectral characteristics of the EEG record frequently did not change from that of wakefulness. Such episodes usually terminated with resumption of normal muscle tone accompanied by full mobility and purposeful behavior (Fig. 15.5B). Less frequently after the onset of some of these episodes, the EEG frequency spectrum transitioned rapidly to that of REM sleep (Fig. 15.5A). The latter episodes, like abrupt arrests in the *orexin*$^{-/-}$ mice, were classified as direct transitions from wakefulness to REM sleep. Abrupt behavioral arrests in the *orexin/ataxin-3* rat thus met the criteria of cataplexy as described for the murine models, except that responses to clomipramine were not tested. There is, however, one important distinction between the murine and rat models of narcolepsy–cataplexy, in that during most of the episodes of abrupt arrest in the rat, at least based on EEG spectral evidence, consciousness appeared to be maintained, whereas this was a short-lived and unusual event in the mouse. Overall, therefore, observations in rodents reflect a spectrum of cataplexy- and REM sleep-related phenomena, similar to that observed clinically (Hishikawa & Shimizu, 1995). In summary, species differences in cataplectic episodes are apparently reflected in the duration of atonia while wakefulness is maintained, as well as in the frequency and rapidity of their transitions to REM sleep.

However, the differences in severity of cataplexy and cataplexy-associated phenomena between orexin- and OX_2R-deficient narcoleptic mice of the same species and genetic background, and under identical experimental conditions, suggest that the cascade of events contributing to cataplexy may not be identical in orexin- and OX_2R-deficient models (Willie et al., 2003). Hence there may also be distinctions across species. This has implications for the extent to which the animal models, including the canines, accurately represent the neurophysiological events generating cataplexy at the neuronal level in narcoleptic patients. More detailed investigation of the rodent models, including extracellular single-unit recordings in hypothalamic and pontine nuclei of freely moving animals, is now required.

Orexin and the gating of REM sleep

Several symptoms of narcolepsy reflect the intrusion of REM sleep, or the features of REM sleep, into wakefulness. For example, orexin-deficient rodents exhibit frequent direct transitions from wakefulness to REM sleep during the dark phase. However, in contrast to the overall fragmentation of wakefulness and non-REM sleep, REM sleep episodes in these animals have a normal, or even slightly increased, duration (Beuckmann et al., 2004; Chemelli et al., 1999; Hara et al., 2001; Willie et al., 2003). Hence the loss of orexin results in the inability to gate the onset of REM sleep appropriately, but once REM sleep is initiated, orexin does not influence the bout duration. By implication, orexin therefore functions in normal animals to inhibit the appearance of REM sleep, particularly when the brain state, including cortical activation, is most similar, as it is during active wakefulness (Beuckmann et al., 2004). Interestingly, after the onset of non-REM sleep, orexin- and orexin-receptor deficient rodents also exhibit reduced latencies to REM sleep during the dark phase (Beuckmann et al., 2004; Chemelli et al., 1999; Hara et al., 2001; Kisanuki et al., 2000, 2001; Willie et al., 2003). This change to sleep architecture is separable from direct transitions to REM sleep, however, since even $OX_1R^{-/-}$ mice show reduced REM sleep latencies despite exhibiting no direct transitions to REM sleep (Kisanuki et al., 2000).

With normal mean bout durations for REM sleep, the increased frequency of REM sleep episodes results in significantly more REM sleep during the active phase in orexin-deficient rodents (Beuckmann et al., 2004; Chemelli et al., 1999; Willie et al., 2003). Narcoleptic patients also show increased REM sleep time (Broughton et al., 1988). Although smaller increases in REM sleep have been observed in $OX_1R^{-/-}$ and $OX_2R^{-/-}$ mice, REM sleep time in $OX1R^{-/-};OX2R^{-/-}$ mice is increased to the same extent as that recorded in $orexin^{-/-}$ mice (Kisanuki et al., 2000, 2001; Willie et al., 2003). During the rest phase, orexin-deficient rodents (Beuckmann et al., 2004; Hara et al., 2001; Willie et al., 2003) and narcoleptic humans (Broughton et al., 1988) exhibit compensatory reductions in REM sleep, indicating intact homeostatic responses to the over-expression of this state during the active phase (Willie & Yanagisawa, 2006).

The onset of REM sleep depends on a balance of activity between the monoaminergic wake-on/REM-off cells exerting an inhibitory influence on the cholinergic wake-off/REM-on cells of the laterodorsal pontine tegmentum (LDT) (Sinton & McCarley, 2004). Electrophysiological studies of the actions of orexin on these cell groups have shown that both OX_1R and OX_2R participate in neuronal activation in these regions (Kohlmeier et al., 2003, 2004; Willie et al., 2003). Hence in normal animals, signaling at both receptors will contribute independently and additively to REM sleep gating. These data thus support the conclusion that disruptions in the orexin signal at either the OX_1R or OX_2R receptor affects this aspect of the narcoleptic phenotype (see above).

Orexin deficiency and abnormal sleepiness

The second constellation of narcoleptic symptoms can be summarized under the rubric of excessive daytime sleepiness, or an inability to regulate wakefulness. As recently reviewed by Mochizuki et al. (2004), at least four explanations have to date been proposed for this sleepiness: a deficit in arousal, an impaired circadian alertness signal, abnormal homeostatic regulation of non-REM sleep, and excessive vigilance state fragmentation. These mechanisms are not mutually exclusive, and there are possible roles for orexin signaling in each of them, as we review in the following sections.

Orexin deficiency and an arousal deficit

Orexin neurons innervate all the major brain regions implicated in the generation of wakefulness including the aminergic and cholinergic brainstem nuclei, hypothalamus, basal forebrain, thalamus, and cortex (Bayer *et al.*, 2002, 2004; Burlet *et al.*, 2002; Eggermann *et al.*, 2001; Eriksson *et al.*, 2001; Hagan *et al.*, 1999; Kohlmeier *et al.*, 2004; Li *et al.*, 2002; Liu *et al.*, 2002; Peyron *et al.*, 1998) (cf. Fig. 15.1). These projections are excitatory, and hence withdrawal of orexin signaling would be expected to result in a deficit in arousal (de Lecea & Sutcliffe, 2005). Indeed, we have noted reduced power in the EEG θ (8–12 Hz) frequency range in *orexin*$^{-/-}$ mice and *orexin/ataxin-3* transgenic rats (Beuckmann *et al.*, 2004; Willie *et al.*, 2005). EEG spectral power in rodents at these frequencies is generated in the hippocampus, driven through the septo-hippocampal system, and dependent on ascending GABAergic and cholinergic innervation from the pontine reticular activating system (Lee *et al.*, 1994; Manns *et al.*, 2003; Vertes & Kocsis, 1997; Vinogradova, 1995). It reflects the engagement of active attentional processes, and correlates with goal-oriented behavior and alertness in the rodent (Bland, 1986; Sutherland and McNaughton, 2000).

Although the EEG spectral data are thus supportive of an inherent arousal deficit, a functional deficit in orexin-deficient rodents has been observed during periods of restricted food availability. Acute food restriction is an important exogenous arousing stimulus; during certain times while fasting, rodents respond by becoming more awake and active (Borbely, 1977; Dewasmes *et al.*, 1989). Although orexin-deficient mice demonstrate only mild deficits in the time spent in wakefulness under normal conditions, they exhibit a significant deficiency in fasting-induced arousal and wakefulness (Mieda *et al.*, 2004a; Yamanaka *et al.*, 2003). The discharge rate of orexin-containing neurons is affected by the concentrations of glucose, leptin, and ghrelin (Yamanaka *et al.*, 2003), and in the whole animal this is likely to translate into an effect of short-term metabolic cues such as the rate of change in leptin and glucose levels on orexin cell activity (Williams *et al.*, 2004). For example, the discharge rate of orexin cells is increased by hypoglycemia (Burdakov *et al.*, 2005), one mechanism by which negative energy balance could increase arousal through the orexin system in the normal animal.

Orexin and the circadian wakefulness signal

The sleepiness associated with narcolepsy may result from impaired circadian influences (Broughton *et al.*, 1998), particularly of the circadian alertness signal which contributes to the timing and consolidation of the sleep period (Dijk & Czeisler, 1994; Edgar *et al.*, 1993). Confirmatory data for this hypothesis was provided by Dantz *et al.* (1994), who, using a forced desynchrony protocol, showed that narcoleptic patients have a normal circadian pacemaker and homeostatic sleep drive, but a deficit in alertness associated with the circadian signal. Although results are more difficult to interpret in an animal with

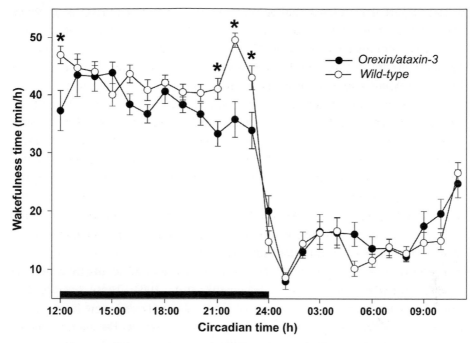

Figure 15.6 The mean hourly distribution of wakefulness time (min/h) in *orexin/ataxin-3* rats and wild-type littermates. Although over the 24 h period there is little total difference in the time spent in wakefulness, it is evident that the transgenic rats spend less time awake during the dark phase, which is denoted by the horizontal bar, especially at the photoperiod boundaries. Note, in particular, the difference at the end of the dark phase. The latter corresponds to a time of maximum orexin levels in the rat, and may be related to a circadian wakefulness signal. Asterisks designate those hours with a significant difference in wakefulness times between the genotypes ($p < 0.05$). Adapted from Beuckmann et al. (2004).

a polyphasic sleep pattern, orexin-deficient rodents similarly exhibit relatively normal timing of sleep-wakefulness under a 12 h light:dark cycle (Beuckmann et al., 2004; Chemelli et al., 1999; Hara et al., 2001; Mochizuki et al., 2004; Willie et al., 2003). They also exhibit relatively normal circadian timing of free-running locomotor activity under prolonged dark:dark conditions (M. Mieda & M. Yanagisawa, unpublished observations). Furthermore, orexin-deficient rodents exhibit an active-phase wakefulness deficit (Beuckmann et al., 2004; Mochizuki et al., 2004; Willie et al., 2003). Notably, however, in *orexin/ataxin-3* transgenic rats (Beuckmann et al., 2004), this wakefulness deficit was found to be concentrated at the photoperiod boundaries, especially at the end of the active phase (Fig. 15.6). This timing corresponds closely with the appearance of the circadian alertness signal in the human (Dijk & Czeisler, 1994). It also correlates with the appearance of the peak of the orexin signal in rat brain, at the end of the active phase of the daily cycle (Fujiki *et al.*, 2001; Taheri *et al.*, 2000; Yoshida *et al.*, 2001). In this regard, Zeitzer *et al.* (2003) have similarly demonstrated that the maximal orexin signal in the squirrel monkey occurs at the end of the active phase, at a time that corresponds with the circadian alertness signal in this species.

Orexin deficiency and abnormal regulation of non-REM sleep homeostasis

Excessive sleepiness in narcolepsy could also result from an abnormal homeostatic regulation of non-REM sleep, with an inappropriately rapid accumulation or expression of sleep pressure (Besset *et al.*, 1994). One method of studying this process is to examine sleep recovery following mild sleep deprivation, typically achieved by the use of gentle handling in rodents. When compared with wild-type mice, *orexin*$^{-/-}$ mice demonstrated a normal dose-dependent response to acute total sleep deprivation with normal decreases in non-REM sleep latencies, a normal increase in non-REM EEG δ power, and subsequently a normal recovery of non-REM sleep deficits (Mochizuki *et al.*, 2004). These authors thus concluded that *orexin*$^{-/-}$ mice appear to have essentially the same homeostatic responses to sleep deprivation as found in wild-type mice. However, using an alternative protocol, when food availability was chronically restricted to a limited period during the light phase every day, wild-type mice maintained the time spent in sleep and wakefulness unchanged over 24 h (Mieda *et al.*, 2004a). But *orexin/ataxin-3* transgenic mice, under these conditions, exhibited significantly reduced wakefulness, despite decreases in food intake and body mass that were identical to those seen in the wild-type mice. In contrast, when food was restricted to a limited period during the dark, active phase, wild-type mice spent more time in food-anticipatory wakefulness, but the *orexin/ataxin-3* transgenic mice exhibited no change to wakefulness prior to the presence of the food. These results suggested that orexin-deficient mice have only a limited capacity to adjust their sleep and wakefulness in response to food restriction. Hence orexin may alter sleep–wake homeostatic set-points in response to metabolic demands even if the neuropeptide does not directly mediate sleep homeostasis in response to sleep deprivation per se.

Orexin and the fragmentation of vigilance states

Sleepiness in narcolepsy has also been considered a subjective phenomenon associated with the instability of boundaries between behavioral states and the constant intrusion of sleep episodes into wakefulness. Under baseline conditions, $OX_2R^{-/-}$, *orexin*$^{-/-}$, and *orexin/ataxin-3* transgenic mice have normal amounts of wakefulness and non-REM sleep during the light and dark phases and over 24 h (Chemelli *et al.*, 1999; Hara *et al.*, 2001; Mochizuki *et al.*, 2004; Willie *et al.*, 2003). *Orexin/ataxin-3* transgenic rats are also similar to their wild-type litter-mates in this regard except that they spend slightly less time awake during the dark phase (Beuckmann *et al.*, 2004). Despite these results, narcoleptic rodents are unable to maintain wakefulness and non-REM sleep episodes for prolonged periods. These decreased mean episode durations are most striking during the active phase, but occur to a lesser extent during the rest phase as well.

After taking account of analysis artifacts caused by direct transitions to REM sleep in *orexin*$^{-/-}$ mice, Mochizuki *et al.* (2004) re-examined the effect of orexin deficiency on sleep and wakefulness. These authors found evidence of short sleep cycles during the light phase, and short bouts of sleep were accompanied by many more transitions between all states, during both the light and dark phases, when compared with wild-type mice. With the exception of direct transitions from wakefulness to REM sleep, *orexin*$^{-/-}$ mice did not exhibit a relative bias for other transitions between wakefulness, non-REM sleep, and the remaining REM sleep. These results thus indicate that one of the primary problems of narcolepsy–cataplexy, the inability to maintain wakefulness during the active phase, is also associated with inability to maintain normal sleep cycles during the rest phase. The latter is consistent with the disturbed nocturnal sleep of narcoleptic patients (Broughton *et al.*, 1988).

These results have led to the conception of orexin as a factor that stabilizes transitions between all vigilance states as well as promoting wakefulness. The neuronal circuitry involved in this proposition has been modeled as a "sleep switch", which provides a mechanistic explanation for organized transitions (Saper *et al.*, 2001). In brief, the model is based on reciprocal innervation between sleep-promoting neurons (Szymusiak *et al.*, 1998) of the hypothalamic ventro-lateral preoptic nucleus (VLPO) and aminergic wake-promoting neurons of the principal arousal nuclei (Chou *et al.*, 2002; Gallopin *et al.*, 2000) (cf. de Lecea, this volume, Fig. 14.4). Mutual inhibition between these two neuronal groups forms a bistable, or flip–flop, switch in the sense used by electrical engineers. This switch could maintain vigilance state stability despite slowly accumulat-ing circadian or homeostatic pressures to the contrary. At a certain point, a threshold is reached and the switch suddenly flips to the opposite pole. As an additional factor, the excitatory influence of orexin on wake-promoting neurons predominates during the active phase, so maintaining this side of the circuit and stabilizing arousal (Burlet *et al.*, 2002; Eggermann *et al.*, 2001; Eriksson *et al.*, 2001; Hagan *et al.*, 1999; Kohlmeier *et al.*, 2004; Li *et al.*, 2002; Liu *et al.*, 2002). Hence the absence of orexin results in poorly maintained wakefulness during the active phase and unregulated switching between vigilance states, and also allows the expression of intermediate states such as cataplexy. Correspondingly, and as additional evidence for this model, selective lesions of the VLPO cause increased wakefulness as well as more fragmented vigilance states during the rest phase (Lu *et al.*, 2000).

Summary of the consequences of orexin signaling deficiency

Although the cause of the presumed loss of orexin-containing neurons in human narcoleptics remains unknown, rodent models have provided valuable information about both the underlying mechanisms of the disorder and the role of orexin in the normal animal. We have noted that the similar inability to maintain wakefulness in orexin- and OX_2R-deficient mice implicates signaling through the OX_2R receptor as critical for the sleepiness and vigilance state instability of narcoleptic mice. However, it is evident that both OX_1R- and OX_2R-dependent pathways must play independent and additive roles in the gating of REM sleep. This follows from the decreases in REM sleep latencies in both $OX_1R^{-/-}$ and $OX_2R^{-/-}$ mice, and from the direct transitions to REM sleep and the significant increases in active phase REM sleep time in $OX_1R^{-/-};OX_2R^{-/-}$ and orexin-deficient mice. Similarly, the milder cataplectic phenotype of $OX_2R^{-/-}$ mice, when compared with that of the $OX_1R^{-/-};OX_2R^{-/-}$ and orexin-deficient mice, implies a significant modulatory role of OX_1R signaling in the triggering of cataplexy.

The interaction of MCH with orexin

The term "orexin" (after the Greek *orexis*, appetite) was chosen to reflect a likely contribution of the neuropeptides to food-seeking behavior: orexin-containing cell bodies had been found uniquely around the LH, an area long known to be involved in feeding, and orexin could also induce this behavior after central administration (Sakurai *et al.*, 1998). The subsequent discovery that orexin increased wakefulness was notable because of the complementary nature of arousal and food-seeking (Willie *et al.*, 2001), a concept that was strengthened by results showing that metabolic state could modulate this effect (see above). Nevertheless, the exact role of orexin in energy homeostasis has remained controversial (Cai *et al.*, 2002; de Lecea *et al.*, 2002; Williams *et al.*, 2004; Willie *et al.*, 2001). In contrast, another LH neuropeptide, MCH, has a well accepted involvement in energy balance (Shimada *et al.*, 1998). It is striking therefore that not only are the orexin and MCH cell body populations in close proximity with axonal contacts between the neurons, but there is also a remarkable convergence of axonal projections and expression of orexin and MCH receptors throughout the neuraxis (Bittencourt *et al.*, 1992; Saito *et al.*, 2001; Steininger *et al.*, 2004; Trivedi *et al.*, 1998).

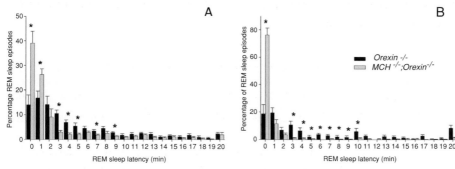

Figure 15.7 Normalized REM sleep latency histograms, expressed as a percentage of all REM sleep episodes, for the *orexin*$^{-/-}$ and *MCH*$^{-/-}$; *orexin*$^{-/-}$ mice under normally fed conditions (A) and during a 24 h period without access to food (B). Note in particular the percentage of REM sleep episodes with zero latency, i.e. the first column in these histograms, representing episodes with direct transition to REM sleep from the preceding wakefulness. The *MCH*$^{-/-}$; *orexin*$^{-/-}$ mice exhibit more of these episodes than the *orexin*$^{-/-}$ mice when normally fed, but this difference is potentiated under conditions of restricted access to food: about 80% of all REM sleep episodes are cataplectic in the double null mice under these conditions. As a result of the 20 s epoch length, the abscissa scale is as follows: 0 min represents REM latencies from 0 to 10 s, 1 min represents latencies from 11 to 70 s, etc. Asterisks, included for REM latencies $\leq$ 10 min, designate those bins that are significantly different between the genotypes ($p < 0.05$).

This anatomical relationship suggested a functional interaction between orexin and MCH, possibly involving vigilance and/or feeding behaviors, which we therefore studied in the double knockout (*MCH*$^{-/-}$; *orexin*$^{-/-}$) mouse (J. T. Willie, C. M. Sinton, E. Maratos-Flier & M. Yanagisawa, manuscript in preparation). Our initial hypothesis of opposing actions of the neuropeptides had experimental support. For example, narcoleptic patients have increased body mass index (Dahmen *et al.*, 2001), and orexin-deficient mice exhibit a decreased metabolic rate and decreased wakefulness during the active phase (Chemelli *et al.*, 1999; Mieda & Yanagisawa, 2002). In contrast, *MCH*$^{-/-}$ mice exhibit a lean phenotype with increased metabolic rate (Shimada *et al.*, 1998); they also sleep less than normal mice during the active phase.

As predicted, *MCH*$^{-/-}$;*orexin*$^{-/-}$ mice displayed an intermediate body weight phenotype, indicating independent and opposing neuromodulatory actions of MCH and orexin on metabolism. Surprisingly, however, rather than expressing an attenuated narcoleptic phenotype, *MCH*$^{-/-}$;*orexin*$^{-/-}$ mice exhibited more severe behavioral state instability during the active phase. When compared with *orexin*$^{-/-}$ mice, the double null mice had about twice as many cataplectic episodes (Fig. 15.7A), they were less able to maintain wakefulness, and they exhibited increased REM sleep time. Under fasting conditions, *MCH*$^{-/-}$; *orexin*$^{-/-}$ mice exhibited even more extreme behavioral state instability with a very high incidence of cataplectic attacks, about four times greater than in the *orexin*$^{-/-}$ mice under these conditions (Fig. 15.7B). In addition, and as in *MCH*$^{-/-}$ mice, *MCH*$^{-/-}$; *orexin*$^{-/-}$ mice also exhibited hyperactivity in response to fasting.

These results indicated that MCH gates arousal and emotionality, especially in response to a motivating or arousing stimulus. Hence, the increased incidence of cataplexy in the *MCH*$^{-/-}$; *orexin*$^{-/-}$ mice might reflect a higher arousal level, which would be sufficient to trigger more cataplectic episodes (Willie *et al.*, 2003). This could be only a partial explanation, however, because these mice also exhibited a greater incidence of sleep attacks, which are distinct from cataplexy (see above) (Willie *et al.*, 2003). Thus extreme vigilance state instability, possibly in addition to increased cataplexy, was a more probable explanation for these results. If so, MCH might participate, with orexin, in the "sleep switch" (Saper *et al.*, 2001) with MCH acting to promote sleep during the active phase. In fact, MCH neurons, like the VLPO neurons, have an inhibitory relationship with pontine cell groups that compose part of the ascending activating system (Bayer *et al.*, 2005; van den Pol *et al.*, 2004). We propose, therefore, that a balance between orexin and MCH activity stabilizes the level of arousal and transitions between sleep and wakefulness in response to a motivating stimulus during the active phase.

Conclusion: integration of hypothalamic arousal systems

In summary, MCH appears to modulate vigilance state transitions during the active phase by providing an inhibitory influence through the "sleep switch", in contrast to the excitatory influence of orexin. We have also shown that this influence is more critical during a period of food restriction, a significant motivational factor. Whether this conclusion is also true under similar motivationally aroused states, when the animal must respond to other needs, remains to be determined, but it is clearly a possibility. To date, we can conclude that the presence of MCH dampens excessive food-seeking behavior and promotes sleepiness when food becomes scarce, whereas orexin enhances such behaviors under these circumstances. Thus the behaviors necessary to cope with changes in energy status are modulated by these hypothalamic circuits, a conclusion supported by findings showing that the activities of both MCH- and orexin-containing cells are coupled to metabolic state (Burdakov *et al.*, 2005). Interestingly, sleep–wakefulness must be included in this range of coping behaviors, and MCH and orexin thus regulate not only overt food-seeking behavior but also vigilance state. It now remains to be determined whether the profound effects of the loss of orexin and MCH on the gating of REM sleep reflects more than an epiphenomenon associated with generalized instability of vigilance states. But the inference from these results is that the expression of REM sleep may be more closely coupled with energy homeostasis than previously considered (Willie *et al.*, 2001).

References

Aldrich, M. S. (1992). Narcolepsy. *Neurology* **42**, 34–43.

Aldrich, M. S. (1998). Diagnostic aspects of narcolepsy. *Neurology* **50**, S2–S7.

Baumann, C. R. & Bassetti, C. L. (2005). Hypocretins (orexins) and sleep-wake disorders. *Lancet Neurol.* **4**, 673–82.

Bayer, L., Eggermann, E., Saint-Mleux, B. *et al.* (2002). Selective action of orexin (hypocretin) on nonspecific thalamocortical projection neurons. *J. Neurosci.* **22**, 7835–9.

Bayer, L., Serafin, M., Eggermann, E. *et al.* (2004). Exclusive postsynaptic action of hypocretin-orexin on sublayer 6b cortical neurons. *J. Neurosci.* **24**, 6760–4.

Bayer, L., Eggermann, E., Serafin, M. *et al.* (2005). Opposite effects of noradrenaline and acetylcholine upon hypocretin/orexin versus melanin concentrating hormone neurons in rat hypothalamic slices. *Neuroscience* **130**, 807–11.

Besset, A., Tafti, M., Nobile, L. & Billiard, M. (1994). Homeostasis and narcolepsy. *Sleep* **17**, S29–34.

Beuckmann, C. T., Sinton, C. M., Williams, S. C. *et al.* (2004). Expression of a poly-glutamine-ataxin-3 transgene in orexin neurons induces narcolepsy-cataplexy in the rat. *J. Neurosci.* **24**, 4469–77.

Bittencourt, J. C., Presse, F., Arias, C. *et al.* (1992). The melanin-concentrating hormone system of the rat brain: an immuno- and hybridization histochemical characterization. *J. Comp. Neurol.* **319**, 218–45.

Bland, B. H. (1986). The physiology and pharmacology of hippocampal formation theta rhythms. *Prog. Neurobiol.* **26**, 1–54.

Borbely, A. A. (1977). Sleep in the rat during food deprivation and subsequent restitution of food. *Brain Res.* **124**, 457–71.

Broughton, R., Dunham, W., Newman, J. *et al.* (1988). Ambulatory 24 hour sleep-wake monitoring in narcolepsy-cataplexy compared to matched controls. *Electroencephalogr. Clin. Neurophysiol.* **70**, 473–81.

Broughton, R., Krupa, S., Boucher, B., Rivers, M. & Mullington, J. (1998). Impaired circadian waking arousal in narcolepsy-cataplexy. *Sleep Res. Online* **1**, 159–65.

Burdakov, D., Gerasimenko, O. & Verkhratsky, A. (2005). Physiological changes in glucose differentially modulate the excitability of hypothalamic melanin-concentrating hormone and orexin neurons in situ. *J. Neurosci.* **25**, 2429–33.

Burlet, S., Tyler, C. J. & Leonard, C. S. (2002). Direct and indirect excitation of laterodorsal tegmental neurons by Hypocretin/Orexin peptides: implications for wakefulness and narcolepsy. *J. Neurosci.* **22**, 2862–72.

Cai, X. J., Liu, X. H., Evans, M. *et al.* (2002). Orexins and feeding: special occasions or everyday occurrence? *Regul. Pept.* **104**, 1–9.

Chabas, D., Taheri, S., Renier, C. & Mignot, E. (2003). The genetics of narcolepsy. *A. Rev. Genomics Hum. Genet.* **4**, 459–83.

Chemelli, R. M., Willie, J. T., Sinton, C. M. *et al.* (1999). Narcolepsy in orexin knockout mice: molecular genetics of sleep regulation. *Cell* **98**, 437–51.

Choo, K. L. & Guilleminault, C. (1998). Narcolepsy and idiopathic hypersomnolence. *Clin. Chest Med.* **19**, 169–81.

Chou, T. C., Bjorkum, A. A., Gaus, S. E. *et al.* (2002). Afferents to the ventrolateral preoptic nucleus. *J. Neurosci.* **22**, 977–90.

Dahmen, N., Bierbrauer, J. & Kasten, M. (2001). Increased prevalence of obesity in narcoleptic patients and relatives. *Eur. Arch. Psychiatry Clin. Neurosci.* **251**, 85–9.

Dantz, B., Edgar, D. M. & Dement, W. C. (1994). Circadian rhythms in narcolepsy: studies on a 90 minute day. *Electroencephalogr. Clin. Neurophysiol.* **90**, 24–35.

Dauvilliers, Y., Carlander, B., Rivier, F., Touchon, J. & Tafti, M. (2004). Successful management of cataplexy with intravenous immunoglobulins at narcolepsy onset. *Ann. Neurol.* **56**, 905–8.

de Lecea, L. & Sutcliffe, J. G. (2005). The hypocretins and sleep. *FEBS J.* **272**, 5675–88.

de Lecea, L., Kilduff, T. S., Peyron, C. *et al.* (1998). The hypocretins: hypothalamus-specific peptides with neuroexcitatory activity. *Proc. Natl. Acad. Sci. USA* **95**, 322–7.

de Lecea, L., Sutcliffe, J. G. & Fabre, V. (2002). Hypocretins/orexins as integrators of physiological information: lessons from mutant animals. *Neuropeptides* **36**, 85–95.

Dewasmes, G., Duchamp, C. & Minaire, Y. (1989). Sleep changes in fasting rats. *Physiol. Behav.* **46**, 179–84.

Dijk, D. J. & Czeisler, C. A. (1994). Paradoxical timing of the circadian rhythm of sleep propensity serves to consolidate sleep and wakefulness in humans. *Neurosci. Lett.* **166**, 63–8.

Edgar, D. M., Dement, W. C. & Fuller, C. A. (1993). Effect of SCN lesions on sleep in squirrel monkeys: evidence for opponent processes in sleep-wake regulation. *J. Neurosci.* **13**, 1065–79.

Eggermann, E., Serafin, M., Bayer, L. *et al.* (2001). Orexins/hypocretins excite basal forebrain cholinergic neurones. *Neuroscience* **108**, 177–81.

Eriksson, K. S., Sergeeva, O., Brown, R. E. & Haas, H. L. (2001). Orexin/hypocretin excites the histaminergic neurons of the tuberomammillary nucleus. *J. Neurosci.* **21**, 9273–9.

Fujiki, N., Yoshida, Y., Ripley, B. *et al.* (2001). Changes in CSF hypocretin-1 (orexin A) levels in rats across 24 hours and in response to food deprivation. *Neuroreport* **12**, 993–7.

Gallopin, T., Fort, P., Eggermann, E. *et al.* (2000). Identification of sleep-promoting neurons in vitro. *Nature* **404**, 992–5.

Gélineau, J. B. E. (1880). De la narcolepsie. *Gazette des Hôpitaux (Paris)*, **53**, 626–8.

Guilleminault, C. & Gelb, M. (1995). Clinical aspects and features of cataplexy. *Adv. Neurol.* **67**, 65–77.

Hagan, J. J., Leslie, R. A., Patel, S. *et al.* (1999). Orexin A activates locus coeruleus cell firing and increases arousal in the rat. *Proc. Natl. Acad. Sci. USA* **96**, 10911–16.

Hara, J., Beuckmann, C. T., Nambu, T. *et al.* (2001). Genetic ablation of orexin neurons in mice results in narcolepsy, hypophagia, and obesity. *Neuron* **30**, 345–54.

Hishikawa, Y. & Shimizu, T. (1995). Physiology of REM sleep, cataplexy, and sleep paralysis. *Adv. Neurol.* **67**, 245–71.

Hoang, Q. V., Bajic, D., Yanagisawa, M., Nakajima, S. & Nakajima, Y. (2003). Effects of orexin (hypocretin) on GIRK channels. *J. Neurophysiol.* **90**, 693–702.

Honda, Y. (1988). Clinical features of narcolepsy: Japanese experiences. In *HLA in Narcolepsy*, ed. Y. Honda & T. Juji, Berlin: Springer-Verlag, pp. 24–57.

Honda, Y., Takahashi, Y., Honda, M. *et al.* (1997). Genetic aspects of narcolepsy. In *Sleep and Sleep Disorders: from Molecules to Behavior*, ed. O. Hayaishi & S. Inoue, New York: Academic Press, pp. 341–58.

International Classification of Sleep Disorders: Diagnostic and Coding Manual (1990). Rochester, MN: American Sleep Disorders Association.

John, J., Wu, M. F., Boehmer, L. N. & Siegel, J. M. (2004). Cataplexy-active neurons in the hypothalamus: implications for the role of histamine in sleep and waking behavior. *Neuron* **42**, 619–34.

Karteris, E., Machado, R. J., Chen, J. *et al.* (2005). Food deprivation differentially modulates orexin receptor expression and signaling in rat hypothalamus and adrenal cortex. *Am. J. Physiol. Endocrinol. Metab.* **288**, E1089–100.

Kisanuki, Y. Y., Chemelli, R. M., Sinton, C. M. *et al.* (2000). The role of orexin receptor type-1 (OX_1R) in the regulation of sleep. *Sleep* **23** (Suppl. 2), A91.

Kisanuki, Y. Y., Chemelli, R. M., Tokita, S. *et al.* (2001). Behavioral and polysomnographic characterization of orexin-1 receptor and orexin-2 receptor double knockout mice. *Sleep* **24** (Suppl.), A22.

Kohlmeier, K. A., Chemelli, R. M., Willie, J. T. *et al.* (2003). Hypocretin/Orexin (H/O) elevates [Ca2+]i in locus ceruleus (LC) neurons via activation of OX_1 and OX_2 receptors. *Sleep*, **26** (Suppl.), A21–2.

Kohlmeier, K. A., Inoue, T. & Leonard, C. S. (2004). Hypocretin/orexin peptide signaling in the ascending arousal system: elevation of intracellular calcium in the mouse dorsal raphe and laterodorsal tegmentum. *J. Neurophysiol.* **92**, 221–35.

Lee, M. G., Chrobak, J. J., Sik, A., Wiley, R. G. & Buzsaki, G. (1994). Hippocampal theta activity following selective lesion of the septal cholinergic system. *Neuroscience* **62**, 1033–47.

Li, Y., Gao, X. B., Sakurai, T. & van den Pol, A. N. (2002). Hypocretin/Orexin excites hypocretin neurons via a local glutamate neuron-A potential mechanism for orchestrating the hypothalamic arousal system. *Neuron* **36**, 1169–81.

Lin, L., Faraco, J., Li, R. *et al.* (1999). The sleep disorder canine narcolepsy is caused by a mutation in the hypocretin (orexin) receptor 2 gene. *Cell* **98**, 365–76.

Liu, R. J., van den Pol, A. N. & Aghajanian, G. K. (2002). Hypocretins (orexins) regulate serotonin neurons in the dorsal raphe nucleus by excitatory direct and inhibitory indirect actions. *J. Neurosci.* **22**, 9453–64.

Lu, J., Greco, M. A., Shiromani, P. & Saper, C. B. (2000). Effect of lesions of the ventrolateral preoptic nucleus on NREM and REM sleep. *J. Neurosci.* **20**, 3830–42.

Manns, I. D., Alonso, A. & Jones, B. E. (2003). Rhythmically discharging basal forebrain units comprise cholinergic, GABAergic, and putative glutamatergic cells. *J. Neurophysiol.* **89**, 1057–66.

Marcus, J. N. & Elmquist, J. K. (2006). Orexin projections and localization of orexin receptors. In *The Orexin/Hypocretin System: Physiology and Pathophysiology*, ed. S. Nishino & T. Sakurai, Totowa, NJ: Humana Press, pp. 21–43.

Marcus, J. N., Aschkenasi, C. J., Lee, C. E. *et al.* (2001). Differential expression of orexin receptors 1 and 2 in the rat brain. *J. Comp. Neurol.* **435**, 6–25.

Mieda, M. & Yanagisawa, M. (2002). Sleep, feeding, and neuropeptides: roles of orexins and orexin receptors. *Curr. Opin. Neurobiol.* **12**, 339–45.

Mieda, M. & Yanagisawa, M. (2006). Rodent models of narcolepsy-cataplexy. In *The Orexin/Hypocretin System: Physiology and Pathophysiology*, ed. S. Nishino & T. Sakurai, Totowa, NJ: Humana Press, pp. 255–66.

Mieda, M., Williams, S. C., Sinton, C. M. *et al.* (2004a). Orexin neurons function in an efferent pathway of a food-entrainable circadian oscillator in eliciting food-anticipatory activity and wakefulness. *J. Neurosci.* **24**, 10493–501.

Mieda, M., Willie, J. T., Hara, J. *et al.* (2004b). Orexin peptides prevent cataplexy and improve wakefulness in an orexin neuron-ablated model of narcolepsy in mice. *Proc. Natl. Acad. Sci. USA* **101**, 4649–54.

Mignot, E. (1998). Genetic and familial aspects of narcolepsy. *Neurology* **50**, S16–S22.

Mignot, E., Lin, L., Rogers, W. *et al.* (2001). Complex HLA-DR and -DQ interactions confer risk of narcolepsy-cataplexy in three ethnic groups. *Am. J. Hum. Genet.* **68**, 686–99.

Mochizuki, T., Crocker, A., McCormack, S. *et al.* (2004). Behavioral state instability in orexin knock-out mice. *J. Neurosci.* **24**, 6291–300.

Nambu, T., Sakurai, T., Mizukami, K. *et al.* (1999). Distribution of orexin neurons in the adult rat brain. *Brain Res.* **827**, 243–60.

Nishino, S., Riehl, J., Hong, J. *et al.* (2000a). Is narcolepsy a REM sleep disorder? Analysis of sleep abnormalities in narcoleptic Dobermans. *Neurosci. Res.* **38**, 437–6.

Nishino, S., Ripley, B., Overeem, S., Lammers, G. J. & Mignot, E. (2000b). Hypocretin (orexin) deficiency in human narcolepsy. *Lancet* **355**, 39–40.

Peyron, C., Tighe, D. K., van den Pol, A. N. *et al.* (1998). Neurons containing hypocretin (orexin) project to multiple neuronal systems. *J. Neurosci.* **18**, 9,996–10,015.

Peyron, C., Faraco, J., Rogers, W. *et al.* (2000). A mutation in a case of early onset narcolepsy and a generalized absence of hypocretin peptides in human narcoleptic brains. *Nat. Med.* **6**, 991–7.

Saito, Y., Cheng, M., Leslie, F. M. & Civelli, O. (2001). Expression of the melanin-concentrating hormone (MCH) receptor mRNA in the rat brain. *J. Comp. Neurol.* **435**, 26–40.

Sakurai, T., Amemiya, A., Ishii, M. *et al.* (1998). Orexins and orexin receptors: a family of hypothalamic neuropeptides and G protein-coupled receptors that regulate feeding behavior. *Cell* **92**, 573–85.

Saper, C. B., Chou, T. C. & Scammell, T. E. (2001). The sleep switch: hypothalamic control of sleep and wakefulness. *Trends Neurosci.* **24**, 726–31.

Shimada, M., Tritos, N. A., Lowell, B. B., Flier, J. S. & Maratos-Flier, E. (1998). Mice lacking melanin-concentrating hormone are hypophagic and lean. *Nature* **396**, 670–4.

Sinton, C. M. & McCarley, R. W. (2004). Neurophysiological mechanisms of sleep and wakefulness: a question of balance. *Semin. Neurol.* **24**, 211–23.

Snider, L. A. & Swedo, S. E. (2004). PANDAS: current status and directions for research. *Mol. Psychiatry.* **9**, 900–7.

Steininger, T. L., Kilduff, T. S., Behan, M., Benca, R. M. & Landry, C. F. (2004). Comparison of hypocretin/orexin and melanin-concentrating hormone neurons and axonal projections in the embryonic and postnatal rat brain. *J. Chem. Neuroanat.* **27**, 165–81.

Sturzenegger, C. & Bassetti, C. L. (2004). The clinical spectrum of narcolepsy with cataplexy: a reappraisal. *J. Sleep Res.* **13**, 395–406.

Sutherland, G. R. & McNaughton, B. (2000). Memory trace reactivation in hippocampal and neocortical neuronal ensembles. *Curr. Opin. Neurobiol.* **10**, 180–6.

Swedo, S. E., Leonard, H. L., Garvey, M. *et al.* (1998). Pediatric autoimmune neuropsychiatric disorders associated with streptococcal infections: clinical description of the first 50 cases. *Am. J. Psychiatry* **155**, 264–71.

Szymusiak, R., Alam, N., Steininger, T. L. & McGinty, D. (1998). Sleep-waking discharge patterns of ventrolateral preoptic/anterior hypothalamic neurons in rats. *Brain Res.* **803**, 178–88.

Taheri, S., Sunter, D., Dakin, C. *et al.* (2000). Diurnal variation in orexin A immunoreactivity and prepro-orexin mRNA in the rat central nervous system. *Neurosci. Lett.* **279**, 109–12.

Taheri, S., Paterno, J., Lin, L. & Mignot, E. (2006). Narcolepsy and autoimmunity. In *The Orexin/Hypocretin System: Physiology and Pathophysiology*, ed. S. Nishino & T. Sakurai, Totowa, NJ: Humana Press, pp. 341–6.

Thannickal, T. C., Moore, R. Y., Nienhuis, R. *et al.* (2000). Reduced number of hypocretin neurons in human narcolepsy. *Neuron* **27**, 469–74.

Trivedi, P., Yu, H., MacNeil, D. J., Van der Ploeg, L. H. & Guan, X. M. (1998). Distribution of orexin receptor mRNA in the rat brain. *FEBS Lett.* **438**, 71–5.

van den Pol, A. N., Acuna-Goycolea, C., Clark, K. R. & Ghosh, P. K. (2004). Physiological properties of hypothalamic MCH neurons identified with selective expression of reporter gene after recombinant virus infection. *Neuron* **42**, 635–52.

Vertes, R. P. & Kocsis, B. (1997). Brainstem-diencephalo-septohippocampal systems controlling the theta rhythm of the hippocampus. *Neuroscience* **81**, 893–926.

Vinogradova, O. S. (1995). Expression, control, and probable functional significance of the neuronal theta-rhythm. *Prog. Neurobiol.* **45**, 523–83.

Westphal, C. F. O. (1877). Eigenthümliche mit einschäfen verbundene Anfälle. *Archiv. Psychiat. Nervenkrank.* **7**, 631–5.

Williams, G., Cai, X. J., Elliott, J. C. & Harrold, J. A. (2004). Anabolic neuropeptides. *Physiol. Behav.* **81**, 211–22.

Willie, J. T. & Yanagisawa, M. (2007). Lessons from sleepy mice: narcolepsy-cataplexy and the orexin neuropeptide system. In *Narcolepsy and Hypersomnia*, ed. C. Bassetti, M. Billiard & E. Mignot, New York, NY: Informa Healthcare, pp. 257–78.

Willie, J. T., Chemelli, R. M., Sinton, C. M. & Yanagisawa, M. (2001). To eat or to sleep? Orexin in the regulation of feeding and wakefulness. *A. Rev. Neurosci.* **24**, 429–58.

Willie, J. T., Chemelli, R. M., Sinton, C. M. *et al.* (2003). Distinct narcolepsy syndromes in Orexin receptor-2 and Orexin null mice: molecular genetic dissection of Non-REM and REM sleep regulatory processes. *Neuron,* **38**, 715–30.

Willie, J. T., Renthal, W., Chemelli, R. M. *et al.* (2005). Modafinil more effectively induces wakefulness in orexin-null mice than in wild-type littermates. *Neuroscience,* **130**, 983–995.

Wu, M. F., John, J., Boehmer, L. N. *et al.* (2004). Activity of dorsal raphe cells across the sleep-waking cycle and during cataplexy in narcoleptic dogs. *J. Physiol.* **554**, 202–15.

Yamanaka, A., Beuckmann, C. T., Willie, J. T. *et al.* (2003). Hypothalamic orexin neurons regulate arousal according to energy balance in mice. *Neuron* **38**, 701–13.

Yoshida, Y., Fujiki, N., Nakajima, T. *et al.* (2001). Fluctuation of extracellular hypocretin-1 (orexin A) levels in the rat in relation to the light-dark cycle and sleep-wake activities. *Eur. J. Neurosci.* **14**, 1075–81.

Zeitzer, J. M., Buckmaster, C. L., Parker, K. J. *et al.* (2003). Circadian and homeostatic regulation of hypocretin in a primate model: implications for the consolidation of wakefulness. *J. Neurosci.* **23**, 3555–60.

16

The relevance of experimental pharmacology to currently available sleep–wake therapeutics

RAFAEL J. SALIN-PASCUAL

Introduction

Determining the underlying therapeutic mechanisms of a drug makes pharmacology a powerful tool for understanding biological phenomena. This chapter reviews the preclinical evidence of the impact of some neurotransmitter systems and related drugs on sleep and wakefulness.

GABA-A and sleep

A series of neurotransmitter systems are responsible for maintaining wakefulness, including norepinephrine (NE), serotonin (5-HT), acetylcholine (ACh), dopamine (DA), excitatory amino acids, hypocretins (i.e. orexins), and histamine (Mendelson 2001; Monti and Jantos 2004; Salin-Pascual et al. 1999; Ursin 2002; Sakurai 2005). Delta sleep, or non-REM sleep, is related to adenosine, GABA, and prostaglandins, among others (Ekimova and Pastukhov 2005; Hayaishi and Matsumura 1995; Johnston 2005; Koyama and Hayaishi 1994). Finally, ACh has a prominent role in rapid eye movement (REM) sleep, together with 5-HT, NE, and hypocretin; these three molecules inhibit cholinergic and cholinoceptive neurons, which are implicated in the initiation of this sleep stage (McCarley 2004; Reinoso-Suarez et al. 2001).

GABA, and molecules that act at GABA-A receptors, have been classically recognized as hypnotics (i.e. benzodiazepines) and anesthetics (i.e. barbiturates). Benzodiazepine (BZD) receptors, a modulatory site on the GABA-A receptor, were

Neurochemistry of Sleep and Wakefulness, ed. J. M. Monti et al. Published by Cambridge University Press. © Cambridge University Press 2008.

discovered in the 1970s. Like other sites on the GABA-A receptor complex, these receptors work allosterically, cooperatively modifying channel permeability to chloride ions. BZDs enhance the GABA inhibitory effect by increasing the time that the chloride channels remain open (Johnston 2005). The GABA-A receptor complex has a pentameric structure, and belongs to the ionotropic receptor class (defined as such because ion channels are the effectors at these receptors). This receptor class includes glycine, serotoninergic (5-HT3), and nicotine receptors. The GABA-A receptor complex comprises five similar but not identical glycoprotein molecules; the differences could have some effect on the overall functioning of the receptor, and a series of subtypes of the receptor consist of various combinations of the different subunits (Johnston 2005).

GABA-A receptors have been identified with α, β, γ, π, ρ, ε, and θ subunits. In rats, there are six α subunits, four β subunits, three γ subunits, and three ρ subunits (Gottesmann 2002; Mölher et al. 1990; Varga et al. 2002; Wafford and Ebert 2006; Jia et al. 2005). GABA as a neurotransmitter is ubiquitous, whereas GABA-A receptors are densely located in certain sleep-related areas such as the hypothalamus. The importance of the hypothalamus in the regulation of wakefulness and sleep has been recently underlined (Jia et al. 2005). Stimulation of the BZD-binding site promotes non-REM sleep in humans, particularly stage II (with increased spindles) at the expense of stages III and IV, and inhibits REM sleep (and its associated eye movements) (Mendelson and Martin 1990; Lancel et al. 1996). In animals, most BZDs and barbiturates increase the intermediate stages of sleep and decrease or suppress REM sleep (Gandolfo et al. 1994). At the level of the central nervous system (CNS), BZDs injected in the dorsal raphe nucleus increase waking (Mendelson et al. 1987), and preoptic area lesions do not prevent the sleep-inducing effect of parenteral triazolam. These data are interpreted as demonstrating a redundancy of sleep-regulating mechanisms in the CNS.

A third generation of hypnotic compounds is primarily composed of the imidazopyridines (e.g. zolpidem) and the cyclopyrrolones (e.g. zopiclone). These compounds also bind to the GABA-A receptor complex, but are structurally different from BZDs. Zolpidem (Depoortere et al. 1986) binds to the $\alpha1$, $\beta2$, and $'\Omega$ subunits, with a preference for the variant $\gamma2L$ (Duncan et al. 1995). Zolpidem induces sleep at lower doses than the BZDs (Depoortere et al. 1986); clinically, this difference translates into a reduction in sleep latency and a more rapid induction of sleep (Lund et al. 1988; Declerck et al. 1992), without significant modifications in sleep architecture. In rats, zolpidem increases non-REM sleep (Depoortere et al. 1995) and decreases REM sleep during the first two hours after administration (Gottesmann et al. 1994), although this effect is not seen after six hours (Gottesmann et al. 1994).

The role of BZDs in sleep is regulated though GABAergic mechanisms. Three areas are important for the sleep-promoting qualities of these compounds: (a) the basal forebrain and preoptic areas (Saper *et al.* 2005a); (b) the centrolateral preoptic nucleus, with its dense projection to the tuberomamillary histaminergic nucleus (Saper *et al.* 2005b); and (c) the suprachiasmatic nucleus (SCN) (Edgar *et al.* 1993). BZDs may facilitate the release of a sleep debt accumulated during wakefulness, rather than induce de novo sleep (Nishino *et al.* 2004).

BZD effects on human sleep are well characterized (Mendelson 2001): (a) decreased sleep latency; (b) decreased awakenings; (c) increased stage II sleep; (d) suppressed stage III and IV sleep; (e) increased REM sleep latency; (f) initial reduction and fragmentation of REM sleep. Discontinuation of BZD treatment after three to four weeks produces a rebound of REM sleep as well as slow-wave sleep (SWS). BZD and non-BZD compounds are pharmacological agents indicated in the management of anxiety, insomnia, and other conditions in which anxiety is the main symptom, and should be considered as symptomatic medications (Nishino *et al.* 2004).

Tolerance and dependence occur with both BZD and non-BZD compounds; abrupt discontinuation results in withdrawal phenomena such as anxiety, agitation, restlessness, and hypertension. Tolerance, especially to the hypnotic effect, is known to occur, so an increase in dose is required to obtain the same effect (Liappas *et al.* 2003).

New compounds with direct action on the GABA-A receptor will be available in the near future. Gaboxadol, a selective extrasynaptic GABA receptor agonist is in the late stage of investigational treatment for insomnia. It acts on a unique GABA-A receptor subtype found exclusively outside the synapse (Wafford and Ebert 2006). Other compounds include non-BZD isomers and remelteon, a melatonin M-1 agonist (Mendelson 2001).

Antidepressants and sleep

Virtually all types of drug that have been shown to be effective in major depression exert profound effects on the functioning of the serotoninergic or noradrenergic systems, or both. Although some treatments have been shown to decrease the sensitivity of certain postsynaptic 5-HT and NE receptors, it is generally believed that it is an enhancement of neurotransmission in these systems that is responsible for the improvement of the core symptoms of depression. For instance, long-term administration of tricyclic antidepressants (TCAs) or monoamine oxidase inhibitors (MAOIs) decreases the density of β-adrenoceptors and cortical 5-HT2 receptors (Blier and Abbott 2003).

Because the effects of these drugs do not occur for at least several weeks, research into mechanisms has focused on specific targets such as signaling pathways coupled to transcription factors and their target genes. Among the most studied are components of the cAMP-regulated pathways such as the

GTP-binding proteins (G-proteins), which couple receptors to adenylyl cyclase, cAMP-dependent protein kinase, and cAMP regulatory element binding protein (CREB) and its phosphorylation (Dumann *et al.* 2004). Agents from the major antidepressant classes (i.e. TCAs, 5-HT reuptake inhibitors, and MAOIs) have all been shown to regulate multiple steps in this pathway (Nibuya *et al.* 1996). Long-term antidepressant treatment increases basal and stimulated adenylyl cyclase activity, increases cAMP-dependent phosphorylation, and increases CREB levels (Thome *et al.* 2000). In contrast, mood stabilizers such as lithium have been shown to decrease or blunt the activity of multiple components of this pathway in rat brain (Dowlatshahi *et al.* 1999). The opposing effects on this pathway may be relevant to their clinical effects. In the rat, long-term antidepressant administration increases levels of CREB mRNA in the CA1, CA3, and dentate gyrus regions of the hippocampus, and leads to increased CREB immunoreactivity and CRE binding activity. This result, found across several different classes of antidepressant, suggests that the upregulation of CREB may be a common target of 5-HT and NE systems, both of which are implicated in the pathophysiology of depression. Long-term administration of electroconvulsive shock (ECS) therapy was also found to increase levels of CREB mRNA, further supporting the potential relevance of changes in CREB levels in the treatment of depression (Dowlatshahi *et al.* 1999; Nibuya *et al.* 1995).

Sleep and depression

The median values of REM sleep latency, total time asleep, and SWS (in minutes and as a percentage of total time asleep) were lower, and REM sleep (percent) values were found to be higher, in depressive disorders than in all other psychiatric conditions. However, the statistical differences between depressed patients and other psychiatric categories were far less evident. Indeed, no sleep variable reliably distinguished depressed patients from those with other psychiatric disorders. The investigators concluded that sleep disturbances are associated with most psychiatric disorders, although the most widespread and most severe disturbances are found in patients with depressive disorders (Van Bemmel 1997).

It is now widely recognized that a number of sleep manipulations improve the symptoms of depression (Gillin 1983; Leibenluft and Wehr 1992). These include total and partial sleep deprivation, selective deprivation of REM sleep, and phase shifting of the sleep–wake cycle. Total and partial sleep deprivation induce an immediate improvement in about 60% of depressed subjects, but this effect is typically reversed by subsequent sleep. If total sleep deprivation is combined with antidepressant medication, starting on the day prior to the sleep deprivation, this sometimes prevents relapse after the recovery sleep (Elsenga and van den Hoofdakker 1993). It has also been reported that the response to sleep deprivation has some predictive value for the response to antidepressant medication (Vogel *et al.* 1968). The therapeutic effects of selective REM sleep deprivation on depression occur in about 50% of patients (Vogel *et al.* 1980; Gillin *et al.* 2001).

All antidepressant drugs have some effects on sleep architecture. Suppression of REM sleep associated with the treatment of depression was such a consistent finding in early studies that it was seen as essential for the antidepressant action. This belief was further supported by the evidence of a correlation between the clinical response and REM sleep suppression as well as a temporal relationship between the onset of clinical response and REM sleep suppression. However, some of the later studies suggested that REM sleep suppression is not necessary for the antidepressant action (Gillin 1983). For example, some studies show evidence of no change or even an increase in REM sleep with the treatment of depression (Gillin *et al.* 2001). Recently, Landolt & Gillin (Landolt and Gillin 2002) have also demonstrated that the antidepressant response to phenelzine treatment does not depend on elimination of REM sleep or inhibition of slow wave activity in non-REM sleep. However, the generalization of some of these studies is limited because of their small sample size.

Electroencephalogram (EEG) sleep studies on the use of antidepressants in depressed patients have not produced clear evidence of the involvement of REM or non-REM sleep in the mechanisms underlying clinical change. Furthermore, the role of the physiological mechanisms of sleep during treatment with antidepressants is still unclear. Further basic sleep research is necessary (Gillin 1983) to interpret the effects of antidepressants on EEG sleep in terms of the physiological processes of sleep.

The sleep-inducing effect of some antidepressants has been used as an additive strategy in depressed patients with complaints of insomnia to negate the side effects of BZDs that could be confused with worsening depressive symptoms, including asthenia, diurnal sedation, and concentration and memory problems. These drugs include trazodone, mianserine, and recently mirtazapine.

Winokur *et al.* (Winokur *et al.* 2000) found that mirtazapine significantly decreased sleep latency and increased total sleep time and sleep efficiency from baseline levels during week 1, with similar results observed after week 2. Mirtazapine did not significantly alter REM sleep parameters. Clinically, the Hamilton Depression Rating Scale and sleep disturbance ratings improved after treatment.

In a recent open clinical trial, patients receiving venlafaxine XR or fluoxetine for six weeks without sleep improvement were randomly assigned to either mirtazapine (7.5 mg) or zolpidem (10 mg). Although both groups improved in terms of their sleep, the patients with either fluoxetine or venlafaxine had a more rapid improvement in depression, as evaluated by the Hamilton depression scale, than the group being treated with zolpidem (Salin-Pascual 2005).

The combination of antidepressants is a common clinical practice. The most usual pharmacological profile is serotoninergic–noradrenergic (96%) and the most popular combinations are selective 5-HT reuptake inhibitor (SSRI) + mirtazapine, SSRI + reboxetine, and SSRI + TCAs (De la Gandara *et al.* 2005).

Antipsychotic medications and sleep

Sleep disturbances in schizophrenia have been well studied. Tandon *et al.* (Tandon *et al.* 1992) examined sleep disturbances in 40 patients with schizophrenia and found that they had a longer sleep latency, a higher number of arousals during sleep, and increased periods of wakefulness after sleep onset compared with those in a non-psychiatric control group, resulting in a lower sleep efficiency rating for the patients with schizophrenia. The control group had 95% sleep efficiency, whereas drug-naïve schizophrenic patients had a 78% sleep efficiency rating and previously treated patients had a 72% sleep efficiency rating.

The sleep disturbances of either never-medicated or previously treated schizophrenic patients are characterized by a sleep-onset and maintenance insomnia. In addition, stage IV sleep, slow wave sleep (i.e. stages III and IV), non-REM sleep duration, and REM latency are decreased (Monti and Monti 2005). In a study that compared non-medicated first-episode schizophrenics with controls, patients with schizophrenia had difficulty initiating sleep, decreased stage IV duration, and reduced REM sleep latency, but they had normal sleep spindles and REM densities. Positive symptoms correlated negatively with REM sleep latency; in a related finding, scores on a clinical scale of severity of the disorder correlated negatively with REM sleep duration and REM density. These results indicated that first-episode and medication-naive schizophrenic patients had difficulties initiating, but not maintaining, sleep. In addition, the data showed that the duration of stage IV and REM sleep latency were reduced in these patients. The fact that measures of REM sleep correlated with a clinical scale of schizophrenia also suggested that REM sleep physiology shared some common features with symptoms of the disease (Polulin *et al.* 2003).

Risperidone may prolong SWS in patients because it has a higher affinity for serotoninergic 5-HT2 receptors than haloperidol. 5-HT2 receptors have been reported to be implicated in modulating the quality of sleep. Olanzapine, another atypical antipsychotic, also has a high affinity for 5-HT2 receptors (Collaborative Working Group on Clinical Trial Evaluations 1998). Thus, although the sedative effects of some antipsychotic medications may have a negative impact on patients, atypical antipsychotics such as risperidone and olanzapine may have the potential to improve the quality of sleep in schizophrenics.

In a previous study from our laboratory, twenty inpatient drug-free schizophrenic patients were studied. Patients slept for five consecutive nights in the sleep unit as follows: one acclimatization night; two baseline nights (the first for sleep disorder screenings); and two olanzapine nights (10 mg olanzapine, one hour before sleep onset). Overall, results showed that sleep continuity variables and total sleep time were improved with olanzapine. Waking time was reduced after the first night of olanzapine administration. The primary sleep architecture changes were a reduction in stage I sleep, while stage II sleep and SWS were significantly enhanced. REM density was also increased by the second olanzapine night. Total sleep improvement after olanzapine treatment was due to the increase in sleep stages II and delta SWS; as noted above, this may be related to the serotoninergic antagonistic properties of olanzapine (Salin-Pascual et al. 1999).

A series of antipsychotics having different selectivity for the dopaminergic D-1 and D-2 receptors were studied for their effects on sleep stages in the rat (Ongini et al. 1993). EEG activity was recorded and classified according to the stages of wakefulness, REM sleep, and non-REM sleep. Total sleep duration, non-REM and REM sleep latencies, and the number and duration of REM sleep episodes were also calculated. The D-1 antagonists SCH 23390 (0.001–0.1 mg/kg s.c.), SCH 39166 (0.01–0.3 mg/kg s.c.) and NNC-756 (0.003–0.1 mg/kg s.c.) markedly enhanced the time spent in sleep through a significant increase of both non-REM and REM sleep. The increase in REM sleep was due to an increase in the number of episodes. In contrast, the selective D-2 antagonists raclopride (0.03–1 mg/kg s.c.) and remoxipride (1–10 mg/kg s.c.) did not affect sleep. Haloperidol (0.1–3 mg/kg p.o.) increased the duration of total sleep by increasing non-REM sleep, without change to REM sleep. The non-selective DA antagonists chlorpromazine (0.3–3 mg/kg s.c.) and clozapine (0.3–3 mg/kg s.c.) produced either no effect or slightly increased non-REM sleep, respectively. Both compounds reduced REM sleep time by reducing the number and duration of episodes. These data thus show that there are differences between D-1 and D-2 antagonists with regard to their effects on sleep and wakefulness. Concomitant enhancement of both total sleep and REM sleep appears to be a specific feature that clearly distinguishes D-1 antagonists from the other DA receptor blockers.

In another study, the effects on sleep of the D-1 antagonist SCH 23390 were compared with those of haloperidol, a D-2 antagonist, in rats. Over a very small dose range (0.003–0.03 mg/kg, s.c.), SCH 23390 significantly increased the time spent in total sleep, including REM and non-REM sleep. The magnitude of the overall change in REM sleep was considerably greater than that of the change in non-REM sleep. Enhancement of the amount of REM sleep was characterized by an increase in the number of episodes without change of the latency to the first period of REM sleep. Haloperidol (0.3–3mg/kg p.o.) increased non-REM sleep but did not affect measures of REM sleep. Considering the small dose range at which SCH 23390 was effective, and the fact that REM and non-REM sleep may be unrelated events, it was suggested that promotion of REM sleep is a specific effect induced by selective blockade of D-1 receptors (Trampus and Ongini 1990; Trampus et al. 1993).

Sleep and sedative effects of the atypical antipsychotics could be related to different mechanisms: antagonism of 5-HT2 receptors, antihistaminic and antimuscarinic effects, and probably an α-1 noradrenergic effect. The difference in the effect on sleep between risperidone and haloperidol may be due to their differential actions on serotoninergic receptors (Trampus and Ongini 1990; Trampus et al. 1993).

Central nervous system stimulants and sleep

Some CNS stimulants have an effect on the same systems that are involved in wakefulness, including glutamate-, NE-, DA-, 5-HT-, histamine-, hypocretin- and ACh-containing neurons. This group includes molecules such as cocaine, amphetamine, and nicotine. The sleep-promoting systems are concentrated in the medial part of the brainstem, dorsal reticular substance of the medulla, anterior hypothalamus, and basal forebrain (Jones 2005). Other stimulants, such as caffeine and theophylline, block some sleep-inducing mechanisms. Modafinil is also a CNS stimulant with an unknown mechanism of action.

Dopamine-acting drugs

Historically, stimulants that increase the activity of catecholamines are the oldest drugs in this group (Jones et al. 1973). Reduction in DA activity has been related to a reduction in wakefulness; lesions of DA cell groups in the ventral tegmentum that project to the forebrain have been shown to induce a marked reduction in behavioral arousal in rats (Jones et al. 1973), and patients with Parkinson's disease, who exhibit consistent DA lesions, experience severe sleep disorders (Rye and Jankovic 2002).

One of the most common psychostimulants, cocaine, is derived from the coca plant (Erythroxylon coca) and has a long history as a stimulant. It has been used for centuries in Bolivia and Peru as a tonic and other preparations to alleviate fatigue (Siegel 1985; Hill et al. 1977).

One class of stimulants, the amphetamines, was synthesized originally as possible alternative drugs for the treatment of asthma and was a principal component of the original Benzedrine™. Amphetamine-like stimulants are known and consumed especially for their activity-sustaining effects (i.e. increased alertness, strength, and endurance). Their wake-promoting properties are evident; objective studies have clearly established their effects on sleep. In rats, cocaine (6 mg/kg, i.p. or p.o.) has been shown to induce a significant increase in sleep latency and a reduction in total sleep time, including a decrease in both non-REM sleep and REM sleep (Schwartz 2004). In humans, cocaine, amphetamines, and methylphenidate also produce decreases in sleepiness, an increased latency to sleep, and a marked decrease in REM sleep associated with an increased latency to the onset of this state. Amphetamine, methylphenidate, and cocaine are known to act by enhancing the amount of the monoamines available within the synaptic cleft of synapses in the CNS. They block the reuptake and also enhance the release of NE, DA and 5-HT (Benerjee *et al.* 2004). There is considerable evidence suggesting that the primary action responsible for their psychostimulant effects is on the CNS DA system (Nehlig 1999).

Thus, amphetamine-like drugs may promote wakefulness primarily by increasing dopaminergic tone. Accordingly, it has been found that intracerebroventricular infusion of D-1 and D-2 receptor agonists in sleeping rats induces a dose-dependent increase in time awake (Benerjee *et al.* 2004).

Caffeine and sleep

Caffeine is the most widely consumed psychoactive substance. Peak plasma caffeine is reached between 15 and 120 minutes after oral ingestion in humans at doses of 5–8 mg/kg. The caffeine half-life ranges from 0.7 to 1.2 h in rodents, from 3 to 5 h in monkeys, and from 2.5 to 4.5 h in humans (Nehlig 1999).

There is consensus that caffeine produces an enhanced vigilance performance on psychomotor tasks and concomitant negative side effects on sleep, particularly when taken at bedtime (Trampus and Ongini 1990). Generally, more than 100–150 mg of caffeine is needed to affect sleep significantly. The most prominent effects are prolonged sleep latency, shortened total sleep time with increases in the light sleep stages at the expense of SWS and REM sleep, sleep fragmentation, and even agitation at higher doses (Landolt *et al.* 2004). EEG studies have shown that sleep is of a lesser quality in the 3–4 h following ingestion of caffeinated coffee, which corresponds to the time required for the liver to metabolize caffeine. It has been suggested that subjects who are sensitive to the effects of coffee might metabolize caffeine more slowly than others (Levy and Zylber-Katz 1983). However, some people seem to have no sleep troubles despite drinking coffee in the evening, an effect that could be attributed to tolerance to its psychoactive effects. In rats, caffeine (12.5–25 mg/kg) decreases the overall duration of sleep and lengthens sleep latency (Levy and Zylber-Katz 1983) whereas, when chronically administered to cats (20 mg/kg), caffeine initially shortened the total sleep duration, but then sleep amounts returned to baseline with repeated exposure (Radulovacki *et al.* 1980; Sinton and Petitjean 1989; Linden 1999).

The mechanism by which caffeine promotes vigilance is related to the antagonism of adenosine. The hypnogenic effects of adenosine were first described in cats by Feldberg & Sherwood in 1954 (Feldberg and Sherwood 1954) and later in dogs by Haulica *et al.* in 1973 (Haulica *et al.* 1973). Since then the sedative effects of parenteral and central administrations of adenosine have been repeatedly demonstrated (Radulovacki *et al.* 1984; Virus *et al.* 1983). Well-known stimulants, such as caffeine and theophylline, antagonize the effects of adenosine by acting as antagonists at adenosine receptors (Fredholm and Lindstrom 1999). Later studies revealed that adenosine analogs promote SWS. Adenosine tends to accumulate in the extracellular space during wakefulness, most notably when the subject is sleep-deprived. At the same time, extracellular adenosine is reduced during sleep (Porkka-Heiskanen *et al.* 1997a). For these reasons it has been proposed that adenosine accumulation could be a substrate for process "S" in the "two model hypothesis of sleep". Neuronal metabolism is high during wakefulness, with increased extracellular adenosine levels that decrease after sleep onset (Porkka-Heiskanen *et al.* 1997b; Maquet *et al.* 1992; Mitchell *et al.* 1993). A circadian rhythm of adenosine similar to that seen in other mammalian species was described in human plasma, with high levels during wakefulness and proportional reductions during sleep (Chagoya de Sanchez *et al.* 1996).

A possible mechanism for the sleep-inducing effects of adenosine is based on results from in vitro electrophysiological studies. Adenosine was found to have a postsynaptic inhibitory effect on basal forebrain neurons, as well as on neurons in the cholinergic laterodorsal tegmental nuclei (LDT). Both cholinergic and non-cholinergic neurons were hyperpolarized by adenosine, an effect that was mediated by an inwardly rectifying K^+ conductance and, in the LDT, also by blockade of the hyperpolarization-activated current. In addition, tonic inhibition of LDT cholinergic neurons via pre-synaptic adenosine A-1 receptors has been demonstrated (Arrigoni *et al.* 2003). These observations support the idea that adenosine might promote sleepiness by inhibiting activity and neurotransmitter release of wakefulness-promoting neurons. The inhibitory effects of adenosine might be exerted on both cholinergic and non-cholinergic neurons. The cholinergic basal forebrain is an important area for mediating the somnogenic effects of adenosine after prolonged sleep deprivation, and the effects of adenosine in this area are mediated by adenosine A-1 receptors (Morairty *et al.* 2004).

An unanswered question about adenosine is how this inhibitory neurotransmitter activates the ventrolateral preoptic area of the hypothalamus (VLPO), which contains a population of sleep-active neurons and is hypothesized to be an important part of the somnogenic process. Whole-cell patch-clamp recordings were obtained from rat brain slices, and drugs were bath applied. VLPO neurons were electrophysiologically heterogeneous, but the data were consistent with the hypothesis that one mechanism by which adenosine might promote sleep is by blocking inhibitory inputs to the VLPO sleep-active neurons (Morairty *et al.* 2004).

As previously proposed, adenosine effects on sleep could also be mediated through the interaction with GABA (Mendelson 2000). In fact, adenosine A-2A receptors have been found on GABAergic cells. In a recent study, the effect of the selective A-2A receptor antagonist KW6002 was investigated on A-2A receptors in the rat nucleus accumbens in vitro and in vivo (Harper *et al.* 2006). Radioligand binding studies confirmed a greater than 50-fold selectivity of KW6002 for A-2A receptors compared with A-1 receptors. Release of [^{3}H]DA from nucleus accumbens slices in vitro was almost doubled in the presence of 300 nM KW6002, while GABA release was inhibited by approximately one-third. In another study, the interactions between A-2A receptors and dopaminergic D-2 receptors on the modulation of depolarization-evoked [^{3}H]GABA release were examined in globus pallidus slices from the rat. The stimulation of release caused by activation of A-2A receptors was blocked when dopaminergic influences were eliminated by three independent methods: (a) antagonism of D-2 receptors with sulpiride; (b) alkylation of these receptors with *N*-ethoxycarbonyl-2-ethoxy-1, 2-dihydroquinoline (EEDQ); and (c) depletion of DA with reserpine. In turn, activation of A-2A receptors modified the response to stimulation of D-2 receptors: the EC$_{50}$ for quinpirole increased nearly one thousand times when A-2A receptors were stimulated. Antagonism of A-2A receptors in the absence of agonists inhibited [^{3}H]GABA release, indicating receptor occupancy by endogenous adenosine (Floran *et al.* 2005).

The interest of our group in adenosine relates to sleep and aging. There are several sleep changes with age: sleep fragmentation, increased time awake, decreases in the length of sleep bouts, and changes in the amplitude of the diurnal rhythms of sleep and REM sleep (Bliwise 2005). Several species, including rats (Shiromani *et al.* 2000), cats (Bowersox *et al.* 1984), monkeys (Pegram *et al.* 1969), and humans (Pegram *et al.* 1969), have a pronounced decline in the amplitude of EEG slow wave activity. This decline in sleep cannot be attributed to a loss of neurons implicated in sleep mechanisms: the number of neurons in the VLPO, one of the regions implicated in generating sleep, is similar in young (3.5 months) and old (21.5 months) rats (Porkka-Heiskanen *et al.* 1997a; Lund *et al.* 1988). Another possibility was a deterioration in the function of the suprachiasmatic nucleus, but that has also been ruled out (Shiromani *et al.* 2000). An alternative explanation could be related to the functioning of the adenosine system. One way to explore this was through the effects of caffeine on the sleep–wake pattern of both animals and humans.

Caffeine is an antagonist at A-1 and A-2A adenosine receptors and is a potent wake-promoting agent. Caffeine (10, 11, 12, 13, 14, 15 mg/kg i.p.) elicited a dose-dependent increase in waking in rats, antagonizing the increase of delta sleep seen after sleep deprivation (Bowersox *et al.* 1984; Pegram *et al.* 1969). Spectral analysis in humans has also shown that delta power is reduced after caffeine (Czeisler *et al.* 1999). Caffeine has been used to promote alertness during prolonged wakefulness. Following 49 h of prolonged wakefulness, various doses of caffeine or placebo were administered to human volunteers in a randomized double-blind design. Wakefulness continued for an additional 12 h. Following caffeine administration, sleep latency, sleepiness scored by the Epworth scale, and reaction time showed dose-related changes that indicated that high does of caffeine had a significant effect on alertness during prolonged wakefulness (Czeisler *et al.* 1999). Similar results have been found in other studies (Schwierin *et al.* 1996; Landolt *et al.* 2004; Kamimori *et al.* 2000; Bardwell *et al.* 2000; Lagarde *et al.* 2000). This effect on alertness may help some patients with excessive somnolence, such as obstructive sleep apnea (OSA) patients. In a naturalistic study, patients with OSA reported significantly greater caffeine consumption than those without OSA (Kamimori *et al.* 2000; Bardwell *et al.* 2000). In cats, caffeine (20 mg/kg per day p.o.) administered chronically produced an initial marked increase in waking. A tolerance phenomenon was later observed and total sleep time was recovered, but animals slept more in stage I of non-REM sleep than in stage II. After caffeine administration ended, an increase of stage II sleep was observed (Lagarde *et al.* 2000). Caffeine at low doses and repeated administration could be effective in dealing with reduced awakening tonic activity, as has been shown during extended wakefulness of more than 24 h (Wurts and Edgar 2000).

To test the possibility that the reduction in sleep with age might be due to changes at the level of the adenosine receptor, the effects of caffeine on sleep in young (3 months), middle-aged (10 months) and old rats (21 months) were examined. It was hypothesized that old rats should be more sensitive to the wake-promoting effects of caffeine compared with young rats. We found that middle-aged and old rats were in fact more sensitive to the alerting effects of caffeine than young rats. We also found that, after sleep deprivation, recovery differed depending on the age of the animals, and that recovery with caffeine was reduced in middle-aged animals but not in the other two groups (Salin-Pascual *et al.* 2000).

The possibility that adenosine production was reduced or deficiently accumulated during wakefulness, which would explain the reduction in SWS, sleep fragmentation, and overall reduced sleep drive in the older animals, was also studied. Microdialysis measurements of adenosine in the basal forebrain were made in old (21.5 months) and young (3.5 months) rats. The older animals had higher adenosine levels than the young rats. Also, when both groups of animals were sleep deprived for 6 h, the older rats had higher amounts of adenosine. Thus, we next asked why the older rats, despite more adenosine, slept less. Changes in the number or sensitivity of adenosine receptors were explored by challenging with an A-1 adenosine agonist. Older rats had a smaller increase in delta sleep than the young rats, supporting the hypothesis of deficits in adenosine receptor mechanisms (Salin-Pascual *et al.* 2000). Higher levels of adenosine in the older animals could thus downregulate or reduce the sensitivity of the adenosine receptor, hence providing an explanation for sleep changes in the older subjects.

Adenosine A-1 receptor density was examined in rat brain by means of quantitative autoradiography to obtain a detailed anatomical overview of the changes during ageing (Murillo-Rodriguez *et al.* 2004). A-1 receptor binding was assessed in young, old, and senescent animals of 3, 24, and 30 months old, respectively. There was a notable age-dependent reduction in adenosine A-1 receptors in most of the brain areas examined, but the magnitude of this reduction varied greatly among regions. Also, whereas some regions displayed a gradual decline in A-1 binding sites across the three age groups, other regions showed a particularly marked decrease between the ages of 24 and 30 months. For example, whereas the hippocampus and thalamus showed a gradual decline in A-1 binding, some cortical and septal regions showed a more abrupt decline after the age of 24 months (Meerlo *et al.* 2004; Singh 1998).

A hypocaloric diet is one of the few methods that has been shown to retard age-related effects (Singh 1998; Algeri *et al.* 1991). However, the effects of such a diet on sleep had never been investigated. We designed a study using 21-month-old male rats that were fed a 60% calorie-reduced diet. Older rats continued to show a significant reduction in delta power (0.3–4 Hz EEG), less sleep following 12 h of total sleep deprivation, and increased sensitivity to caffeine compared with young rats (3 months) fed a similar diet. These results indicate that caloric restriction is unable to prevent the decline in sleep that occurs with aging (Salin-Pascual *et al.* 2002).

Insomnia is defined as difficulty falling asleep, difficulty remaining asleep, and early morning awakening/or non-restorative sleep (Thorphy 1990). In addition, insomnia could be categorized as a symptom or a disease, in both cases with a significant impact on an individual's physical and social performance, ability to work, and quality of life (Billiard and Bentley 2004). The possibility that insomnia patients may have a low homeostatic drive for sleep was explored recently in a study by administering a caffeine challenge (200 mg) to six primary insomniac patients, compared with normal volunteers (Salin-Pascual *et al.* 2006). Both groups were studied as follows: one night of baseline recordings, followed by the multiple sleep latency test (MSLT), one night of total sleep deprivation, and the following day another test of the MSLT coupled with caffeine or placebo under a crossover design where each subject was his or her control. The MSLT consists of a series of four naps every two hours at 10:00, 12:00, 14:00 and 16:00 h during which subjects are instructed to remain with eyes closed during the 30 min nap duration. Insomnia patients had significantly less delta sleep and total sleep time than normal volunteers. After one night of total sleep deprivation and under caffeine administration, the insomniacs had a significantly longer sleep latency and less total sleep time in the MSLT compared with normal volunteers, in whom caffeine was unable to reverse the reduced sleep latencies and the increase in total sleep time.

The importance of adenosine deaminase in the duration and intensity of sleep in humans has been noted recently (Rétey *et al.* 2005). Animal studies suggest that sleep needs are genetically controlled, and this also seems to apply in humans. Probably, a genetic variant of adenosine deaminase, which is associated with the reduced metabolism of adenosine to inosine, specifically enhances deep sleep and slow wave activity during sleep. Thus low activity of the catabolic enzyme for adenosine results in elevated adenosine, and deep sleep. In contrast, insomnia patients could have a distinct polymorphism of more active adenosine deaminase resulting in less adenosine accumulation, insomnia, and a low threshold for anxiety. This could also explain interindividual differences in anxiety symptoms after caffeine intake in healthy volunteers. This could affect the EEG during sleep and wakefulness in a non-state-specific manner.

Recent evidence indicates that sleep induced by adenosine, an endogenous sleep-promoting substance, requires activation of brain A-2A receptors. The hypothesis that adenosine could activate VLPO sleep-active neurons via A-2A adenosine receptors in rat brain slices was recently examined (Gelopin *et al.* 2005). Following the initial in vitro identification of these neurons as uniformly inhibited by NE and ACh, it was established that the VLPO nucleus comprises two intermingled subtypes of sleep neuron, differing in their firing responses to 5-HT, inducing either inhibition (Type-1 cells) or excitation (Type-2 cells).

Although caffeine is known to mobilize intracellular calcium, to inhibit phosphodiesterase activity, and to increase in vitro 5-HT and NE concentrations in the brainstem (Garrett and Griffiths 1997; Berkowitz *et al.* 1970; Carter *et al.* 1995; Solinas *et al.* 2002), it is now widely accepted that the mechanism of action of caffeine on wakefulness, at least at the dose range produced by voluntary caffeine intake, is via the antagonism of adenosine receptors.

The caffeine-induced increase of cortical ACh release is dose-dependent, and the increased cortical cholinergic activity, resulting from the blockade of A-1 receptors, may thus provide a basis for the psychostimulant effects of caffeine (Swerdlow *et al.* 1986). The wake-promoting effects of caffeine could also be due to the blocking of adenosine receptors on GABA neurons, which reinforces the inhibition of VLPO neurons that are specifically active during sleep (Solinas *et al.* 2002). Thus, by blocking the firing-rate cessation normally induced by adenosine, caffeine reinforces arousal by two different and complementary mechanisms: (1) stimulation of ACh neurons in the basal forebrain and (2) reinforcement of the inhibition exerted on sleep-promoting neurons. Despite the ability of caffeine to increase vigilance, which is an important reason for caffeine use, it has been suggested that the dopaminergic system also could contribute to the widespread consumption of caffeine-containing beverages (Swerdlow *et al.* 1985). However, although it has been shown that caffeine induces DA and glutamate release in the shell of the nucleus accumbens, these actions are not thought to contribute to its psychoactive effects (Swerdlow *et al.* 985; Swerdlow and Koob 1985).

Modafinil and wakefulness

The wake-promoting mechanism of action of modafinil remains unknown, despite numerous reports of its pharmacological action in the brain. Early studies highlighted the absence of an interaction between modafinil and the DA system (Duteil *et al.* 1990; Scammell *et al.* 2000; Akaoka *et al.* 1991; Lin *et al.* 1992). It also was established that the mixed D-1/D-2 antagonist haloperidol did not block the arousing effect of modafinil, whereas it consistently decreased the amphetamine-induced increase in wakefulness (Ferraro *et al.* 1997). Modafinil also showed a low affinity for DA reuptake sites (Mignot *et al.* 1994). It has been suggested, therefore, that the arousing effects of modafinil could be related to NE neurotransmission, given that the arousal produced by modafinil was blocked by α1 and β adrenergic receptor antagonists (Akaoka *et al.* 1991) and that modafinil affected the firing of locus coeruleus noradrenergic neurons (Lin *et al.* 1992). Using c-Fos immunocytochemistry in cats, it has been shown that amphetamine and methylphenidate do not share the same pattern of c-Fos activation with modafinil (Lin *et al.* 1996). Indeed, whereas the use of amphetamine and methylphenidate induced labeled neurons mainly in the cortex and the striatum, modafinil-induced wakefulness was associated mainly with activated neurons in the anterior hypothalamus, emphasizing therefore that modafinil induces wakefulness by mechanisms distinct from those of amphetamine and methylphenidate. Despite a confirmation of c-Fos immunoreactivity in the anterior hypothalamus in modafinil-treated rats (Engber *et al.* 1998), a recent study involving c-Fos labeling in modafinil-treated rats highlighted c-Fos activation mainly in the tuberomammillary nucleus and in hypocretin/orexin neurons of the perifornical area, and to a lesser extent, in the central nucleus of the amygdala, the striatum, and the cingulate cortex (Eugber *et al.* 1998). Thus, these authors concluded that modafinil may exert its arousing effects via an activation of these two regions implicated in the promotion of normal wakefulness. However, modafinil is efficient in promoting wakefulness in narcoleptic patients, despite the fact that narcoleptic patients exhibit a marked reduction in hypocretin-1 in cerebrospinal fluid (Nishino *et al.* 2000) and in the number of hypocretin neurons (Peyron *et al.* 2000; Thannickal *et al.* 2000). This discrepancy is likely explained by the fact that modafinil may also generate waking by increasing both dopaminergic and serotoninergic neurotransmission in the cortex, and by increasing NE release in the hypothalamus (de Saint *et al.* 2001).

Nicotine and sleep

The role of nicotine and nicotine receptors in the sleep–wake cycle is complex because most neurotransmitter systems modified by nicotine are also involved in sleep–wake regulation (i.e. ACh, 5-HT, DA, NE). Different variables such as dose, animal model, and time and route of administration change the way in which sleep is modified by nicotine. For example, nicotine given intravenously (Domino and Yamammoto 1965), subcutaneously (Jewel and Norton 1966), or through microinjections into the mPRF (medial pontine reticular formation) (Velazquez-Moctezuma *et al.* 1990) increases REM sleep in cats. In contrast, the administration of repeated doses of subcutaneous nicotine to rats resulted in a decrease of REM sleep and non-REM sleep and an increase in wake time in a dose-dependent fashion (Salin-Pascual *et al.* 1999). Also in this study, we noted that the effects of nicotine on sleep can be prevented by pretreatment with the nicotinic receptor antagonist mecamylamine (0.5 mg/kg, i.p.), suggesting that the effects of nicotine on sleep are modulated by nicotinic receptors (Salin-Pascual *et al.* 1999). Although systemic administration of nicotine activates all neuronal systems involved in the maintenance of arousal (Yu and Wecker 1994), a primary mode of action for the promotion of wakefulness is likely to be through stimulation of cholinergic neurotransmission in the basal forebrain.

However, nicotine also has been shown to stimulate the hypothalamic–pituitary–adrenal axis in rodents, leading to elevated plasma levels of adrenocorticotropic hormone and corticosterone (Andersson *et al.* 1983; Cam *et al.* 1979), which are known to exert a wake-promoting effect. However, studies in humans have shown that only intense smoking is able to activate the hypothalamic–pituitary–adrenal axis (Gilbert *et al.* 1992; Kirschbaum *et al.* 1992). Nicotine patches, in addition to their use in nicotine suppression and craving, have been used to explore the relationship between sleep and nicotine in human volunteers. Gillin *et al.* (Gillin *et al.* 1994) reported that transdermal nicotine evoked a dose-dependant decrease in REM sleep and an increase in wakefulness in normal volunteers. In contrast, Salin-Pascual *et al.* (Salin-Pascual *et al.* 1995) found that acute administration of nicotine via transdermal patches increased REM sleep in patients suffering from major depression. Cats behave almost identically to human volunteers. Transdermal nicotine patches were administered at three different doses (17.5, 35, and 52.5 mg) to cats chronically instrumented for sleep and ponto-geniculo-occipital spike (PGO) recordings. Both total sleep time as well as REM sleep was reduced, and PGO activity was abolished by all doses of nicotine (Vazquez *et al.* 1996). PGO activity is regulated by 5-HT activity, and depletion of 5-HT by reserpine or para-chlorophenylalanine (PCPA) produces continuous PGO activity, even during wakefulness. In contrast, drugs that increase 5-HT in the CNS reduce PGO activity as well as REM sleep (Simon *et al.* 1973). Thus the PGO suppression in cats by nicotine was explained as an increase in the activity of 5-HT at the pontine level, an effect that was subsequently confirmed (Mihailescu *et al.* 998).

In humans, an increase in REM sleep has been reported in nicotine addicts on withdrawal nights compared with nights when cigarettes were available (Kalese *et al.* 1970). Increased dreaming is also among the commonly reported side effects associated with transdermal nicotine treatment in smokers. Transdermal nicotine patches have been associated with early morning awakenings and reduced total REM sleep (Salin-Pascual and Drucker-Colín 1998). On recovery nights after nicotine patches were removed, REM latency and sleep stage II were significantly reduced, whereas REM sleep time and REM sleep percentage increased. Mood and subjective recall of dreaming were not affected.

Transdermal nicotine patches had a different effect on sleep in major depressive disorder patients. Compared with normal volunteers, a 17.5 mg patch produced an increase in REM sleep time without changes in other sleep stages in depressed patients; these patients also had a short-term improvement in mood (Salin-Pascual and Drucker-Colín 1998). This finding was supported by another study, in which depressed patients and normal volunteers received nicotine patches for four continuous nights. Of importance is that REM sleep enhancement was linked to improvement in mood scores. The increase in REM sleep could be related to a release of ACh mediated by nicotine autoreceptors that may indirectly activate the muscarinic postsynaptic M2 receptor, which is believed to be hypersensitive in depression, thus resulting in enhanced REM sleep (Sitaram and Gillin 1980). The main conclusions regarding the relationship of nicotine and sleep are thus that exogenous administration of nicotine promotes wakefulness in normal subjects, but may produce an increase of REM sleep time, as well as transitory mood improvement, in depressed patients.

Sleep fragmentation in the third part of the sleep period has been reported to be associated with nicotine addiction (Gourlay *et al.* 1999), and was hypothesized to be an early manifestation of nicotine withdrawal. Staner *et al.* (Staner *et al.* 2006) provided evidence in support of this hypothesis when they showed that a 24 h patch was better than a 16 h patch in terms of sleep continuity and the promotion of delta slow waves. The main effects of nicotine withdrawal on sleep are awakenings. Recent work also indicates that such awakenings affect the cardiovascular system by providing repetitive bursts of sympathetic nervous system activation, possibly contributing to elevated levels of cardiovascular and cerebrovascular morbidity. Pharmacological treatments designed to facilitate smoking cessation are ineffective for sustained abstinence in many smokers. This may be related to the associated sleep disturbances. Indeed, preliminary evidence suggests that nicotine replacement therapy (NRT) or bupropion can result in disrupted sleep, particularly in women. However, a better understanding of the role that nicotine withdrawal and bupropion or NRT treatment, independently or in combination, might play in sleep disturbances, will only be possible with more knowledge of the sleep disorders themselves (Colrain *et al.* 2004; West 2003).

The pharmacology of hypocretins and sleep

Hypocretins (i.e. orexins) are two peptides comprising 33 and 28 amino acids. The cell bodies are located predominantly in the lateral hypothalamus and surrounding regions. In the Doberman canine narcolepsy model, in which the disease is presented with an autosomal recessive pattern, a mutation was detected in the hypocretin-2 receptor. Failures in the hypocretin system have been confirmed as a key factor in narcolepsy by other findings in laboratory animals and humans (Mignot 2004; Saper *et al.* 2005a,b). Currently, no agonists or antagonists are available. The pharmacology of this system could be affected through either the input to, or output from, the hypocretin system.

Intraventricular injections of hypocretin directly into the brain enhance arousal (Saper *et al.* 2005a). Loss of the peptide or its receptors can result in narcolepsy in rodents, dogs, and humans (van den Pol 1999; Peyron *et al.* 1998). Axons from the hypocretin cells project widely throughout the CNS with a high level of innervation in some select brain regions, specifically in wake-related centers (i.e. locus coeruleus, posterior hypothalamus, and the LDT/PPT). One region that receives a dense hypocretinergic innervation is the locus coeruleus (LC). Most LC neurons synthesize NE and, similarly to the hypocretin neurons, send axons to many regions of the brain including the lateral hypothalamus. NE-containing axons are found in apparent contact with hypocretin neurons (Baldo *et al.* 2003).

Hypocretin neurons also send excitatory projections to regions of the brain that synthesize DA and NE, both of which also play a role in arousal (Kaslin *et al.* 2004). The central noradrenergic system is involved in the control of arousal (Mallick *et al.* 2002). LC neurons fire fastest during wakefulness, slow down during non-REM sleep, and stop firing almost completely during REM sleep (Aston-Jones *et al.* 1991).

Recent studies have revealed that the hypocretin neurons receive serotoninergic, noradrenergic, cholinergic, GABAergic, and glutamatergic regulation (Bayer *et al.* 2005; Sakurai *et al.* 2005; Winsky-Sommerer *et al.* 2004; Yamanaka *et al.* 2003). The activity of hypocretin neurons has also been reported to be influenced by corticotropin-releasing factor (CRF) (158), glucagon-like peptide-1 (GLP-1) (Acuna-Goycolea and van den Pol 2004), neuropeptide Y (NPY) (Fu *et al.* 2004), ghrelin, leptin, and glucose (Yamanaka *et al.* 2003). Hypocretin agonists and antagonists may soon be developed, benefiting patients with excessive somnolence, including that associated with narcolepsy, major depression, night-eating syndrome, and obstructive sleep apnea.

Conclusions

Advances in neurosciences and in the understanding of the pathophysiology of alterations in sleep are fundamental for the development of new medications. Basic research is also paramount to provide an integral vision of the mechanisms of action of medications, and to the development of new biochemical hypotheses. However, understanding the pathophysiology does not necessarily reveal the causes of the illness. Nevertheless, that knowledge can help the patient by relieving the symptoms or curing the disorder, and thus research continues to play an important role in the advance of the pharmacology of sleep.

References

Acuna-Goycolea C., van den Pol A. (2004). Glucagon-like peptide 1 excites hypocretin/orexin neurons by direct and indirect mechanisms: implications for viscera-mediated arousal. *J. Neurosci.* **24**, 8141–52.

Akaoka H., Roussel B., Lin J. S., Chouvet G., Jouvet M. (1991). Effect of modafinil and amphetamine on the rat catecholaminergic neuron activity. *Neurosci. Lett.* **123**, 20–2.

Algeri S., Biagini L., Manfridi A., Pitsikas N. (1991). Age-related ability of rats kept on a life-long hypocaloric diet in a spatial memory test. Longitudinal observations. *Neurobiol. Aging* **12**, 277–82.

Andersson K., Siegel R., Fuxe K., Eneroth P. (1983). Intravenous injections of nicotine induce very rapid and discrete reductions of hypothalamic catecholamine levels associated with increases of ACTH, vasopressin and prolactin secretion. *Acta Physiol. Scand.* **118**, 35–40.

Arrigoni E., Chamberlin N. L., Saper C. B., McCarley R. W. (2003). The effects of adenosine on the membrane properties of basal forebrain cholinergic neurons. *Sleep.* **26**, 45.

Aston-Jones G., Chiang C., Alexinsky T. (1991). Discharge of noradrenergic locus coeruleus neurons in behaving rats and monkeys suggests a role in vigilance. *Prog. Brain Res.* **88**, 501–20.

Baldo B. A., Daniel R. A., Berridge C. W., Kelley A. E. (2003). Overlapping distributions of orexin/hypocretin- and dopamine-beta-hydroxylase immunoreactive fibers in rat brain regions mediating arousal, motivation, and stress. *J. Comp. Neurol.* **464**, 220–37.

Bardwell W. A., Ziegler M. G., Ancoli-Israel S. *et al.* (2000). Does caffeine confound relationships among adrenergic tone, blood pressure and sleep apnoea? *J. Sleep Res.* **9**, 269–72.

Bayer L., Eggermann E., Serafin M. *et al.* (2005). Opposite effects of noradrenaline and acetylcholine upon hypocretin/orexin versus melanin concentrating hormone neurons in rat hypothalamic slices. *Neuroscience* **130**, 807–11.

Benerjee D., Vitiello M. V., Grunstein R. R. (2004). Pharmacotherapy for excessive daytime sleepiness. *Sleep Med. Rev.* **8**, 339–54.

Berkowitz B. A., Tarver J. H., Spector S. (1970). Release of norepinephrine in the central nervous system by theophylline and caffeine. *Eur. J. Pharmacol.* **10**, 64–71.

Billiard M., Bentley A. (2004). Is insomnia best categorized as a symptom or a disease? *Sleep Med.* **5**, S35–S40.

Blier P., Abbott F. V. (2001). Putative mechanisms of action of antidepressant drugs in affective and anxiety disorders and pain. *J. Psychiatry Neurosci.* **26**, 37–43.

Bliwise D. L. (2005). Sleep in normal aging and dementia. *Sleep* **16**, 40–81.

Bowersox S. S., Baker T., Dement W. C. (1984). Sleep-wakefulness patterns in the aged cat. *Electroencephalogr. Clin. Neurophysiol.* **58**, 240–52.

Cam G. R., Bassett J. R., Cairncross K. D. (1979). The action of nicotine on the pituitary-adrenal cortical axis. *Arch. Int. Pharmacodyn. Ther.* **237**, 49–66.

Carter A. J., O'Connor W. T., Carter M. J., Ungerstedt U. (1995). Caffeine enhances acetylcholine release in the hippocampus in vivo by a selective interaction with adenosine A1 receptors. *J. Pharmacol. Exp. Ther.* **273**, 637–42.

Chagoya de Sanchez V., Hernandez-Munoz R., Suarez J. *et al.* (1996). Temporal variations of adenosine metabolism in human blood. *Chronobiol. Int.* **13**, 163–77.

Collaborative Working Group on Clinical Trial Evaluations. (1998). Measuring outcome in schizophrenia: differences among the atypical antipsychotics. *J. Clin. Psychiatry* **59**(Suppl. 12), 3–9.

Colrain I. M., Trinder J., Swan G. E. (2004). The impact of smoking cessation on objective and subjective markers of sleep: review, synthesis, and recommendations. *Nicotine Tob. Res.* **6**, 913–25.

Czeisler C. A., Duffy J. F., Shanahan T. L. *et al.* (1999). Stability, precision and near-24-hour period human circadian pacemacker. *Science* **284**, 2177–81.

De la Gandara J., Aguera L., Rojo J. E., Ros S., de Pedro J. M. (2005). Use of antidepressant combinations: which, when and why? Results of a Spanish survey. *Acta Psychiatr. Scand.* **428**(Suppl.), 32–6.

de Saint H. Z., Orosco M., Rouch C., Blanc G., Nicolaidis S. (2001). Variations in extracellular monoamines in the prefrontal cortex and medial hypothalamus after modafinil administration: a microdialysis study in rats. *Neuroreport* **2**, 3533–7.

Declerck A. C., Ruwe F., O'Hanlon J. F., Wauquier A. (1992). Effects of Zolpidem and flunitrazepam on nocturnal sleep of women subjectively complaining of insomnia. *Psychopharmacology* **106**, 497–501.

Depoortere H., Françon D., van Luijtelaar E. L. J. M., Drinkenburg W. H. I. M., Coenen A. M. L. (1995). Differential effects of midazolam and zolpidem on sleep-wake states and epileptic activity in WAG/Rij rats. *Pharmacol. Biochem. Behav.* **51**, 571–6.

Depoortere H., Zivkovic B., Lloyd K. G. *et al.* (1986). Zolpidem, a novel nonbenzodiazepine hypnotic. I. Neuropharmacological and behavioral effects. *J. Pharmacol. Exp. Ther.* **237**, 649–58.

Domino E. F., Yamammoto K. (1965). Nicotine effect on the sleep cycle of the cat. *Science* **150**, 637–8.

Dowlatshahi D., MacQueen G. M., Wang J. F., Reiach J. S., Young L. T. (1999). G-protein-coupled cyclic AMP signaling in postmortem brain of subjects with mood disorders: effects of diagnosis, suicide, and treatment at the time of death. *J. Neurochem.* **73**, 1121–26.

Dumann R. S., Malberg J., Nakawa S., D'Sa C. (2004). Neuronal plasticity and survival in mood disorders. *Biol. Psychiatry.* **48**, 732–9.

Duncan G. E., Breese G. R., Criswell H. E. *et al.* (1995). Distribution of (3H) zolpidem binding sites in relation to messenger RNA encoding the K1, L2 and Q2 subunits of GABAA receptors in rat brain. *Neuroscience* **64**, 1113–28.

Duteil J., Rambert F. A., Pessonnier J. *et al.* (1990). Central alpha 1-adrenergic stimulation in relation to the behaviour stimulating effect of modafinil; studies with experimental animals. *Eur. J. Pharmacol.* **180**, 49–58.

Edgar D. M., Dement W. C., Fuller C. A. (1993). Effect of SCN lesions on sleep in squirrel monkeys: evidence for opponent processes in sleep-wake regulation. *J. Neurosci.* **13**(3), 1065–79.

Ekimova I. V., Pastukhov I. (2005). [GABA-ergic mechanisms of the ventrolateral preoptic area of the hypothalamus in regulation of sleep and wakefulness and temperature homeostasis in pigeon Columba livia]. *Zh. Evol. Biokhim. Fiziol.* **41**, 356–63.

Elsenga S., van den Hoofdakker R. H. (1993). Clinical effects of sleep deprivation and clomipramine in endogenous depression. *J. Psychiatr. Res.* **17**, 361–74.

Engber T. M., Koury E. J., Dennis S. A. *et al.* (1998). Differential patterns of regional c-Fos induction in the rat brain by amphetamine and the novel wakefulness-promoting agent modafinil. *Neurosci. Lett.* **241**, 95–8.

Feldberg W., Sherwood S. L. (1954). Behaviour of cats after intraventricular injections of eserine and DFO. *J. Physiol.* **125**, 488–500.

Ferraro L., Antonelli T., O'Connor W. T. *et al.* (1997). Modafinil: an antinarcoleptic drug with a different neurochemical profile to d-amphetamine and dopamine uptake blockers. *Biol. Psychiatry* **2**, 1181–3.

Floran B., Gonzalez B., Floran L., Erlij D., Aceves J. (2005). Interactions between adenosine A(2a) and dopamine D2 receptors in the control of [(3)H]GABA release in the globus pallidus of the rat. *Eur. J. Pharmacol.* **520**(1–3), 43–50.

Fredholm B. B., Lindstrom K. (1999). Autoradiographic comparison of the potency of several structurally unrelated adenosine receptor antagonists at adenosine A1 and A(2A) receptors. *Eur. J. Pharmacol.* **380**, 197–202.

Fu L. Y., Acuna-Goycolea C., van den Pol A. N. (2004). Neuropeptide Y inhibits hypocretin/orexin neurons by multiple presynaptic and postsynaptic mechanisms: tonic depression of the hypothalamic arousal system. *J. Neurosci.* **24**, 8741–51.

Gandolfo G., Scherschlicht R., Gottesmann C. (1994). Benzodiazepines promote the intermediate stage at the expense of paradoxical sleep in the rat. *Pharmacol. Biochem. Behav.* **49**, 921–7.

Garrett B. E., Griffiths R. R. (1997). The role of dopamine in the behavioral effects of caffeine in animals and humans. *Pharmacol. Biochem. Behav.* **57**, 533–41.

Gelopin T., Luppi P.-H., Cauli B. *et al.* (2005). The endogenous somnogen adenosine excites a subset of sleep-promoting neurons via A2A receptors in the ventrolateral preoptic nucleus. *Neuroscience* **00**, 1377–90.

Gilbert D. G., Meliska C. J., Williams C. L., Jensen R. A. (1992). Subjective correlates of cigarette-smoking-induced elevations of peripheral betaendorphin and cortisol. *Psychopharmacology* **106**, 275–81.

Gillin J. C. (1983). The sleep therapies of depression. *Prog. Neuropsychopharmacol. Biol. Psychiatry* **7**, 351–64.

Gillin J. C., Lardon M., Ruiz C., Golshan S., Salin-Pascual R. J. (1994). Dose-dependent effects of transdermal nicotine on early morning awakening and rapid eye movement sleep time in non-smoking normal volunteers. *J. Clin. Psychopharmacol.* **14**, 264–7.

Gillin J. C., Smith-Vaniz A., Schnierow B. *et al.* (2001). An open-label, 12-week clinical and sleep EEG study of nefazodone in chronic combat-related posttraumatic stress disorder. *J. Clin. Psychiatry* **62**, 789–96.

Gottesmann C. (2002). GABA mechanisms and sleep. *Neuroscience* **111**, 231–9.

Gottesmann C., Trefouret S., Depoortere H. (1994). Influence of Zolpidem, a novel hypnotic, on the intermediate stage and paradoxical sleep in the rat. *Pharmacol. Biochem. Behav.* **47**, 359–62.

Gourlay S. G., Forbes A., Marriner T., Mc Nei J. J. (1999). Predictor of adverse experiences during transdermal nicotine therapy. *Drug Saf.* **20**, 545–55.

Harper L. K., Beckett S. R., Marsden C. A., McCreary A. C., Alexander S. P. (2006). Effects of the A(2A) adenosine receptor antagonist KW6002 in the nucleus accumbens in vitro and in vivo. *Pharmacol. Biochem. Behav.* in press.

Haulica I., Ababei L., Branisteanu D., Topoliceanu F. (1973). Letter. Preliminary data on the possible hypnogenic role of adenosine. *J. Neurochem.* **4**, 1019–20.

Hayaishi O., Matsumura H. (1995). Prostaglandins and sleep. *Adv. Neuroimmunol.* **5**, 211–16.

Hill S. Y., Mendelson W. B., Bernstein D. A. (1977). Cocaine effects on sleep parameters in the rat. *Psychopharmacology* **51**, 125–7.

Jewet R. E., Norton S. (1966). Effects of some stimulants and depressant drugs on the sleep cycle of the cat. *Exp. Neurol.* **15**, 463–74.

Jia F., Pignataro L., Schofield C. M. *et al.* (2005). An extrasynaptic GABA-A receptor mediates tonic inhibition in thalamic VB neurons. *J. Neurophysiol.* **94**(6), 4491–501.

Johnston G. A. (2005). GABA(A) receptor channel pharmacology. *Curr. Pharm. Des.* **11**, 1867–85.

Jones B. E. (2005). From waking to sleeping: neuronal and chemical substrates. *Trends Pharmacol. Sci.* **26**, 578–86.

Jones B. E., Bobillier P., Pin C., Jouvet M. (1973). The effect of lesions of catecholamine-containing neurons upon monoamine content of the brain and EEG and behavioral waking in the cat. *Brain Res.* **58**, 57–177.

Kales J., Allen C., Preston T. A., Tan T. L., Kales A. (1970). Changes in REM sleep and dreaming with cigarette smoking and following withdrawal. *Association of Professional Sleep Societies Meeting. Abstracts Book*, **7**, 347–8.

Kamimori G. H., Penetar D. M., Headley D. B. *et al.* (2000). Effect of three caffeine doses on plasma catecholamines and alertness during prolonged wakefulness. *Eur. J. Clin. Pharmacol.* **56**, 537–44.

Kaslin J., Nystedt J. M., Ostergard M., Peitsaro N., Panula P. (2004). The orexin/hypocretin system in zebrafish is connected to the aminergic and cholinergic systems. *J. Neurosci.* **24**, 2678–89.

Kirschbaum C., Wust S., Strasburger C. J. (1992). 'Normal' cigarette smokingincreases free cortisol in habitual smokers. *Life Sci.* **50**, 435–42.

Koyama Y., Hayaishi O. (1994). Modulation by prostaglandins of activity of sleep-related neurons in the preoptic/anterior hypothalamic areas in rats. *Brain Res. Bull.* **33**, 367–72.

Lagarde D., Batejat D., Sicard B. *et al.* (2000). Slow-release caffeine: a new response to the effects of a limited sleep deprivation. *Sleep* **23**, 651–61.

Lancel M., Faulhaber J., Holsboer F., Ruppert R. (1996). Progesterone induces changes in sleep comparable to those of agonists GABAA receptor modulations. *Am. J. Physiol.* **34**, E763–72.

Landolt H. P, Gillin J. C. (2002). Different effects of phenelzine treatment on EEG topography in waking and sleep in depressed patients. *Neuropsychopharmacology* **27**, 462–9.

Landolt H.-P., Retey J. V., Tonz K. *et al.* (2004). Caffeine attenuates waking and sleep electroencephalographic markers of sleep homeostasis in humans. *Neuropsychopharmacology* **29**(10), 1933–9.

Landolt H.-P., Retey J. V., Tonz K. *et al.* (2004). Caffeine attenuates waking and sleep electroencephalographic markers of sleep homeostasis in humans. *Neuropsychopharmacology* **29**, 1933–9.

Leibenluft E., Wehr T. (1992). Is sleep deprivation useful in the treatment of depression? *Am. J. Psychiatry* **149**, 156–68.

Levy M., Zylber-Katz E. (1983). Caffeine metabolism and coffee-attributed sleep disturbances. *Clin. Pharmacol. Ther.* **33**, 770–5.

Liappas I. A., Malitas P. N., Dimopoulos N. P., Gitsa O. E., Liappass Ch. K. (2003). Zolpidem dependence case series: possible neurobiological mechanisms and clinical management. *J. Psychopharmacol.* **17**, 131–5.

Lin J. S., Hou Y., Jouvet M. (1996). Potential brain neuronal targets for amphetamine-, methylphenidate-, and modafinil-induced wakefulness, evidenced by c-fos immunocytochemistry in the cat. *Proc. Natl. Acad. Sci. USA* **93**, 14128–33.

Lin J. S., Roussel B., Akaoka H. *et al.* (1992). Role of catecholamines in the modafinil and amphetamine induced wakefulness, a comparative pharmacological study in the cat. *Brain Res.* **591**, 319–26.

Linden J. M. (1999). Purinergic systems. In: Siegel GL, Agranoff BW, Albers RW, Fisher SK, Uhler MD, eds, *Basic Neurochemistry: Molecular, Cellular and Medical Aspects*. Philadephia, PA: Lippincott-Raven, 347–62.

Lund R., Rüther E., Wober W., Hippius, H. (1988). Effects of Zolpidem (10 and 20 mg), lormetazepam, triazolam and placebo on night sleep and residual effects during the day. In: Sauvanet J. P., Langer S. Z., Morselli P. L (eds.), *Imidazopyridines in Sleep Disorders*. New York, NY: Raven Press, pp. 193–203.

Mölher H., Malherbe P., Draguhn A. *et al.* (1990). GABA-A-receptor subunits: functional expression and gene localisation, in *GABA and Benzodiazepine Receptor Subtypes*, ed. Biggio G., Costa E. New York, NY: Raven Press, pp. 23–34.

Mallick B. N., Majumdar S., Faisal M. *et al.* (2002). Role of norepinephrine in the regulation of rapid eye movement sleep. *J. Biosci.* **27**, 539–51.

Maquet P., Dive D., Salmon E. *et al.* (1992). Cerebral glucose utilization during stage 2 sleep in man. *Brain Res.* **571**, 149–53.

McCarley R. W. (2004). Mechanisms and models of REM sleep control. *Arch. Ital. Biol.* **142**(4): 429–67.

Meerlo P., Roman V., Farkas E. *et al.* (2004). Ageing-related decline in adenosine A1 receptor binding in the rat brain: an autoradiographic study. *J. Neurosci. Res.* **178**, 742–8.

Mendelson W. (2000). Sleep-inducing effects of adenosine microinjections into the medial preoptic area are blocked by flumazenil. *Brain Res.* **852**, 479–82.

Mendelson W. B. (2001). Neurotransmitters and sleep. *J. Clin. Psychiatry* **62**, Suppl: 105–8.

Mendelson W. B., Martin J. V., Perlis M., Wagner R. (1987). Arousal induced by injection of triazolam into the dorsal raphe nucleus of rats. *Neuropsychopharmacology* **1**, 85–8.

Mendelson W. B., Martin J. V. (1990). Effects of muscimol and flurazepam on the sleep EEG in the rat. *Life Sci.* **47**, 99–101.

Mignot E. (2004). Sleep, sleep disorders and hypocretin (orexin). *Sleep Med.* **5**(Suppl.) **1**, S2–S8.

Mignot E., Nishino S., Guilleminault C., Dement W. C. (1994). Modafinil binds to the dopamine uptake carrier site with low affinity. *Sleep* **17**, 436–7.

Mihailescu S., Palomero-Rivero M., Meade-Huerta P., Maza-Flores A., Drucker-Colin R. (1998). Effects of nicotine and mecamylamine on rat dorsal raphe neurons. *Eur. J. Pharmacol.* **360**, 31–6.

Mitchell J. B., Lupica C. R., Dunwiddie T. V. (1993). Activity-dependent release of endogenous adenosine modulates synaptic responses in the rat hippocampus. *J. Neurosci.* **13**, 3439–47.

Monti J. M., Jantos H. (2004). Microinjection of the nitric oxide synthase inhibitor L-NAME into the lateral basal forebrain alters the sleep/wake cycle of the rat. *Prog. Neuropsychopharmacol. Biol. Psychiatry* **28**, 239–47.

Monti J. M., Monti D. (2005). Sleep disturbance in schizophrenia. *Int. Rev. Psychiatry* **17**, 247–53.

Morairty S., Rainnie D., McCarley R., Greene R. (2004). Disinhibition of ventrolateral preoptic area sleep-active neurons by adenosine: a new mechanism for sleep promotion. *Neuroscience* **123**, 451–7.

Murillo-Rodriguez E., Blanco-Centurion C., Gerashchenko D., Salin-Pascual R. J., Shiromani P. J. (2004). The diurnal rhythm of adenosine levels in the basal forebrain of young and old rats. *Neuroscience* **123**, 361–70.

Nehlig A. (1999). Are we dependent upon coffee and caffeine? A review on human and animal data. *Neurosci. Biobehav.* **23**, 563–676.

Nibuya M., Morinobu S., Duman R. S. (1995). Regulation of BDNF and trkB mRNA in rat brain by chronic electroconvulsive seizure and antidepressant drug treatments. *J. Neurosci.* **15**, 7539–47.

Nibuya M., Nestlr E. J., Duman R. S. (1996). Chronic antidepressant administration increases the expression of cAMP response element binding protein (CREB) in rat hippocampus. *J. Neurosci.* **16**, 2365–72.

Nishino S., Mishima K., Mignot E., Dement W. C. (2004). Sedative-hypnotics, in *Textbook of Psychopharmacology*, ed. Schatzberg A. F., Nemeroff C. B. Washington, DC: American Psychiatric Publishing, Inc., pp. 651–70.

Nishino S., Ripley B., Overeem S., Lammers G. J., Mignot E. (2000). Hypocretin (orexin) deficiency in human narcolepsy. *Lancet* **355**, 39–40.

Ongini E., Bonizzoni E., Ferri N., MIlani S., Tramous M. (1993). Differential effects of dopamine D-1 and D-2 receptor antagonist antipsychotics on sleep-wake patterns in the rat. *J. Pharmacol. Exp. Ther.* **266**, 726–31.

Pegram V., Bert J., Naquet R. (1969). The ontogeny of EEG sleep patterns in the baboon. *Psychophysiology* **6**, 228.

Peyron C., Faraco J., Rogers W. *et al.* (2000). A mutation in a case of early onset narcolepsy and a generalized absence of hypocretin peptides in human narcoleptic brains. *Nat. Med.* **6**, 991–7.

Peyron C., Tighe D. K., van den Pol A. N. *et al.* (1998). Neurons containing hypocretin (orexin) project to multiple neuronal systems. *J. Neurosci.* **18**, 9,996–10,015.

Polulin J., Daoust A. M., Forest G., Stip E., Godbout R. (2003). Sleep architecture and its clinical correlates in first episode and neuroleptic-naive patients with schizophrenia. *Schizophr. Res.* **62**, 147–53.

Porkka-Heiskanen T., Strecker R. E., Björkum A. A. *et al.* (1997b). Adenosine a mediator of the sleep-inducing effects of prolonged wakefulness. *Science* **276**, 1265–8.

Porkka-Heiskanen T., Strecker R. E., Thakkar M., McCarley R. W. (1997a). Brain extracellular adenosine level during sleep waking and prolonged wakefulness. *Soc. Neurosci. Abstr.* **23**, 312.

Rétey J. V., Adam M., Honegger E. *et al.* (2005). A functional genetic variation of adenosine deaminase affects the duration and intensity of deep sleep in humans. *PNAS* **102**, 15676–81.

Radulovacki M., Virus R. M., Djuricic-Nedelson M., Green R. D. (1984). Adenosine analogs and sleep in rats. *J. Pharmacol. Exp. Ther.* **228**, 268–74.

Radulovacki M., Walovitch R., Yanick G. (1980). Caffeine produces REM sleep rebound in rats. *Brain Res.* **201**, 497–500.

Reinoso-Suarez F. de A. I., Rodrigo-Angulo M. L., Garzon M. (2001). Brain structures and mechanisms involved in the generation of REM sleep. *Sleep Med. Rev.* **5**(1), 63–77.

Rye D. B., Jankovic J. (2002). Emerging views of dopamine in modulating sleep/wake state from an unlikely source: PD. *Neurology* **58**, 341–6.

Sakurai T. (2005). Roles of orexin/hypocretin in regulation of sleep/wakefulness and energy homeostasis. *Sleep Med. Rev.* **9**, 231–41.

Sakurai T., Nagata R., Yamanaka A. *et al.* (2005). Input of orexin/hypocretin neurons revealed by a genetically encoded tracer in mice. *Neuron* **46**, 297–308.

Salin-Pascual R. J. (2005). Comparative study between mirtazapine vs. zolpidem in isomnia associated with major depression management. *Rev. Mex. Neurosci.* **6**, 212–17.

Salin-Pascual R. J., de la Fuente J. R., Galicia-Polo L, Drucker-Colin R. (1995). Effects of transdermal nicotine on mood and sleep in nonsmoking major depressed patients. *Psychopharmacology* **121**, 476–9.

Salin-Pascual R. J., Drucker-Colín R. (1998). A novel effect of nicotine on mood and sleep in major depression. *Neuroreport* **9**, 57–60.

Salin-Pascual R. J., Herrera-Estrella M., Galicia-Polo L., Laurrabaquio M. R. (1999). Olanzapine acute administration in schizophrenic patients increases delta sleep and sleep efficiency. *Biol. Psychiatry* **46**, 141–3.

Salin-Pascual R. J., Moro-Lopez M. L., Gonzalez-Sanchez H., Blanco-Centurion C. (1999). Changes in sleep after acute and repeated administration of nicotine in the rat. *Psychopharmacology* **145**, 133–8.

Salin-Pascual R. J., Moro-Lopez M. L., Gonzalez-Sanchez H., Blanco-Centurion C. (1999). Changes in sleep after acute and repeated administration of nicotine in the rat. *Psychopharmacology* **145**, 133–8.

Salin-Pascual R. J., Upadhyaya U., Shiromani P. J. (2002). Effects of hypocaloric diet on sleep in young and old rats. *Neurobiol. Aging* **23**, 771–6.

Salin-Pascual R. J., Valencia-Flores M., Campos R. M., Castaño A., Shiromani P. J. (2006). Caffeine challenge in insomnia patients after total sleep deprivation. *Sleep Med.* **7**, 141–5.

Salin-Pascual R. J., Wagner D., Upadhyaya U., Shiromani P. J. (2000). Caffeine decreases sleep in middle-aged and old rats but not young rats. *Sleep* **23**, A53.

Saper C. B., Lu J., Chou T. C., Gooley J. (2005b). The hypothalamic integrator for circadian rhythms. *Trends Neurosci.* **28**(3), 152–7.

Saper C. B., Lu J., Chou T. C., Gooley J. (2005a). The hypothalamic integrator for circadian rhythms. *Trends Neurosci.* **28**, 152–7.

Saper C. B., Scammell T. E., Lu J. (2005a). Hypothalamic regulation of sleep and circadian rhythms. *Nature* **437**(7063), 1257–63.

Saper C. B., Scammell T. E., Lu J. (2005b). Hypothalamic regulation of sleep and circadian rhythms. *Nature* **437**, 1257–63.

Scammell T. E., Estabrooke I. V., McCarthy M. T. *et al.* (2000). Hypothalamic arousal regions are activated during modafinil-induced wakefulness. *J. Neurosci.* **20**, 8620–8.

Schwartz J. R. (2004). Pharmacologic management of daytime sleepiness. *J. Clin. Psychiatry* **65**(Suppl. 16), 46–9.

Schwierin B., Borbely A. A., Tobler I. (1996). Effects of N6-cyclopentyladenosine and caffeine on sleep regulation in the rat. *Eur. J. Pharmacol.* **300**, 163–71.

Shiromani P. J., Lu J., Wagner D. *et al.* (2000). Compensatory sleep response to 12 h wakefulness in young and old rats. *Am. J. Physiol. Regul. Integ. Comp. Physiol.* **278**, R125–33.

Siegel R. K. (1985). New patterns of cocaine use: changing doses and routes. *NIDA Res. Monogr.* **61**, 204–20.

Simon R. P., Gershon M. D., Brooks D. C. (1973). The role of the raphe nuclei in the regulation of ponto-geniculo-occipital wave activity. *Brain Res.* **148**, 105–19.

Singh M. A. (1998). Combined exercise and dietary intervention to optimize body composition in aging. *Ann. NY Acad. Sci.* **854**, 378–93.

Sinton C. M., Petitjean F. (1989). The influence of chronic caffeine administration on sleep parameters in the cat. *Pharmacol. Biochem. Behav.* **32**, 459–62.

Sitaram N., Gillin J. C. (1980). Development and use of pharmacological probes of the CNS in man: evidence of cholinergic abnormalities in primary affective disorders. *Biol. Psychiatry* **15**, 925–55.

Solinas M., Ferre S., You Z. B. *et al.* (2002). Caffeine induces dopamine and glutamate release in the shell of the nucleus accumbens. *J. Neurosci.* **22**, 6321–4.

Staner L., Luthringer R., Dupon D., Aubin H. J., Lagrue G. (2006). Sleep effects of a 24-h versus a 16-h nicotine patch: a polysomnographic study during smoking cessation. *Sleep Med.* **7**, 147–54.

Swerdlow N. R., Koob G. F. (1985). Separate neural substrates of the locomotor-activating properties of amphetamine, heroin, caffeine and corticotrophin releasing factor (CRF) in the rat. *Pharmacol. Biochem. Behav.* **23**, 303–7.

Swerdlow N. R., Vaccarino F. J., Amalric M., Koob G. F. (1986). The neural substrates for the motor-activating properties of psychostimulants: a review of recent findings. *Pharmacol. Biochem. Behav.* **25**, 233–48.

Swerdlow N. R., Vaccarino F. J., Koob G. F. (1985). Effects of naloxone on heroin-, amphetamine- and caffeine-stimulated locomotor activity in the rat. *Pharmacol. Biochem. Behav.* **23**, 499–501.

Tandon R., Shipley J. E., Taylos S. *et al.* (1992). Electroencephalographic sleep abnormalities in schizophrenia. Relationship to positive/negative symptoms and prior neuroleptic treatment. *Arch. Gen. Psychiatry* **49**, 185–94.

Thannickal T. C., Moore R. Y., Nienhuis R. *et al.* (2000). Reduced number of hypocretin neurons in human narcolepsy. *Neuron* **27**, 469–74.

Thome J., Sakain N., Shin K. *et al.* (2000). cAMP response element-mediated gene transcription in upregulated by chronic antidepressant. *J. Neurosci.* **20**, 4030–6.

Thorphy M. J. (1990). *International Classification of Sleep Disorders: Diagnostic and Coding Manual.* Rochester, MN: American Sleep Disorders Association.

Trampus M., Ferri N., Adami M., Ongini E. (1993). The dopamine D1 receptor agonists, A68930 and SKF 38393, induce arousal and suppress REM sleep in the rat. *Eur. J. Pharmacol.* **235**, 83–7.

Trampus M., Ongini E. (1990). The D1 dopamine receptor antagonist SCH 23390 enhances REM sleep in the rat. *Neuropharmacology* **29**, 889–893.

Ursin R. (2002). Serotonin and sleep. *Sleep Med. Rev.* **6**, 55–69.

Van Bemmel A. L. (1997). The link between sleep and depression: the effects of antidepressants on EEG sleep. *J. Psychosom. Res.* **42**, 555–64.

van den Pol A. N (1999). Hypothalamic hypocretin (orexin): robust innervation of the spinal cord. *J. Neurosci.* **19**, 3171–82.

Varga V., Sik A., Freund T. F., Kocsis B. (2002). GABA(B) receptors in the median raphe nucleus: distribution and role in the serotonergic control of hippocampal activity. *Neuroscience* **109**(1), 119–32.

Vazquez J., Guzmán-Marín R., Salin-Pascual R. J., Drucker-Colín R. (1996). Transdermal nicotine on sleep and PGO spikes. *Brain Res.* **737**, 317–20.

Velazquez-Moctezuma J., Shalauta M. D., Gillin J. C., Shiromani P. J. (1990). Microinjection of nicotine in the medial pontine reticular formation elicits REM sleep. *Neurosci. Lett.* **115**, 265–8.

Virus R. M., Djuricic-Nedelson M., Radulovacki M., Green R. D. (1983). The effects of adenosine and 2′-deoxycoformycin on sleep and wakefulness in rats. *Neuropharmacology* **22**, 1401–4.

Vogel G. W., Traub A. C., Bem-Horin P., Meyers G. M. (1968). REM deprivation. II. The effects on depressed patient. *Arch. Gen. Psychiatry* **18**(3), 301–11.

Vogel G. W., Vogel F., McAbee R. S., Thurmond A. J. (1980). Improvement of depression by REM sleep deprivation, new findings and a theory. *Arch. Gen. Psychiatry* **37**, 247–53.

Wafford K. A., Ebert B. (2006). Gaboxadol – a new awakening in sleep. *Curr. Opin. Pharmacol.* **6**(1), 30–6.

West R. (2003). Bupropion SR for smoking cessation. *Expert Opin. Pharmacother.* **4**, 533–40.

Winokur A., Sateia M. J., Boyd Hayes J. *et al.* (2000). Acute effects of mirtazapine on sleep continuity and sleep architecture in depressed patients: a pilot study. *Biol. Psychiatry* **48**, 75–7.

Winsky-Sommerer R., Yamanaka A., Diano S. *et al.* (2004). Interaction between the corticotropin-releasing factor system and hypocretins (orexins): a novel circuit mediating stress response. *J. Neurosci.* **24**, 11439–48.

Wurts S. W., Edgar D. M. (2000). Caffeine during sleep deprivation: sleep tendency and dynamics of recovery sleep in rats. *Pharmacol. Biochem. Behav.* **65**, 155–62.

Yamanaka A., Muraki Y., Tsujino N., Goto K., Sakurai T. (2003). Regulation of orexin neurons by the monoaminergic and cholinergic systems. *Biochem. Biophys. Res. Commun.* **303**, 120–9.

Yu Z. J., Wecker L. (1994). Chronic nicotine administration differentially affects neurotransmitter release from rat striatal slices. *J. Neurochem.* **63**, 186–94.

Index